Second Edition

VETERINARY MICROBIOLOGY

Second Edition

VETERINARY
MICROBIOLOGY

Dwight C. Hirsh
N. James MacLachlan
Richard L. Walker

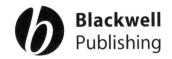

Blackwell
Publishing

Dwight C. Hirsh, DVM, PhD, is emeritus professor, Department of Pathology, Microbiology and Immunology, University of California-Davis.

N. James MacLachlan, DVM, PhD, is professor, Department of Pathology, Microbiology and Immunology, University of California-Davis.

Richard L. Walker, DVM, PhD, MPVM, is professor of clinical diagnostic bacteriology, California Animal Health and Food Safety Laboratory, University of California-Davis.

Blackwell Publishing Professional
2121 State Avenue, Ames, Iowa 50014, USA

Orders:	1-800-862-6657
Office:	1-515-292-0140
Fax:	1-515-292-3348
Web site:	www.blackwellprofessional.com

Blackwell Publishing Ltd
9600 Garsington Road, Oxford OX4 2DQ, UK
Tel.: +44 (0)1865 776868

Blackwell Publishing Asia
550 Swanston Street, Carlton, Victoria 3053, Australia
Tel.: +61 (0)3 8359 1011

Printed on acid-free paper in the United States of America

First edition, ©1999 Blackwell Science, Inc.
Second edition, ©2004 Blackwell Publishing

Library of Congress Cataloging-in-Publication Data
Veterinary microbiology / [edited by] Dwight C. Hirsh,
   N. James MacLachlan, Richard L. Walker.—2nd ed.
      p. ; cm.
   Includes bibliographical references and index.
   ISBN-13: 978-0-8138-0379-1
   ISBN-10: 0-8138-0379-9 (alk. paper)
   1. Veterinary microbiology.
   [DNLM: 1. Animal Population Groups—microbiology.
   2. Veterinary Medicine. QW 70 V586 2004] I. Hirsh,
   Dwight C. II. MacLachlan, Nigel James. III. Walker,
   Richard L., DVM.
SF780.2.V48 2004
636.089′69041—dc22
                                                2004008413

The last digit is the print number: 9 8 7 6 5 4 3

Dedications

To Lucy, Dwight, and Elizabeth for years of patience and understanding; and to the memory of my brother, Harry.
—*Dwight C. Hirsh*

To Ken and Marion for lighting the fire of inquisitiveness.
—*N. James MacLachlan*

To Dee Dee and Mary for their support, understanding, and focus on what is really important.
—*Richard L. Walker*

Contents

Contributors

Alex A. Ardans, DVM, MS
Professor, Department of Medicine and Epidemiology;
Director, California Animal Health and Food Safety
  Laboratory System
School of Veterinary Medicine
University of California
Davis, California

Udeni B. R. Balasuriya, BVSc, PhD
Associate Research Molecular Virologist
Department of Pathology, Microbiology and
  Immunology
School of Veterinary Medicine
University of California
Davis, California

Bradd C. Barr, DVM, PhD
Professor, Department of Pathology, Microbiology, and
  Immunology;
California Animal Health and Food Safety Laboratory
School of Veterinary Medicine
University of California
Davis, CA 95616

Ernst L. Biberstein, DVM, PhD
Professor Emeritus, Department of Pathology,
  Microbiology, and Immunology
School of Veterinary Medicine
University of California
Davis, California

Anthony E. Castro, DVM, PhD
Department of Veterinary Sciences
Pennsylvania State University
University Park, Pennsylvania

Bruno B. Chomel, DVM, PhD
Associate Professor, Department of Population Health
  and Reproduction
School of Veterinary Medicine
University of California
Davis, California

Richard M. Donovan, PhD
Viral and Rickettsial Disease Laboratory
California Department of Health Services
Richmond, California

Janet E. Foley, DVM, PhD
Assistant Professor, Department of Medicine and
  Epidemiology
School of Veterinary Medicine
University of California
Davis, California

James G. Fox, DVM
Professor and Director, Division of Comparative Medicine
Massachusetts Institute of Technology
Cambridge, Massachusetts

Frederick J. Fuller, PhD
Professor, Department of Population Health and
  Pathobiology
College of Veterinary Medicine
North Carolina State University
Raleigh, North Carolina

Laurel J. Gershwin, DVM, PhD
Professor, Department of Pathology, Microbiology, and
  Immunology;
Chief, Clinical Immunology, Virology, and Microbiology
  Service
Veterinary Medical Teaching Hospital
School of Veterinary Medicine
University of California
Davis, California

Dwight C. Hirsh, DVM, PhD
Professor Emeritus, Department of Pathology,
  Microbiology, and Immunology
School of Veterinary Medicine
University of California
Davis, California

Rickie W. Kasten, PhD
Department of Population Health and Reproduction
School of Veterinary Medicine
University of California
Davis, California

Rance B. LeFebvre, PhD
Professor, Department of Pathology, Microbiology, and
  Immunology
School of Veterinary Medicine
University of California
Davis, California

N. James MacLachlan, DVM, PhD
Professor, Department of Pathology, Microbiology, and
   Immunology
School of Veterinary Medicine
University of California
Davis, California

John F. Prescott, Vet MB, PhD
Professor, Department of Pathobiology
University of Guelph
Ontario, Canada

Jeffrey L. Stott, PhD
Professor, Department of Pathology, Microbiology, and
   Immunology
School of Veterinary Medicine
University of California
Davis, California

Richard L. Walker, DVM, PhD, MPVM
Professor, Department of Pathology, Microbiology, and
   Immunology;
Section Head, Bacteriology
California Animal Health and Food Safety Laboratory
   System
School of Veterinary Medicine
University of California
Davis, California

Yuan Chung Zee, DVM, PhD
Professor Emeritus, Department of Pathology,
   Microbiology, and Immunology
School of Veterinary Medicine
University of California
Davis, California

Preface

This book is intended for veterinary students, to accompany and supplement their first courses in pathogenic bacteriology-mycology and virology (Parts I through III), as well as subsequent courses dealing with infectious diseases (Part IV). The focus includes pathogenic mechanisms and processes in infectious diseases; methods of diagnosis; and principles of resistance, prevention, and therapy. A working knowledge of general microbiology is assumed.

Beyond serving as a resource for students, the book is also meant to serve as a convenient reference for veterinarians and veterinary scientists whose main line of activity and expertise is outside the areas of microbiology.

The book is divided into four sections. Part I deals with the general characteristics of the host–parasite relationship, laboratory diagnosis of conditions involving an infectious etiology, antimicrobial treatment, and prevention of infectious disease.

Parts II (bacteria and fungi) and III (viruses) present the infectious agents that affect the veterinary species. The chapters dealing with the bacterial agents are grouped mainly by morphology, and their gram-staining characteristics. The fungal agents are grouped mainly by morphologic characteristics (yeast, mold). The viruses are grouped along taxonomic grounds.

Part IV deals with the infectious agents in the context of the host. This section is organized by organ system. Each organ system is discussed first as a microbial habitat, followed by discussion of those infectious agents that mainly affect that particular system.

The content and organization of this book varies somewhat from the last edition of *Veterinary Microbiology* (1999). Most notable is the organization of the infectious agents discussed in Part II, the bacteria and fungi. These agents are now discussed without regard to major organ system, but along more traditional grounds (i.e., morphology and gram reaction in the case of the bacterial agents, and yeast vs. mold for the fungal agents). A major change in the content of this edition is the addition of Part IV, which deals with the infectious agents along more clinically useful lines. In addition, we have eliminated references from the end of each chapter. Aside from a space-saving device, almost universal access to the Internet and virtual libraries make such references redundant.

We gratefully acknowledge Natalie Karst, whose help is much appreciated. Special thanks go to Dede Andersen and Tad Ringo of Blackwell Publishing, who have been unbelievably patient and extremely helpful in getting our effort to press.

PART I

Introduction

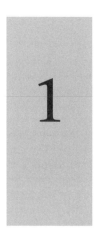

Parasitism and Pathogenicity

ERNST L. BIBERSTEIN

Veterinary microbiology deals with microbial agents affecting animals. Such agents are characterized according to their ecologic arrangements: *parasites* live in permanent association with, and at the expense of, animal hosts; *saprophytes* normally inhabit the inanimate environment. Parasites that cause their host no discernible harm are called *commensals*. The term *symbiosis* usually refers to reciprocally beneficial associations of organisms. This arrangement is also called *mutualism*.

Pathogenic organisms are parasites or saprophytes that cause disease. The process by which they establish themselves in a host individual is infection, but infection need not be followed by clinical illness. The term *virulence* is sometimes used to mean pathogenicity but sometimes to express degrees of pathogenicity.

Some Attributes of Host–Parasite Relationships

Many pathogenic microorganisms are host-specific in that they parasitize only one or a few animal species. The cause of equine strangles, *Streptococcus equi* subspecies *equi*, is essentially limited to horses. Others—certain *Salmonella* types, for example—have a broad host range. The basis for this difference in host specificity is incompletely understood, but it may in part be related to the need for specific attachment devices between host (receptors) and parasite (adhesins).

Some agents infect several host species but with varying effects. The plague bacillus *Yersinia pestis* behaves as a commensal parasite in many, but by no means all, small rodent species but causes fatal disease in rats and humans. Evolutionary pressure may have produced some of these differences, but not others: *Coccidioides immitis*, a saprophytic fungus requiring no living host, infects cattle and dogs with equal ease; yet it produces no clinical signs in cattle but frequently causes progressive fatal disease in dogs.

Potential pathogens vary in their effects on different tissues in the same host. The *Escherichia coli* that is commensal in the intestine can cause severe disease in the urinary tract and peritoneal cavity.

Some microorganisms that are commensal in one habitat may turn pathogenic in a habitat that is pathologically altered or otherwise compromised. Thus, oral streptococci, which occasionally enter the bloodstream, may colonize a damaged heart valve and initiate bacterial endocarditis. In the absence of such a lesion, however, they would be cleared uneventfully via the macrophage system. Similarly, the frequent entrance of intestinal bacteria into vascular channels normally leads to their disposal by humoral and cellular defense mechanisms. In immunoincompetent hosts, however, such entrance may lead to fatal septicemia.

Transfer to a new host or tissue, or a change in host resistance, are common ways that commensal parasites are converted into active pathogens. *Commensalism* is the stable form of parasitic existence. It ensures survival of the microorganism, which active disease would jeopardize by killing the host or evoking an active immune response. Either effect deprives the agent of its habitat. Evolutionary selective pressure therefore tends to eliminate host–parasite relationships that threaten the survival of either partner. It does so by allowing milder strains of the pathogen, which permit longer survival of the host and thereby facilitate their own dissemination, to replace the more lethal ones. It also favors a resistant host population by screening out highly susceptible stock. The trend is thus toward commensalism. Most agents causing serious disease have alternative modes of survival as commensals in tissues or hosts not subject to disease (e.g., plague) or in the inanimate environment (e.g., coccidioidomycosis). Others cause chronic infections lasting months or years (tuberculosis, syphilis), during which their dissemination to other hosts ensures their survival.

Criteria of Pathogenicity—Koch's Postulates

The presence of a microorganism in diseased individuals does not prove its pathogenic significance. To demonstrate the causal role of an agent in a disease, the following qualifications or "postulates" formulated by Robert Koch (1843–1910) should be satisfied:

1. The suspected agent is present in all cases of the disease.
2. The agent is isolated from such disease and propagated serially in pure culture, apart from its natural host.
3. Upon introduction into an experimental host, the isolate produces the original disease.

4. The agent can be reisolated from this experimental infection.

These postulates are ideals that are not satisfied in all cases of infectious diseases. The presence of some microorganisms cannot be demonstrated at the time of disease, especially in affected tissues (e.g., tetanus, botulism). Others lose virulence rapidly after isolation (e.g., *Leptospira* spp.), while still others, though indispensable for pathogenesis, require undetermined accessory factors (e.g., *Pasteurella*-related pneumonias). For some human viral pathogens (e.g., Cytomegalovirus), no experimental host is known, and some agents (e.g., *Mycobacterium leprae*) have not been grown apart from their natural hosts.

Elements in the Production of an Infectious Disease

Effective transmission through indirect contact occurs by ingestion; inhalation; or mucosal, cutaneous, or wound contamination. Airborne infection takes place largely via droplet nuclei, which are 0.1 to 5mm in diameter. Particles of this size stay suspended in air and can be inhaled. Larger particles settle out but can be resuspended in dust, which may also harbor infectious agents from nonrespiratory sources (e.g., skin squames, feces, saliva). Arthropods may serve as mechanical carriers of pathogens (e.g., *Shigella, Dermatophilus*) or play an indispensable part in the life cycles of disease-producing agents (plague, ehrlichioses, viral encephalitides).

Attachment to host surfaces requires interaction between the agent's adhesins, which are usually proteins, and the host's receptors, which are most often carbohydrate residues. Examples of bacterial adhesins are fimbrial proteins (*Escherichia coli, Salmonella* spp.), P-1 protein of *Mycoplasma pneumoniae*, and afimbrial surface proteins (some streptococci). Examples of host receptor substances include fibronectin for some streptococci and staphylococci, mannose for many *E. coli* strains, and sialic acid for *M. pneumoniae*.

Attachment is inhibited by normal commensal flora that occupy or block available receptor sites and discourage colonization by excreting toxic metabolites, bacteriocins and microcins. This "colonization resistance" is an important defense mechanism and may be assisted by mucosal antibody and other antibacterial substances (defensins, lysozyme, lactoferrin, organic acids).

Penetration of host surfaces is a variable requirement among pathogens. Some agents, having reached a primary target cell population, penetrate no farther (e.g., enterotoxigenic *E. coli*). Others traverse surface membranes after inducing cytoskeletal rearrangements, resulting in "ruffles" that entrap adhered bacteria or passage between epithelial cells (e.g., *Salmonella, Yersinia*). Inhaled facultative intracellular parasites like *Mycobacterium tuberculosis* are taken up by pulmonary macrophages, in which they may multiply and travel via lymphatics to lymph nodes and other tissues. Percutaneous penetration occurs mostly through injuries, including arthropod bites.

Dissemination takes place by extension, aided perhaps by such bacterial enzymes as collagenase and hyaluronidase, which are produced by many pathogens. Microorganisms are also spread via lymph and blood vessels, the bronchial tree, bile ducts, nerve trunks, and mobile phagocytes.

Growth in or on host tissue is a prerequisite of pathogenesis for all pathogenic organisms, except the few that produce toxins in foodstuffs prior to ingestion. In order to multiply to pathogenic levels, they must be able to neutralize host defense efforts. Relevant adaptations of various bacteria include firm attachment to prevent mechanical removal; repulsion or nonattraction of phagocytes; and interference with phagocytic function by capsules and cell walls, by leukotoxic activity, or by prevention of phagocytic digestion. Some bacteria digest or divert antibodies and deplete complement. Some destroy the vascular supply to tissue, shutting out defensive resources and suspending antimicrobial activity in the affected area.

With host defenses neutralized, microbial growth can proceed if nutritional supplies are adequate and the pH, temperature, and oxidation-reduction potential (Eh) are appropriate. Iron is often a limiting nutrient. Microbial ability to appropriate iron from iron-binding host proteins (transferrin, lactoferrin) is a factor in virulence. Gastric acidity accounts for the resistance of the stomach to most pathogenic bacteria, although expression of alternative sigma factors when bacteria are in stationary phase results in an RNA polymerase that transcribes genes whose products help the pathogen resist an acidic environment (e.g., *Salmonella, E. coli*). The high body temperature of birds may explain their resistance to some diseases (e.g., anthrax, histoplasmosis), while low Eh requirements account for the restriction of anaerobic growth to devitalized (i.e., nonoxygenated) tissues or tissues in which simultaneous aerobic growth has lowered the Eh.

Pathogenic Action

Microbial disease manifests itself either as direct damage to host structures and functions by exotoxins or viruses, or as damage due to host reactions such as those triggered by endotoxin or immune responses.

Direct Damage

Exotoxins are bacterial proteins, which are often freely excreted into the environment. The differences between endotoxins and exotoxins are shown in Table 1.1.

Two types of exotoxins exist. One acts extracellularly or on cell membranes, attacking intercellular substances or cell surfaces by enzymatic or detergent-like mechanisms. It includes, for example, bacterial hemolysins, leukocidins, collagenases, and hyaluronidases, which may play an ancillary role in infections.

The other type of exotoxin consists of proteins or polypeptides that enter cells and enzymatically disrupt cellular processes. These usually consist of an A fragment, which has enzymatic activity, and a B fragment, which is responsible for binding the toxin to its target cell. Exotoxins are encoded chromosomally, on plasmids, or on bacterio-

Table 1.1.   Exo- and Endotoxins Compared

Exotoxins	Endotoxins
Often spontaneously diffusible	Cell-bound as part of cell wall
Proteins or polypeptides	Lipopolysaccharide (lipid A is toxic component)
Produced by gram-positive and gram-negative bacteria	Limited to gram-negative bacteria
Produce a single, pharmacologically specific effect	Produce a range of effects, largely due to host-derived mediators
Each is distinct in structure and reactivity according to its bacterial species of origin	All similar in structure and effect regardless of bacterial species of origin
Lethal in minute amounts (mice = nanograms)	Lethal in larger amounts (mice = micrograms)
Labile to heat, chemicals, storage	Very stable to heat, chemicals, storage
Convertible to toxoids (= nontoxic, immunogenic toxin-derivatives); elicit antitoxin production	Not convertible to toxoids

phages. The function the toxins serve the bacteria is not known.

Viruses produce injury by destroying the cells in which they replicate or by altering cell function, appearance, and growth characteristics.

Endotoxins are lipopolysaccharides, which are part of the gram-negative cell wall. They consist of polysaccharide surface chains, which may be virulence factors and somatic (O) antigens; a core polysaccharide; and lipid A, where the toxicity resides.

Lipopolysaccharides bind to lipopolysaccharide-binding protein (a serum protein), which in turn transfers it to the blood phase of CD14. The CD14-LPS complex binds to Toll-like receptor proteins on the surface of macrophage cells triggering the release of proinflammatory cytokines. These substances elicit manifestations of endotoxemia, including fever, headache, hypotension, leukopenia, thrombocytopenia, intravascular coagulation, inflammation, endothelial damage, hemorrhage, fluid extravasation, and circulatory collapse. Many of these result from 1) activation of the complement cascade and 2) production of arachidonic acid metabolites: prostaglandins, leukotrienes, and thromboxanes. The phenomena produced by endotoxins closely resemble aspects of gram-negative septicemias, but most of them can also be duplicated by peptidoglycans of gram-positive bacteria.

Immune-Mediated Damage

Tissue damage due to immune reactions is considered elsewhere (see Chapter 2). Complement-mediated responses (such as inflammation) and reactions resembling immediate-type allergic phenomena can occur in response to endotoxins or to peptidoglycan without preceding sensitization.

Specific immune responses participate in the pathogenesis of many infections, particularly chronic granulomatous infections such as tuberculosis. Lesions are due to cell-mediated hypersensitivity, which is established in the early weeks of infection. Cell-mediated responses intensify inflammatory responses and tissue destruction upon subsequent encounters with the agent or its protein through the release of effector substances from T lymphocytes (e.g., cytokines, perforins).

Immune mechanisms apparently contribute to anemias seen in anaplasmosis, and the haemotrophic mycoplasmas. The antibody response to hemoparasitism does not distinguish between the parasite and the host erythrocyte. Both are removed by phagocytosis.

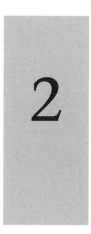

2

Immune Responses to Infectious Agents

Laurel J. Gershwin

The immune response to infectious agents is comprised of a series of innate and acquired mechanisms that work together to prevent infection, if possible, and to control the pathogenic effects of organisms that are able to evade the initial innate immune defenses. In recent years there have been significant advances in understanding several heretofore unappreciated innate defenses. Direction of immune responses for appropriate anti-pathogen responses by immunomodulatory cytokines and appropriate mechanisms of antigen presentation are now well defined. This chapter emphasizes the current knowledge defining how the immune system customizes the response depending upon the type of pathogen encountered.

Innate Immunity

Anatomic Features, Physiological Processes, and Normal Flora

Traditionally, innate immunity has been considered to be composed of anatomic features, physiological functions, microbiological barriers (the normal flora), fluid phase components, and cellular constituents. For example, the mucosa-covered nasal turbinates form an initial "sticky" barrier to remove larger particles from the inhaled air. Smaller particles that gain access to the respiratory tract encounter the ciliated epithelium and mucus blanket that effectively produces a mucociliary apparatus; this works to remove inhaled material from the lower respiratory tract. Within the gastrointestinal tract, peristalsis and the vomit reflex have similar effects on removal of undesired material from the body. The flushing action of the bladder is important in preventing urine stasis, which predisposes to bacterial infection.

The normal flora plays an important role in prevention of colonization by more virulent organisms. These bacteria and fungi establish a unique relationship with the host, a relationship that begins as the microbiologically sterile fetus begins its journey down the birth canal. Acquisition of bacteria and fungi begins immediately, with infection (colonization) of all exposed surfaces, including mucosal surfaces (alimentary canal, upper respiratory tract, and distal genitourinary tract), with microorganisms from the birth canal and from the mother's immediate environment. The association of microbe with the host is not haphazard but rather is an association that depends upon 1)

receptors (usually in the form of carbohydrates that are part of glycoproteins on the surface of the host cell) and adhesins on the microbe cell surface, 2) the chemicals in the immediate environment of the microbe–host interaction, in part due to products secreted by competing microorganisms (e.g., microcins, bacteriocins, and volatile fatty acids) and in part due to products secreted by the host (e.g., acid environment of the stomach, defensins secreted by Paneth cells, the contents of bile in the upper small intestine, or the content of sebum on the skin), and 3) the availability of nutrient substances.

The establishment of the normal flora is a dynamic one, with replacement at various exposed locations with microbes more capable of living at a particular site (niche) than the ones preceding. In addition, the immune system appears to play some role, since it has been shown that members of the normal flora are very poorly immunogenic in the host from which the microbes are isolated. This suggests that immune responses to microbes attempting to colonize a particular location (niche) will result in the blockage of association between adhesin (microbe) with receptor (host). If a microbe cannot associate, then it will be replaced with one that will. This occurs until a strain of microbe is encountered that is more similar to the host than its predecessor, which is subsequently "accepted" as part of the normal flora of that particular animal. The result is an ecosystem composed of numerous species of bacteria and fungi that are associated with an abundance of niches, each of which is occupied with a particular species of microbe most suited to live at that location. This "occupation" results in a barrier to colonization (infection) by microbes that are not members of the normal flora, thus the term *colonization resistance*.

Cellular Responses in Innate Defense

The innate phase of the immune response has been described as a "speed bump" for pathogens. There are several cell types that participate in innate defense. The phagocytic cell is of particular importance in defense against bacterial pathogens. There are primarily two types of phagocytes in mammals, the polymorphonuclear leukocyte (neutrophil) and the macrophage. While the neutrophil's main role is removal of foreign material and the killing and subsequent removal of bacteria, the macrophage plays a dual role by acting as an antigen presenting cell for initiation of an acquired immune response. A third type of cell that is important in the innate response against viruses is the natural killer cell.

The Neutrophil. The polymorphonuclear leukocyte, *neutrophil*, is a bone-marrow–derived end-cell that normally comprises 30% to 70% percent of the total leukocytes in the peripheral blood of various species. The neutrophil is a granulocytic leukocyte and contains two types of granules: primary or azurophilic granules and secondary or specific granules. Neutrophils spend only about 12 hours in circulation, then go into the tissues where they survive for an additional two to three days. Within the bone marrow there is a large storage compartment for neutrophils. A bacterial infection within the body causes a rapid mobilization of this pool and the neutrophils accumulate at the site of the infectious process. They are attracted by the chemotactic factors, C3a and C5a, which are generated subsequent to activation of the complement system. The process of neutrophil accumulation begins by *adherence* of the circulating neutrophils to the vascular endothelium (margination), *extravasation* into tissue spaces, and *chemotaxis* of the cells toward the focus of injury. Invading microorganisms are ingested by neutrophils in a process called *phagocytosis* (Figs 2.1 and 2.2).

Phagocytosis of bacteria by neutrophils involves several steps. First, initial recognition and binding occur. This process is made more efficient by the presence of opsonins consisting of immunoglobulin and/or complement components. Opsonization coats the surface of a particle, neutralizing the net negative charges, which might otherwise cause the neutrophil and bacterial cell to repel each other. In addition, on the cell membrane of the neutrophil, receptors are present for antibody (Fc receptors) and for complement (CR). These receptors facilitate firm attachment of the opsonized bacterium to the neutrophil. Next, pseudopodia form around the organism and then fuse to form a *phagocytic vacuole* containing the organism. Some organisms are more readily engulfed than others. For example, the presence of a polysaccharide capsule causes an organism to be resistant to phagocytosis. After engulfment, lysosomal granules fuse with the phagosome membrane to form the *phagolysosome*. The eventual elimination of the engulfed organism occurs within this structure.

Bacterial killing is accomplished by a series of metabolic and enzymatic events. Metabolic activity increases within a neutrophil during phagocytosis. Oxygen consumption increases and light energy is emitted (chemiluminescence). This metabolic or *respiratory burst* involves oxidation of glucose by the hexosemonophosphate shunt. Bactericidal products are generated. Superoxide radicals are produced and converted to H_2O_2 by superoxide dismutase. Hydrogen peroxide is toxic for bacteria that lack catalase. The enzyme myeloperoxidase, present in azurophil granules, catalyzes the oxidation of halide ions to hypohalite, which is also toxic to microorganisms. Thus the myeloperoxidase-hydrogen-peroxide-halide system is efficient in bacterial killing. Susceptible organisms are killed within minutes. Inside the primary granules of neutrophils, enzymes released during degranulation act on proteins, lipids, carbohydrates, and nucleic acids to degrade the killed bacterial cells. Some of these enzymes are collagenase, elastase, acid phosphatase, phospholipase, lysozyme, hyaluronidase, acid ribonuclease, and deoxyribonuclease. *Lysozyme* can cleave glycosyl bonds in the bacterial cell wall, making the cell susceptible to lysis. Also, lysosomes contain cationic peptides (defensins) that form lethal pores in bacteria as well as fungal cell walls.

FIGURE 2.1.   *Neutrophil response to an infectious agent: A. Neutrophils are present in the circulation. B. Neutrophils express adhesin molecules (CD18) and adhere to the endothelial cells in the blood vessel. This process is called* margination. *C. Neutrophils pass through the endothelial cells by diapedesis. D. Neutrophils, now extravascular, respond and move along a chemotactic gradient.*

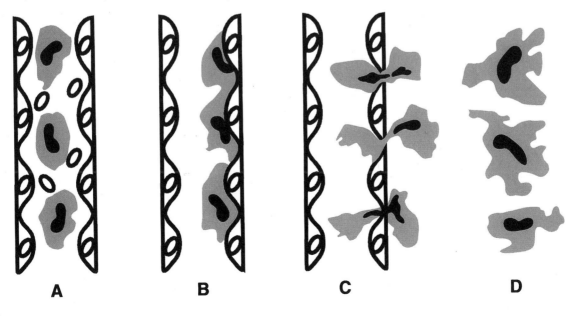

A   **B**   **C**   **D**

FIGURE 2.2.   *The process of phagocytosis: A. A bacterium is opsonized by antibody. The antibody binds to an Fc receptor on a phagocyte. B. The phagocyte begins to engulf the attached bacterium. C. The phagosome containing the bacterium fuses with lysosomes in the phagocyte cytoplasm to form a phagolysosome. D. The bacterium is killed and digested. E. The bacterial breakdown products are eliminated from the cell. Some parts of the bacterium will remain on macrophage membrane associated MHC class II to be used in antigen presentation to T cells.*

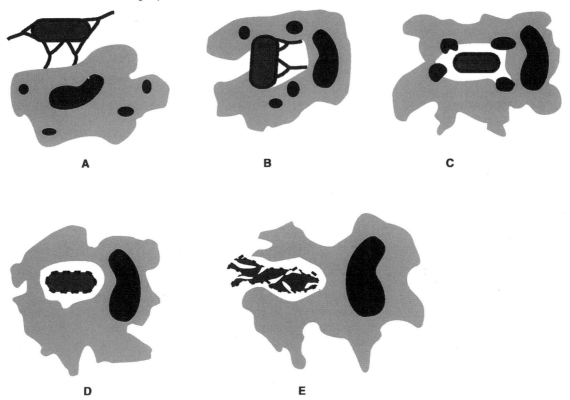

Macrophage. The macrophage is a mononuclear cell derived from the bone marrow. For several days after release from the bone marrow, it circulates as a blood *monocyte* before going into the tissues, where it becomes a functional macrophage. Free macrophages are present in many parts of the body and are named accordingly, for example, alveolar macrophages (lung) and peritoneal macrophages. Fixed macrophages line sinus cavities that filter blood. These include the Kupffer cells (liver), Langerhans cells (skin), histiocytes (connective tissue), mesangial cells (kidneys), and sinus-lining cells of the spleen, lymph nodes, and bone marrow. Some of these macrophages are important in antigen processing for induction of an immune response (described later in this chapter).

The macrophage differs from the neutrophil in that it has a longer life span in tissue and can reuse phagolysosomes. In addition, macrophages stimulated by cytokines (e.g., interferon) or microbial products (e.g., lipopolysaccharide) result in activation of nitric oxide synthase that catalyzes the production of nitric oxide (NO) from l-arginine. NO is toxic to many bacteria, especially those residing within macrophages (e.g., *Salmonella, Listeria*). The macrophage is similar to the neutrophil in that toxic oxygen metabolites are generated for bacterial killing and the lysosomes contain potent hydrolytic enzymes and

cationic peptides (defensins). While the neutrophil responds to a stimulus rapidly, the macrophage is not present until later in an infectious process, often after 8 to 12 hours. In some instances, neutrophils may eliminate an organism before macrophages arrive in any great number. When tissue destruction has occurred as a result of an inflammatory response, macrophages are attracted to the area by products from dying neutrophils and bacteria. They phagocytose the debris and remove it. In some instances, macrophages may engulf particulate material that they are unable to digest. When this occurs, the macrophage may migrate to a mucosal surface such as the respiratory or gastrointestinal tract for elimination from the body.

Some microorganisms are more easily killed by phagocytes than others. Bacteria that have polysaccharide capsules are less readily engulfed than unencapsulated counterparts. Opsonizing antibody or complement components must be present to coat such organisms before phagocytes can engulf them (as described above) Some microorganisms are readily phagocytosed, but are able to grow intracellularly. For example, microorganisms such as *Listeria monocytogenes* and *Mycobacterium tuberculosis* are not killed after phagocytosis by macrophages. Organisms may produce factors that inhibit phagolysosome fusion or even escape the phagolysosome into the cytoplasm, thus preventing exposure to enzymatic degradation. These organisms require macrophage activation by interferon γ, a product of both NK cells and activated T helper 1 cells.

Natural Killer (NK) Cells. Natural killer cells are a central and important component of the innate immune response to viruses and some bacteria. The NK cell is a distinct lineage of lymphocyte that, unlike the T and B lymphocyte, does not have a specific receptor for antigen—i.e., they do not rearrange genes encoding membrane receptors. Yet, this cell type is able to recognize and target cells for destruction. NK cells comprise from 5–20% of lymphocytes in the peripheral blood and more than 90% of lymphocytes in the placenta. Their function includes cell mediated immunity, antibody-dependent cellular cytotoxicity, production of interferon γ early in infection, and secretion of a variety of other cytokines. In the adult mammal NK cells develop within the bone marrow from hematopoietic cell precursors. NK cells are responsive to several cytokines and they secrete cytokines, including interferon γ, and tumor necrosis factor α (TNFα). The NK cell response is coordinated and modulated by cytokines that include interferons α and β and Interleukins 2, 12, 15, and 18. Recently a variety of receptors have been identified on NK cells. These receptors allow the NK cell to either kill a target cell, or to turn off the potential killing response. Inhibitory receptors expressed on NK cells include the killer immunoglobulin-like receptor (KIR). This receptor binds to MHC class I molecules on body cells and facilitates an inhibitory response through activation of intracellular tyrosine–based inhibitory motifs. This function prevents the powerful killing capacity of the NK cell from acting on normal body cells. In contrast, when a cell lacks MHC class I, the NK cell recognizes the absence and begins the process of killing that target cell.

The NK cell is particularly effective in eliminating tumor cells and cells infected with some viruses. A number of viruses (and some tumor cells) down-regulate cellular MHC class I molecule synthesis. These viruses effectively evade the acquired T cytotoxic cell (CD8) response (detailed later in this chapter) by removing the MHC molecule that presents antigen to cytotoxic T cells. However, the NK cell targets these cells that display the "missing self" appearance. NK cells are important in elimination of herpes viruses. For example, in human beings that lack NK cells, the diseases varicella zoster and cytomegalovirus infection (both herpes viruses) are often fatal, whereas the normal individual is able to successfully recover from these infections. The mechanism by which the NK cell kills the target involves secretion of perforin molecules that are able to poke holes in the cell membrane, permitting caustic granzymes entry to the cytosol.

The early production of interferon γ by NK cells is helpful in initiating a T helper 1 type response (described later in this chapter) that activates macrophages for more efficient killing of some bacteria. Other killing mechanisms include antibody-dependent cellular cytotoxicity (ADCC). NK cells display the cell membrane receptor CD16, a low-affinity IgG receptor. By using this receptor to bind IgG, the NK cell is able to participate in ADCC, killing cells that are recognized by the attached immunoglobulin. In this way the NK cell collaborates with the acquired immune system to eliminate infected cells.

Gamma-Delta T Cells. T cells that display membrane receptors called *γδ chains* (gamma-delta T cells) constitute a small percentage of the circulating pool of lymphocytes in nonruminant species. In ruminants, however, gamma-delta T cells may represent up to 30% of the circulating lymphocyte pool. In most species, gamma-delta T cells are present in the lamina propria underlying mucosal epithelia, strategically beneficial sites for cells involved in host defense.

Functional studies in mouse models and also data from human beings has demonstrated a role for these cells in defense against mycobacterial pathogens. The role of gamma-delta T cells in innate defense against *Mycobacterium tuberculosis* appears to be most important early in the infection. Activation of these cells by *M. tuberculosis* antigens is dependent on accessory cells, such as alveolar macrophages, which provide co-stimulatory molecules. The ligands on the mycobacterium that stimulate the gamma-delta T cells have recently been shown to be small phosphate-containing molecules. The major effector functions of gamma-delta T lymphocytes in defense against *M. tuberculosis* is in cytokine secretion and in cytotoxic effector cell function. These cells produce interferon γ, TNFα, and a small amount of IL-2.

Gamma-delta T cells have a role in limiting viral replication in some viral diseases. In mouse models of influenza virus infection these cells accumulate in the lung presumably to resolve the pneumonic process. In both mouse models and in human patients the role of gamma-delta T cells in resolution of herpes simplex-1 infection has been demonstrated.

Toll-like Receptors. Toll-like receptors (TLR) are a primitive mechanism of innate immunity. They are defined as pattern-recognition receptors and are present on a variety of immune and other cells. Originally described in Drosophila, these molecules and their signaling pathways are important for detection of invading pathogens in fruit flies, mammals, and plants. There are 10 known TLR in mammals. Each TLR recognizes a specific component of a pathogen. For example, TLR1, 2, and 6 recognize various microbial components. TLR2 recognizes lipoproteins, lipoteichoic acid from gram-positive bacteria, and lipoarabinomannan from mycobacteria. TLR3 recognizes double-stranded RNA, and is therefore important in viral recognition. TLR4 has a role in transducing the signals of lipopolysaccharide (LPS) from gram-negative bacteria. TLR5 is activated by flagellin, its specific ligand. Thus, TLR5 is important in the response to flagellated bacteria, but not to those that are not. When the basolateral surface of the intestinal epithelium is exposed to flagellin an inflammatory response occurs. This is the site of expression of the TLR5. TLR7 is activated by certain synthetic compounds that have anti-viral activity. TLR9 recognizes bacterial CpG motifs in DNA. These motifs have recently been identified as important immune modulators (stimulating a T_{H1} response).

Recognition of viruses by TLR has been reported for some viruses. TLR4 binds to one of the major surface proteins on respiratory syncytial virus (RSV), an important pathogen of human children and bovine calves. In an experimental mouse model with mutated TLR4, RSV was found to be cleared less efficiently than from mice that have normal TLR4. Other viruses, such as mouse mammary tumor virus, have been shown to bind TLR4 to envelope proteins. In addition, signaling through TLR3 and TLR7 has been shown to induce synthesis of alpha and beta interferons.

Other studies with TLR mutant mice have demonstrated the importance of these receptors in resistance to bacterial infection. TLR4-mutant mice are highly susceptible to infection with the gram-negative bacteria, *Salmonella typhimurium*. Whereas, mice defective in TLR2 are highly sensitive to infection with gram-positive bacteria, *Streptococcus pneumoniae*.

Acquired Immunity

Generation of the Immune Response

The initial step required for initiation of an acquired immune response is presentation of an antigen to T lymphocytes.

Antigen Presentation. There are several cell types that are capable of antigen presentation: dendritic cell, macrophage, B lymphocyte, and specialized cells in the skin called *Langerhan's cells*. Of these cell types, the dendritic cell is considered to be a "professional antigen presenting cell" and as such is most efficient at antigen presentation. It is currently believed that the dendritic cell involved in primary antigen presentation is responsible for determining what type of immune response is generated in response to the pathogen. Subsets of dendritic cells are responsive to different cytokines; they in turn produce cytokines that influence the T cell response towards a humoral (T_{H2}) or a cellular (T_{H1} response). For example, production of Interleukin 12 (IL-12) by dendritic cells is required for initiation of a T_{H1} response in T lymphocytes. Binding of TLR by dendritic cells and phagocytes that present antigen influences the type of response that is induced, so that it is appropriate for the type of pathogen that is invading the host.

The process of antigen presentation occurs either by the extracellular (phagocytic) pathway, or by the endocytic (cytosolic) pathway. Inactivated and killed organisms, once digested and processed in a phagosome, are bound to (major histocompatibility) MHC class II molecules and are brought to the cell surface for presentation to CD4 T (helper) lymphocytes.

Recognition of the antigen/MHC class II complex by a T cell with the same MHC class II is referred to as *MHC-restriction* and is a characteristic of the acquired immune response. Production of IL-2 by the T cell occurs after binding with the antigenic peptide and co-stimulatory molecules. Interleukin-2 is a T cell growth factor that facilitates clonal expansion of the participating T cell. These T cells, which are phenotypically CD4 and functionally called *helper T cells*, produce additional cytokines to influence the development of B cells, which are specific for the antigen. Under the influence of T cell–produced IL-4, B cells develop and mature into plasma cells secreting antibodies. Helper T cells produce predominantly IL-4 (T helper 2 cells or T_{H2}), which facilitate production of IgG_1 and IgE.

Another subset of T helper cells responds to presented antigen by making other cytokines. These cytokines are important in activation of macrophages for killing facultative intracellular bacteria and for supporting other cell-mediated responses. T helper type 1 cells produce interferon γ and IL-2, in addition to IL-12. As noted above, the initial production of IL-12 by the dendritic cell or NK cell can prejudice the T helper cell response towards T_{H1}. This response may be initiated through TLR binding to the dendritic cell.

Antigen presentation for intracellular pathogens follows the endocytic pathway through the cytosol. When a virus is replicating in the cytosol, viral proteins are processed and united with MHC class I molecules. These peptide-MHC complexes are then sent to the surface of the cell where they are bound by the CD8 cytotoxic T cells.

Effector Function. The ultimate result of antigen presentation to CD4 T lymphocytes is the development of an immune response. As stated above this response is mediated by the type of cytokine environment that has been created. If the T_{H2} cytokines are present, and for most pathogens there are usually some, there will be a humoral (antibody) response. When the pathogen has skewed the T helper cell response towards T_{H1} cytokine production (this occurs with facultative intracellular bacteria and viral pathogens), cytokines are produced to activate macrophages and CD8 T cells to become more effective killers.

Humoral Immunity (The Antibody Response). The initial introduction of antigen to a host followed by presentation of antigenic peptides to CD4 T cells results in stimulation of these cells to become T helper type 2 cells secreting cytokines that assist B cells in differentiating into cells that become antibody producing plasma cells. Production of Interleukin 4 (IL-4) by these T_{H2} cells results in expansion of B cell clones specific to the different epitopes on the antigen. The B cells also recognize antigenic epitopes on the microbe and in addition develop binding of co-stimulatory molecules on the T cell. Then under the influence of T cell cytokines, these B cells differentiate into antibody-producing plasma cells (Fig 2.3).

The first antibody to be produced is IgM and it appears in the circulation 7 to 10 days after initiation of the immune response. Next, IgG appears but does not rise to very high titers in this primary immune response. Subsequent encounters with antigen result in a secondary or anamnestic response. In the secondary response, the kinetics of antibody appearance in the circulation are more rapid and the quantity of antibody produced is greater. Most importantly, the isotype that predominates in the secondary response is predominantly IgG. The longer half-life of IgG facilitates the maintenance of an antibody titer higher for a longer duration of time. Often evaluation of the immune response (IgG versus IgM) to a disease agent can yield important information as to the chronicity of the exposure. It is a well-accepted diagnostic procedure to obtain acute and convalescent serum samples to be evaluated for antibody titer and isotype. Generally, when a disease agent is responsible for clinical signs two to three weeks after the initial appearance of signs, the titer will have increased by at least fourfold if the agent was involved in the infectious process. In an initial exposure to a disease agent, IgM is the predominant isotype, while a second or tertiary exposure (or vaccination) will elicit mostly IgG.

Effector Functions of Antibody. Antibodies can neutralize virus, bacteria, and soluble toxins. Some isotypes of antibody (IgG, IgM) can lyse target cells after activating the complement cascade. Antibodies can facilitate phagocytosis by acting as opsonins to help phagocytes adhere to microbes. The antibody response that is important in defense against bacterial disease depends on the pathogenic mechanisms involved, the site of the infectious process, and the isotype of the antibody elicited (Table 2.1). In a disease caused by an extracellular toxin, such as tetanus, antitoxin antibodies are important to neutralize and bind the toxin before it can bind to cellular sites and initiate clinical signs. This mechanism is important in diseases such as tetanus, anthrax, and botulism—all toxin-mediated diseases. In some instances, when a nonimmune host is at risk of developing a toxin-mediated disease, immediate administration of antitoxin (a solution containing antibodies to the toxin) is required to prevent the disease. In order to eliminate infectious agents, antibodies serve as opsonins as well as initiating the complement cascade (activation through the classical pathway). Opsonins lead to increased uptake by phagocytic cells, whereas complement activation leads to initiation of inflammation and generation of compounds that are detrimental to the infectious agent (e.g., membrane attack complex), as bacteria that

have capsules are particularly resistant to engulfment by phagocytes unless they have opsonins present.

Generally, the IgE response is limited to parasitic infections and hypersensitivity reactions to various environmental allergens, such as pollens and grasses. Occasionally, IgE is elicited in response to vaccination against some bacterial and viral pathogens. When this occurs, very serious adverse responses, such as anaphylactic shock, can result. Often there is a hereditary predisposition toward IgE production and these individuals are at increased risk of having such a vaccine reaction. For immunity to parasite infections, IgE may assist in the phenomenon of "self cure," in which large numbers of nematodes are purged from the gut by mast cell mediator–induced smooth muscle contraction. Alternatively, some infestations are controlled by antibody dependent cellular cytotoxicity (ADCC), in which IgE binds to eosinophils by low-affinity Fc receptors and facilitates release of major basic protein and other caustic enzymes on the parasite surface.

Table 2.1.   Effector Functions of Antibody

Isotype	Site of Action	Effector Functions
IgM	Intravascular	Complement fixation, agglutination
IgG	Intravascular	Complement fixation, neutralization
	Tissue spaces	Opsonization, ADCC[a]
IgA	Secretions: respiratory, GI, salivary	Neutralization on mucosal surfaces
IgE	Subcutaneous Submucosal	Mast-cell sensitization, ADCC

[a]Antibody-dependent cellular cytotoxicity

IgA is a very desirable response to infectious agents that affect mucosal surfaces. Since secretory IgA (SIgA) is protected by a secretory component from digestion in the gut by proteolytic enzymes, it is the most efficient antibody to be active in the environment of the gastrointestinal lumen. There it can neutralize viruses and bacteria to prevent their respective attachment to cellular receptors. Similarly, SIgA is effective within the secretions of the respiratory tract. Before a virus or a bacterium can infect a cell it must first bind to a cell surface protein that acts as a receptor for the infectious agent. Thus, binding of the infectious agent by antibody can inhibit binding to the receptor, and thus lower the infectivity of the agent. For example, influenza virus expresses a hemagglutinin that binds to certain glycoproteins expressed on epithelial cells in the respiratory tract. Binding of antibodies to the hemagglutinin prevents entry of the virus into these cells, and disease is prevented.

Antibodies are most effective against viruses that undergo a viremic phase, when there are numerous virus particles in the extracellular environment. Viruses such as influenza virus, for example, are neutralized by antibodies specific for the major surface antigens (hemagglutinin and neuraminidase). Other viruses—herpes virus, for example—remain very closely associated with cells and do not present much opportunity for antibody-mediated inactivation. The IgA isotype is especially effective on mucosal surfaces and functions to neutralize viruses before entry into the body. Secretory IgA is an extremely effective defense against respiratory and gastrointestinal viruses, as well as viruses that cause systemic disease but enter via the oral route. Virus neutralization occurs because the antibody binds to surface determinants of the virus and prevents the virus from binding to the cellular receptors to which it must attach in order to initiate the infectious process.

The relative importance of antibody and cell-mediated immune response depends upon the pathogenesis of the disease. For example, bacteria that produce potent exotoxins, such as *Clostridium tetani,* require antibodies to neutralize the toxin. Heavily encapsulated bacteria, such as *Klebsiella pneumonia,* require opsonizing antibodies for effective removal of the bacteria and ultimate killing by phagocytes. In contrast, bacteria that are capable of living within phagocytes, such as *Listeria monocytogenes,* are not effectively killed by an antibody, and require the T_{H1} response for effective elimination. Similarly, viral infections that produce viremia, such as influenza, are handled well by an appropriate antibody response; compared with herpes viruses that are cell-associated and require a cell-mediated immune response for effective control.

Cell-Mediated Immunity. Cell-mediated immune responses mediated by T cells involve two different mechanisms: macrophage activation and cytotoxic T cell activity (Table 2.2).

Killing of Facultative Intracellular Bacteria by Activated Macrophages. A variety of bacteria have the ability to prevent phagosome-lysome fusion. Bacteria that fall into this category include *Brucella, Mycobacterium, Listeria, Salmonella, Rhodococcus equi,* and others. When this occurs, the macrophage is often killed by the bacteria, rather than the ex-

Table 2.2.   Effector Functions of Cell-mediated Immune Responses

Effector Cell	Target	Mechanism
CD8	MHC class I with peptide	Perforin, granzymes, fas-fas ligand, TNFα
CD4/T_{H1}	Macrophage with intracellular organisms	Interferon γ–mediated activation of macrophage
NK Cell	Cells lacking MHCI	Perforin-mediated

pected opposite response. In the presence of CD4 T lymphocytes that make the so-called T helper cytokines, the macrophage is armed and able to circumvent the bacteria and to kill. The cytokines induce lysosomal fusion and increase macrophage bacteriocidal activity. Macrophages are activated following the production of interferon γ by these T_{H1} cells. This subset of T helper cells is stimulated subsequent to the production of IL-12 by infected macrophages and NK cells. Thus, the "arming" of macrophages results in destruction of the infectious agent that the macrophage previously had been unable to destroy (Fig 2.4).

Killing of Virus-Infected Cells by Cytotoxic T Cells. Pathogens, such as viruses, that live and grow inside of cells are best contained by elimination of the cell in which they are reproducing. Virus proteins made in the cytosol are able to associate with surface molecules of the cell for presentation to T cells. Cytotoxic T cells (CD8) recognize an antigenic peptide that is held in the groove formed by the chains of the MHC class I molecule on the cell surface. All nucleated cells have MHC class I on their surface and are therefore able to bind and present antigen from inside the cell in this manner. Recognition of the combination of MHC class I and antigenic determinant by cytotoxic T cells (by way of a specific T cell receptor) results in the release of perforins that make small pores in the cell membrane. This allows destructive enzymes called *granzymes* to enter the cytoplasm. In addition, tumor necrosis factor α is produced. Death of the cell is facilitated by the interaction of Fas-Fas ligand system, stimulating apoptosis. One CD8 T cell can repeatedly kill infected target cells, programming one to die, and then moving on to the next cell to kill it (Fig 2.5). The cytotoxic T cell is an efficient way to decrease viral progeny in an infected host.

Effector Cells Can Use Antibody to Bind Target Cells. Antibody dependent cellular cytotoxicity (ADCC) occurs when antibody binds to a cell that has receptors for the Fc portion of immunoglobulin G or E. The Fc receptor for the gamma chain is CD21 and the low affinity IgE receptor is CD23. These molecules are present on several types of effector cells, including neutrophils, macrophages, NK cells and eosinophils. The attachment of antibody to a cell that previously had no receptor for antigen renders it antigen-specific and capable of binding antigen. Besides NK cells, eosinophils and macrophages can also become involved in ADCC. ADCC is an effective method of killing cells infected with microorganisms (viral, bacterial, or fungal) as well as parasites. In the case of parasites, the eosinophil re-

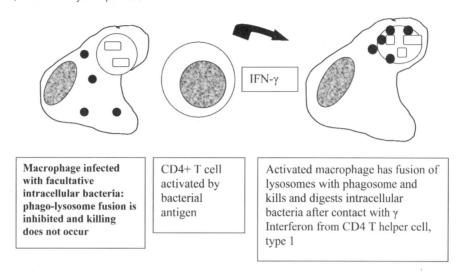

FIGURE 2.4.   *Destruction of an intracellular infectious agent by activated macrophages stimulated by T helper cells.*

| Macrophage infected with facultative intracellular bacteria: phago-lysosome fusion is inhibited and killing does not occur | CD4+ T cell activated by bacterial antigen | Activated macrophage has fusion of lysosomes with phagosome and kills and digests intracellular bacteria after contact with γ Interferon from CD4 T helper cell, type 1 |

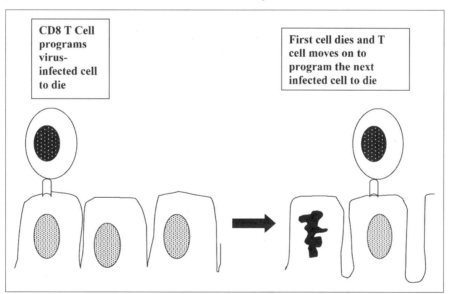

FIGURE 2.5.   *Destruction of a virus-infected cell by CD8 T cell.*

| CD8 T Cell programs virus-infected cell to die | First cell dies and T cell moves on to program the next infected cell to die |

leases granules containing major basic protein rendering the cuticle of the parasite permeable.

Evaluation of Immune Responses to Infectious Agents

The use of serological assays to evaluate exposure to or infection with bacterial and viral pathogens has been a mainstay for control of infectious diseases. In addition, for some infections, such as those with mycobacterial species,

the in vivo skin testing for cell-mediated responses has been of even greater use. For determination of recent infection status, serum samples are obtained during acute illness and again 2 to 3 weeks later. These acute and convalescent samples are then assayed for antibody titer using one of the methods described in Table 2.3. When the titer has increased at least fourfold (two dilutions), seroconversion has occurred and the disease agent for which the titers are specific is confirmed as having stimulated a recent response. Table 2.3 lists the common types of immunodiagnostic tests and some examples of disease for which the method has been/is being used.

Table 2.3.   Assay Methods for Infectious Diseases

Type of Assay	Application/Example
Precipitin in gel	Coggin's test for antibody to equine infectious anemiavirus (EIA)
Complement fixation	Antibody titer to *Brucella abortus*
Agglutination	Antibody titer to bacteria/*Salmonella*
Indirect Immunofluorescence	Antibody titer to canine distemper virus (CDV)
Direct Immunofluorescence	Antigen detection in cells: CDV, feline leukemia virus (FeLV)
Virus neutralization	Functional titer of antibody that prevents viral infection; equine influenza, bovine respiratory syncytial virus
ELISA	Detection of antigen (FeLV, parvovirus) or antibody against viral, bacterial, fungal, and protozoan antigens

Antibody-Based Serology

The current trend for immunodiagnosis utilizes the solid phase-binding assays, such as the enzyme-linked immunosorbent assay (ELISA). These assays are generally more sensitive than assays based on precipitin formation or complement fixation. Depending on the disease to be diagnosed, ELISA can be designed to detect antigen (as in feline leukemia virus and canine parvovirus infections) or antibody. ELISA has the advantage that the format is easily adaptable to either a quick (positive or negative) read-out or a titer determination.

Cell-Mediated Immunity-Based Diagnostics

For those pathogens that induce a strong T helper 1 type immune response with production of associated cytokines (e.g., interferon γ), an intradermal skin test with antigen from the pathogen can often be used to demonstrate exposure or infection. Recently, in vitro correlates have been used for some diseases. *Mycobacterium bovis* infection can be diagnosed with intradermal infection of tuberculin. Within 48 to 72 hours of antigen injection, erythema and induration at the site are apparent in infected patients. Infection with *Mycobacterium avium* subspecies *pseudotuberculosis* (Johnes disease agent) can be detected by in vitro incubation of patient lymphocytes with antigen and subsequent analysis of interferon γ levels in the culture supernatant. Infection by additional organisms that are among the group called *facultative intracellular pathogens* can be detected using similar testing strategies.

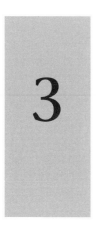

3 Laboratory Diagnosis

Dwight C. Hirsh   Yuan Chung Zee

Anthony E. Castro

Bacteria and Fungi

A key decision made early in the diagnostic workup is whether the patient's condition has an infectious etiology. This decision is important because drugs used to treat conditions with noninfectious etiologies—corticosteroids, for example—are often contraindicated for treatment of conditions with an infectious one, for which antibiotics are appropriate.

One of the first major goals of the microbiology laboratory is to isolate clinically significant microorganisms from an affected site and, if more than one type of microorganism is present, to isolate them in approximately the same ratio as occurs in vivo. Whether an isolate is "clinically significant" or not depends upon the circumstances of isolation. For example, the isolation of large numbers of a particular microorganism from a normally sterile site in the presence of an inflammatory cytology would be interpreted as significant.

Attention must be given to the site cultured as well as to the method of obtaining the sample for culture. The determination of significance is made a great deal easier if the sample is obtained from a normally sterile site. Obtaining a sample from the alimentary canal, and expecting meaningful answers, may be unrealistic unless one is looking for the presence or absence of a particular microorganism, for example, *Salmonella* or *Campylobacter*.

Sample Collection

Care must be given to how the sample is collected; if not, interpretation of results may be difficult. Most infectious processes arise subsequent to the contamination of a compromised surface or site by microorganisms that are also a part of the flora occurring on a contiguous mucosal surface. In other words, microorganisms isolated from an affected site are often similar (if not identical) to those found as part of the normal flora of the patient.

Transport of Samples

The sooner the sample is processed in the microbiology laboratory, the better. Realistically, the time between sample collection and processing may range from minutes to hours. Sample drying (all microorganisms) and exposure to a noxious atmosphere (oxygen for obligate anaerobes) are the major dangers in not analyzing samples promptly. For this reason, it is important that the sample be kept moist (for a syringe full of exudate, this is obviously not an important consideration) and, if conditions warrant (see below), air excluded. Moistness is maintained by placing the sample in a transport (holding) medium composed of a balanced salt solution usually in a gelled matrix. Because this medium does not contain any nutrient material, microorganisms in the sample multiply poorly if at all (and thereby relative numbers and ratios are preserved) but remain viable for a time, at least for overnight (exactly how long depends upon the microorganism involved—beta hemolytic *Streptococcus*, for example, does not survive as long as *Escherichia coli*). Swabs should always be placed in transport medium, regardless of the time elapsed between processing and collection. Fluids that may contain anaerobic bacteria (e.g., exudate from draining tracts, peritoneal and pleural effusions, abscess material) should be cultured immediately. If this material is contained in a syringe, then the air should be expelled and a sterile stopper placed over the needle. If a swab is used to collect the sample, it should be placed in an anaerobic transport medium. If a syringe full of sample cannot be processed immediately, the syringe should be emptied into an anaerobic transport medium and held at room temperature. Similarly placed swabs are treated in the same manner. Do not refrigerate samples suspected of containing anaerobes because some species do not tolerate reduced temperatures.

Demonstration of an Infectious Agent

The presence of an infectious agent is accomplished by examination of stained smears made from a portion of the clinical sample, culture techniques, molecular/immunological methods, or a combination of these methods.

Direct Smears. Information obtained from examination of a stained smear is valuable because it may be the first indication (and sometimes the only one) that an infectious agent is present. Also, what is seen (shape, staining characteristics) will help guide the choice of therapy 24 hours before culture results are available. At least 10^4 microorganisms/ml or gram of material must be present in order to be readily detected microscopically.

As is the case with a sample obtained from a normally

sterile site, the presence of bacteria in bladder urine is a significant finding. However, interpretation of the results of analysis of urine samples obtained by catheter or by "catch" is difficult because of the confounding presence of flora flushed from the distal urethra. Finding bacteria by direct smear in concentrated (the preferred) or unconcentrated urine obtained by percutaneous aspiration of bladder urine is a significant finding. Demonstration of 1 bacteria/oil field in a drop of unconcentrated urine (which has been allowed to dry and then stained) represents about 10^5 to 10^6 bacteria/ml of urine.

Two types of stains are available, the gram stain and Romanovsky-type stains such as Wright's or Giemsa. Each type of stain has advantages and disadvantages. The gram stain is useful in that the shape and the gram-staining characteristics of the agent are seen. The disadvantage of the gram stain is that the cellular content of the sample is not readily discerned. On the other hand, a Romanovsky-type stain gives the observer a feeling for the cellular nature of the sample and whether or not there is an infectious agent present. Cytologic evaluation of the sample is very important in assessing the significance of the microorganism seen and subsequently grown.

Culture Techniques. Media are inoculated with a portion of the specimen. Inoculation should be performed in a semiquantitative fashion (especially samples of bladder urine obtained by catheter or catch).

Determination of the relative numbers of microorganisms in a sample greatly helps interpretation of significance. Colonies of microorganisms growing on all four quadrants of a petri plate indicate that there are large numbers of microorganisms in the sample. If a sample yielded one or two colonies growing on the plate, the significance of these colonies and thus the question as to the infectious etiology of the condition would be in doubt. "Enrichment" prior to plating of a sample obtained from a normally sterile site should never be done because one microorganism can grow to numbers that equal many thousands in a very short period of time. Obviously more credence will be given to a process from which thousands of microorganisms were isolated than to a sample from which one was isolated. An important exception to this general "rule" is whether the presence or absence of a particular microorganism is significant, e.g., *Salmonella* in a fecal specimen. From a clinical perspective, the use of enrichment broths, other than for the determination of the presence or absence of a particular species of bacterium, is more trouble than it is worth. Too often, enrichment culture results lead to the unnecessary workup and treatment of a contaminating microorganism.

Determination of significance is aided by the cytology of the sample obtained from the affected site. Isolation (demonstration) of numerous microorganisms from a normally sterile site without the presence of inflammatory cells should be viewed with suspicion. The one exception to this rule is cryptococcal infection wherein the sample may contain a large number of yeast cells but very few inflammatory cells (the cryptococcal capsule is immunosuppressive). The isolation or demonstration of a "significant number" of microorganisms from a normally sterile site

without evidence of an inflammatory response can be explained by contaminated collection devices; contamination of the collection device from a contiguous, normally nonsterile site; contamination of the medium inoculation device in the microbiology laboratory; or contamination of the medium before inoculation. Collection devices (e.g., catheters) sterilized by liquid disinfectants quite often become contaminated by microorganisms able to live in such fluids (*Pseudomonas* is notorious for this).

Plates may be streaked in any fashion as long as individual colonies are produced after incubation. Assessing relative numbers is very subjective, and every laboratory has its own way of doing this. Relative numbers of microorganisms may be reported by noting how much growth occurs on the surface of the plate. Obviously, growth of one colony (the offspring of one bacterium) vs. growth of colonies over the whole plate would be viewed differently with respect to clinical significance. Determination of the actual numbers of bacteria present is only important when analyzing urine obtained by "catch" or catheter because of the problem of contamination of the sample by bacteria in the distal urethra. In this instance, disposable calibrated loops containing 0.001 or 0.01 ml of urine are used to inoculate appropriate media (blood/MacConkey, for example). Greater than 10^5 bacteria/ml of urine obtained by catheter or "catch" is considered significant (i.e., the bacteria are more likely to be coming from the bladder rather than the distal urethra).

Aerobic Bacteria. The standard medium inoculated for the isolation of facultative microorganisms is a blood agar plate. Many laboratories include a MacConkey agar plate as well (or as a "split" plate with blood agar on half and MacConkey agar on the other half). MacConkey agar is useful because enteric microorganisms (members of the Family Enterobacteriaceae, e.g., *Escherichia coli*, *Klebsiella*, *Enterobacter*) grow very well, as does the nonenteric *Pseudomonas*. Most other nonenteric gram-negative rods and all gram-positive microorganisms do not grow well on this medium. *Bordetella* grows as tiny pinpoint colonies after 24 hours; but after 48 hours of incubation, the colonies will be quite large. Assessing the growth on MacConkey agar will help greatly in determining the presence or absence of enteric organisms, the group of bacteria most difficult to deal with therapeutically.

Anaerobic Bacteria. Anaerobic bacteria grow on blood agar that is specially prepared by ridding the medium as much as possible of oxygen and its products. The plates come from the manufacturer in sealed pouches designed to exclude air. After anaerobic plates are inoculated, they should be placed in a container of flowing oxygen-free CO_2 or placed directly into an anaerobic environment. (Note that anaerobic blood plates that have been removed from their pouches should be stored in flowing oxygen-free CO_2 or in an anaerobic environment.)

When to inoculate media for anaerobic incubation depends upon the source of the sample. Processing samples for anaerobes is time-consuming and expensive. The most common sites or conditions that contain anaerobic bacteria are draining tracts; abscesses; pleural, pericardial, and peritoneal effusions; pyometra; osteomyelitis; and lungs. Anaerobic culture of sites that contain a population of anaerobic bacteria as part of the normal flora is wasteful (e.g., feces, vagina, distal urethra, oral cavity). An exception would be culture of duodenal aspirates for assessment of bacterial overgrowth. In this instance, the relative numbers found are what are sought (overgrowth is usually considered present when the total number of bacteria, anaerobes and aerobes, exceeds 10^8/ml of contents). Anaerobic culture of the urinary tract is not routinely performed because the recovery of these microorganisms from this site is extremely rare.

Molecular/Immunologic Methods. Sometimes it is important to determine the presence or absence of a particular microorganism as quickly as possible so that appropriate measures can be taken to deal with the problem. This is especially true when infectious agents are suspected that pose a threat to other animals, including human care givers (e.g., *Salmonella, Leptospira*). Likewise, some infectious agents take so long to grow in culture that formulation of a rational therapeutic strategy is difficult (e.g., some fungal agents, *Mycobacterium*). Still others are hard to detect because they are difficult to culture (e.g., *Leptospira*, rickettsiae) or have not been cultured in artificial media (e.g., *Clostridium piliformis, Lawsonia intracellularis*). In these instances, various techniques are available.

Immunologically based techniques make use of antibodies specific for the microorganism in question. These antibodies are usually immobilized on a solid support and are used to trap the agent. The presence of the trapped agent is then detected with specific antibody that has been labeled in some way (usually with a color reagent). Some kits making use of this approach are commercially available (e.g., *Salmonella*).

Molecular techniques utilizing DNA probes specific for a segment of DNA that is unique to the microorganism in question, or the polymerase chain reaction (PCR) using specific DNA primers, have been designed for a number of agents.

Virus

General Considerations

The diagnosis of viral diseases traditionally has been both tedious and time-consuming, but increasingly is expedited by modern technologies such as the polymerase chain reaction. Prompt and accurate diagnosis of viral diseases is therefore essential for an effective course of disease prevention and control.

Proper methods of collecting and processing clinical specimens and a complete history are vital to the successful isolation of viruses. Tissues that are extensively autolyzed or poorly stored usually do not yield infectious virus because of the susceptibility of most viruses to detrimental environmental conditions. Viral isolation and/or identification should be attempted in the following conditions:

1. During outbreaks of vesicular disease in livestock (e.g., foot-and-mouth disease in cattle, pigs, sheep, or goats).
2. During outbreaks of disease in large animal populations such as feedlots, poultry houses, or catteries

where many animals are at risk and prompt, accurate diagnosis is critical to the institution of control methods (such as vaccination).
3. In instances of potentially zoonotic diseases like rabies, West Nile fever, equine encephalomyelitis, particularly when human exposure has ocurred.
4. In determining the etiology of new disease, or in defining uncharacterized aspects of existing ones.

Tissues for virus isolation should be collected from recently dead animals whenever possible (Tables 3.1 and 3.2). Collection of appropriate specimens during the acute phase of the disease, and inclusion of additional submissions from similarly affected animals, enhances the likelihood of isolating viruses. The following factors should be considered in selecting clinical specimens: 1) type of disease (e.g., respiratory—lung or trachea, or vesicular—vesicle or skin biopsy), 2) the age and species of host, 3) the nature of the lesions in affected animals, and 4) the size of carcasses (able to be shipped on ice?). The following is a systematic approach for the rapid laboratory diagnosis of a viral-caused disease in animals:

1. Examination (gross and histologic) of the diseased animal/tissues as a presumptive diagnosis for a viral etiology.
2. Measurement of the development of viral-specific antibodies (acute and convalescent sera) during clinical disease.
3. Immunohistochemical staining of tissue sections with virus-specific antibodies to detect individual viral antigens in the tissue.
4. Examination of feces, plasma, or serum by immunoassays that detect specific viral antigens (e.g., rotavirus in feces, feline leukemia virus in serum, bovine respiratory syncytial virus in lung).
5. Examination of positive- or negative-stained specimens by electron microscopy to identify the morphology of virus. This diagnostic procedure is limited by the concentration of viral particles required for detection ($>10^5$/ml).
6. Isolation or amplification of infectious virus in cell cultures and identification of the virus propagated from clinical submission.

Many viral diseases do not kill the host, but the host may serve as a reservoir of virus and disseminate the virus to other contact animals. Serological assays can sometimes be used to determine which animals carry specific viruses and which animals are susceptible to infection.

It is to be emphasized that merely isolating a virus from an animal does not necessarily implicate that virus as the causative agent of any disease that is occurring in that animal. It is very important to confirm that the isolated virus produces a similar disease in the same or related species, which may even involve the inoculation of susceptible or nonimmune animals. When two or more viruses are isolated from a specimen, a clear interpretation of the role of each isolate in the disease process is also necessary. Finally, it must be remembered that vaccine strains of viruses can also be reisolated from vaccinated animals, and can be confused with true field strains.

Table 3.1.   Suggested Specimens from Mammalian Species for Virus Isolation and Identification

Type of Illness or Infection	Common Name or Associated Virus	Other Infections	Clinical Specimens to Collect	Diagnostic Identification Tests
Respiratory	Adenovirus (bovine, porcine, canine)		Nasal and ocular secretions, feces, lung, brain, tonsil	VI (CPE), HA, CF, FA, VN
	Infectious canine hepatitis (adenovirus)		Spleen, liver, lymph nodes, kidney, blood	VI (CPE), HA, FA, VN
	Bovine viral diarrhea (mucosal disease) (pestivirus)	Genital, abortions, enteric	Nasal secretions, oral lesions, lung, spleen, blood, mesenteric lymph nodes, intestinal mucosa, vaginal secretions, fetal tissues, unclotted blood	VI (CPE and virus interference), FA, VN
	Infectious bovine rhinotracheitis (herpesvirus)	Central nervous system (CNS), genital, abortions	Nasal and ocular secretions, lung, tracheal swab, tracheal segment, brain, vaginal secretions, serum, aborted fetus, liver, spleen, kidney	VI (CPE), FA, VN
	Feline rhinotracheitis (herpesvirus)		Nasal and pharyngeal secretions, conjunctival membranes, liver, lung, spleen, kidney, salivary gland, brain	VI (CPE and inclusions), FA
	Equine rhinopneumonitis (herpesvirus)	Genital, abortions	Placenta, fetus, lung, nasal secretions, lymph nodes	FA, VI (ECE and CPE), VN
	Influenza (equine, porcine) (orthomyxovirus)		Nasal and ocular secretions, lung, tracheal swab	VI (ECE), HA, HI
	Parainfluenza (bovine, equine, porcine, ovine, canine) (paramyxovirus)		Nasal and ocular secretions, lung, tracheal swab	VI (ECE), HA, HI, VN
	Bovine respiratory syncytial virus (pneumovirus)		Trachea, lung, nasal secretions, clotted blood	VI (CPE), FA, ELISA
	Bovine herpesvirus 4 (Movar, DN599)	Abortions (?)	Trachea, lung, nasal secretions, fetus, clotted blood	VI (CPE), FA, VN
	Reovirus (bovine, equine, canine, feline)		Feces, intestinal mucosa, nasal and pharyngeal secretions	VI, HA, HI
	African horse sickness (orbivirus)[a]		Whole blood in anticoagulant, lesion material, nasal and pharyngeal secretions	VI (CPE and mice), VN
	Malignant catarrhal fever[a] (herpesvirus)		Whole blood in anticoagulant, lymph nodes, spleen, lung	VI (CPE), ELISA, FA, VN, EM
	Pseudorabies[a] (herpesvirus)	CNS, genital, abortions	Nasal secretions, tonsil, lung, brain (midbrain, pons, medulla), spinal cord (sheep and cattle), spleen (swine), vaginal secretion, serum	VI (CPE and rabbits), VN, ELISA, FA
	Canine herpesvirus		Kidney, liver, lung, spleen, nasal, oropharyngeal, and vaginal secretions	VI (CPE and inclusions), FA, VN
	Porcine inclusion body rhinitis (cytomegalovirus)		Turbinate, nasal mucosa	EM, VI (CPE), FA, VN
	Equine rhinovirus		Nasal secretions, feces	VI (CPE), VN
	Maedi-Visna, ovine progressive pneumonia (retrovirus, lentivirus)	CNS	CSF, whole blood, salivary glands, lung, mediastinal lymph nodes, choroid plexus, spleen	VI (CPE and sheep), VN, CF
	Bovine rhinovirus		Nasal secretions	VI (CPE), VN
	Rift valley fever[a] (bovine, ovine) (phlebovirus)		Whole blood in anticoagulant, fetus, liver, spleen, kidney, brain	VI (CPE and mice), VN, CF, FA
Enteric	Bovine enterovirus		Feces, oropharyngeal swab	VI (CPE), VN
	Transmissible gastroenteritis (coronavirus)		Feces, nasal secretions, jejunum, ileum	VI (newborn pigs), FA, EM
	Neonatal diarrheas			
	1. Rotaviruses		Feces, small intestine	VI (CPE with trypsin), ELISA, FA, EM
	2. Parvoviruses	Abortion	Feces, intestinal mucosa, regional lymph nodes, brain, heart	VI (CPE), FA, EM, HA, HI, VN

Table 3.1. Continued

Type of Illness or Infection	Common Name or Associated Virus	Other Infections	Clinical Specimens to Collect	Diagnostic Identification Tests
	3. Coronaviruses		Feces, small intestine	VI (CPE with trypsin), FA, EM
	Picornavirus SMEDI (enterovirus)		Feces, intestine, brain, tonsil, liver	VI (CPE), VN, EM
	Polioencephalitis (Teschen, Talfan) (enterovirus)	CNS	Brain, intestine, feces	VI (CPE), VN
	Rinderpest[a] (morbillivirus)		Blood in anticoagulant, spleen, mesenteric lymph nodes	VI (CPE and cattle), AGID, CF, VN
	Peste des petits ruminants[a] (morbillivirus)		Blood in anticoagulant, spleen, mesenteric lymph nodes	VI (CPE and goats), VN, CF, AGID
Central nervous system (CNS)	Rabies (lyssavirus)		Brain, salivary gland	VI (mice and inclusions), FA, VN
	Equine encephalomyelitis (VEE,[a] EEE, WEE)[b] (alphavirus)		Whole blood, brain, cerebrospinal fluid, nasal and pharyngeal secretions, pancreas	VI (ECE and mice), HA, HI, VN, CF
	Louping ill encephalomyelitis[a] (flavivirus)		Whole blood, brain, cerebrospinal fluid	VI (ECE and CPE), FA, VN, HI
	Hemagglutinating encephalomyelitis virus (coronavirus)		Brain, spinal cord, tonsil, blood	VI (CPE), HA, HAD, VN, FA
	Caprine arthritis encephalitis (retrovirus, pentivirus)	Arthritis	Blood, spinal cord	VI (CPE), AGID, ELISA
	Japanese B encephalitis[a] (flavivirus)		Brain, CSF	VI (ECE and mice), IgM, VN, CF, HI, FA, ELISA
	Borna disease (unclassified)		Brain, spinal cord	VI (ECE and rabbits), FA, CF
	Prion diseases[a]		Brain	VI (mice and sheep), MI (?)
Mucous membranes and skin	Poxviruses 1. swine pox (suipoxvirus) 2. vaccinia (orthopoxvirus) 3. cowpox (orthopoxvirus) 4. sheep and goat pox[a] (capripoxvirus)		Lesion scrapings, lesions, vesicular fluids, crusts, liver, spleen	VI (ECE, CPE, and rabbits), HA, HI, VN, FA, EM
	Foot-and-mouth[a] disease (Aphthovirus)	Enteric	Lesion material, tonsil, vesicular fluid, hoof lesions, esophageal-pharyngeal (ep) fluids, all tissues	VI (CPE and neonatal mice), CF, VN, FA, AGID, ELISA
	Bovine mammillitis (herpesvirus)		Lesion scrapings, lesions, teat swab, fluid exudates from lesion	VI (CPE), VN
	Vesicular stomatitis[a] (vesiculovirus)		Vesicular fluid, epithelial covering of lesions, whole blood, regional lymph nodes, tongue swab	VI (CPE), VN, CF
	Vesicular exanthema of swine[a] (calicivirus)		Vesicular fluid, epithelial covering of foot lesion, tonsil lymph node, serum, oral and nasal lesions	VI (CPE), CF, VN, AGID
	Swine vesicular disease[a] (enterovirus)		Vesicular fluid, epithelial covering of lesion, oral or nasal lesions	VI (CPE), VN, FA, AGID
	Papillomaviruses	Neoplasia	Lesion material, warts, skin scraping	EM, cell transformation, FA
	Contagious ecthyma ORF (parapoxvirus)		Scabs, lesions on lip	VI (ECE and CPE), VN, AGID, FA, EM
	Bovine papular stomatitis (parapoxvirus)		Lesion biopsy, scraping muzzle, mouth, teats	VI (ECE and CPE), EM
Genital and/or abortions	Enteroviruses	CNS, respiratory	Vaginal secretions, serum from dam or sow, nasal swab, tonsil, brain (swine), feces (cattle and swine)	VI (CPE), VN
	Parvovirus (swine)		Vaginal secretions, serum from dam or sow, lung (mummified fetus)	VI (CPE), FA, HA, HI

Table 3.1.   Continued

Type of Illness or Infection	Common Name or Associated Virus	Other Infections	Clinical Specimens to Collect	Diagnostic Identification Tests
Hemorrhage syndrome (viremia)	Bluetongue, Epizootic hemorrhagic disease of deer, Ibaraki (orbivirus)	Hemorrhagic syndrome, (viremia), respiratory	Serum from dam, fetal heart, heparinized blood, spleen, bone marrow, lymph nodes, lung, semen	VI (CPE and ECE), CF, AGID, FA, VN, EM
	Equine viral arteritis (Pestivirus)		Whole blood, nasal and pharyngeal secretions, placenta, fetus, spleen, nostril, lymph nodes, conjunctival sac, semen	VI (CPE), CF, AGID, FA
	Border disease (hairy shaker) (pestivirus)	CNS	Brain, spleen, blood, bone marrow	VI (CPE and interference), FA, VN
	Akabane[a] (Bunyavirus)		Placenta, fetal muscle, nerve tissues	VI (CPE and suckling mice), FA, VN, HI, HA
	Hog cholera[a] (pestivirus)		Tonsil, spleen, liver, brain, lymph nodes	VI (pigs), FA, VN
	Equine infectious anemia (retrovirus, Pentivirus)		Whole blood, spleen, lymph nodes	VI (CPE and horses), FA, VN, CF, ELISA, AGID
	African swine fever[a] (Iridovirus)		Blood in anticoagulant, spleen, liver, tonsil, lymph nodes	VI (CPE and pigs), HAD, HA, CF, FA, RIA (radioimmunoassay), ELISA, IEOP (immunoelectro-osmophoresis)
	Nairobi sheep disease[a] (Nairovirus)		Spleen, blood (plasma), mesenteric lymph nodes	VI (intracerebral suckling mice), FA
	Rift valley fever[a] (phlebovirus)		Fetus, blood in anticoagulant, liver, spleen, kidney, brain, serum	VI (CPE and suckling hamsters or mice), VN, CF, AGID, HI, FA
Neoplasia	Retrovirus (bovine, feline) (oncovirinae)	Immunodeficiency, leukemia, anemia	Lymph nodes, metastatic growths, blood in anticoagulant, serum	VI, reverse transcriptase, EM, ELISA, FA, Western immunoblot

AGID = agar gel immunodiffusion, CF = complement fixation, COFAL = complement-fixation for avian leukosis, CPE = cytopathic effect, ECE = embryonating chicken eggs, EM = electron microscopy, FA = immunofluorescence, HA = hemagglutinin, HAD = hemadsorption, HI = hemagglutination inhibition, RIA = radioimmunoassay, VI = virus isolation, VN = virus neutralization, MI = molecular/immunologic.
[a] Reportable disease or a foreign animal disease in United States.
[b] VEE = Venezuelan equine encephalomyelitis, EEE = eastern equine encephalomyelitis, WEE = western equine encephalomyelitis.

Isolation of Virus from Clinical Specimens

Cultivation in Tissue Culture.   Viruses are isolated from clinical specimens by inoculating susceptible primary or continuous cell cultures derived from the host or related species, embryonated eggs, or laboratory animals. Specimens submitted for viral isolation should be placed in virus transport media (e.g., a balanced salt solution containing antibiotics) in sealed containers for safety in handling. They should be clearly identified by appropriate labeling, and submitted on ice (4°C) or frozen (−20°C).

Specimens should be collected from live animals during acute phases of the disease. Depending on the specific disease process, excretions or secretions, swabs of body orifices or liquids (lymph or blood), and tissue collected by biopsy are all suitable specimens for viral isolation. In the laboratory, tissue specimens are processed as a 10% or 20% (w/v) homogenate in a balanced salt solution along with antibiotics. Heavily contaminated specimens may be filtered to remove other microorganisms. Virus isolation should be conducted in cell cultures free of contaminating agents such as noncytopathic bovine viral diarrhea virus or mycoplasma.

To isolate virus, tissue homogenates are placed onto cellular monolayers and absorbed 1 hour or longer at 35°C to 37°C, and the inoculum is left on or removed and fresh media added. Inoculated and uninfected cell cultures are observed for 7 to 10 days. Viral cytopathic effect (CPE) in cells is usually evident between 24 and 72 hours for most cytopathic viruses (Fig 3.1). However, for most clinical material containing low concentrations of virus, several (>3) blind cell passages are recommended.

After a virus has been demonstrated at limiting dilution to replicate in a cell by CPE or other parameters, infectious virus is released from cells by three cycles of freeze–thaw or sonication, followed by centrifugation and storage to maintain maximum infectivity. Each virus isolated should be identified as to species of origin, morphologic type, passage level, and host cell used for propagation.

Embryonated Eggs.   A number of mammalian viruses, and many avian viral pathogens can be isolated in embryonating chicken eggs (ECE). A key to successful viral isolation in ECE is the route of inoculation (Fig 3.2). Candled ECE that die within 24 hours after inoculation are considered traumatic deaths. Subsequent deaths of inoculated ECE are placed at 4°C for several hours (to avoid hemorrhages)

Table 3.2. Suggested Specimens from Avian Species for Virus Isolation and Identification

Type of Illness or Infection	Common Name or Associated Virus	Other Infections	Clinical Specimens to Collect	Diagnostic Identification Tests
Respiratory	Newcastle disease VVND[a] (paramyxovirus)	CNS	Tracheal or cloacal swabs, lung, spleen, liver, kidney, bone marrow	VI (ECE, CPE), VN, HA, HI
	Avian influenza[a] (fowl plague virus) (orthomyxovirus)	Drop in egg production, enteric	Trachea, lung, air sac, sinus exudate, liver, spleen, blood, cloacal swab	VI (ECE), HA, HI, AGP, VN
	Infectious bronchitis (coronavirus)	Nephrosis, drop in egg production	Lung, trachea, tracheal swabs	VI (ECE tracheal ring cultures), VN, HA, HI, EM
	Herpesvirus of 1. psittacines (Pacheco's Disease) 2. cranes 3. pigeons 4. owls 5. falcons		Liver, spleen, intestine	VI (ECE, birds), VN, FA, EM
	Laryngotracheitis (herpesvirus)		Trachea or tracheal exudate, lung	VI (ECE, CPE), AGP, VN, FA
	Avian adenovirus	Eggdrop syndrome, hepatitis, enteritis	Trachea, lung, air sacs, intestine, feces	VI (ECE, CPE), AGP, VN, FA
Enteric	Coronaviral enteritis of turkeys		Intestine, bursa of Fabricius, ceca	VI (ETE), FA, VN
	Reovirus		Intestine, feces	EM, VI
Central nervous system	Avian encephalomyelitis (enterovirus)		Brain	VI (chicks, ECE), VN, FA
	Alphavirus infections (eastern and western equine encephalitis viruses)		Serum, brain, heart, spleen, liver	VI (ECE, mice, CPE), VN, CF, HI
	Turkey meningoencephalitis (flavivirus)		Brain, spleen, serum	VI (ECE, mice, CPE), VN, HI
Mucous membranes and skin	Avipoxvirus 1. Pigeon pox 2. Canary pox 3. Fowl pox 4. Turkey pox		Nodular skin lesions, scab	VI (ECE, CPE), AGP, HA, VN, FA, immunoperoxidase
Hemorrhagic syndrome (viremia)	Viral arthritis (reovirus)		Synovial fluid from tibiotarsal or tibiofemoral joints, spleen swab	VI (CPE, ECE), AGP, VN, FA
	Duck plague (duck virus enteritis) (herpesvirus)		Liver, spleen, blood	VI (CPE, EDE), VN
	Hemorrhagic enteritis of turkeys or marble spleen of pheasants (adenovirus, type 2)		Intestinal contents, spleen	VI (CPE, poults), AGP, EM
	Turkey viral hepatitis (unclassified)		Liver	VI (ECE)
	Infectious bursal disease (Birnavirus)	Immunosuppression	Spleen, bursa	VI (ECE), VN, AGP
	Fledgling disease (papovavirus)		Bone marrow, kidney, heart, spleen	VI (CPE), VN, EM, FA
	Chicken anemia agent (parvovirus)	Immunosuppression, pancytopenia	Spleen, bursa, thymus, blood	VI (chicks), EM, VN, ELISA
Neoplasia	Leukosis and sarcomas (retrovirus, oncovirinae)		Whole blood, plasma, cloacal swabs, meconium, albumin, embryos, tumors	RT, VI (CPE, cell transformation, ECE), ELISA, FA, COFAL
	Reticuloendotheliosis (retrovirus, oncovirinae)	Immunosuppression, lymphoma	Spleen, tumor tissue, heparinized blood	VI (CPE, ETE), FA, RT, AGP, VN
	Marek's disease (herpesvirus)		Blood, tumor, kidney, spleen, feathers	VI (CPE, ECE), AGP, VN, FA

AGID = agar gel immunodiffusion, AGP = agar gel precipitin, CF = complement fixation, COFAL = complement-fixation for avian leukosis, CPE = cytopathic effect, ECE = embryonating chicken eggs, EDE = embryonating duck eggs, EM = electron microscopy, ETE = embryonating turkey eggs, FA = immunofluorescence, HA = hemagglutinin, HAD = hemadsorption, HI = hemagglutination inhibition, RIA = radioimmunoassay, RT = reverse transcriptase, VI = virus isolation, VN = virus neutralization, VVND = velogenic viscerotropic Newcastle disease.

FIGURE 3.1.   *Cytopathic effect (syncytial) on bovine fetal kidney cells by the herpes virus of malignant catarrhal fever (X200).*

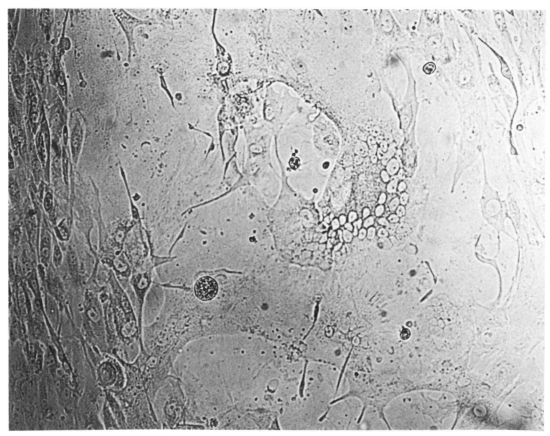

FIGURE 3.2.   *The chicken embryo (10 to 12 days old) and routes of inoculation to reach the various cell types (as indicated). For chorioallantoic membrane inoculation, a hole is first drilled through the egg shell and shell membrane; the shell over the air sac is then perforated, causing air to enter between the shell membrane and the chorioallantoic membrane, creating an artificial air sac, where the sample is deposited. The sample comes in contact with the chorionic epithelium. Yolk sac inoculation is usually carried out in younger (6-day-old) embryos, in which the yolk sac is larger. (Reproduced with permission from Davis BD et al. Microbiology. 2nd ed. Hagerstown, MD: Harper and Row, 1977.)*

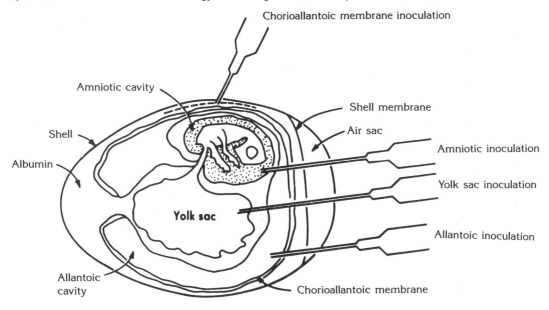

prior to collection of fluids or visual examination of the embryos and egg membranes. Embryos that are stunted, deformed, edematous, or hemorrhagic, and membranes that contain lesions (i.e., pocks) should be homogenized in a sterile balanced saline as a 10% (w/v) suspension and repassaged in ECE or cell cultures. To avoid toxicity, a dilution of the inoculum is done.

Animal Inoculation. The inoculation of susceptible laboratory animals remains a useful procedure for the identification procedure for the identification of some viral pathogens, particularly those that are highly fastidious and difficult to propagate in other systems.

Identification of Viruses or Viral Antigens in Clinical Specimens

Electron Microscopy. Electron microscopy (EM) can be used to rapidly identify the morphology and size of any virus present in a specimen or isolated in cell culture of ECE. Tentative diagnosis of viral diseases can be made by EM on thin sections of affected tissues and cell-free homogenates of clinical specimens. The use of EM for diagnosis is limited, however, because the method is not very sensitive ($>10^5$ virus particles/ml are required to see a single viral particle on a 200 mesh grid), and viruses from different species have similar morphology and size.

Immune Electron Microscopy. Immune electron microscopy (IEM) enhances detection of viruses in tissues, cells, or fecal specimens by reacting specific immune sera with

virus. In IEM, specific antibody to a virus, preferably polyclonal, is mixed with virus for 1 hour to produce antigen-antibody complexes. These immune complexes are centrifuged at 1000 X g onto Formvar-coated grids, then stained with 4% PTA, pH 7.0 and examined by EM. The reaction of viral fluids with specific acute or convalescent serum as viewed by EM determines if a virus is associated with a specific disease. This procedure has been used successfully for viruses associated with infectious diarrhea.

Immunofluorescence. Immunofluorescence is a visible fluorescence accentuated by ultraviolet light as a specific antibody covalently bound to a fluorochrome (e.g., fluorescein isothiocyanate, rhodamine) that combines with a fixed antigen. This technique provides a sensitive and rapid method for detecting and identifying specific viruses in either tissues or cell cultures (Fig 3.3). Immunofluorescence is detectable by either a direct or indirect procedure. The direct immunofluorescence test employs a virus-specific antibody labeled with fluorescein that combines with a specific viral antigen located in cells or tissues. The indirect test requires the use of a fluorescein-labeled antiserum to a virus-specific immunoglobulin.

Immunohistochemical staining uses the same approach, except that the virus-specific antibody is either directly or indirectly labeled with an enzyme. The presence of the enzyme is determined by addition of its substrate, and the reaction detected by a color change. The advantage of immunohistochemical staining over immunofluorescence is that a fluorescent microscope is not required,

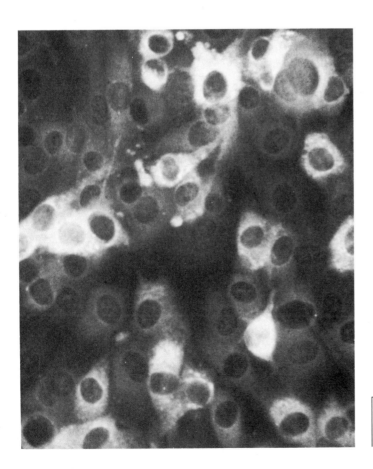

FIGURE 3.3. *Cytoplasmic immunofluorescence in fetal bovine lung cells produced by BVD virus (X200). (Reproduced with permission from Castro AE. Bov Pract 1984;19:61.)*

and the use of an enzyme-enhancement step greatly increases the sensitivity of the procedure.

Nucleic Acid Hybridization. Molecular hybridization techniques have led to the synthetic production of viral DNA probes that are highly specific for individual viruses. These probes are labeled with various detection systems that allow identification of the presence of individual viruses, either in tissues or in extracts of them.

Polymerase Chain Reaction. The relatively recent development of the polymerase chain reaction (PCR) has revolutionized the rapid diagnosis of many viral diseases. The importance of the procedure lies in its ability to amplify small amounts of viral DNA or RNA even from contaminated specimens, and on its ability to be conducted on a large scale so that vast numbers of samples can simultaneously be evaluated. Furthermore, technical developments such as real-time PCR allow the quantitation of template that is present in a sample, which is reflective of the viral load. The PCR assay is based on the cyclic synthesis of a DNA segment limited by two specific oligonucleotides that are used as primers to specifically amplify portions of the viral genome. Properly run, the PCR assay is both sensitive and specific, although the identification of viral nucleic acid does not prove that infectious virus was present, so PCR-positive samples often should be subjected to traditional virus isolation procedures.

Enzyme-Linked Immunosorbent Assay. The enzyme-linked immunosorbent assay (ELISA) is a rapid, highly sensitive immunoassay adapted to measure viral antigen or antibody (see Chapter 2). ELISAs have been developed for numerous avian viral pathogens (e.g., avian laryngotracheitis virus, avian encephalitis, Newcastle disease virus, infectious bronchitis virus, and reovirus), and increasingly are being developed to detect viruses that infect other species of domestic animals.

Serologic Detection of Viruses

Most viruses usually elicit an immune response in the host; thus the detection of a humoral (antibody) or cellular response is often used to determine prior infection of an animal with a viral pathogen. Serologic assays measure humoral immunity in animals, and assays for measuring cellular immunity to viruses are used infrequently in veterinary diagnostic medicine.

Viruses have certain antigens that are type- or group-specific and that in part determine the serologic assay used. Serologic diagnosis of virus infections typically requires the collection of paired samples: an acute (at or prior to the onset of clinical signs) and a convalescent serum (10 to 28 days later). A fourfold or greater rise in antibody titer (the reciprocal of the serum dilution) indicates recent or ongoing viral infection. Antibody levels in single serum samples are more difficult to interpret, although the presence of antibody is indicative of prior exposure (or resulting from the passive transfer of maternal antibodies in young animals) which is especially important in chronic diseases with a carrier state like bovine leukemia virus in

cattle, equine infectious anemia, and equine arteritis virus infection of stallions.

Serology can help to rapidly establish a diagnosis when viral isolation procedures are negative. Serology can also be used to definitively rule out the presence of specific viruses in a given disease outbreak, whereas a negative viral isolation cannot.

Serum Virus Neutralization (SN) Test. Most viruses produce a visible cytopathic effect (CPE) in cell cultures. CPE is used to determine the presence of protective or virus-neutralizing antibodies in a serum. To quantify the amount of neutralizing antibody, serum from an animal is serially diluted by twofold dilutions and mixed with a known amount of virus (generally 50 to 300 infectious doses of virus-$TCID_{50}$) for 1 hour at 37°C prior to inoculation of a volume of the mixture into animals, embryonating chicken eggs (ECE) or cell cultures. The SN test is very specific and highly sensitive, but it is time-consuming and expensive. The SN can be used to confirm recent infection of animals if paired sera are evaluated.

Hemagglutination Inhibition (HI) Test. Viruses that possess a hemagglutinin protein (HA) will agglutinate erythrocytes, a fact that has been used to quantify the amount (titrate) of these viruses that are present in a sample. The HI test can be used to identify or type a virus through the inhibition of hemagglutination by virus-specific antiserum.

Hemadsorption-Inhibition (HAD-I) Test. The HAD-I test is based on the ability of certain virus-infected cells (monolayers) to attract specific erythrocytes to their surface. The presence of hemadsorbing erythrocyte clusters on a cellular monolayer indicates that viral protein (hemagglutinin) has accumulated on the surface of the cell membrane. The hemadsorption phenomenon can be inhibited by pretreatment of virus-infected cells for 30 minutes, usually at ambient temperature with twofold dilutions of antisera followed by the addition of 0.05% to 0.5% erythrocytes. Antibody (Ab) can be quantified by comparing the observed washed virus-infected cell monolayers that contain adhered clumped erythrocytes on the surface of the cell (Ab negative) with the cell monolayers that contain free-floating erythrocytes (Ab positive).

Complement Fixation. Complement fixation (CF) tests employ the cascade of complement in reactions of viral antigens that fix complement—usually guinea pig—when combined to antibody. Although CF has been used in early test tube assays to detect virus (e.g., leukemia viruses), virus-infected cells, or virus-specific antibody, the complexity of the assay and the time required have led to its replacement by simpler procedures.

Immunodiffusion. The immunodiffusion (ID) procedure is routinely used as a diagnostic tool to monitor the spread of specific viral pathogens in various animal diseases (e.g., bluetongue, equine infectious anemia, bovine leukosis, caprine arthritis, encephalitis, infectious bursal disease). The basis of the test is the ability of certain soluble viral antigens to diffuse in a semisolid medium (agar) with the formation of a precipitin line with specific antisera.

Immunoelectroosmophoresis combines the diffusion procedure with the principle of movement of charged protein molecules in an electrical field. Since most viral antigens assume an electrically negative charge, application of an electrical current moves the viral particle to the anode. Following electrical migration, the antigen can be elucidated by the use of a positive antiserum that migrates toward the cathode. This technique has been used to detect antigens of African swine fever virus.

Radioimmunoassay. The radioimmunoassay (RIA) is an exquisitely sensitive method for quantifying antigens or antibodies when one component is radio-labeled. Although RIA has an advantage for detecting minute amounts of antibodies, the need for a scintillation counter to measure radioactivity and very pure reagents limits use of this assay to appropriately equipped diagnostic laboratories.

Enzyme-Linked Immunosorbent Assay (ELISA). ELISAs are highly specific and sensitive immunoassays in which the specificity of the reaction can be enhanced by increasing the level of purification of the antigen or antibody employed. The ELISA can detect nanogram levels of IgG-, IgM-, and IgA-type antibodies. ELISAs can be made quantitative if appropriate standard curves are developed. Numerous commercially available assays for avian and mammalian viruses provide qualitative information on antibody to various viruses, whereas others detect the viruses themselves in clinical specimens. The blocking ELISA evaluates the ability of a test serum to displace the binding of a virus protein-specific antibody to its antigen.

Western Immunoblot Assay. The Western immunoblot assay can detect antibodies to a full range of viral proteins as revealed on a strip of nitrocellulose paper as discrete bands by electrophoresis. When a serum sample is applied to the nitrocellulose strip, antibodies from animals infected with a specific virus bind to the specific viral proteins at the appropriate positions. These bands become dark and distinct when the nitrocellulose paper is treated with a reagent (Fig 3.4). Because it provides a full viral antibody profile of the serum sample, this test is the most specific viral diagnostic test currently available.

FIGURE 3.4. *Western immunoblot of bluetongue virus proteins using serum obtained before and after natural infection with BTV serotype 17. Virus proteins identified are given in the right margin; LMW represents three low molecular weight virus proteins that have not been previously defined; X represents an additional noncharacterized virus protein; P designates specific BTV protein; NS is the nonstructural virus protein. Lanes A and B represent pre- and postinfection serum, respectively. Immune complexes were detected in lane B using a biotin-avidin-enzyme probe, e.g., biotin-labeled rabbit antisheep IgG in association with peroxidase-labeled avidin. (Reproduced with permission from MA Adkison and JL Stott.)*

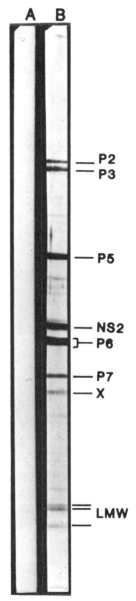

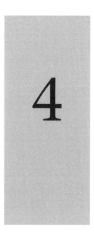

4 Antimicrobial Chemotherapy

JOHN F. PRESCOTT

Antimicrobial drugs exploit differences in structure or biochemical function between host and parasite. Modern chemotherapy is traced to the work of Paul Ehrlich, who devoted his life to discovering agents that possessed *selective toxicity*. The first clinically successful broad-spectrum antibacterial drugs were the sulfonamides, developed in 1935 as a result of Ehrlich's work with synthetic dyes. It was, however, the discovery of penicillin by Fleming and its development by Chain and Florey in World War II that led to the subsequent discovery of further *antibiotics*, chemical substances produced by microorganisms that at low concentrations inhibit or kill other microorganisms. The chemical modification of many of the drugs discovered early in the antibiotic revolution has led to the development of new and powerful antimicrobial drugs with properties distinct from their parents. Antibiotics and their derivatives have more importance as antimicrobial agents than do the fewer synthetic antibacterial drugs. By contrast, antiviral drugs are all chemically synthesized. The term antimicrobial will be used throughout to include both antibiotics and synthetic antimicrobial drugs.

Important milestones in the development of antimicrobial drugs are shown in Figure 4.1. The therapeutic use of antimicrobial drugs in veterinary medicine has followed their use in human medicine because of the high cost of their development.

Classification of Antimicrobial Drugs

Antimicrobial drugs can be classified in a number of ways:

1. *Spectrum of activity against class of microorganism.* Penicillins are narrow spectrum because they inhibit only bacteria; sulfonamides, trimethoprim, and lincosamides are broader because they inhibit both bacteria and protozoa. Polyenes only inhibit fungi.
2. *Antibacterial activity.* Some antibiotics are narrow-spectrum in that they inhibit only gram-positive (bacitracin, vancomycin) or mainly gram-negative bacteria (polymyxin), whereas broad-spectrum drugs such as tetracyclines inhibit both gram-positive and gram-negative bacteria. Other drugs such as penicillin G or lincosamides are most active against gram-positive bacteria but will inhibit some gram-negatives.

3. *Bacteriostatic or bactericidal.* This distinction is an approximation that depends on drug concentrations and the organism involved. For example, penicillin is bactericidal at high concentrations and bacteriostatic at lower ones. The distinction between bactericidal and bacteriostatic is critical in certain circumstances, such as the treatment of meningitis or of septicemia in neutropenic patients.
4. *Pharmacodynamic activity.* Antibacterial action is concentration- or time-dependent (see below under dosing considerations).
5. *Mechanism of action.* Like pharmacodynamic activity, this is dependent on the drug class, and is discussed below. This is probably the most useful of the classifications, since it determines the previous four classification approaches.

Mechanism of Action of Antimicrobial Drugs

The marked structural and biochemical differences between eukaryotic and prokaryotic cells give greater opportunity for selective toxicity of antibacterial drugs compared to antifungal drugs because fungi, like mammalian cells, are eukaryotic. Developing selectively toxic antiviral drugs is particularly difficult because viral replication depends largely on the metabolic pathways of the host cell. This chapter mainly discusses antibacterial drugs.

The mechanisms of action of antibacterial drugs fall into four categories: 1) inhibition of cell wall synthesis, 2) damage to cell membrane function, 3) inhibition of nucleic acid synthesis or function, and 4) inhibition of protein synthesis (Fig 4.2).

Inhibition of Cell Wall Synthesis

Antibiotics that interfere with cell wall synthesis include penicillins and cephalosporins (beta-lactam antibiotics), cycloserine, bacitracin, and vancomycin. The bacterial cell wall is a thick envelope that gives shape to the cell. This tough wall outside the cell membrane is a major difference between bacteria and mammalian cells. In gram-positive bacteria it consists largely of a thick layer of peptidoglycan, which gives the cell rigidity and maintains a high internal osmotic pressure of about 20 atmospheres. In gram-negative bacteria this layer is thinner and the internal

FIGURE 4.1. *Milestones in antimicrobial therapy.*

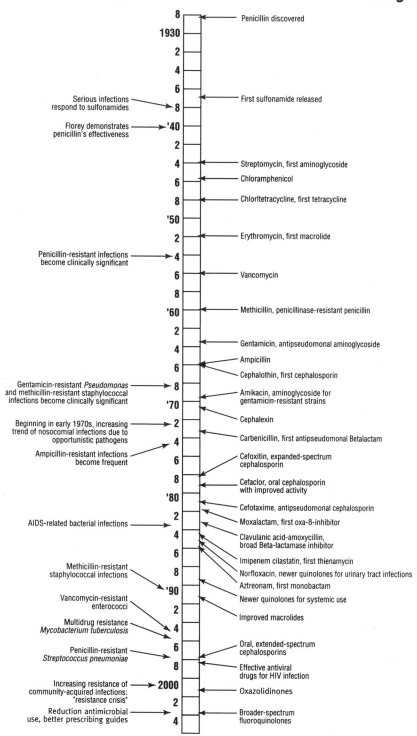

Human Infectious Disease

Antibacterial Agents

Penicillin discovered

First sulfonamide released

Serious infections respond to sulfonamides

Florey demonstrates penicillin's effectiveness

Streptomycin, first aminoglycoside

Chloramphenicol

Chlorltetracycline, first tetracycline

Erythromycin, first macrolide

Penicillin-resistant infections become clinically significant

Vancomycin

Methicillin, penicillinase-resistant penicillin

Gentamicin, antipseudomonal aminoglycoside

Ampicillin

Cephalothin, first cephalosporin

Gentamicin-resistant *Pseudomonas* and methicillin-resistant staphylococcal infections become clinically significant

Amikacin, aminoglycoside for gentamicin-resistant strains

Cephalexin

Beginning in early 1970s, increasing trend of nosocomial infections due to opportunistic pathogens

Carbenicillin, first antipseudomonal Betalactam

Ampicillin-resistant infections become frequent

Cefoxitin, expanded-spectrum cephalosporin

Cefaclor, oral cephalosporin with improved activity

Cefotaxime, antipseudomonal cephalosporin

AIDS-related bacterial infections

Moxalactam, first oxa-ß-inhibitor

Clavulanic acid-amoxycillin, broad Beta-lactamase inhibitor

Imipenem cilastatin, first thienamycin

Methicillin-resistant staphylococcal infections

Norfloxacin, newer quinolones for urinary tract infections

Aztreonam, first monobactam

Vancomycin-resistant enterococci

Newer quinolones for systemic use

Improved macrolides

Multidrug resistance *Mycobacterium tuberculosis*

Penicillin-resistant *Streptococcus pneumoniae*

Oral, extended-spectrum cephalosporins

Effective antiviral drugs for HIV infection

Increasing resistance of community-acquired infections: "resistance crisis"

Oxazolidinones

Reduction antimicrobial use, better prescribing guides

Broader-spectrum fluoroquinolones

osmotic pressure correspondingly lower. Peptidoglycan consists of a polysaccharide chain made up of a repeating disaccharide backbone of alternating N-acetylglucosamine-N-acetylmuramic acid in beta-1,4 linkage, a tetrapeptide attached to the N-acetylmuramic acid, and a peptide bridge from one tetrapeptide to another, so that the disaccharide backbone is cross-linked both within and between layers. The cross-linkage between transpeptides gives the cell wall remarkable strength. Several enzymes are involved in transpeptidation reactions.

FIGURE 4.2. *Mechanisms of action of antibacterial drugs.*

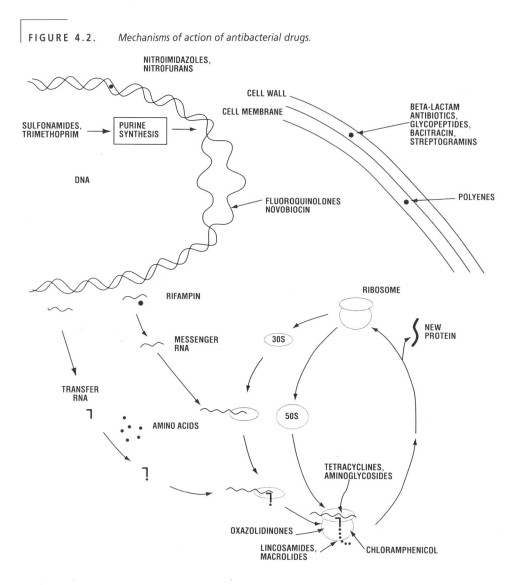

The effect of beta-lactam antibiotics (penicillins and cephalosporins) is to prevent the final cross-linking in the cell wall, inhibiting division and creating weak points. Among the targets of these drugs are penicillin-binding proteins (PBPs), of which there are three to eight in bacteria; many of these PBPs are transpeptidase enzymes. They are responsible for the formation and remodeling of the cell wall during growth and division. Different PBPs have different affinities for drugs, explaining the variation in the spectrum of action of different beta-lactam antibiotics. Degradative mechanisms are also involved in cell wall production. These are carried out by autolysins, and some penicillins act partly by decreasing normal inhibition of the autolysins.

The action of beta-lactam antibiotics is thus to block peptidoglycan synthesis, which severely weakens the cell wall, and to promote the action of the autolysins, which lyse the cell. Beta-lactams are active only against actively growing cells. The greater activity of some beta-lactams against gram-positive bacteria is the result of the greater quantity of peptidoglycan and higher osmotic pressure in gram-positive bacteria, the impermeability of some gram-

negative bacteria because of their lipopolysaccharide and lipid exterior, and the presence of beta-lactamase enzymes in many gram-negative organisms. The remarkable activity against gram-negatives of some of the newest penicillins and cephalosporins is the result not just of their improved ability to enter gram-negative cells and bind PBPs, but to their ability to resist a variety of beta-lactamase enzymes found in the periplasmic space of gram-negative bacteria. More recently, beta-lactamase–inhibiting drugs with no intrinsic antibacterial activity, such as clavulanic acid and sulbactam, have been combined with amoxicillin or ticarcillin to expand the spectrum of activity of these latter compounds by neutralizing enzymes that might otherwise degrade them.

Bacitracin and vancomycin inhibit the early stages in peptidoglycan synthesis. They are active only against gram-positive bacteria.

Penicillins. Sir Alexander Fleming's observation that colonies of staphylococci lysed on a plate that had become contaminated with a *Penicillum* fungus was the discovery that led to the development of antibiotics. In 1940, Chain,

Florey, and their associates succeeded in producing thera-peutic quantities of penicillin from *Penicillium notatum*. Almost a decade later, penicillin G became widely avail-able for clinical use. In the years that followed, this antibi-otic was found to have certain limitations: its relative in-stability to stomach acid, its susceptibility to inactivation by penicillinase, and its relative inactivity against most gram-negative bacteria. Isolation of the active moiety, 6-aminopenicillanic acid, in the penicillin molecule has re-sulted in the design and development of semisynthetic penicillins that overcome some of these limitations.

The development of the cephalosporin family, which shares with penicillin the beta-lactam ring, has led to a re-markable array of drugs with improved ability to penetrate different gram-negative bacterial species and to resist beta-lactamase enzymes. In recent years, other naturally occur-ring beta-lactam antibiotics have been described that lack the bicyclic ring of the classical beta-lactam penicillins and cephalosporins. Many of these new drugs have potent anti-bacterial activity and are highly resistant to beta-lactamase enzymes.

Clinically important penicillins can be divided into six groups:

1. Benzyl penicillins and its long-acting forms. Injec-table penicillins, highest activity against gram-positive organisms, but susceptible to acid hydrolysis and beta-lactamase inactivation (e.g., penicillin G).
2. Orally absorbed penicillins, spectrum similar to benzyl penicillins (e.g., penicillin V).
3. Antistaphylococcal isoxazolyl penicillins. Relatively resistant to staphylococcal beta-lactamases (e.g., cloxacillin, methicillin).
4. Extended-spectrum penicillins: Aminopenicillins (e.g., amoxicillin, ampicillin).
5. Antipseudomonal penicillins: Carboxy- and ureido-penicillins (e.g., carbenicillin, piperacillin, ticarcillin).
6. Beta-lactamase resistant penicillins: Temocillin.

Antimicrobial Activity. Penicillin G is the most active of the penicillins against gram-positive aerobic bacteria such as non–beta-lactamase–producing coagulase-positive sta-phylococci, beta-hemolytic streptococci, *Bacillus anthracis* and other gram-positive rods, corynebacteria, *Erysipelo-thrix, Listeria,* and against most anaerobes. It is moderately active against the more fastidious gram-negative aerobes such as *Haemophilus, Pasteurella,* and some *Actinobacillus,* but it is inactive against members of the family *Enterobac-teriaceae, Bordetella,* and *Pseudomonas.* The penicillinase-resistant isoxazolyl penicillins (oxacillin, cloxacillin me-thicillin, and nafcillin) are resistant to coagulase-positive staphylococcal penicillinase, but are less active than peni-cillin G against other penicillin-sensitive gram-positive bacteria. Most gram-negative bacteria are resistant to them. Ampicillin and amoxicillin are slightly less active than penicillin G against gram-positive and anaerobic bacteria and are also inactivated by penicillinase produced by coagulase-positive staphylococci. They have considerably greater activity against gram-negative bacteria. They are in-effective against *Pseudomonas aeruginosa.* Carbenicillin and ticarcillin resemble ampicillin in spectrum of activity with the notable difference of having activity against *P. aerugi-*

nosa. Temocillin is highly resistant to beta-lactamases in-cluding extended-spectrum cephalosporinases, and has broad-activity against members of the family *Enterobac-teriaceae,* including otherwise resistant isolates. *Myco-plasma* and mycobacteria are resistant to penicillins.

Resistance. In gram-positive bacteria (particularly coagulase-positive staphylococci), resistance is mainly through production of extracellular beta-lactamase (peni-cillinase) enzymes that break the beta-lactam ring of most penicillins. Resistance in gram-negative bacteria results, in part, from a wide variety of beta-lactamase enzymes and also from low bacterial permeability or lack of penicillin-binding protein receptors. Most or all gram-negative bacte-ria express low levels of species-specific chromosomally mediated beta-lactamase enzymes within the periplasmic space, and these sometimes contribute to resistance.

Plasmid-mediated beta-lactamase production is wide-spread among common gram-negative bacteria. The en-zymes are constitutively expressed and cause high-level re-sistance. The majority are penicillinases rather than cephalosporinases. The most widespread are TEM-type beta-lactamases, which readily hydrolyze penicillin G and ampicillin rather than methicillin, cloxacillin, or carbeni-cillin. The less widespread OXA-type beta-lactamases hy-drolyze isoxazolyl penicillins (oxacillin, cloxacillin, and related compounds). SHV-type beta-lactamases are found particularly in *Klebsiella pneumoniae* but may be found in other members of the family *Enterobacteriaceae.*

A major recent advance has been the discovery of broad-spectrum inhibitors of beta-lactamase (e.g., clavulanic acid, sulbactam). These drugs have weak antibacterial activity but show extraordinary synergism when administered with penicillin G, ampicillin, amoxicillin or ticarcillin be-cause they irreversibly bind the beta-lactamase enzymes of resistant bacteria.

Absorption, Distribution, and Excretion. The penicillins are organic acids that are generally available as the sodium or potassium salt of the free acid. Apart from the isoxazolyl penicillins and penicillin V, acid hydrolysis limits the sys-temic availability of most penicillins from oral prepara-tions. Both ampicillin and amoxicillin are relatively stable in acid.

The penicillins are predominantly ionized in the blood plasma, have relatively small apparent volumes of distribu-tion, and have short half-lives (0.5 to 1.2 hours) in all species of domestic animals. After absorption, penicillins are widely distributed in body fluids. Because of their high degree of ionization and low solubility in lipid, they attain only low intracellular concentrations and do not penetrate well into transcellular fluids. The relatively poor diffusibil-ity of penicillins across cell membranes is reflected in their milk-to-plasma concentration ratios (0.3). The relatively low tissue levels attained may, however, be clinically effec-tive because of the high sensitivity of susceptible bacteria to penicillins and their bactericidal action. Ampicillin and amoxicillin, in addition to having a wider spectrum of an-timicrobial activity, penetrate cellular barriers more read-ily than penicillin G. Their somewhat longer half-lives might be attributed to enterohepatic circulation. Penetra-tion to cerebrospinal fluid (CSF) is usually poor but is en-hanced by inflammation. In addition, active removal of penicillin from CSF is diminished by inflammation. The penicillins are eliminated almost entirely by renal excretion, which results in very high levels in the urine. The renal excretion mechanisms include glomerular filtration and mainly proximal tubular secretion.

Adverse Effects. Penicillins are remarkably free of toxic effects, even at doses grossly in excess of those recommended. The major adverse effect is acute anaphylaxis; milder hypersensitivity reactions (urticaria, fever, angioneurotic edema) are more common. All penicillins are cross-sensitizing and cross-reacting. Anaphylactic reactions are less common after oral penicillin administration than after parenteral administration. Many of the acute toxicities reported in animals are the toxic effects of the potassium or procaine with which the penicillin is combined. The use of penicillin in guinea pigs invariably causes fatal *Clostridium difficile* colitis, and use of ampicillin in rabbits causes fatal *C. spiroforme* colitis.

Cephalosporins. Cephalosporins are natural or semisynthetic products of the fungi *Cephalsporium* spp.; the related cephamycins are derived from the actinomycetes type of bacteria. The nucleus of the semisynthetic cephalosporins, 7-aminocephalosporanic acid, bears a close structural resemblance to that of the penicillins, which accounts for a common mechanism of action and other properties shared by these two classes of drugs. They are bactericidal. Like the penicillins, cephalosporins have short half-lives, and most are excreted unchanged in the urine. Attachment of various R groups to the cephalosporanic acid nucleus has resulted in compounds with low toxicity and high therapeutic activity. Though not an ideal description, the classification of cephalosporins as belonging to generations relates to their increasing spectrum of activity against gram-negative bacteria because of improved penetration of cells and their progressive resistance to the beta-lactamases of gram-negative bacteria.

Antimicrobial Activity. The first-generation cephalosporins (e.g., cephalothin, cephalexin, cephaloridine, and cefadroxil) have a similar spectrum of activity to ampicillin, with the notable difference that beta-lactamase-producing staphylococci are susceptible. They are active against a variety of gram-positive bacteria such as coagulase-positive staphylococci, many streptococci (except enterococci), corynebacteria, and gram-positive anaerobes (*Clostridium*). Among gram-negative bacteria, *Haemophilus* and *Pasteurella* are susceptible, as are some *Escherichia coli*, *Klebsiella*, *Proteus,* and *Salmonella*. *Enterobacter* and *P. aeruginosa* are resistant. Many anaerobic bacteria, except members of the *Bacteroides fragilis* group, are susceptible. The second-generation cephalosporins (e.g., cefamandole, cefoxitin, and cefuroxime) have increased resistance to gram-negative beta-lactamases and thus broader activity against gram-negative bacteria as well as against bacteria susceptible to the first-generation drugs. They are active against some strains of *Enterobacter* and against cephalothin-resistant *E. coli, Klebsiella*, and *Proteus*. Some *B. fragilis* are susceptible. Like the first-generation cephalosporins, these drugs are not active against *P. aeruginosa* or *Serratia*. The third-generation cephalosporins (e.g., cefotaxime, moxalactam, and cefoperazone) are characterized by reduced activity against gram-positive bacteria, modest activity against *P. aeruginosa*, and remarkable activity against members of the family *Enterobacteriaceae*. Some third-generation cephalosporins (e.g., ceftazidime) are highly active against *P. aeruginosa* at the expense of activity against members of the family *Enterobacteriaceae*. Fourth-generation cephalosporins (e.g., cefepime, cefpirome) have very broad-spectrum activity and are stable to hydrolysis by many beta-lactamases.

Resistance. Methicillin-resistant coagulase-positive staphylococci are resistant to all generations of cephalosporins. Plasmid-mediated resistance to first-, second-, and third-generation drugs has been described in gram-negative bacteria. Emergence of resistance in *Enterobacter, Serratia*, and *P. aeruginosa* during treatment with third-generation drugs results from derepression of inducible, chromosomal beta-lactamase enzymes, which in turn results in broad-spectrum resistance to beta-lactam antibiotics. In addition, plasmid-mediated resistance to third-generation cephalosporins is increasingly reported. It can involve either TEM- or SHV-beta-lactamases or other beta-lactamase families including CTX-M1, which hydrolyses cefotaxime. These beta-lactamases are inhibited by clavulanic acid. More recently, broad-spectrum cephalosporinases (cephamycinases), CMY-2 beta-lactamases, have been recognized on plasmids of *E. coli* and *Salmonella*; these are not inhibited by clavulanic acid.

Absorption, Distribution, and Excretion. Cephalosporins are water-soluble drugs. Of the first-generation cephalosporins, cephalexin, and cephadroxil are relatively acid-stable and sufficiently well absorbed from the intestine to be administered orally to dogs and cats, but not to herbivores. Other first-generation cephalosporins must be administered parenterally although they are often painful on intramuscular injection and irritating on intravenous injection. Second- and third-generation cephalosporins are sometimes available for oral use and could be given to dogs and cats by this route rather than parenterally. Following absorption from injection sites, cephalosporins are widely distributed into tissue and body fluids. Third-generation cephalosporins penetrate cerebrospinal fluid moderately well, and because of their high activity against gram-negative bacteria have particular potential application in the treatment of meningitis.

Adverse Effects. Cephalosporins are relatively nontoxic antibiotics in humans. Allergic reactions occur in 5% to 10% of human patients who are hypersensitive to penicillin. Intravenous and intramuscular injections of some drugs are an irritant.

Other Beta-Lactam Antibiotics. The last 20 years have seen the discovery of other naturally occurring beta-lactam antibiotics. These include the cephamycins, clavulanic acid, thienamycin, the monobactams (such as aztreonam), the carbapenems (such as imipenem), the PS-compounds, and the carpetimycins—all compounds with the basic beta-lactam ring but without the bicyclic ring structure of the classical beta-lactams. All are highly resistant to beta-lactamases, and many possess potent antibacterial properties or are used in combination with earlier beta-lactams (ampicillin, amoxicillin, ticarcillin) for their potent beta-lactamase inhibitory effects (clavulanic acid, sulbactam, tazobactam). Carbapenems (biapenem, imipenem-cilastatin, meropenem) have exceptional activity against clinically important aerobic and anaerobic bacteria, with the greatest activity of all antimicrobials against gram-negative bacteria.

Damage to Cell Membrane Function

Antibiotics that damage cell membrane function include the polymyxins, the polyenes (amphotericin, nystatin), the imidazoles (miconazole, ketoconazole, itraconazole, fluconazole, clotrimazole), and monensin. The cell membrane lies beneath the cell wall, enclosing the cytoplasm. It controls the passage of materials into or out of the cell. If its function is damaged, cellular contents (proteins, nucleotides, ions) can leak from the cell and result in cell damage and death.

Polymyxins. The structure of the polymyxins is such that they have well-defined separate hydrophilic and hydrophobic sectors. Polymyxins act by binding to membrane phospholipids, which results in structural disorganization, permeability damage, and cell lysis. The polymyxins are selectively toxic to gram-negative bacteria because of the presence of certain phospholipids in the cell membrane and because the outer surface of the outer membrane of gram-negative bacteria consists mainly of lipopolysaccharide. Parenteral use is associated with nephrotoxic, neurotoxic, and neuromuscular blocking effects. The major clinical applications are limited to the oral treatment of gram-negative bacterial infections.

Polyenes. The polyenes are selectively active against fungi since they only affect membranes containing ergosterol. Polyenes inhibit the formation of membrane lipids, forming pores through which the vital contents of the cytoplasm are lost. See the section on antifungal therapy, below.

Imidazoles. Imidazoles interfere with the biosynthesis of sterols and bind cell membrane phospholipids to cause leakage of cell contents. They are active against the fungal cell membrane. See the section on antifungal therapy, below.

Inhibition of Nucleic Acid Function

Examples of drugs that inhibit nucleic acid function are nitroimidazoles, nitrofurans, nalidixic acid, the fluoroquinolones (ciprofloxacin, danofloxacin, difloxacin, enrofloxacin, orbifloxacin, sarafloxacin), novobiocin, rifampin, sulfonamides, trimethoprim, and 5-flucytosine. Because the mechanisms of nucleic acid synthesis, replication, and transcription are similar in all cells, drugs affecting nucleic acid function have poor selective toxicity. Most act by binding to DNA to inhibit its replication or transcription. Drugs with greater selective toxicity are the sulfonamides and trimethoprim, which inhibit the synthesis of folic acid.

Nitroimidazoles. Nitroimidazoles, such as metronidazole and dimetridazole, possess antiprotozoal and antibacterial properties. Activity within bacterial cells is due to the unidentified, reduced products of the drug, which are only seen in anaerobes or microaerophiles. Nitroimidazoles cause extensive DNA strand breakage either by inhibiting the DNA repair enzyme, DNase 1, or by forming complexes with the nucleotide bases that the enzyme does not recognize. Nitroimidazoles are bactericidal to anaerobic gram-negative and many gram-positive bacteria and are active against protozoa such as *Tritrichomonas fetus, Giardia lamblia,* and *Histomonas meleagridis*. Chromosomal resistance may cause slight increases in minimum inhibitory concentrations (MIC) but, as is the case for nitrofurans, plasmid-encoded resistance is rare. Nitroimidazoles are generally well absorbed after oral administration, but parenteral injection is highly irritating. They are well distributed throughout body tissues and fluids, including brain and cerebrospinal fluid. Excretion is through the urine. The most serious potential hazard is the controversial report of carcinogenicity in laboratory animals. For this reason, these drugs are not used in food animals.

Nitrofurans. Like the nitroimidazoles, the nitrofurans are antiprotozoal but have wider antibacterial activity; they are most active under anaerobic conditions. After entry into the cell, bacterial nitroreductases produce uncharacterized unstable reduction products, which differ with each type of nitrofuran. These products cause strand breakage in bacterial DNA. The nitrofurans are synthetic 5-nitrofuraldehyde derivatives with broad antimicrobial activity. Toxicity and low tissue concentrations limit their use to the local treatment of infections and to the treatment of urinary tract infections.

Fluoroquinolones. Fluoroquinolones (ciprofloxacin, danofloxacin, difloxacin, enrofloxacin, orbifloxacin, sarafloxacin) are active against gram-negative bacteria. They cause selective inhibition of bacterial DNA synthesis by inhibiting DNA gyrase (topoisomerase II) and DNA topoisomerase IV. DNA gyrase is involved in packing (supercoiling) DNA into bacterial cells whereas topoisomerase IV is involved in relaxing supercoiled DNA. Fluoroquinolones are bactericidal drugs. Nalidixic acid (a quinolone rarely used because of toxicity) is most active against gram-negative bacteria except *P. aeruginosa*, but the newer fluoroquinolone derivatives are broader spectrum and active against some gram-positive bacteria, including mycobacteria. Activity against *Mycoplasma* and rickettsia is also an important attribute of the newer fluoroquinolones. The fluoroquinolones are rapidly absorbed after oral administration and have half-lives varying from 4 to 12 hours. They are widely distributed in tissues, and may be concentrated, for example in the prostate. Penetration into cerebrospinal fluid is about half that of serum, which makes these drugs useful to treat meningitis. They are being introduced rapidly into veterinary use, particularly for use against gram-negative bacteria and *Mycoplasma*. One drawback is the fairly rapid development of chromosomally mediated resistance, which in *Campylobacter jejuni* and *P. aeruginosa* can produce high-level resistance after single nucleotide mutations but is more gradual in other bacteria, usually as the result of cumulative rather than individual nucleotide mutations. Resistance can also result from decreased permeability of the cell wall as well as from acquisition or enhanced activity of an efflux pump that actively transports fluoroquinolones from the cell.

Rifampin. Rifampin, which has particular activity against gram-positive bacteria and mycobacteria, has remarkable selectivity of inhibition of bacterial DNA-dependent ribonucleic acid (RNA) polymerase. Rifampin prevents initiation of transcription. Resistance develops rapidly as the result of chromosomal mutation, so that this drug is rarely used on its own but rather is used in combination with other antimicrobial drugs.

Sulfonamides and Trimethoprim. Sulfonamides are synthetic drugs with broad antibacterial and antiprotozoal properties. They interfere with the biosynthesis of folic acid and prevent the formation of purine nucleotides. Sulfonamides are functional analogues of para-aminobenzoic acid and compete with it for the same enzyme, tetrahydropteroate synthetase, forming nonfunctional folic acid analogues and inhibiting bacterial growth. Selective toxicity of sulfonamides occurs because mammalian cells have lost their ability to synthesize folic acid but rather absorb it from the intestine, whereas bacteria must synthesize it. In the bacterial cell, preformed folic acid is progressively exhausted by several bacterial divisions.

Other drugs affect folic acid synthesis by interfering with the enzyme dihydrofolate reductase. One example is trimethoprim, which is selectively toxic to bacteria rather than to mammalian cells because of greater affinity for the bacterial enzyme. The enzyme inhibits the conversion of dihydrofolate to tetrahydrofolate, producing with sulfonamides a sequential blockade of folic acid synthesis.

Sulfonamides. The sulfonamides constitute a series of weak organic acids that enter most tissues and body fluids. The degree of ionization and lipid solubility of the large number of individual sulfonamides influences absorption, determines capacity to penetrate cell membranes, and can affect the rate of elimination. Sulfonamides exert a bacteriostatic effect against both gram-positive and gram-negative bacteria and can also inhibit other microorganisms (some protozoa). They are available in a wide variety of preparations for either oral or parenteral use. They have largely been abandoned because of widespread resistance, difficulties in administration, and the existence of better alternatives. Certain individual sulfonamides are combined with trimethoprim in fixed ratio (5:1) combination preparations that have the advantage of both synergistic and bactericidal effects.

Individual sulfonamides are derivatives of sulfanilamide, which contains the structural prerequisites for antibacterial activity. The various derivatives differ in physicochemical and pharmacokinetic properties and in degree of antimicrobial activity. The sodium salts of sulfonamides are readily soluble in water, and parenteral preparations are available for intravenous administration. Certain sulfonamide molecules are designed for low solubility (e.g.,

phthalylsulfathiazole) so that they will be slowly absorbed; these are intended for use in the treatment of enteric infections.

Antimicrobial Activity. Sulfonamides are broad-spectrum antimicrobial drugs. They are active against aerobic gram-positive cocci and some rods and some gram-negative bacteria, including members of the family *Enterobacteriaceae.* Many anaerobes are sensitive.

Resistance. Resistance to sulfonamides in pathogenic and nonpathogenic bacteria isolated from animals is widespread. This situation reflects their extensive use in human and veterinary medicine for many years. Sulfonamide resistance may occur as a result of mutation causing overproduction of para-aminobenzoic acid (PABA) or as a result of a structural change in the dihydrofolic acid-synthesizing enzyme with a lowered affinity for sulfonamides. Most often, sulfonamide resistance is plasmid-mediated.

Absorption, Distribution, and Excretion. Most sulfonamides are rapidly absorbed from the gastrointestinal tract and distributed widely to all tissues and body fluids, including synovial and cerebrospinal fluid. They are bound to plasma proteins to a variable extent. In addition to differences among sulfonamides in extent of binding, there is variation among species in binding of individual sulfonamides. Extensive (80%) protein binding serves to increase half-life. They enter cerebrospinal fluid well.

Sulfonamides are eliminated by a combination of renal excretion and biotransformation processes in the liver. This combination of elimination processes contributes to the species variation in the half-life of individual sulfonamides. While a large number of sulfonamide preparations is available for use in veterinary medicine, many of these are different dosage forms of sulfamethazine. This sulfonamide is most widely used in the food-producing animals and can attain effective plasma concentrations (within the range 50 to 150 µg/ml) when administered either orally or parenterally. Due to their alkalinity, most parenteral preparations should only be administered by intravenous injection. Prolonged-release oral dosage forms of sulfamethazine are available.

Adverse Effects. The sulfonamides can produce a wide variety of side effects, some of which may have an allergic basis whereas others are due to direct toxicity. The more common adverse effects are urinary tract disturbances (crystalluria, hematuria, or even obstruction) and hematopoietic disorders (thrombocytopenia and leukopenia). Some adverse effects are associated with particular sulfonamides. Sulfadiazine and sulfasalazine given for long periods to dogs to control chronic hemorrhagic colitis have caused keratoconjunctivitis sicca.

Trimethoprim-Sulfonamide Combinations. Trimethoprim is combined with a variety of sulfonamides in a fixed ratio. The combination produces a bactericidal effect against a wide range of bacteria, with some important exceptions, and also inhibits certain other microorganisms. Veterinary preparations contain trimethoprim combined with sulfadiazine or sulfadoxine in the 1:5 ratio. Other antibacterial diaminopyrimidines combined with sulfonamides for use in animals include baquiloprim and ormetoprim.

Antimicrobial Activity. Trimethoprim-sulfonamide combinations have a generally broad spectrum and usually bactericidal action against many gram-positive and gram-negative aerobic bacteria, including members of the family *Enterobacteriaceae*. The combination is active against a large proportion of anaerobic bacteria, at least under in vitro conditions. *Mycoplasma* and *P. aeruginosa* are resistant.

Synergism occurs when the microorganisms are sensitive to both drugs in the combination. When bacteria are resistant to sulfonamides, synergism may still be obtained in up to 40% of cases, even when bacteria are only moderately susceptible to trimethoprim. Because of differences between the trimethoprim and sulfonamide in distribution pattern and processes of elimination, the concentration ratios of the two drugs will differ considerably in tissues and urine from the ratio in the plasma. This variation is not important since the synergistic interaction occurs over a wide range of concentration ratios of the two drugs.

Resistance. Resistance to sulfonamides is due to structural alteration in the dihydrofolic acid synthesizing enzyme (dihydropteroate synthetase), whereas resistance to trimethoprim usually results from plasmid-encoded synthesis of a resistant dihydrofolate reductase enzyme. Bacterial resistance to the combination has progressively developed with use of these preparations in animals.

Absorption, Distribution, and Elimination. Trimethoprim is a lipid-soluble organic base that is approximately 60% bound to plasma proteins and 60% ionized in the plasma. This combination of physicochemical properties enables the drug to distribute widely, to penetrate cellular barriers by nonionic diffusion, and to attain effective concentrations in most body fluids and tissues, including brain and cerebrospinal fluid. Hepatic metabolism is the principal process for elimination of trimethoprim. The half-life and fraction of the dose that is excreted unchanged in the urine vary widely among different species. The drug is well absorbed following oral administration in dogs, cats, and horses or from injection sites in these and other species.

Adverse Effects. Serious side effects are uncommon; those that do occur can usually be attributed to the sulfonamide component. Oral trimethoprim-sulfonamide has the advantage over other oral antimicrobials of causing little disturbance among the normal intestinal anaerobic microflora.

Inhibition of Protein Synthesis

Examples of drugs that inhibit protein synthesis are tetracyclines, aminoglycosides (amikacin, gentamicin, kanamycin, neomycin, streptomycin, tobramycin, and others), aminocyclitols (spectinomycin), chloramphenicol, lincosamides (clindamycin, lincomycin), and macrolides (azithromycin, clarithromycin, erythromycin, tylosin, tiamulin, and others). Because of the marked differences in ribosomal structure, composition, and function between prokaryotic and eukaryotic cells, many important antibacterial drugs selectively inhibit bacterial protein synthesis. Antibiotics affecting protein synthesis can be divided into those affecting the 30S ribosome (tetracyclines, aminoglycosides, aminocyclitols) and those affecting the 50S ribosome (chloramphenicol, macrolides, lincosamides).

Tetracyclines. Tetracyclines interfere with protein synthesis by inhibiting the binding of aminoacyl tRNA to the recognition site. The various tetracyclines have similar antimicrobial activity but differ in pharmacologic characteristics.

Antimicrobial Activity. Tetracyclines are broad-spectrum drugs active against gram-positive and gram-negative bacteria, including rickettsia and chlamydia, some mycoplasmas, and protozoa such as *Theileria*. Tetracyclines have good activity against many gram-positive bacteria, the more fastidious nonenteric bacteria such as *Actinobacillus, Bordetella, Brucella, Haemophilus*, some *Pasteurella*, and many anaerobic bacteria, but their activity against these bacteria and against members of the family *Enterobacteriaceae* are limited by acquired resistance. *Pseudomonas aeruginosa* is resistant, except in urinary tract infections where, because of their high concentrations, tetracyclines may be drugs of choice.

Resistance. Widespread resistance to the tetracyclines has considerably reduced their usefulness. Such resistance is high level and usually plasmid- and transposon-mediated. Cross-resistance between tetracyclines is complete.

Adverse Effects. Tetracyclines are generally safe antibiotics with a reasonably high therapeutic index. The main adverse effects are associated with their severely irritant nature, with disturbances in gastrointestinal flora, with their ability to bind calcium (cardiovascular effects, teeth or bone deposition), and with the toxic effects of degradation products on liver and kidney cells. Their use in horses has largely been abandoned because of a tendency to produce broad-spectrum suppression of the normal intestinal flora and fatal superinfection with *Salmonella* or *Clostridium difficile*.

Chloramphenicol and Florfenicol. Chloramphenicol and florfenicol are broad-spectrum, generally bacteriostatic drugs that bind the 50S ribosome, distorting the region and inhibiting the peptidyl transferase reaction. They are stable, lipid-soluble, neutral compounds.

Antimicrobial Activity. Chloramphenicol and florfenicol are active against gram-positive and gram-negative bacteria, including chlamydia and rickettsia, and some mycoplasmas. Most gram-positive and many gram-negative pathogenic aerobic and anaerobic bacteria are susceptible, though resistance is increasing in members of the family *Enterobacteriaceae*. Florfenicol is less active against members of the family *Enterobacteriaceae* but has high activity against *Haemophilus, Mannheimia haemolytica*, and *Pasteurella*. The drugs are generally bacteriostatic.

Resistance. Most resistance is the result of plasmid-encoded acetylase enzymes.

Absorption, Distribution, and Excretion. In dogs, cats, and preruminants, chloramphenicol is well absorbed from the intestine; in ruminants the drug is inactivated after oral administration. Because of its low molecular weight, lipid solubility, and modest plasma protein binding, the drug is well distributed in most tissues and fluids, including the cerebrospinal fluid and aqueous humor. The half-life of chloramphenicol varies widely in animals from a low of 1 hour in horses to 5 or 6 hours in cats. In neonates the half-life is considerably longer. The drug is mainly eliminated by glucuronide conjugation in the liver.

Adverse Effects. The fatal aplastic anemia seen in 1 in 25,000 to 40,000 humans treated with chloramphenicol does not occur in animals, although prolonged high dosing may cause reversible abnormalities in bone marrow activity. The potential for nondose-related fatal aplastic anaemia in humans has led to its prohibition for use in food animals in most countries because of fear of the presence of drug residues in meat products. Florfenicol does not have this effect and so has selective use for food animals.

Aminoglycosides.   The aminoglycosides are bactericidal. The mode of action of streptomycin is best understood. Streptomycin has a variety of complex effects in the bacterial cell: a) it binds to a specific receptor protein in the 30S ribosomal subunit, distorting the codon–anticodon interactions at the recognition site and causing misreading of the genetic code so that faulty proteins are produced; b) it binds to "initiating" ribosomes to prevent the formation of 70S ribosomes; and c) it inhibits the elongation reaction of protein synthesis. The other aminoglycosides act similarly to streptomycin in causing mistranslation of the genetic code and in irreversible inhibition of initiation, although the extent and type often differ. They have multiple binding sites on the ribosome, whereas streptomycin has only one, and can also inhibit the translocation step in protein synthesis. Spectinomycin is a bacteriostatic aminocyclitol antibiotic that is believed to inhibit polypeptide chain elongation at the translocation step.

The aminoglycoside antibiotics are polar organic bases. Their polarity largely accounts for the similar pharmacokinetic properties that are shared by all members of the group. Chemically, they consist of a hexose nucleus to which amino sugars are attached by glycosidic linkages. All are potentially ototoxic and nephrotoxic. The newer aminoglycosides are more resistant to plasmid-mediated enzymatic degradation and are less toxic than the older compounds. Amikacin > tobramycin > gentamicin > neomycin = kanamycin > streptomycin in potency, spectrum of activity, and stability to plasmid-mediated resistance. This activity mirrors the chronology of introduction of the drugs, with streptomycin being the oldest of the aminoglycosides.

Antimicrobial Activity. Aminoglycosides are particularly active against gram-negative bacteria as well as against mycobacteria and some mycoplasma. Anaerobic bacteria are usually resistant. As a general rule, gram-positive bacteria are resistant to older drugs (streptomycin, neomycin) but may be inhibited by newer drugs (gentamicin, amikacin). A particularly useful property is the activity of newer aminoglycosides against *P. aeruginosa*. Their bactericidal action on aerobic gram-negative bacilli is markedly influenced by pH; they are most active in an alkaline environment. Increased local acidity secondary to tissue damage may account for the failure of an aminoglycoside to kill usually susceptible microorganisms at infection sites or in abscess cavities. Combinations of aminoglycosides with penicillins are often synergistic; the concurrent administration of the newer beta-lactam antibiotics with gentamicin or tobramycin has been used to treat serious gram-negative infections, for example, those caused by *P. aeruginosa*.

Resistance. Most clinically important resistance is caused by a variety of R plasmid-specified degradative enzymes located in the periplasmic space. Certain of these enzymes inactivate only the older aminoglycosides (streptomycin, or neomycin and kanamycin), but others are broader spectrum. The remarkable property of amikacin is its resistance to many of the enzymes that inactivate other aminoglycosides. Plasmid-mediated resistance to streptomycin is widespread and commonly linked to sulfonamides, tetracyclines, and ampicillin. Chromosomal resistance to streptomycin, but not to the other aminoglycosides, develops fairly readily during treatment.

Absorption, Distribution, and Excretion. Aminoglycosides are poorly absorbed from the gastrointestinal tract, bind to a low extent to plasma proteins, and have limited capacity to enter cells and penetrate cellular barriers. They do not readily attain therapeutic concentrations in transcellular fluids, particularly cerebrospinal and ocular fluid. Poor diffusibility can be attributed to their low degree of lipid solubility. Their apparent volumes of distribution are relatively small, and their half-lives are short (2 hours) in domestic animals. Even though these drugs have a small volume of distribution, selective binding to renal tissue (kidney cortex) occurs. Elimination takes place entirely by renal excretion (glomerular filtration), and unchanged drug is rapidly excreted in the urine. Impaired renal function decreases their rate of excretion and makes adjustment of the maintenance dosage necessary to prevent accumulation with attendant toxicity.

Major changes are taking place in recommendations for intramuscular dosage with aminoglycosides, which is moving from three times daily to a single daily dosage. This has the effect of increasing therapeutic efficacy, since antibacterial activity depends on both peak concentrations and total concentration, and of reducing toxicity, since the nephrotoxic effects depend on a threshold effect, concentrations above which have no further action. This dramatically changed understanding of aminoglycoside dosage may increase the use of the less toxic members.

Adverse Effects. All aminoglycosides can cause varying degrees of ototoxicity and nephrotoxicity. The tendency to produce vestibular or cochlear damage varies with the drug: neomycin is the most likely to cause cochlear damage and streptomycin to cause vestibular damage. Nephrotoxicity (acute tubular necrosis) occurs in association with prolonged therapy and excessive trough concentrations of the aminoglycoside (particularly gentamicin) in plasma. The aminoglycosides can produce neuromuscular blockage of the nondepolarizing type, which causes flaccid paralysis and apnea. This is most likely to occur in association with anesthesia.

Aminocyclitols.   Spectinomycin is an aminocyclitol antibiotic with a spectrum of activity and mechanism of action similar to that of kanamycin but without the toxic effects of the aminoglycosides. It is normally bacteriostatic and is not particularly active on a weight basis. Its activity against gram-negative bacteria is unpredictable because of naturally resistant strains. Chromosomal resistance develops readily but does not cross-react with aminoglycosides. Plasmid resistance is uncommon but often extends to streptomycin. The drug has most of the pharmacokinetic properties of aminoglycosides but appears to penetrate cerebrospinal fluid better. It has been used in agricultural practice to treat salmonellosis and mycoplasma infections.

Macrolides. Macrolide antibiotics are bacteriostatic with activity particularly against gram-positive bacteria and mycoplasma. They bind to 50S ribosome in competition with chloramphenicol and inhibit the translocation step of protein synthesis. The precise mechanism of action is unknown. Macrolide antibiotics (azithromycin, clarithromycin, erythromycin, tylosin, tiamulin, and spiramycin) have action and pharmacokinetic properties similar to the lincosamides. Like the lincosamides they are lipid soluble, basic drugs that are concentrated in tissue compared to serum and penetrate cells well.

Antimicrobial Activity. Erythromycin has an antibacterial spectrum similar to penicillin G, but it includes activity against penicillinase-producing coagulase-positive staphylococci, *Campylobacter, Leptospira, Bordetella,* rickettsia, chlamydia, some mycoplasma, and atypical mycobacteria. It may be bactericidal at high concentrations. Tylosin and spiramycin are less active than erythromycin against bacteria but more active against a broad range of mycoplasma. Tiamulin has better activity than the other macrolides against anaerobes, including *Brachyspira hyodysenteriae*, and is distinguished for its remarkable activity against mycoplasmas. Azithromycin and clarithromycin are particularly active against non-tuberculous mycobacteria. The activity of these two drugs against a variety of intracellular bacteria not only depends on their intrinsic activity but also on the often remarkable concentration of the drugs in cells, including macrophages. Azithromycin may concentrate 200–500 fold inside macrophages compared to its serum concentrations.

Resistance. One-step chromosomal resistance to erythromycin develops fairly readily, even during treatment, but is generally unstable. Plasmid-mediated resistance is common. Cross-resistance between erythromycin and lincosamides and other macrolides is common. There is little information about resistance of veterinary pathogens to tylosin. Development of resistance to tiamulin appears to be relatively uncommon; organisms resistant to tiamulin show one-way cross-resistance with other macrolides.

Absorption, Distribution, and Excretion. Erythromycin stearate and estolate are well absorbed after oral administration, but the base is not. Intramuscular injection of erythromycin is very irritating. The absorption of tylosin from the intestine varies with the formulation. Tiamulin is well absorbed. These drugs are well distributed through body tissues and fluids, except the cerebrospinal fluid. Tissue concentrations often exceed serum concentrations, notably for azithromycin and clarithromycin, which are therefore often dosed once a day or less frequently. In the case of spiramycin, such tissue concentration is extreme and is associated with tissue binding. A large proportion of these drugs is degraded in the body, but some is excreted through the kidney and the liver.

Adverse Effects. Macrolides are generally safe drugs though painful on injection. Their potential for causing irreversible diarrhea in adult horses means that they should be avoided in this species. Tylosin and tiamulin administered intravenously to calves may produce severe nervous depression. The drugs should not be given orally to ruminants because of their potential for disturbing the rumen flora.

Lincosamides. Lincomycin and clindamycin have antibacterial activity mainly against gram-positive aerobic bacteria and against anaerobic bacteria. The drugs bind the 50S ribosomal subunits at binding sites that overlap with those of chloramphenicol and the macrolides. They inhibit the peptidyl transferase reaction. The lincosamides, lincomycin and clindamycin, are products of an actinomycete with activity and mechanism of action similar to that of the macrolides. Lincomycin is most commonly used in veterinary medicine, although it is less active on a weight basis than clindamycin. Lincosamides are active against gram-positive aerobic and all anaerobic bacteria, and against mycoplasmas, but most gram-negative aerobes are resistant. Clindamycin is more active than lincomycin against anaerobes and may be bactericidal. Chromosomal stepwise resistance develops fairly readily, and plasmid-mediated resistance is common. Cross-resistance between lincosamides is complete and commonly occurs also with macrolides. Lincomycin is readily absorbed after oral or intramuscular administration. Food delays and reduces absorption. The absorption of different clindamycin compounds is variable. The lincosamides are widely distributed in body tissues and fluids, including the prostate and milk, but cerebrospinal fluid concentrations are low. They penetrate intracellularly because of their lipophilic properties. Most excretion is through the liver. The major adverse effect of lincosamides is their ability to cause fatal diarrhea in horses, rabbits, guinea pigs, and hamsters. In rabbits, fatal diarrhea results from proliferation of *Clostridium spiroforme* or *C. difficile*. Oral lincosamides at low concentrations produce severe ruminal disturbances in adult ruminants.

Antimicrobial Susceptibility and Drug Dosage Prediction

The use of antimicrobial drugs in treating infections depends on the relation of the quantitative susceptibility of the microorganism to tissue concentrations of drug. The antimicrobial susceptibility of many veterinary pathogens is predictable and clinical experience has established effective dosages for infections caused by these organisms. In many bacteria, however, the presence of various mechanisms for acquiring resistance means that susceptibility to a particular antibacterial drug may need to be tested.

Antimicrobial Susceptibility Testing

There are two general methods for antimicrobial susceptibility testing in vitro: the dilution method and the diffusion method. The dilution method gives quantitative information on drug susceptibility while the diffusion method gives qualitative (or at best semiquantitative) information. The tests must be performed under standardized conditions. The description of a bacterium as susceptible or resistant to an antimicrobial drug depends ultimately on clinical success or failure of treatment. Quantitative information on susceptibility is obtained in the laboratory under artificial circumstances, which cannot easily take into account host defenses, the dynamics of drug disposition, or the dynamics of interaction of a varying drug concentration with a bacterium in the host environment. Nevertheless, infections caused by bacteria classified as resistant in susceptibility tests rarely respond successfully to treatment, except under exceptional circumstances. Infections caused by bacteria classified as susceptible can be predicted to do so, depending on the clinical circumstances, nature of the infection, appropriate dosage, and a variety of other factors—some of which are discussed below.

Dilution Antimicrobial Tests. Antimicrobial drugs of known potency are prepared in doubling dilutions of concentrations similar to those achievable in the tissues of patients given usual drug dosages. The highest dilution at which there is no visible bacterial growth following inoculation and incubation is the minimum inhibitory concentration (MIC), which is usually less than the minimum bactericidal concentration (MBC) for drugs (Table 4.1).

The advantage of determining quantitative susceptibility of an organism is that this information can be related to knowledge of drug concentrations in particular tissues in the prediction of appropriate drug dosage. In medical practice, MIC results are usually interpreted by the system of categories suggested by the U.S. National Committee for Clinical Laboratory Standards (NCCLS). These interpretative guidelines take into account the inherent susceptibility of the organism to each drug, the pharmacokinetic and pharmacodynamic properties of the particular drug, dosage, site of infection, and drug toxicity. These categories are 1) susceptible, meaning that the infecting organism is usually inhibited by concentrations of a particular antibiotic attained in tissues by usual dosage; 2) intermediately susceptible, meaning that the infecting organism is inhibited by blood or tissue concentrations achieved with maximum dosage; and 3) resistant, meaning that it is resistant to normally achievable and tolerated concentrations of antimicrobial drugs. A fourth category, *flexible*, has recently been introduced by the NCCLS Subcommittee on Veterinary Antimicrobial Susceptibility Testing (1999). This indicates the availability in the United States of the U.S. Food and Drug Administration flexible label, which allows veterinarians to adjust the dose, within a given range, based on the MIC of the pathogen.

Diffusion Antimicrobial Tests. A standard concentration of a pure culture of the pathogen is placed on appropriate agar and individual filter paper discs containing known concentrations of individual antibiotics are placed on the agar, which is incubated for 18 hours at 35°C. The zone of inhibition around each disc is measured and the measurement is referred to a chart that classifies the organism as being susceptible, resistant, or intermediately susceptible to the particular antibiotic in each disc. Standards for performing these tests are defined. Under standard conditions, there is a linear inverse relationship between the diameter of the zone of growth inhibition and MIC. The

Table 4.1.   Minimum Concentration of Tetracycline Inhibitory to Selected Veterinary Pathogens

	Minimum Inhibitory Concentration (µg/ml)	
	MIC$_{50}$*	MIC$_{90}$*
Bordetella bronchiseptica	2	2
Brucella canis	0.25	0.25
Corynebacterium pseudotuberculosis	0.25	0.25
Escherichia coli	4.0	64.0
Klebsiella pneumoniae	2.0	64.0
Mycoplasma canis	4.0	8.0
Pasteurella multocida	0.5	0.5

*Highest MIC$_{50}$ of 50% of isolates tested, MIC$_{90}$ of 90% of isolates tested. The MIC of different organisms varies with strain and species.

interpretation of zone diameters as susceptible, resistant, or intermediate relates to serum drug concentrations of antibiotics in different animal species commonly achievable under standard dosage regimens. From these drug concentrations, MIC breakpoints have been selected and extrapolated to zone diameters in providing the interpretative standards. A specialized modified diffusion system is the E test, which is a modified diffusion concentration gradient strip system that gives quantitative results.

Design of Drug Dosage and Pharmacodynamic Properties

Pharmacokinetic descriptions of drug disposition in different animal species, when combined with quantitative susceptibility (MIC) data and knowledge of the pharmacodynamic properties of the antimicrobial, allow prediction of reasonable drug dosage in animals.

Pharmacokinetic properties include the route of administration, rate of absorption, rate of distribution, volume of distribution, and route and rate of elimination. Pharmacodynamic properties include concentration versus time in the tissue and other body fluids, as well as at the site of infection, toxicologic effect, and antimicrobial effect at the site of infection. The pharmacodynamic effects at the site of infection include the MIC, MBC, concentration-dependent killing effect, post-antibiotic effect, sub-MIC effect, post-antibiotic leukocyte enhancement (PALE) effect, as well as first exposure effect. For some ("concentration-dependent") antimicrobials (aminoglycosides, fluoroquinolones), killing is a function of antimicrobial concentration relative to MIC, a function that may persist long after drug concentrations are below MIC. For these drugs the total amount of the drug above MIC ("area under the curve") is also important. For other ("time-dependent") antimicrobials (beta-lactams, chloramphenicol, lincosamides, macrolides, tetracyclines, trimethoprim-sulfonamides), bacterial inhibition is a function of the time that tissue concentrations exceed MIC; these drugs therefore have to be dosed to maintain concentrations at the site of infection above MIC. For these drugs, the total amount of drug above MIC is not important since no additional killing occurs with increased concentrations (and indeed for some drugs killing may actually decrease at high concentrations). The maximum interval of drug dosing should preclude resumption of bacterial growth.

Factors Affecting Tissue Drug Concentrations. *Dosage.* The dosage regimen is made up of the *size* of the dose, which is limited by drug toxicity, and the dosage *interval*, which is determined by the half-life of the drug. The dosage interval required to maintain therapeutic tissue concentrations by intravenous dosing should not exceed twice the half-life for most antibiotics, but giving drugs by other routes lengthens the dosage interval.

Routes of Administration. Antibacterial drugs can be administered by a wide variety of routes—for example, intravenous, intramuscular, oral, subcutaneous, intramammary, intrauterine, or respiratory:

1. Intravenous injection of a drug gives immediate high serum drug concentrations, which rapidly decline as the drug is distributed. Intravenous dosing may be the only way to exceed the MIC of some pathogens, but frequent dosing by this route is generally impractical in veterinary medicine.
2. Intramuscular injection is commonly used in veterinary medicine because it gives good serum concentrations within 1 to 2 hours of administration. The major advantage is that intramuscular injection gives the highest serum concentration of all routes other than intravenous, although subcutaneous injection is a reasonable alternative. Drug formulation can be prepared to give slow release of the drug after intramuscular injection and thus prolong dosage intervals to reduce handling of animals.
3. The oral administration of antimicrobial drugs is limited to monogastric and preruminant animals and to young foals. The oral dose is generally several times greater than the parenteral dose because the drug is less well absorbed. Although the oral route is often the easiest way to administer drugs, it is not always the most reliable. Some drugs (aminoglycosides, polymyxins) are not absorbed from the intestine, others are destroyed by stomach acidity (benzyl penicillin), and absorption may be impaired by food (as occurs with ampicillin, tetracyclines, lincomycin). Administration of antibiotics in water is nevertheless a particularly simple, convenient, and inexpensive way to treat livestock because it involves little if any handling of animals and avoids the expense of mixing antibiotics in feed.
4. Infections of the udder, female genital tract, external ear canal, and skin are commonly treated by local application of antibiotics. High drug concentrations are obtained without systemic toxic effects. The concentration of free drug in the serum largely determines the concentration in tissue fluids, since penetration of drugs into interstitial fluids in most tissues of the body is through pores in capillary endothelium.

Physicochemical Properties of the Drug. These characteristics largely determine the extent of the distribution of a drug in the body. Most antimicrobial drugs distribute well in extravascular tissue fluids, principally the interstitial fluid. They penetrate capillary endothelium through pores that admit molecules with a molecular weight of less than about 1000. Passage across biological membranes such as into tissue cells or across nonfenestrated capillary endothelium depends on drug ionization, lipid solubility, molecular weight, and the amount of free drug present. Lipid-soluble and nonionized drugs such as the macrolides and chloramphenicol distribute well and even concentrate in tissue, whereas ionized and weakly lipid-soluble drugs such as penicillins and aminoglycosides distribute poorly. These physicochemical differences largely determine the pharmacokinetic characteristics of the drugs; thus, aminoglycosides and penicillins have small apparent volumes of distribution and short half-lives after intravenous injection and are eliminated through the urinary tract, whereas macrolides and tetracyclines have large apparent volumes of distribution and longer half-lives and are eliminated in part through the liver. Penetration of special sites in the body such as the central nervous system, eye, and prostate (which among other differences lack capillary pores) is only by low molecular weight, lipid-soluble, nonionized drugs.

Protein Binding of Drug. In general, serum protein binding of drugs up to 90 percent is of little clinical importance. Aminoglycosides and polymyxin bind extensively to intracellular constituents and thus are inactivated by pus.

Excretion Mechanisms. These determine the concentration of drugs in the organs of excretion. Remarkably high concentrations of drugs may be achieved in urine or bile.

Physiological Barriers. Anatomic-physiologic barriers in the brain, cerebrospinal fluid, eye, and mammary gland reduce the entry of drugs from the blood. Inflammation reduces but does not abolish these barriers.

Duration of Treatment. Although it is axiomatic that a drug must be present for adequate time at the site of infection, the variables affecting time of treatment have not been defined. The response of different types of infection to antibiotics varies, and clinical experience with different types of infection is important in assessing response to treatment. In general, if no response to treatment is observed after two days, diagnosis and treatment should be reassessed. Treatment should be continued for 48 hours after symptoms have resolved, depending on the severity of infection. For serious infections, treatment should last 7 to 10 days. Some uncomplicated infections, such as cystitis in females, have been successfully treated with single doses of antibiotics.

Use of Antibacterial Combinations

Combinations of drugs sometimes have dramatic success where individual drugs fail. An outstanding early example is the use of penicillin-streptomycin combinations in enterococcal endocarditis in humans. However, early studies of the outcome of combination treatment of pneumococcal meningitis in humans showed the serious clinical effects of mixing bacteriostatic and bactericidal drugs. The importance of antagonistic interactions between drugs is greatest in those infections or patients where immune defenses are poor—meningitis, endocarditis, or chronic os- teomyelitis—or where immunodeficiencies are present, and where a bactericidal action is needed. If a bacterio- static drug is mixed with a bactericidal drug, then the former may neutralize the latter, which may be crucial for clear- ance of infection from certain sites or infections (menin- gitis, endocarditis, chronic osteomyelitis). In other pa- tients or diseases, because of the complexity of the host-bacterial–antimicrobial interaction, it is harder to de- tect either synergistic or antagonistic effects clinically, and it is likely that antagonistic effects of drugs are "laboratory artifacts" with no clinical meaning.

A drug combination is *additive* if the combined effect of several drugs is the sum of their independent activities measured separately, *synergistic* if the combined effect is significantly greater than their independent effects, and *antagonistic* if it is significantly less than their independent effects. Synergism and antagonism are not absolute char- acteristics; such interactions are often difficult to predict, vary with bacterial species and strains, and may occur only over a narrow range of concentrations. No single in vitro method detects all such interactions. The methods used to determine in vitro interactions are generally time- consuming and are not often available in the laboratory.

Antimicrobial combinations are frequently synergistic if they involve the following mechanisms: 1) sequential inhibition of successive steps in metabolism (e.g., trimethoprim-sulfonamide combination), 2) sequential inhibition of cell wall synthesis (e.g., vancomycin- penicillin, mecillinam-ampicillin), 3) facilitation of drug entry of one antibiotic by another (e.g., beta-lactam- aminoglycoside, polymyxin-sulfonamide), 4) inhibition of inactivating enzymes (e.g., ampicillin-clavulanic acid), and 5) prevention of emergence of resistant populations (e.g., erythromycin-rifampin combination against *Rhodo- coccus equi*).

As suggested earlier, to some extent antagonism be- tween antibiotic combinations is a laboratory artifact that depends on the method of measurement and is thus, with some exceptions, unimportant clinically. The antagonistic effects of some combinations are, however, detected clini- cally. Antagonism may occur if antimicrobial combina- tions involve the following mechanisms: 1) inhibition of bactericidal activity (e.g., bacteriostatic and bactericidal drugs used to treat meningitis where, depending on the time-dose relation, bactericidal effects are prevented), 2) competition for drug binding sites (e.g., macrolide- chloramphenicol combinations, which are of unclear clinical significance), 3) inhibition of cell permeability mechanisms (e.g., chloramphenicol or tetracycline- aminoglycoside combinations, which are of unclear clini- cal significance), and 4) derepression of resistance en- zymes (e.g., new third-generation cephalosporin antibi- otics with older beta-lactam drugs).

Resistance to Antibacterial Drugs

The potential for mutation and for genetic exchange be- tween all types of bacteria, combined with the short bacte- rial generation time, is of major importance in limiting the use of antimicrobial drugs in controlling infection in ani- mals and humans. The use of antimicrobial drugs does not induce resistance in bacteria but rather eliminates the sus- ceptible bacteria and leaves the resistant bacteria already present in the population. The exposure of animals to an- timicrobials is the basis of selection for the evolution and spread of resistance genes and resistant bacteria. The ge- netic processes involved in the development of resistance in bacteria are precisely those involved in the evolution of bacteria generally. What has surprised people has been the speed and scale with which resistance has emerged in many bacterial pathogens, a phenomenon that seems to have increased in recent years.

Resistance to antimicrobial drugs can be classified as constitutive or acquired.

Constitutive Resistance

Microorganisms may be resistant to certain antibiotics be- cause the cellular mechanisms required for antibiotic sus- ceptibility are absent from the cell. *Mycoplasma*, for exam- ple, are resistant to benzyl penicillin G because they lack a cell wall.

Acquired Resistance

Acquired, genetically based resistance can arise because of chromosomal mutation or, more importantly, through the acquisition of genetic material. Chromosomal muta- tions tend to produce changes in bacterial cell structures, whereas plasmid-mediated resistance tends to encode syn- thesis of enzymes that modify antibiotics. Chromosomal resistance is often a gradual, stepwise process, whereas plasmid resistance is often high-level, all-or-none, resist- ance. Examples of important mechanisms of resistance are 1) enzymatic inactivation of antibiotics, 2) failure of bacte- rial permeability, 3) alteration in target receptors, 4) devel- opment of by-pass mechanisms in metabolic pathways, 5) development of enzymes with low drug affinity, and 6) removing antimicrobial drugs from the cell through ef- flux pumps.

Chromosomal Mutation to Resistance. Chromosomal mutation to resistance is generally a minor problem. Mu- tations to antibiotic resistance are spontaneous events in- volving changes in chromosomal DNA sequences unin- fluenced by the presence of antibiotics. Such mutations may lead to other changes that leave the cell at a disadvan- tage so that, in the absence of antibiotic selection, these mutants may gradually be lost. Mutation to antibiotic re- sistance can be dramatic, as in the case of single-step mu- tation to streptomycin resistance where MIC increases a thousandfold, or gradual, as in the case of chromosomal resistance to penicillin where a series of mutational events may gradually increase the MIC of the organisms. These differences occur because when antibiotics affect one tar- get site, chromosomal mutation is a single-step process, whereas when several targets are affected, mutation to re- sistance is a multistep process.

The rate of mutation differs for, and is characteristic of, each antibiotic. Sometimes antibiotics are used in combi- nation to overcome the possibility of mutation to resistance—the chance of mutation to resistance to two antibiotics is the product of the chances of mutation for each antibiotic alone. In veterinary medicine, mutational resistance has limited the use of streptomycin, novobiocin, rifampin, and, to a lesser extent, erythromycin. It appears to be increasingly limiting the use of fluoroquinolones. Interestingly, for fluoroquinolones, there are differences between species in the importance of single-step mutations in the development of resistance. For *Campylobacter jejuni* and *Pseudomonas aeruginosa*, a single mutation at a particular site in the *gyrA* DNA gyrase gene can lead to clinical resistance whereas in *E. coli* a single mutation may lead to only a slight reduction in susceptibility.

A chromosomal mutation resulting in multiple antibiotic resistance has been described for clinically relevant bacteria. The region involved, the Mar (multiple antibiotic resistance) locus, controls efflux systems resulting in resistance to a variety of drugs without modification of the drugs.

Transferable Drug Resistance. Genetic exchange as a cause of antibiotic resistance is of major importance in veterinary medicine. Unlike chromosomal resistance, which occurs in individual bacteria, transfer of genetic material produces *epidemic* or *infectious* resistance, often to several antibiotics at one time and even, though rarely, in the absence of antibiotic selection. The extrachromosomal DNA molecules responsible for antibiotic resistance are usually plasmids, which in this context are sometimes called *R factors* (or *R plasmids*). The plasmid DNA responsible for resistance can reproduce itself within a cell and spread to other cells by transduction, conjugation, transposition, or integrons:

1. *Transduction.* A process by which plasmid DNA is incorporated by a bacterial virus and then transferred to another bacterium. An example is transfer of a beta-lactamase gene from penicillin resistant to susceptible staphylococci. The importance of transduction in spread of antimicrobial resistance has probably been underestimated but the narrow specificity of bacteriophages may have limited their role in resistance transfer.

2. *Conjugation.* This refers to plasmid-mediated transfer of resistance. In this common process of gene transfer, a donor bacterium synthesizes a sex pilus, which attaches to a recipient bacterium in a mating process and transfers copies of plasmid genes to the recipients. The donor retains copies of the plasmid genes but the recipient has now become a potential donor. Conjugation can occur not only between species of the same genera but also across genera and families, so that similar plasmids can be found in a wide range of unrelated bacteria. Plasmids are often partly constructed from transposons and integrons (see below).

3. *Transposition.* Short DNA sequences known as *transposons* ("jumping genes") can transpose from plasmid to plasmid, plasmid to chromosome, or chromosome to plasmid. A transposon copy usually remains at the original site. The frequency of transposition is characteristic of the particular transpo-

son and bacterium. The importance of transposition as a key element in resistance transfer is that transposition is independent of the recombination process of the bacterial cell—homology with the interacting DNA is not required. Plasmids from diverse sources often possess *identical* antibiotic inactivating genes because of transposons. There are a variety of different types of transposons that carry resistance genes; some transposons may even cause conjugation. Some transposons may contain integrons (see below). The simplest form of a transposon is a resistance gene flanked on either side by an *insertion sequence*, the smallest form of mobile genetic element. Because of the widespread nature of insertion sequences in bacteria, there is essentially no gene in bacterial genomes that cannot be mobilized and moved to other bacterial genomes as a transposon.

4. *Integrons.* Integrons are increasingly recognized as widespread genetic elements associated with multiple drug resistance in gram-negative enteric bacteria. An integron consists of an integrase gene and a site-specific integration site into which the integrase can insert antimicrobial drug resistance *cassettes*. Over nine types of integrons and over 60 different gene cassettes have been identified in gram-negative enteric bacteria, with some integrons containing as many as seven different resistance genes on their cassettes. In addition, some bacteria may carry cassettes in their genomes which have not incorporated into integrons but may be assumed to be capable of so doing. Integrons (with or without resistance-gene cassettes) may be found in the chromosome or in plasmids.

Clinical Importance of Antimicrobial Drug Resistance

Acquired drug resistance has become a major problem in pathogenic bacteria of veterinary importance. It is common in many species, although some bacteria, particularly gram-positive bacteria such as many streptococci and corynebacteria, have remained highly susceptible to commonly used drugs. As a result, in many cases diseases produced by these bacteria have declined considerably in importance, to be replaced by diseases produced by bacteria that have the ability to evolve more readily. Acquired resistance to penicillins is frequent in coagulase-positive staphylococci, and acquired multiple antibiotic resistance to many common antibiotics seriously limits their use in members of the family *Enterobacteriaceae* such as *Salmonella* and *E. coli*. Acquired resistance is increasingly observed in nonenteric bacteria such as *Pasteurella*, *Bordetella*, and *Haemophilus* and has been identified in virtually every pathogenic bacterial genus as well as in the normal flora.

There is to some extent a causal relationship between antimicrobial drug use and the development of resistance but its importance varies with different pathogens and essentially reflects their ability to adapt to changing circumstances, i.e., to evolve. The development of resistance has been particularly well documented among enteric bacteria in veterinary medicine. The intestine is a major site of transfer of antibiotic resistance both because of the vast numbers of bacteria present, the use of oral antimicrobial drugs, and because of the opportunities for spread of these bacteria between intensively reared animals kept under unhygienic conditions in close association with their manure. While the spread of drug resistance is not so well documented in individual companion animals such as horses and dogs, analogies to the situation on farms are useful in understanding how spread occurs.

Where multiple drug resistance is encoded on a plasmid or an integron, the use of any antimicrobial to which resistance is encoded by one of the genes present will help maintain the entire collection of genes.

Intestinal Escherichia coli. Extensive study of antimicrobial resistance in intestinal *E. coli* in animals has provided information on the mechanisms and ecology of antimicrobial resistance. These studies have shown the relationship between the extent of resistance and the degree of antimicrobial use. For example, resistance in *E. coli* from adult ruminants at pasture is slight, whereas it is pronounced in intensively reared animals where antibiotic use is common. These *E. coli* may be resistant to up to 10 clinically useful drugs as a result of plasmid-mediated resistance. Among enterotoxigenic *E. coli* from farm animals, plasmid-mediated resistance to tetracyclines, sulfonamides, and streptomycin is now practically universal, and is increasingly common to ampicillin and neomycin. Antibiotic-resistance encoding plasmids in enterotoxigenic *E. coli* in swine and calves may also include genes for virulence determinants such as toxin production or adhesins. Although an unexplored area, antibiotic use may thus potentially promote the transfer of virulence genes between bacteria.

Within the intestine, R plasmids are found in *E. coli* and in the more dominant anaerobic flora of the large bowel. Within a short time of treating an animal with an antibiotic, the *E. coli* and much of the anaerobe population become resistant to that antibiotic, principally because of selection of resistant strains but also because of enhanced transfer of R plasmids. In the absence of antimicrobials, conditions in the large bowel seem to prevent the transfer of R factors. Short-term oral use of antimicrobials is followed by high levels of *E. coli* resistance, which fall once the antimicrobials are removed because the majority of R plasmid bearing *E. coli* are not good intestinal colonizers. However, the continuous presence of antimicrobials is associated with extensive resistance, which persists long after the antimicrobial is removed since resistant *E. coli* that are good intestinal colonizers have been selected.

Salmonella Typhimurium. Multiple antimicrobial resistance is a major problem in *Salmonella* Typhimurium and is often the result of chromosomally incorporated integrons. Among *S.* Typhimurium strains, clones of certain phage types are characterized by the presence of multiple-antimicrobial resistant integrons. The extent of resistance is most marked among calf isolates because the extensive use of antimicrobials in some types of calf rearing and the nature of salmonellosis in calves apparently provide an opportunity for the development and spread of resistant *Salmonella.* Recently, a multiply resistant and highly viru-

lent clone of *S.* Typhimurium DT 104 (a particular phage type) has disseminated widely through cattle on a global basis and has spread from this basic reservoir into other animal species and to humans. This isolate has a florfenicol and tetracycline resistance encoding gene flanked by two integrons carrying a beta-lactamase and streptomycin resistance gene cassette. This cluster of genes form part of a larger, distinctive, region called *Salmonella* genomic island 1, which may have been a plasmid that has integrated into the chromosome; this island has also been identified in other *Salmonella* serovars, including Agona.

Hospital-Acquired Resistant Infections

Acquired antimicrobial resistance in resident hospital bacteria is a major problem in human hospitals and is increasingly recognized in veterinary hospitals. There is a causal relationship between antimicrobial use in hospitals and the development of resistance in bacteria. Colonization of patients by resistant opportunist bacteria is hard to prevent because of shared air spaces and environment, utensils, and veterinary staff. In addition, patients with serious illnesses may be treated with broad-spectrum antimicrobial drugs, thus removing the normal colonization resistance of the body, including the large intestine, provided by the normal microbial flora, which are destroyed by such drugs. These patients may also be immunosuppressed by their illnesses or by treatment by immunosuppressive drugs. Under such circumstances these patients can readily be colonized by bacteria that are either intrinsically resistant to many antimicrobial drugs (e.g., *Acinetobacter* spp., *Citrobacter* spp., *Enterococcus* spp.) or that have acquired resistance.

Public Health Aspects of Antimicrobial Resistance in Animal Pathogens

The use of antimicrobial agents in animals, particularly in intensively reared livestock, can result in antimicrobial-resistant bacteria reaching the human population through a variety of routes. The scale of the contribution via these routes has not been determined and indeed, because of the complexity of resistance in bacterial pathogens, would be hard to determine precisely.

Most antimicrobial resistance in human pathogens comes from antimicrobial use in human medicine. However, antimicrobial-resistant bacteria of animal origin, such as *Enterococcus* spp. and *E. coli*, can colonize the intestines of people. Heavily exposed humans (e.g., farmers who use feed containing antimicrobials, slaughterhouse workers, cooks, and other food handlers) often have a higher incidence of resistant *E. coli* in their feces than the general population. Contamination of meat by intestinal bacteria at slaughter is extensive and an important route by which resistant bacteria reach people. While many of these bacteria are nonpathogenic, many pathogenic bacterial species from the intestines of animals cause zoonotic infections in humans (e.g., *Salmonella, Campylobacter jejuni*) and these infections may be harder to treat because of acquired resistance. The nonpathogenic bacteria of animals acquired by humans are a potential source of resistance genes for human pathogenic bacteria other than the zoonotic bacteria. These bacteria may reach humans not only through the food chain but also through water contaminated by resistant bacteria of animal origin.

The topic of the contribution of antimicrobial use in food animals for growth promotion and disease prophylactic purposes to resistance in human pathogens has been the subject of repeated review over many years, but the last seven years has seen the issue subject to the most intense scrutiny. The major driving force for the renewed debate on the prudence of using antimicrobial drugs in food animals for growth promotion and disease prophylactic purposes has been the alarming increase in resistance in human pathogens, particularly those causing "community-acquired" (e.g., *Streptococcus pneumoniae*) infections rather than hospital-acquired infections. This has led to a total reappraisal of the use of all antimicrobial drugs in all circumstances. Another factor driving the change is evidence from Europe that vancomycin-resistant *Enterococcus faecium* (VRE), a serious and essentially untreatable hospital-acquired pathogen of immunocompromised human patients, were being selected in intensively reared farm animals by the use of avoparcin, a glycopeptide antimicrobial drug used as a growth promoter and disease prophylactic. These VREs were almost universal in the intestines of treated animals and were found in a small proportion of healthy humans in Europe. By contrast, they were not present in healthy humans in the United States, where the drug was not used. These findings were a demonstration of the scale of the movement of resistant bacteria from animals to humans, which was clearly measurable. Another driving factor was the entry of Sweden into the European Union in 1999. Since Sweden had banned the use of all antimicrobial drugs as growth promoters and disease prophylactics for many years, in order to bring its practices into line with those of other European Union (EU) countries it either had to change its regulations or to change those of the EU. It used the VRE evidence to persuade the EU to change policies on the use of antimicrobial growth promoters, most of which (avoparcin, bacitracin, spiramycin, tylosin) were banned in Europe in late 1999. This ban has withstood court challenge and seems certain to remain. A similar ban has occurred in Australia, and seems likely in Canada and Japan.

In the United States, there has also been extensive reexamination of the use of antimicrobials in animals. One notable decision was to reverse the approval of fluoroquinolones for treatment of *E. coli* septicemia in chickens because of the rapid development of fluoroquinolone-resistance in *C. jejuni*. It was estimated that as many as 14,000 people annually treated for campylobacteriosis had their treatment affected because they were infected with resistant bacteria acquired from fluoroquinolone-treated chickens. In addition, the Center for Veterinary Medicine of the U.S. Food and Drug Administration has recently developed a guidance document for the evaluation of the impact of resistance as part of the regulatory approval of new antimicrobial drugs. The document takes into account the relative importance of different antimicrobial drug classes in human medicine and analyzes the risks of production of resistance and its acquisition by humans, depending on the proposed usage of the drug. The Center for Veterinary Medicine intends to reassess the safety of all antimicrobial drugs used in food animals in a prioritized manner depending on the type of risk analysis proposed for new drug approvals.

It seems likely that antimicrobial drugs important in human medicine will be removed from use as growth promoters or long-term disease prophylactics throughout the world. This is in keeping with the important prudent-use principle that antimicrobial drugs should only be used when the benefits are clear and substantial.

Control of Antimicrobial Resistance

Avoiding the use of a drug is the best way to control antimicrobial resistance. Most major national veterinary medical associations have published prudent-use guidelines for the optimal use of antimicrobial agents that are readily available on their web sites. Prudent use is defined as optimizing the efficacy of antimicrobial drug use while minimizing the development and spread of resistance. Although these guidelines are general in scope, they are increasingly supplemented by species or veterinary practice-type guidelines that are sometimes case-specific. Further refinement of such guidelines will occur into the future.

Antifungal Chemotherapy

The susceptibility of fungi to different drugs is often, but not always, predictable. Fungal drug susceptibility testing is technically complex and simple methods paralleling the disk diffusion antibacterial susceptibility test are not generally available.

Antifungal Agents for Topical Use

Many chemicals have antifungal properties and are used for topical treatment of fungal infections of the skin and sometimes of the mucosal surfaces. These include phenolic antiseptics such as hexachlorophene; iodides; quaternary ammonium antiseptics; 8-hydroxyquinoline; salicylamide; propionic, salicylic, and undecanoic acids; and chlorphenesin. Among the more effective topical broad-spectrum antifungal drugs are natamycin (a polyene antimicrobial), clotrimazole (an imidazole compound), nystatin (a polyene antimicrobial), and ketoconazole and miconazole (see below).

Antifungal Agents for Systemic Use

The recent development of the imidazoles (ketoconazole, itraconazole, and fluconazole) has been a major advance in systemic fungal therapy because of their oral administration, relative lack of toxicity, and effectiveness. The earlier major antifungal drug for systemic use, amphotericin

B, had the disadvantages of toxicity and requiring intravenous administration, but it did have the advantage of fungicidal activity.

Griseofulvin. Griseofulvin is a fungistatic antimicrobial that inhibits mitosis and is active only against dermatophytes (ringworm fungi). Resistance in some dermatophytes has been reported to develop during treatment. Griseofulvin is effective against ringworm fungi only if administered orally. The drug is incorporated into keratin in the basal cells of the epidermis and reaches the superficial dead and parasitized keratinized epithelium through progressive maturation of the basal cells.

Amphotericin. Amphotericin B is a polyene antimicrobial, like nystatin, which binds ergosterol, the principal sterol of the fungal membrane, causing leakage of the cell contents. It is a broad-spectrum, generally fungicidal antimicrobial. It is active against *Blastomyces dermatitidis*, *Histoplasma capsulatum*, *Cryptococcus neoformans*, *Candida* spp., *Sporothrix schenckii*, and *Coccidioides immitis*. Strains of filamentous fungi, though commonly susceptible, vary from extreme susceptibility to resistance. Amphotericin B must be administered intravenously. Renal toxicity is an inevitable side effect of such treatment and must be monitored; the effect is reversible if the drug is stopped. Amphotericin is the most important drug available for treating systemic mycoses caused by dimorphic fungi and by yeasts. Its prime place is increasingly being challenged by the imidazoles, which are less toxic and easier to administer. The drug is given by slow intravenous injection, usually every other day over 6 to 10 weeks. Lipid formulations containing amphotericin B, though expensive, show great promise clinically because of lower kidney toxicity.

Flucytosine. 5-flucytosine is deaminated in the fungal cell to 5-fluorouracil, which is incorporated into messenger RNA to produce garbled codons and faulty proteins. It has a narrow spectrum of activity, which includes most *Cryptococcus neoformans* and many *Candida*, but most filamentous fungi are resistant. Resistance develops readily during treatment. Therefore, flucytosine is often used only in combination with other drugs, usually amphotericin.

Imidazoles: Ketoconazole, Miconazole, Itraconazole, Fluconazole. Imidazoles interfere with the biosynthesis of ergosterol and bind fungal cell membrane phospholipids to cause leakage of cell contents. Ketoconazole, miconazole, itraconazole, and fluconazole are fungistatic against a wide range of yeasts, dimorphic fungi, and dermatophytes; they also have some antibacterial and antiprotozoal activity. Ketoconazole, itraconazole, and fluconazole appear to be more active than miconazole and are the favored drugs for systemic administration because they can be given orally rather than intravenously. Ketoconazole, itraconazole, and fluconazole appear to produce few significant adverse effects in humans and animals, but liver damage has been reported in people given ketoconazole. They appear to be an effective treatment for many systemic fungal infections in dogs and cats, but there has been little experience with their use in other animal species. They have the disadvantage of fungistatic action; prolonged treatment may be necessary in serious infections to prevent the relapses that have occurred, and this is expensive.

Antiviral Chemotherapy

Antiviral Drugs

The development of nontoxic chemicals for therapeutic use in viral diseases is far more difficult than the development of antibacterial drugs, but the long-term prospects for antiviral chemotherapy in animals are encouraging. Human immunodeficiency virus (HIV) infection in people has led to the development and introduction of antiviral drugs effective against retroviruses. Viral replication depends largely on the active participation of the metabolic pathways of the host cell, and the balance between preventing viral replication and wrecking cellular metabolism is delicate. Only a relatively small number of useful drugs have been described, and their spectrum of antiviral activity is often narrow. Work has concentrated on selective drugs that use virally encoded enzymes either as specific targets for inhibition or to activate drugs within virally infected cells. Recently these have included many drugs preferentially phosphorylated by virus-specific thymidine kinase and further phosphorylated by cellular enzymes; the resulting triphosphates of these second generation antiviral drugs inhibit viral DNA polymerase, act as bogus substrates for this enzyme, or both.

Basic antiviral targets include the following:

1. Inhibition of viral attachment to cells (immunoglobulins, receptor homologues)
2. Inhibition of uncoating of viruses (amantadine, rimantadine)
3. Inhibition of DNA or RNA synthesis
4. Nucleoside analogues (idoxuridine, vidarabine, trifluridine; acyclovir, ganciclovir, ribavirin; foscarnet
5. Inhibition of reverse transcriptase (zidovudine)
6. Inhibition of mRNA translation (antisense oligonucleotides, interferons)
7. Inhibitors of posttranslational modification (protease inhibitors, glycosylation inhibitors)

Antiviral drugs are generally only effective prophylactically or in the early stages of disease when viral replication is occurring. Rapid diagnosis is therefore required. Although no antiviral drugs have been approved for veterinary use, Table 4.2 summarizes the potential of currently available medical antiviral compounds for topical and systemic use in animals. The desirable characteristics of veterinary antiviral compounds are broad-spectrum efficacy, low cost, ease of administration, and lack of drug residues. Few of the antiviral drugs available possess these characteristics, although some of the immunomodulators may have them.

Table 4.2. Potential Topical and Systemic Application of Antiviral Drugs in Veterinary Medicine

Drug	Topical	Systemic	Possible Veterinary Use
Acyclovir	+	+	Herpes infections
Amantadine		+	Equine influenza prophylaxis
2-deoxy-D-glucose	+		Herpes infections
Foscarnet	+	+	Herpes infections
Ganciclovir		+	Cytomegalovirus infections
Idoxuridine	+		Herpes infections
Interferon		+	Feline herpes, feline leukemia, feline infectious peritonitis
Methisazone	+		Bovine vaccinia or pseudocowpox
Ribavirin	+	+	Influenza, parainfluenza, bovine herpes, canine distemper, feline infectious peritonitis, feline calicivirus
Vidarabine	+	+	Canine herpes
Zidovudine		+	Feline leukemia virus, equine infectious anemia, feline immunodeficiency virus

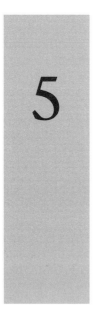

5

Antimicrobial Drugs: A Strategy for Rational Use and the Ramifications of Misuse

DWIGHT C. HIRSH

Antimicrobial drugs are used to treat (therapeutic) or prevent (prophylactic) disease produced by infectious bacterial agents. Most of the discussion that follows will deal with therapeutic use of these drugs, though comment will be made regarding prophylactic use when appropriate. Further, the discussion will deal only with bacterial agents.

Strategy for Rational Use

The decision to use antimicrobial drugs therapeutically involves the determination of whether there is an infectious agent present. Some consideration (though this rarely occurs) should be given to whether the infectious process actually poses a threat of sufficient seriousness to outweigh the risks of use of these drugs (discussed below), and whether the infectious process will resolve without their use. The same comment should be made about prophylactic use: consideration should be given as to whether there is an unacceptably high prevalence of infectious complications following a certain procedure to justify use of antimicrobial drugs.

Central to the decision to use antimicrobial drugs is the demonstration that an infectious agent is part of the disease process under consideration. The gold standard for this determination, of course, is the result of microbiological culture. Strict application of this standard is unrealistic, however, because the decisions to use antimicrobial drugs are made several days before culture data are available. Therefore, as an aid in determining that a particular process has an infectious component, certain clues are used. The Infection Control Committee at the Veterinary Medical Teaching Hospital, University of California, has drawn up guidelines to be used as aids in the decision-making process (Table 5.1).

The following scheme is used to justify the therapeutic use of an antimicrobial drug *the day the patient is first seen*. The whole purpose of the exercise is to answer the following questions: Is there an infectious agent present? What is the best antimicrobial drug to use?

Is There an Infectious Agent Present?

Apart from having the results of bacteriologic culture in hand, this question can be answered by experience (e.g., all similar cases have had an infectious component) or microbiologically. It is the microbiological aspect of the decision process that will be the focus of the discussion here. Unless noted otherwise, all subsequent remarks will be focused on infectious processes involving normally sterile (or nearly sterile) sites.

One of the most rewarding methods that can be used to determine the presence or absence of an infectious agent is the direct smear (see Chapter 3). Examination of a direct smear answers two very important questions: Is there an infectious agent present? And, if so, what is the agent likely to be? Answers to both of these questions help justify the use of an antimicrobial agent, and, what is equally important, help determine which one is likely to be effective.

After it has been demonstrated that an infectious agent is present, i.e., microorganisms are seen in the direct smear, the next step in the process is to make an educated guess as to their identity. This is the most important step in the process in the rational use of antimicrobial drugs—to have in mind what it is you are going to be treating. Experience and retrospective data are keys to this determination, and allow the clinician to formulate a "microbiological differential list" with the proper hierarchy. By noting the shape of the microorganisms seen in the direct smear, certain members of the differential list can be "ruled in" or "ruled out." Generally, bacteria come in two shapes: rods and cocci. Filamentous forms (*Actinomyces, Nocardia*) are treated as a separate category. Of course, if no infectious agents are seen but other clues point to infectious process, a microbiological differential list is still constructed, but it will be more difficult to "rule in" or "rule out" certain microorganisms or groups of microorganisms because of the lack of visual clues.

More sophisticated methods involve the detection of prokaryotic (bacterial) DNA in a normally sterile site. A polymerase chain reaction (PCR) that uses universal

Table 5.1.   Guidelines for Rational Use of Antimicrobial Agents

1. Demonstration of an infectious agent

or

2. Clinical data (at least two of the following)
   a. Fever
   b. Leukocytosis
   c. Localized inflammation
   d. Components of the sample
   e. Radiographic evidence
   f. Elevated serum fibrinogen

primers for prokaryotic DNA allows for this determination. The disadvantage to such a determination is the lack of an "isolate" to identify and to test for susceptibility to antimicrobial agents.

Observation of bacteria in a direct smear may seem to result in the formulation of a microbiological differential list of endless possibilities. Experience and retrospective data allow for the paring down of the list, keeping only the most common in proper hierarchical order. For example, in samples from dogs, *Bordetella* is almost never found except from the respiratory tract, and here it is not commonly found in samples obtained from the lower tract of patients with clinical signs of pneumonia. Likewise, in samples from dogs, *Pseudomonas* is hardly ever found in locations other than the external ear or the lower urinary tract. *Bordetella* or *Pseudomonas* would be very unlikely candidates for rod-shaped bacteria in a sample of exudate from the peritoneal cavity of a dog. Aside from "common microbiological sense," there are other clues that are helpful. For example, misshapen or long, slender rods are almost always members of the anaerobe group (especially if seen in malodorous fluid obtained from a normally sterile site).

Alimentary Canal—A Special Case. Seeing a microorganism in a normally sterile site does not pose much of a problem in determining whether there is an infectious process present. Infectious diseases of normally contaminated sites (mouth, vagina, gastrointestinal canal), however, pose special problems. The alimentary canal is the only contaminated site where the direct smear can help determine whether there is an infectious bacterial disease. There are three conditions in which direct smear can aid in the diagnosis and treatment: 1) diarrhea associated with *Campylobacter*, 2) *Helicobacter*-associated conditions of stomach and intestinal canal, and 3) *Brachyspira* (*Serpulina*)-associated diseases. In the first condition, the observation in stained (e.g., Wright-Giemsa) smears of curved rods, in the second, the observation of helical-shaped rods, and in the third, the observation of spirochetal shapes suggest that an infectious agent may be associated with the abnormal signs observed. In all three instances, the presence of a microorganism with a unique characteristic gives the visual clue necessary to make an educated guess as to the etiology of the abnormal signs. More sophisticated techniques (PCR) have been shown to be useful in determining the presence of other pathogenic microorganisms, e.g., *Clostridium difficile* or the genes encoding its toxins.

What Is the Best Antimicrobial Agent to Use?

If an infectious agent is observed in the direct smear, the answer to the first question posed above has been answered. If none are seen, yet the other clues are present pointing to an infectious process (see Table 5.1), the first question has also been answered in the affirmative. The next step in the decision-making process is "what antimicrobial drug should be used?" To answer this question, it is important to have in mind the "microbiological target." Depending upon the site from which the sample was obtained and what was seen in the direct smear, an educated guess can be made as to the identity of the agent(s) involved. Retrospective data are used to suggest what antimicrobial agents would be effective for the microorganisms on the microbiological differential list. Then, depending upon distribution, toxicity, and expense, a final choice is made.

The next day, the microbiology laboratory should be able to furnish information that is useful in determining the appropriateness of first-day choice of antimicrobial agent(s). The laboratory can, for instance, tell you whether a rod-shaped bacteria seen in direct smear is a member of the family *Enterobacteriaceae* (enteric group) which is an extremely important piece of information since members of this group are unpredictable with respect to susceptibility patterns (due to the propensity of this group of microorganisms to possess resistance-encoding genes, see Chapter 4 and below) and, as a consequence, more expensive and more toxic antimicrobial drugs are used if their presence is likely.

Obligate anaerobic bacteria pose a special challenge. It is important to suspect their presence early because the methods used to confirm them are lengthy; and, just as importantly, most laboratories do not perform susceptibility tests on them. Even if they did, the results would not be available for at least a week after sample submission. There are, however, some clues that help determine whether members of this group are present. A major clue is odor. If an exudate or fluid smells fetid, there is a good chance that obligate anaerobes are present. Without smell, an educated guess can also be made as to their presence depending upon the site from which the sample was obtained and the shape of the microorganism (misshapen, slender rods).

Ramifications of Misuse of Antimicrobial Agents

In addition to obvious benefits derived from antimicrobial agents, there are risks involved with their use. These risks involve the patient as well as others that share the same environment, including ourselves. The risks concern resistance to antimicrobial agents.

Resistance

In general, there are two mechanisms whereby bacteria become resistant: mutation and acquisition of genes encoding the resistant phenotype. Mutations occur randomly (i.e., they are unrelated to the presence of the drug). If a mutational event involves DNA encoding a target for a particular antimicrobial drug, then resistance to that drug may result. Other mutational events may have more "global" effects, however. For instance, the chromosomal gene encoding the transcriptional activator residing in the Mar (multiple antibiotic resistance) locus results in multiple drug resistance. The mechanism for this phenomenon is the deregulation of control of chromosomal genes governing the flux of drugs across the bacterial cell wall. Thus, the "multidrug resistance" phenotype is due to changes in the transport systems of the cell wall, leading to resistance to just about any clinically useful antibiotic (e.g., fluoroquinolones, beta-lactams, tetracyclines, and chloramphenicol). Drugs are pumped out of the bacterial cell before they reach therapeutically useful concentrations. This phenotype has been described for *Escherichia coli, Salmonella, Pseudomonas aeruginosa, Proteus vulgaris, Klebsiella,* and *Campylobacter.*

The major way in which bacteria become resistant, however, is through the acquisition of DNA that encodes resistance to antimicrobial drugs. These genes may contain the information for enzymes that inactivate certain antimicrobials by acetylation or phosphorylation (aminoglycoside and chloramphenicol modifying enzymes), for enzymes that inactivate by breaking bonds (beta-lactamases and cephalosporinases that inactivate penicillin/ampicillin and cephalosporins, respectively), or for proteins that are involved with transport of an antimicrobial (tetracyclines), or they may encode a target protein different from the native (susceptible) one (a different tetrahydrofolate reductase is responsible for trimethoprim resistance).

DNA encoding these various enzymes can be acquired by bacteria in several ways: 1) they can take up DNA from their environment (called *transformation*); 2) they may become "infected" by a bacterial virus that contains the resistance genes the virus had acquired from a previously resistant bacterial host (called *transduction*); or 3) they can "receive" it from other bacteria by a sexual process (called *conjugation*). Although there are examples of each of these occurring in nature, the most common method of DNA acquisition is through conjugation, at least for the acquisition of resistance genes by bacteria in an environment containing antimicrobial drugs.

Acquired DNA may exist within the bacterial cell separate from the chromosome (extrachromosomally). This extrachromosomal DNA is called a *plasmid.* If the plasmid contains genes encoding resistance to antimicrobial drugs, then these plasmids are called *R plasmids.* R plasmids may encode information for conjugation, and if so, such plasmids are transmissible and therefore have the capacity to move from one bacterium to another, either within a family (e.g., *E. coli* to *E. coli,* or *E. coli* to *Salmonella*) or outside of a family (e.g., *E. coli* to *Pasteurella*). This transmissibility has been noted for gram-positive and gram-negative bacteria, for obligate aerobes, and for facultative and obligate anaerobes. It appears to be most clinically relevant among members of the family *Enterobacteriaceae* (e.g., *E. coli, Salmonella, Klebsiella*).

A particular bacterium may contain a number of different plasmids, several of which may be R plasmids. The number of resistance genes encoded on a plasmid is variable, from two (which seems to be about the minimum) to more than seven. The genes encoding resistance to almost all of the commonly used antimicrobial drugs are found on plasmid DNA. The exceptions are resistance to the fluoroquinolones, the polymyxins, and metronidazole. Consequently, after conjugation, a susceptible strain of bacteria may have acquired resistance to a number of antimicrobial agents and have the potential to pass these resistance genes on to yet another, while keeping a copy for themselves.

In addition to being mobile by means of conjugation, resistance genes are mobile in their own right. Mobile genes, called *transposable genetic elements* or *transposons,* move from one piece of DNA to another. Most often, the information encoding resistance to a particular antimicrobial agent is on a transposon. The importance of this is that, in the hospital environment where bacteria are exposed to a number of different antimicrobial agents (and by definition they will have acquired the gene necessary to cope with *each* of these antimicrobials), the genetic pool of resistance genes is very large. And since the genes themselves are mobile, they would have the tendency to insert themselves on any number of plasmids, forming plasmids with many and varied resistance genes. Bacteria (both gram-positive and gram-negative) containing such R plasmids would be extremely difficult to kill or suppress with antimicrobial drugs if they were to become involved with a disease process.

Another mechanism whereby bacteria may become resistant is through "trapping" of segments of resistance-encoding DNA (called cassettes) by segments of DNA (integrons) residing in the chromosome, on a plasmid, or within a transposon. Integrons contain the DNA needed for the insertion of the cassette (an integrase), a recognition unit that is "recognized" by the cassette, and a promoter (the cassettes do not usually have one). There are many types of cassettes, but the most commonly occurring are those that contain resistance-encoding genes. Several cassettes containing several resistance encoding genes can associate with a particular integron, of which a bacterium may have many. Integrons are very common in gram-negative bacteria, and have been reported in some gram-positive species.

Integrons containing antimicrobial resistance-encoding genes, and R plasmids seem to be quite common among members of the family *Enterobacteriaceae.* It is extremely difficult; therefore, to predict which resistance genes will be present, especially if the R plasmid has been "constructed" from the resistance gene pool in a hospital environment. For this reason, a major effort should be made in "ruling out" or "ruling in" members of this group on the microbiological differential list for a particular site or condition.

Within 24 to 48 hours after the initiation of antimicrobial therapy, dramatic changes occur in one of the major host defense systems of the patient, the normal flora. These changes are reflected in the replacement of the normal flora with bacteria resistant to the antimicrobial drug being used. To understand why this is a risk, it is important to understand the role of the normal flora as a host defense barrier.

The Risk

Colonization resistance (see Chapter 2) is a term that describes the innate immunity afforded the host by its normal flora. It is the normal flora and the mechanisms whereby the normal flora is maintained that protect the host from colonization (infection) by extraneous microorganisms. This is an important concept since prevention of colonization by agents with pathogenic potential (e.g., *Salmonella*) or prevention of colonization by resistant strains of microorganisms is key to minimizing the risk we and our patients take in living in an environment contaminated by microorganisms.

Colonization resistance can be decreased by a number of outside influences, principally stress, and by antimicrobial agents. If the colonization resistance is decreased sufficiently, then replacement will occur (a surface does not go unoccupied!).

Antimicrobial agents decrease colonization resistance (hospitalized dogs were 38 times more likely to have acquired resistant *Salmonella* if they were first given an antibiotic). Within 24 to 48 hours after administration of an antimicrobial, the normal flora is depressed to the degree that resistant strains start to recolonize since those microorganisms that replace the normal flora will be resistant to the antimicrobial drug administered. These resistant strains may be a part of the normal flora (e.g., normal, unmedicated dogs periodically shed large numbers of R plasmid containing *E. coli* in their feces—the reason for this is unknown) or from the animal's environment. In either case, the replacement strain will be resistant to the antimicrobial being used. Having resistant bacteria occupying a surface is not harmful in itself, unless the resistant strain has the ability to invade the host cell to which it has gained access. But as mentioned above, if a normally sterile site contiguous to the recolonized surface becomes compromised, bacteria (now resistant bacteria) will contaminate, and the resulting disease will be more difficult to treat. This recolonization effect is the reason behind the recommendation that prophylactic use of antimicrobial agents extend no longer than 24 to 48 hours.

Colonization resistance is reduced by the stress of illness and the stress of new social/environmental experiences. These changes occur secondary to changes in the normal flora. What appears to transpire are changes in the elements responsible for the maintenance of the stable, normal flora. Although these changes have been defined most precisely in the oral cavity, there are data that suggest that they also occur in the intestinal canal. In the oral cavity, the epithelial cells are coated with fibronectin, a glycoprotein. Fibronectin contains receptors for streptococci, the most abundant microorganism found on the buccal, lingual, and gingival surfaces. It is the streptococci that exclude other, potentially more dangerous microbes from associating with the oral cavity (most would agree that these would be microorganisms belonging to the enteric group such as *E. coli* or *Klebsiella*). The amount of fibronectin coating these cells decreases in the stressed animal, leaving available underlying attachment sites (for gram-negative microorganisms) either on the cells themselves or on gly-coproteins that coat the cells after fibronectin is gone. It should be noted, too, that if the animal is treated with antimicrobials as well, the streptococci would also be removed since the oral streptococci are very susceptible to most antimicrobial agents. There is recent evidence that shows that some gram-negative enteric bacteria possess adhesins for receptors on fibronectin, underscoring the importance of keeping the normal flora intact. The resulting change from a flora composed of relatively innocuous bacteria (nonhemolytic streptococci) to one with pathogenic *potential* (members of the enteric group) becomes an important issue if compromise occurs in a normally sterile contiguous site (e.g., the lung).

Risk to Others

Antimicrobial agents select bacteria that contain genes encoding resistance to that particular drug. Because the genes encoding resistance are almost always found on R plasmid DNA, antimicrobial use selects for resistance genes to other antibiotics as well. In the hospital environment where antimicrobials are used, the environment is contaminated with microorganisms containing very mobile genetic material encoding resistance to a variety of antimicrobial agents. We are a part of this environment, and therefore also partake in this gene pool. Even with an intact colonization resistance, we are transiently colonized with bacteria derived from animals placed in our care. Transient colonization is enough for conjugation and subsequent passage of resistance genes to our resident normal flora. If by chance the host human is also being medicated with antimicrobials, the chance of colonization with resistant animal strains increases, as does the possibility of passage of an R plasmid.

Summary

In outlining the rational use of antimicrobial agents, this chapter emphasizes the importance of two questions: Is there an infectious component to the disease process under consideration? And, if so, what antimicrobial drug would be effective? The direct smear is a tool that is useful in ascertaining whether an infectious component exists. Once it has been reasonably established that there is an infectious component, a "microbiological differential list" (in hierarchical order) is created and further shaped depending upon visual clues obtained from the direct smear. Experience and retrospective susceptibility data are used to determine which antimicrobial drugs would be effective for the most likely of the constituents of the microbiological differential list. A final choice is made after considering distribution, toxicity, and cost.

Antimicrobial drugs should be treated as an environmental pollutant. They exert very powerful selective pressures on the gene pool in which we all partake. In addition to being potent selective agents, antimicrobials are a risk to those patients receiving them by diminishing host defense barriers.

6 Vaccines

N. James MacLachlan   Dwight C. Hirsh

Introduction

Vaccines are substances that are used to elicit immune responses to prevent or minimize disease produced by infectious agents. Vaccines can be composed of the infectious agent itself (either live or killed), a portion of the agent that induces a protective immune response (subunit vaccine), or a product of the agent. Products containing a killed bacterial agent are more properly called *bacterins*. Products that have toxic activities are called *toxins*, and toxins that have been inactivated are called *toxoids*.

To be effective, vaccines must elicit an immune response that interferes with the "life style" of the infectious agent.

Humoral Immunity

Antibodies function immunologically by binding to epitopes on the surface of the infectious agent and/or one of its products. By binding to the surface of an infectious agent, antibodies interfere with attachment to host target cells by stearic interference and/or by changing the charge or hydrophobicity of the surface of the agent, and trigger the complement cascade generating products that are opsonic and products that are damaging to agents that have surface membranes. Antibodies that bind to products of infectious agents can block the attachment of the product to receptors on cellular targets and/or change the configuration of the product resulting in a change in binding affinity.

Cell-Mediated Immunity

Cell-mediated immunity is an immune response that results in the generation of "activated" macrophages and/or specific cytotoxic T lymphocytes. This aspect of the immune response concerns agents that live inside of cells, which are thus protected from interaction with the elements of the humoral components of the system.

Activated macrophages are mononuclear phagocytic cells that have come in contact with Interleukin 1 (IL-1) and interferon γ (INF-gamma). Such cells have increased phagocytic and enzymatic activity, contain increased amounts of nitric oxide, and have increased production of cytokines, such as tumor necrosis factor (TNF) and IL-1, and increased expression of MHC class I (MHC-II). This increase in activity is thought to be responsible for the destruction of infectious agents that nonactivated mononuclear cells cannot destroy following uptake. Some term this immune state (i.e., activation of macrophages) *cellular hypersensitivity*.

Cytotoxic T lymphocytes recognize affected host cells (e.g., cells infected with virus or bacteria). In so doing, these lymphocytes secrete substances that result in the death of the affected host cell. If the affected host cell contained an infectious agent, that agent would now be liberated and in contact with other host immune participants (e.g., antibody, complement, activated macrophages).

Generation of the Immune Response

Antigens that are processed by antigen-processing cells via the exogenous pathway elicit antibodies. Thus, extracellular bacteria (live or killed), inactivated viral particles, portions (subunits) of virus, and products are processed by the exogenous pathway. Epitopes are presented to the immune system in context of MHC-II by an antigen-presenting cell that secretes IL-1 and little, if any, IL-12. T helper cells (T_{H2} subset of CD4 lymphocytes) respond to this stimulus by secreting cytokines that trigger an antibody response (IL-4, IL-5, IL-13).

Some infectious agents replicate within cells. If the agent multiplies within a mononuclear phagocyte, then antigens are processed by way of the exogenous and/or endogenous pathways (see below). As outlined above with extracellular antigens, antigens of intracellular agents are presented in context of MHC-II, but the antigen-presenting cell secretes IL-1 and IL-12. IL-12 stimulates T helper cells (T_{H1} subset) while turning off cells of the T_{H2} subset. T_{H1} cells secrete INF-gamma, resulting in the activation of mononuclear phagocytic cells. Some of these "intracellular" agents (some viruses, bacteria, fungi) replicate in the cytoplasm of mononuclear phagocytic cells. Antigens from these agents are also processed by the endogenous pathway, as are antigens liberated within nonphagocytic cells, so that epitopes are presented to the immune system in context of MHC-I. Epitopes presented in this fashion are recognized by CD8 cytotoxic lymphocytes. These lymphocytes function by lysing infected targets, i.e., cells expressing epitope-MHC-I complexes.

DNA Vaccines

DNA vaccines are those in which the gene encoding the antigen in question is inserted into a plasmid vector that has a strong promoter (e.g., cytomegalovirus immediate/early promoter; SV40 early promoter) that will result in expression of the target gene, a termination sequence (polyA tail), and a number of cytidine-phosphate-guanosine (CpG) motifs. The function of the CpG motif (a motif common in bacterial genomes) is to direct the antigen processing cell to secrete lymphokines that favor T_{H1} lymphocytes. The construct is administered in any number of ways (intramuscular, intradermally, upon a mucosal surface), but intramuscularly is the most common. Myocytes that become transfected serve as antigen-presenting cells and express antigen in context of MHC-I (turn on CD8 T lymphocytes). It is unclear how antigen is expressed in context of MHC-II (for CD4 T lymphocytes). Possibilities include MHC-II antigen-presenting cells (macrophages/dendritic cells/B lymphocytes) becoming transfected, or transfected myocytes transferring the plasmid construct to MHC-II antigen-presenting cells.

DNA vaccines have been successful in eliciting protective immune responses (both humoral and cellular) to a variety of bacterial, viral, and protozoal microorganisms; however, commercial DNA vaccines are not yet available in veterinary medicine.

Adjuvants

Adjuvants are used to influence the nature of the immune response elicited by an antigen. The response is influenced at various stages, depending upon the adjuvant. Some adjuvants function as depots, so that antigen is slowly released over an extended period of time to maximize the immune response. Examples include water/oil emulsions, minerals/salts (bentonite, aluminum), and inert particles (microspheres). Other adjuvants direct activity to the processing step in the initiation of the immune response. Examples include "immune stimulating complexes" (ISCOMs) composed of cholesterol-phospholipid structures that contain the immunogen, and liposomes (lipid vesicles). "Targeting" various components by using various cytokines as adjuvants can influence immune responses. For example, IL-1 activates T lymphocytes, IL-12 and INF-gamma influence the helper T lymphocyte subset selection, and granulocyte macrophage colony-stimulating factors activate macrophages and increase efficiency of antigen processing.

Viral Vaccines

Immunization of animals with viral vaccines is critical to the prevention of many viral diseases. The basis of an effective vaccine is its ability to induce an immune response or responses capable of eliciting protection to subsequent field exposure to pathogenic viruses. A multitude of vaccine preparations have been developed and used over the years, with variable success. The success of a potential vaccine hinges primarily on safety and efficacy; however, economics also continue to dictate vaccine design, development, and ultimate production on a commercial basis.

Various approaches to vaccination have been employed over the years. These include 1) administering live virulent virus in an anatomical site so that the target tissue or tissues are not infected, 2) administering live virulent virus to animals at a time of relative resistance to disease expression, 3) concurrent administration of live virulent virus and immune serum, which no longer is acceptable for obvious reasons, 4) use of live avirulent viral strains (e.g., attenuated or "modified live" viruses), and 5) use of inactivated virus. In recent years, additional approaches to vaccine development have become available. These include subunit, synthetic peptide, and recombinant products. Regardless of vaccine type, the desired result is to induce immune responses specific for viral antigens expressed on the virion surface or on the surface of infected cells, so that the immunized host is immune when exposed to the virulent virus. The rational development of an efficacious viral vaccine requires an understanding of viral pathogenesis, of protective immune responses induced following infection, and of their protein specificities. The latter point is of obvious importance for developing recombinant and synthetic peptide vaccines.

Concerning pathogenesis, the following three general types of viral infections occur:

1. Infections that are confined to the mucosal surfaces of the respiratory or gastrointestinal tracts. In such instances, local immunity in the form of secretory antibody (e.g., IgA) is important. The role of cell-mediated immunity (CMI) is less well characterized in such infections.
2. Infections that begin at mucosal surfaces but then cause a systemic infection with viremia, and subsequent infection of distant target tissues. In these infections, both immunity at the mucosal surface as well as systemic immunity are important.
3. Infections that gain direct entry into the host's circulation via insect bite (arthropod-borne viruses), inadvertent inoculation, or a traumatic break in an epithelial surface. In such infections, systemic immunity is the primary line of defense.

These mechanisms of viral infection and subsequent dissemination must be considered in vaccine development. Modified live (attenuated) and inactivated (killed) virus vaccines dominate the veterinary vaccine market (Table 6.1).

Live Attenuated Viral Vaccines

The attenuated viral vaccines include artificially attenuated (modified-live) strains of virus or naturally occurring viruses with reduced virulence for the host. The origin of these naturally attenuated isolates may be the natural host, or a closely related virus isolated from a different host; for example, the cowpox virus was initially used to vaccinate humans against smallpox. The major requirements of such an approach are that it induce adequate immunity and that the attenuation (lack of virulence) of the vaccine strain be stable. The majority of vaccines currently used today in veterinary medicine are attenuated viruses. The most common approach to viral attenuation is the development of host-range mutants. Other approaches in-

Table 6.1.   Types of Viral Vaccines

I. Live Viral Vaccines
  A. Attenuation for low virulence of viruses that produce natural diseases.
  B. Host-range mutants—use of different viral strains infecting different host species that are related antigenically to the virus strain that produces a natural disease in the original host.
  C. Recombinant heterologous viral vector vaccines—construction of an infectious viral recombinant that expresses protective antigen(s) of another virus that produces a natural disease. Construction of a recombinant virus with insertion of genes with known antiviral activities or with known immunoregulatory functions.
  D. Recombinant homologous viral strains attenuated by targeted mutations on deletions of genes coding for specific virulence factors that produce a natural disease.
  E. Nonreplicating recombinant viral vector vaccines capable of replicating to high titer in vitro but unable to grow efficiently in vivo.
II. Inactivated Viral Vaccines
  A. Inactivated viral vaccines by chemical methods.
  B. Inactivated viral vaccines by physical methods.
  C. Purified viral antigens using monoclonal antibody immunoaffinity chromatography.
  D. Cloned viral protein subunit vaccines produced in eukaryotic or prokaryotic cells by recombinant DNA technology.
  E. Synthetic viral polypeptide vaccines representing immunologically urpident domains of viral surface antigens.
  F. Direct injection of plasmid DNA encoding viral protective antigens into tissues in vivo.
  G. Use of anti-idiotypic antibodies as antigens to induce an antiviral antibody response.

clude development of temperature-sensitive and cold-adapted mutants (missense mutations), deletion mutants, and recombinant viruses.

Host-range mutants are developed by serial passage in a host system different from the natural host to be vaccinated, usually laboratory animals, embryonated chicken eggs, or, increasingly, cell cultures. Upon serial passage in these systems, viruses often lose their virulence for the natural host due to accumulation of mutations in the viral genome that result in changes in virus-specified proteins. The basis of attenuation of many modified live virus vaccines, however, is poorly characterized and the possibility of reversion to virulence after growth in the natural host is always a concern.

Conditional lethal mutants have been generated with the intent that such viruses would exhibit limited replication in the host and so serve as vaccines. Temperature-sensitive mutants are typically created by mutagenesis and phenotypically selected on the basis of temperature. Cold-adapted mutants are generated by propagation at successively lower temperatures, the end product being incapable of replication at normal temperatures. The cold-adapted mutants typically acquire multiple mutations in genes encoding virulence and are relatively more stable than temperature-sensitive mutants.

A unique approach to expression of cloned viral genes is the use of heterologous viral expression vectors. Vaccinia virus has widely been used as an infectious vaccine expression vector because it is a virus that has widely been used as a human vaccine and the fact that at least 22 kilobases of the vaccinia genome can be deleted without loss of infectivity. The latter attribute gives researchers ample space in which to insert foreign cloned genes and has the potential to permit insertion of multiple foreign viral genes for the purpose of designing multivalent and multiviral vaccines. A major potential advantage of such infectious vaccine vectors is the potential for induction of cellular immunity by inserting expressed viral proteins into the host cell membrane in context with histocompatibility antigens.

Construction of deletion mutants is another potential mechanism of virus attenuation; thus, the selective deletion of genes that express factors for virulence, persistence, or immunosuppression can often be accomplished without compromising viral replication. This approach requires a thorough understanding of the virus and the pathogenesis of the disease it causes; a deletant vaccine has been developed to prevent pseudorabies in swine. The thymidine kinase gene is deleted in the pseudorabies vaccine strain, which is able to induce an immune response without producing disease. Furthermore, the genes encoding virus glycoproteins gpI, gpIII, or gpx are deleted in the vaccine strain. The presence of antibody to these specific virus antigens can be used to differentiate field-strain infected animals from vaccinated animals, an important advance in defining the epidemiology and control of this disease.

Nonreplicating recombinant viral vectors that are not capable of replication in vivo but that can express foreign proteins during abortive infections can induce humoral and cell-mediated immunity in immunized hosts. Experimental studies show that dogs or cats are resistant to wild-type rabies viral challenge when inoculated with avian pox-rabies glycoprotein recombinant viruses. This type of viral vaccine has the distinct advantage of being safe in the immunosuppressed host.

There are advantages and disadvantages to attenuated viral vaccines. Table 6.2 lists the general characteristics of live attenuated as compared to killed viral vaccines. A major advantage of live viral vaccines is their ability to replicate within the host and thereby elicit both humoral and cellular immune responses. In the case of viral infections attaching primarily to the mucosal surfaces of the respiratory and gastrointestinal tracts, administering attenuated viruses by the nasal or oral routes stimulates local immunity. Economic considerations also favor attenuated vaccines due to the lower cost of production and the typical absence of a requirement for adjuvants, immunopotentiating agents, and the need for multiple immunizations.

While attenuated viral vaccines continue to provide the mainstay of veterinary vaccines, there are a variety of potentially serious disadvantages to their use. Significantly, only a fine line separates modification and loss of immunogenicity. Thus, modified live vaccine strains of virus require a compromise between loss of virulence of the virus and loss of its immunogenicity because many viruses

Table 6.2. Relative Advantages and Disadvantages of Live vs. Inactivated Virus Vaccines

Criteria	Live	Inactivated
Immunity	Long	Short
Adjuvant	No	Yes
Safety	Variable	Usually very safe
Complications (potential)	Reversion to virulence, spread to susceptible animals	Sensitization
Potential contamination	Possible	Minimal
Interference	Possible	Minimal
Cost	Minimal	Significant
Immunomodulation	Not required	Required
Vaccine marker	Possibly genetic marker	Serologic marker
Stability	Poor	Good
CMI induction	Yes	No
Local secretory immunity	Yes	No
Reassortment/recombination	Possible	No
Persistent	Yes	No

exhibit reduced immunogenicity as they become attenuated. Furthermore, accurate assessment of viral attenuation can often be difficult since consistent experimental reproduction of clinical disease is difficult with certain viruses. In such instances, a vaccine virus considered to be attenuated may produce clinical disease under special circumstances involving stress, physiologic imbalance, or concurrent infections with other organisms. Viruses that exhibit a wide host range are also problematic. Virus attenuated for one animal species may retain virulence for more susceptible species, and since attenuated viruses cause an active infection, transmission to other species may occur.

A major concern in the use of attenuated viruses is reversion to virulence. This phenomenon has plagued vaccine development and licensing over the years. Reversion to virulence is a more serious possibility with those viruses that enjoy a wide host range or that are biologically transmitted by arthropod vectors. While the virus may appear stable in the host for which the vaccine was intended, reversion to virulence may occur in the vector or in other species. Vaccination of pregnant animals must also be of concern, since attenuated viruses may be pathogenic for the developing fetus. Vaccinating animals with reduced immunologic responsiveness can result in expression of clinical disease.

Additional negative features of attenuated virus vaccines include 1) the potential for reassortment (viruses with segmented genomes) or recombination between vaccine strains or with wild-type virus to create new viruses, 2) lack of a vaccine marker for serologic differentiation of vaccine and wild-type virus exposure, 3) development of persistent infections, 4) poor stability of vaccine virus, especially in hot tropical areas, and 5) replication interference between viruses in multivalent vaccines. Viruses that exhibit continued antigenic drift present another dilemma since new isolates must be continually attenuated and tested for safety and efficacy.

Inactivated Virus Vaccines

Many inactivated vaccines have been developed for use in veterinary medicine. Virus inactivation has most commonly employed formalin, beta-propiolactone, acetylethyleneimine, or binaryethyleneimine. Additional methods include ultraviolet light, gamma irradiation, psoralen compounds, and ozone gas. The primary advantage of killed virus vaccines is safety—many potential disadvantages of live-virus vaccines are eliminated since no virus replication occurs. Virus for inactivation has been produced in laboratory animals, embryonated chicken eggs, and, most commonly today, in cell cultures. From an economic viewpoint, viruses that grow to high titer in cell cultures and exhibit first-order inactivation kinetics provide the best candidates for vaccine preparation. Adjuvants are typically required to induce good immunity with killed viral products, and multiple doses are usually required. With the continued development of better adjuvants and immunopotentiating complexes (ISCOMs), inactivated vaccines will prove more effective. Inactivated vaccines are also relatively stable under adverse conditions, and their potential for strain interference in multivalent preparations is reduced compared to attenuated vaccines.

There are, however, certain disadvantages associated with the use of inactivated virus vaccines. Most inactivating agents are toxic, and some are carcinogenic. Unlike live virus, inactivated vaccine virus is not quantitatively amplified, so it requires adjuvant and multiple inoculations. Furthermore, such preparations do not induce strong cellular immunity, since inducing such responses requires that the antigen be presented in association with histocompatibility antigens on cell surfaces (processed via the endogenous pathways, see above). Nor are such vaccines associated with development of local secretory immunity, due to the usual parenteral route of vaccination.

The success of viral inactivation depends on the inactivant and viral characteristics. While most viruses can be successfully inactivated, the retention of critical antigenic integrity is variable. Antigens responsible for inducing protective immunity must be preserved. A possible complication of inactivated vaccine use is the potential for animal sensitization such that an exacerbated clinical disease is experienced upon exposure to virulent field virus. This sensitization is not well understood, but it is apparently immunologically precipitated by an unbalanced immune response such as humoral vs. cellular immunity, immune response to nonneutralizing epitopes, or preferential stimulation of IgE.

Development of subunit vaccines is currently an area of extensive research; it includes purification of viral subunits, recombinant technology, and peptide synthesis. The basis of a subunit vaccine is an immunogenic protein (or peptide sequences) capable of eliciting protective immunity. Such proteins would typically be found on the virion surface and contain epitopes capable of inducing neutralizing antibody. Vaccines can be prepared by disruption of the virus followed by protein purification. The potential cost of such preparations has precluded their commercial development, but recent biotechnological advances have offered alternatives via recombinant DNA and peptide synthesis technologies.

The approach to developing recombinant vaccines involves insertion of DNA that contains the desired viral genomic coding sequences into an appropriate expression vector. The viral or complementary DNA (cDNA) is inserted into a plasmid or bacteriophage followed by infection of susceptible prokaryotic cells such as *Escherichia coli;* yeast cells, or mammalian cells. Multiple strategies have been used to construct vaccine expression vectors, and most include a strong promoter (constitutive or inducible). Following infection of the cell with the plasmid, the cloned cDNA can be expressed and the desired gene product purified for vaccine use. Recent attention has also been focused on the inoculation of plasmid DNA encoding viral antigens directly into animals. Such DNA vaccines offer the hypothetical advantage of having viral glycoproteins expressed on the surface of transfected cells and inducing immunity without interference from passively acquired viral antibodies.

Synthetic peptide vaccines have also been developed. As with cloned viral vaccines, the successful development of synthetic peptide vaccines requires extensive knowledge of the viral proteins involved in inducing protective immunity. Two basic approaches are available for determining critical peptide sequences: 1) indirectly, from nucleotide sequences derived from cloned viral genes, and 2) directly, by sequencing purified peptides. Immunologically based peptide and epitope mapping to determine the regions involved in protective immunity facilitate the latter approach. An additional approach to determining critical peptide sequences is based upon the projected tertiary structure of the viral protein, with the areas that demonstrate hydrophilic characteristics serving as candidate sequences. One major drawback of synthesizing peptide vaccines is the potential for critical epitopes to be formed by the tertiary structure (an epitope formed by juxtaposition of two separated peptide sequences). Such epitopes confound attempts to deduce the peptide sequence and realize such complex configurations in the synthetic product.

The use of anti-idiotypic antibodies as immunogens to stimulate the production of viral neutralizing antibodies has also been explored. The advantage of this type of immunogen may overcome viral variability problems by inducing broadly neutralizing antibodies. However, this type of vaccine induces only antibody responses, not cell-mediated responses.

Toxoids, Bacterins, and Bacterial Vaccines

As with viral vaccines, the basis of an effective toxoid, bacterin, or bacterial vaccine is the ability to induce an immune response or responses capable of eliciting protection from field exposure to the pathogenic microorganism. Most of the principles outlined above with respect to viral vaccines apply to products designed to induce protective immunity to bacterial agents. The development of an efficacious product depends on understanding the pathogenesis of the bacterial disease that is to be prevented.

In general terms, diseases produced by bacteria can be grouped into three categories: 1) those that result from as-sociation with a bacterial toxin, 2) those that result from the sequelae of extracellular multiplication of the bacterial agent, and 3) those that result from the sequelae of intracellular multiplication.

Toxoids

Bacterial toxins are of two kinds: exotoxins and endotoxins. Endotoxins are strictly defined as the lipopolysaccharide portion of the gram-negative cell wall (it is the lipid A portion that is specifically responsible for the "toxic" manifestations). Muramyl dipeptide, which is present in gram-positive cell walls and to a lesser extent in gram-negative, also has "toxic" properties. We have used quotation marks around "toxic" because both endotoxin and muramyl dipeptide elicit their "toxic" activities by inducing the production of a variety of cytokines by host cells. It is the degree of vigor of the host response that defines the toxicity. Exotoxins are proteins that interact with host cells (usually after binding to a specific receptor) resulting in deregulation of host cell function without undue harm to the cell, interference of the normal physiology of the host cell(s), or death of the host cell.

Antibodies elicited to various epitopes on toxins that result in neutralization are sometimes called *antitoxins*. As mentioned previously, an antibody may block interaction between a toxin and its cellular receptor or change the configuration of the toxin so that it no longer has an effect on the host cell. Antibodies to exotoxins have been shown to be efficacious in preventing disease. Antibodies to endotoxins have had mixed results as far as preventing disease.

Toxoids are toxins without toxic activity that can elicit an immune response, i.e., antibodies (see above for explanation). Toxoids can be produced by chemical inactivation of the native toxin or by manipulations of the gene encoding the toxin so that the toxin is inactivated. For example, in the case of A-B toxins (see Chapter 8), where the A subunit is responsible for the toxic activity of the toxin and the B subunits are responsible for binding of the toxin to the host, the gene encoding the A subunit can be eliminated and a toxoid produced that is composed of B subunits. Antibody to lipopolysaccharide (endotoxin) is elicited by immunization with mutants (called "rough" mutants) that produce very little of the O-repeat unit of the lipopolysaccharide (see Chapter 8).

The main advantage of toxoids is that they are safe. Toxoids administered parenterally elicit antibody (IgM and IgG) that interferes with toxin-host cell interactions that are not at a mucosal surface. On the other hand, the administration of toxoids on a mucosal surface elicits antibody (sIgM and sIgA) that interferes with toxin-host cell interaction at the mucosal surface. The main disadvantage of toxoids used for immunization by way of a mucosal surface is their extremely short half-life.

Bacterins

Bacterins are killed pathogenic bacteria. They are usually produced by chemical killing of the infectious agent, with the aim to preserve bacterial structures expressing epitopes important in eliciting a protective immune response. The immune response is almost always antibody (see above for explanation).

The advantage of bacterins is that they are safe. If administered parenterally, the antibody elicited (IgM and IgG) will be effective if the bacterin is made from a pathogen that has an extracellular life style. If the bacterin is administered by way of a mucosal surface, the antibody elicited (sIgM and sIgA) will interfere with interactions of pathogen with host cells. The disadvantage is that the main immune response is antibody so that only antibody-mediated protection will occur. Thus, bacterins administered parenterally are not as effective against intracellular pathogens. Bacterins placed on a mucosal surface have extremely short half-lives, a serious disadvantage. Another disadvantage is that the pathogen is usually grown in vitro, and epitopes expressed in vivo may not be expressed, which can result in a product that may elicit antibodies with inappropriate specificities.

Bacterial Vaccines

Bacterial vaccines are composed of attenuated versions of the pathogen; i.e., they are live but reduced in virulence.

Attenuation may be accomplished in a number of ways: selection of a naturally occurring attenuated strain, repeated passage on artificial media, or elimination of a virulence trait by mutation of the gene encoding the trait.

The major advantages of bacterial vaccines are directly related to their being alive. Live vaccines not only have longer half-lives than their dead counterparts (regardless of location), they will express epitopes that may only be expressed in vivo, thus eliciting antibody to epitopes that the pathogen will also express following infection. Another advantage is that live vaccines will elicit antibody and cellular hypersensitivity (see above for explanation). A major disadvantage is that live vaccines may produce disease, for example, through reversion to the virulent phenotype. Also, if the vaccinated host has reduced resistance, then the vaccine is more apt to produce disease.

PART II

Bacteria and Fungi

7

Family *Enterobacteriaceae*

Dwight C. Hirsh

Members of the family *Enterobacteriaceae* ("enterics") cause disease in both food animals (e.g., neonatal diarrhea and salmonellosis) and companion animals (e.g., urinary tract infections, abscesses). Approximately 35 genera comprise the family, but only a few are consistently involved with disease of animals (Table 7.1).

Descriptive Features

Morphology and Staining

Members of the family are similar in morphology and staining characteristics, being pleomorphic, gram-negative, non-spore-forming rods that measure 2 to 3 μm by 0.4 to 0.6 μm (for an example of gram-negative rods, see Fig 74.2A). It is difficult to tell members of one genus from those of another by visual observation.

Cellular Anatomy and Composition

The cell wall is typically gram-negative and consists of inner and outer membranes separated by peptidoglycan. Various proteins are found in each membrane, some traversing both. Capsules, flagella, and various adhesins are sometimes present.

The capsule (K-antigens) is the outermost structural component of the bacterial cell. Capsules of enteric organisms are composed of carbohydrates. The various types of carbohydrates, together with the types of linkages between the sugars, form the antigenic determinants that define capsular antigens. Encapsulated enteric bacteria are relatively hydrophilic, a characteristic imparted by the capsule.

The somatic antigens (O-antigens) are composed of antigenic determinants formed by the different configurations of sugar types, and the linkages between sugars found in the O-repeat portion of the lipopolysaccharide (Figs 7.1 and 7.2).

Flagella, which are cellular organelles used for locomotion, are composed of protein subunits (flagellin). Depending upon the type of flagellin, different antigenic determinants are formed. These antigenic determinants comprise the H-antigens. In cells of most *Salmonella* and some other species, one or the other of two sets ("phases") of antigenic determinants are possible. In culture, spontaneous phase variation occurs, that is, a shift from phase 1 to 2 or vice versa. The antigens of both phases, if present, help define the serotypes.

Fimbriae or pili are protein adhesins that are composed of subunits—pilin—and assembled in various configurations using different pilin molecules, which results in the generation of different types defined by their affinity for various carbohydrates. The most commonly found fimbriae have affinity for mannose-containing compounds. These fimbriae are called *type 1* or *common fimbriae* (also termed F1). Type 1 fimbriae have not been conclusively shown to be virulence determinants. On the other hand, a variety of other virulence-associated fimbriae have been described that agglutinate erythrocytes in the presence of mannose. Examples of such mannose resistant (MR) hemagglutinins are F4 (K88) and F5 (K99), two virulence-associated adhesins that are important in the pathogenesis of enteric disease produced by certain strains of *Escherichia coli*.

Most members of the family possess mucopeptide antigens in common, the so-called enterobacterial common antigen.

Cellular Products of Medical Interest

Cellular products of medical interest common to all or most of the members of the family are endotoxins and various siderophores.

Endotoxin. Endotoxin is the term given the lipopolysaccharide (LPS) that is part, and extrudes from, the outer membrane of the gram-negative cell wall (see Fig 7.2). The lipid portion of this substance is embedded in the outer membrane and has the toxic properties associated with endotoxin. The most important constituent of LPS as far as the toxic manifestations of the molecule are concerned is the lipid portion, called *lipid A*. LPS binds to lipopolysaccharide-binding protein (a serum protein), which in turn transfers it to the blood phase of CD14. The CD14-LPS complex binds to Toll-like receptor proteins (see Chapter 2) on the surface of macrophage cells triggering the release of proinflammatory cytokines. It is these cytokines that are responsible, in part, for the abnormal signs associated with endotoxin.

Siderophores. Siderophores (Greek for "iron bearing") are iron-carrying molecules (catechols or hydroxamates) of bacterial origin. They function in the solubilization and transport of ferric ions. There is very little free iron in hosts; nearly all is associated with the iron-binding proteins (ferritin, transferrin, and lactoferrin). Since iron is an absolute requirement for almost all bacteria, parasitic strains, especially invasive ones, must compete for iron.

Table 7.1.   Members of the Family *Enterobacteriaceae* Important in Veterinary Medicine

Citrobacter	*Providencia*
Enterobacter	*Salmonella*
Escherichia	*Serratia*
Klebsiella	*Shigella*
Morganella	*Yersinia*
Proteus	

FIGURE 7.1.   *Anatomy of an enterobacterial cell showing localization of cell surface antigens of* Escherichia coli. *Only one of many peritrichous flagella is shown. (Reproduced by permission of Barnum DA, et al. Colibacillosis. CIBA Veterinary Monograph Series 1967;2:8.)*

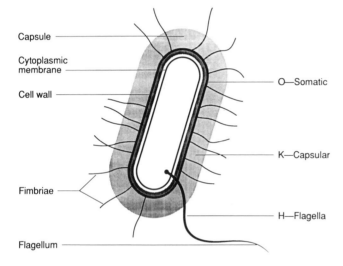

FIGURE 7.2.   *Molecular organization of the outer membrane of gram-negative bacteria. The chains of rectangles represent the O-repeat units determining O-antigen specificity. They are attached to the polysaccharide core (irregular shapes), which is linked to lipid A (fringed oblongs). These three components constitute the lipopolysaccharide (LPS) of the gram-negative cell wall. With the underlying zone of phospholipid (fringed circles), LPS makes up the outer membrane, an asymmetric bilayer that also contains proteins: A—outer membrane protein A; PP—pore protein; BP—nutrient-binding protein. Interior to the outer membrane lies the periplasmic space (PPS); the peptidoglycan layer (PG); and the cytoplasmic membrane (CM) with carrier protein (CP). (Reproduced by permission of Lugentberg B, Van Alphen L. Molecular architecture and functioning of the outer membrane of Escherichia coli and other gram-negative bacteria. Biochim Biophys Acta 1983;737:94.)*

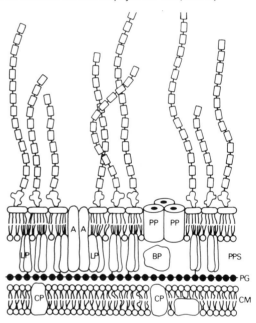

Most utilize siderophores that remove iron from the iron-binding proteins of the host.

Growth Characteristics

Members of this group of microorganisms are facultative anaerobes. They utilize a variety of simple substrates for growth. Under anaerobic conditions, they are dependent upon the presence of fermentable carbohydrate. Under aerobic conditions, the range of suitable substrates includes organic acids, amino acids, and carbohydrates.

The end products of sugar fermentation are useful in making an identification. Almost all members of this group ferment glucose to pyruvic acid via the Embden-Meyerhof pathway. Some, such as *E. coli* and *Salmonella*, produce succinic acid, acetic acid, formic acid, and ethanol by way of the mixed acid fermentation pathway. Others, such as *Klebsiella* and *Enterobacter*, produce butanediol from pyruvic acid, thereby reducing the relative amounts of acidic by-products.

An important diagnostically useful biochemical characteristic of all the members of the family *Enterobacteriaceae*

is the absence of cytochrome c, making them oxidase-negative.

Resistance

Sunlight, drying, pasteurization, and the common disinfectants kill members of the family *Enterobacteriaceae*. In moist, shaded environments, such as pastures, manure, litter, and bedding, they can survive for many months. Though many are susceptible to broad-spectrum antimicrobial agents, their susceptibility is not accurately predictable and can change rapidly through acquisition of R plasmids, or resistance-encoding DNA cassettes (which may insert into numerous integrons located in the genome and in plasmids) (see Chapters 4 and 5).

Variability

Variability of one isolate of enteric as compared to another within the same species or genus depends upon the genetic basis for the trait under consideration. Differences in the capsular, somatic, or flagellar antigens account for variability among isolates of the same genus and species. Some variation among members of the same genus and species in the family, as well as among members of different genera and species, is accounted for by the presence of genes residing on plasmids encoding certain phenotypic traits. Such traits as resistance to antimicrobial agents, production of toxin, or secretion of hemolysin may be plasmid encoded and will vary depending on the presence or absence of a particular plasmid.

Transition from the smooth to the rough phenotype occurs with all members of the family. Likewise, change in the O-antigens has been shown to occur following lysogeny by certain bacteriophages (lysogenic conversion).

Susceptibility to various bacteriophages (phage typing) is sometimes useful in demonstrating differences in isolates (strains) of the same genus and species. Phage typing is a useful epidemiological tool.

Laboratory Diagnosis

The family is composed of a large number of related, facultatively anaerobic, oxidase-negative, nitrate reducing gram-negative rods. No clear divisions exist between the recognized genera. Differentiation within the family is accomplished by a combination of cultural, biochemical, and serologic tests. A number of manuals deal exclusively with this family, and because of the extreme clinical importance and prevalence of these organisms, an increasing number of programmed and/or computerized identification schemes are commercially available.

Morphology and Staining

All are gram-negative rods. All look similar in the gram-stained smear.

Cultural Characteristics

Methods used to isolate enteric pathogens vary depending upon whether the source of the sample is intestinal or extraintestinal. When the source is extraintestinal, isolating any of the family from normally sterile sites is significant. A culture medium with wide appeal is used. The medium for this purpose is an agar medium containing red blood cells (usually sheep or cow). Incubation is at 35–37°C.

When the source is intestinal, two consistently pathogenic genera may occur in fecal samples: *Salmonella* and *Shigella*. Though pathogenic strains of *E. coli* might be present, there is no easy way to determine a pathogenic strain from normally occurring, nonpathogenic strains of *E. coli.*

All enteric media are devised to favor the identification of *Salmonella, Shigella,* or both. The bases of the media are as follows:

1. An inhibitory substance, usually a bile salt or a dye. These substances inhibit gram-positive organisms from growing.
2. A substrate utilized or not by *Salmonella, Shigella,* and by few others.
3. A pH indicator to tell if the substrate has been changed.

The following are useful selective media for isolating enteric pathogens.

MacConkey Agar.
Inhibitor: Bile salts and crystal violet (inhibit gram-positive microorganisms).
Substrate: Lactose—*Salmonella, Shigella,* and *Proteus* do not ferment lactose.
Neutral red: If lactose is fermented (acid), colonies will be pink; if lactose is not fermented (peptides digested—basic), colonies will be colorless.
Usefulness: Very permissive medium. *Salmonella* and *Shigella* readily grow on this medium (as do most other enterics and *Pseudomonas*).

Xylose Lysine Deoxycholate (XLD) Agar.
Inhibitor: Bile salts.
Substrate: 1) Xylose—not fermented by *Shigella* (*Salmonella* ferments xylose). 2) Lysine—isolates that ferment xylose, but not lactose and sucrose, and are lysine decarboxylase-negative (*Proteus mirabilis*) produce colonies that will be amber-orange. *Salmonella* decarboxylates lysine. The ratio of xylose to lysine is such that an alkaline pH predominates (more decarboxylation). *Shigella* does not decarboxylate lysine. 3) Lactose and sucrose—*Salmonella* and *Shigella* do not ferment these sugars rapidly. 4) Ferric salt—colonies of organisms producing H_2S (*Salmonella; Proteus*) will have black centers (iron sulfide).
Phenol red: Acid colonies (non-*Salmonella* or non-*Shigella*) will be yellow. Alkaline colonies (possible *Salmonella* or *Shigella*) will be red.
Usefulness: An excellent all-purpose medium for both *Salmonella* and *Shigella*.

Hektoen Enteric (HE) Agar.
Inhibitor: Bile salts.
Substrate: Lactose and salicin—*Salmonella, Shigella,* and some species of *Proteus* and *Providencia* are lactose-negative and salicin-negative.
Ferric salt: Organisms producing H_2S will form black-centered colonies.
Bromthymol blue: Fermentors of salicin and/or lactose will form yellow to orange colonies; isolates not fermenting these sugars will form green or blue-green colonies.
Usefulness: Excellent for *Salmonella* and *Shigella*.

Brilliant Green Agar.
Inhibitor: Brilliant green dye (suppresses the growth of most members of the family except *Salmonella*).
Substrate: Lactose and sucrose—*Salmonella* (and some strains of *Proteus*) does not ferment these sugars. Neither does *Shigella*, but *Shigella* grows poorly (if at all) on this medium.
Phenol red: If sugars are not fermented (alkaline), colonies will be red; if sugars are fermented (acid), colonies will be yellow-green (due to the color of the background dye).
Usefulness: Excellent for isolating *Salmonella*.

Enrichment Media. At times, the numbers of *Salmonella* or *Shigella* in fecal samples may be too low ($<10^4$/gm) to be detected on the primary plating media discussed above. Therefore, in addition to being plated directly to a selective medium, the fecal sample is also placed in an enrichment medium. To detect *Salmonella* by utilizing enrichment methods, at least 100 salmonellae/gm are needed.

For *Salmonella*, enrichment may be achieved by incubating feces for 12 to 18 hours in selenite F broth. During this time, the growth of organisms other than *Salmonella* is suppressed, whereas growth of *Salmonella* is not. After the 12 to 18 hours have elapsed, an aliquot of the broth is streaked onto a plate of selective medium (e.g., brilliant green agar).

Enrichment for *Shigella* is not easy because it is rather sensitive to commonly used inhibitory substances found in selenite F and tetrathionate broths. An enrichment broth called *gram-negative* (or *GN broth*) is used in the same manner as selenite is used for *Salmonella*.

Members of the genus *Pseudomonas* (especially *P. aeruginosa*) may be found in feces, but this is probably an insignificant finding. *Pseudomonas* (not a member of the family *Enterobacteriaceae*) will grow on enteric media. This microorganism does very little to the substrates other than the peptides and peptones and thus mimics *Salmonella* and *Shigella* on selective media. *Pseudomonas* is oxidase-positive, a useful distinction.

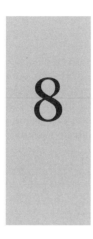

8

Enterobacteriaceae: Escherichia

Dwight C. Hirsh

The genus *Escherichia*, a member of the family *Enterobacteriaceae* is composed of several species, but only *E. coli* is an important pathogen of animals. This species, the major facultative gram-negative species comprising the normal flora of the gastrointestinal tract, is the cause of septicemic disease in foals, calves, piglets, puppies, and lambs; of diarrhea in newborn farm animals; and of edema disease in pigs. It may also be opportunistic in almost all animal species (e.g., in urinary tract disease, abscesses, and pneumonia).

Descriptive Features

Cellular Anatomy and Composition

The anatomy of the members of the genus *Escherichia* is typical for the family *Enterobacteriaceae*. They may possess capsules (K antigens), flagella (H antigens), or adhesins (fimbria or pili), and all possess a typical gram-negative cell wall composed of lipopolysaccharides (O-antigen) and proteins.

Cellular Products of Medical Interest

Adhesins. Adhesins (also known as *fimbria* or *pili*) are proteins that mediate adherence to target cells in the gastrointestinal tract and to cells comprising the niche for the strain. Because of their relative hydrophobicity, adhesins may also promote association with the membrane of phagocytic cells. Adhesins are important virulence factors when the microbe is on mucosal surfaces. *Escherichia coli* produces many different types of adhesin, most being linked with strains associated with a specific disease. Almost all of the adhesins promote adherence to glycoproteins on the surface of epithelial cells of the intestinal tract:

1. F4, F5, F6, F41. The fimbrial adhesins F4 (formerly known as K88), F5 (K99), F6 (987P), F17, and F41 are used by enterotoxigenic *E. coli* to adhere to target cells in the small intestine. F4, F5, and F6 are usually plasmid-encoded, while F41 is chromosomal.
2. F17. The protein F17 (like CS31A) is a plasmid-encoded adhesin responsible for adherence of septicemic ("invasive") strains of *E. coli* to their small intestine target cells.
3. CS31A. The protein CS31A (like F17) is a plasmid-encoded adhesin responsible for adherence of septicemic ("invasive") strains of *E. coli* to the small intestine target cells.
4. AAF. The adhesin AAF (*aggregative adherence fimbriae*) is responsible for the adherence of enteroaggregative *E. coli* to their small intestinal epithelial cell targets.
5. Bfp. The Bfp adhesin (for *bundle forming pilus*, due to its propensity to tangle together and form "bundles" when viewed under the electron microscope) is responsible for the adherence of enteropathogenic *E. coli* to their small intestinal epithelial cell targets.
6. Curli. Curli are adhesins that promote adherence to extracellular matrix proteins.
7. OmpA. OmpA (outermembrane protein A) is a putative adhesin used by enterohemorragic *E.coli* in adherence to large intestinal epithelial cell targets.

Capsule. Capsular polysaccharides (K-antigens) are important for those microorganisms (such as invasive strains of *E. coli*) that come in contact with elements of the innate immune system of the host. Capsular substances protect the outer membrane from the membrane attack complex of the complement cascade, and inhibit the microbe from attachment to, and ingestion by, phagocytic host cells. The capsule is thought to endow a degree of hydrophilicity relative to the membrane of phagocytic cells. Most capsules are negatively charged, as are the membranes of phagocytic cells.

Cell Wall. The cell wall of the members of this genus is one typical of gram negatives. The lipopolysaccharide (LPS) in the outer membrane is an important virulence determinant. Not only is the lipid A component toxic (endotoxin), but the length of the side chain in the O-repeat unit hinders the attachment of the membrane attack complex of the complement system to the outer membrane. LPS binds to lipopolysaccharide-binding protein (a serum protein), which in turn transfers it to the blood phase of CD14. The CD14-LPS complex binds to Toll-like receptor proteins (see Chapter 2) on the surface of macrophage cells triggering the release of proinflammatory cytokines

Enterotoxins. Enterotoxins are usually plasmid-encoded proteins. *Escherichia coli* produces at least three: labile toxin (LT), stable toxin (ST), and Enteroaggregative *E. coli*

heat-stable enterotoxin 1 (EAST1). These protein exotoxins affect the control of cyclic nucleotide activity within the "target" cell, which results in deregulation of water and electrolyte secretion by the affected host cell:

1. Labile toxin (LT). LT affects the adenylyl cyclase system. LT is composed of two subunits, A and B. The B subunit is a multimer that binds to gangliosides on the surface of the intestinal host cell, followed by translocation of the A subunit across the host cell membrane. The A subunit, after activation, cleaves nicotinamide from nicotinamide adenine dinucleotide (NAD) and then couples the remaining ribosyl adenine diphosphate onto the G regulatory protein of the adenylyl cyclase enzyme system. The result is deregulation of adenylyl cyclase, causing overproduction of cyclic AMP (cAMP) followed by opening of chloride channels in crypt cells (so-called cystic fibrosis transmembrane conductance regulator chloride channels) and the blockage of NaCl absorption in apical tip cells. As a consequence, water and electrolytes (chloride, sodium, and bicarbonate ions) are lost into the intestinal lumen. These events lead to diarrhea, hypovolemia, metabolic acidosis, and, if the acidosis is severe, hyperkalemia. There are two serologically distinct subclasses of LT. LTI is plasmid-encoded and neutralized by anticholera toxin antibodies; LTII is neither. LTI has been isolated from *E. coli* affecting humans (LTh-l) and swine (LTp-l). LTII has been isolated from cattle, water buffalo, humans, and food.

2. Stable toxin (ST). There are two kinds of ST: STa and STb. The genes encoding STa are located on a transposable element. The genes for STb are not. STa causes fluid accumulation in the intestines of suckling mice and piglets; STb causes fluid accumulation only in piglets and weaned pigs. The toxins are not related antigenically. STa affects the guanylyl cyclase system by deregulating cyclic GMP (cGMP) synthesis, resulting in fluid and electrolyte accumulation in the bowel lumen subsequent to blockage of sodium and chloride ion (and thus water) absorption (tip cells) and loss of chloride ions (crypt cells). The receptor for STa is a membrane-bound guanylyl cyclase. This receptor, when bound, results in the synthesis of cGMP. Increase in intracellular cGMP leads to the opening of chloride channels with the resultant flow of chloride and water into the intestinal lumen. The STa receptor is normally the target for guanylin (a 15 amino acid paracrine regulator), which is produced by goblet cells. Guanylin appears responsible for hydration of mucus that is also produced by goblet cells. STa and guanylin have common C-termini. STb binds to a sulfatide receptor followed by synthesis of cAMP activating a G regulatory protein. This leads to an increase in intracellular calcium concentration, which in turn activates protein kinase C. Protein kinase C phosphorylates proteins composing the chloride channels resulting in loss of chloride and water into the intestinal lumen, as well as the phosphorylation of the membrane-associated ion transport proteins resulting in blockage of absorption of NaCl. In wild strains of enterotoxigenic *E. coli*, STa is more commonly found.

3. Enteroaggregative *E. coli* heat-stable enterotoxin 1 (EAST1) is an enterotoxin similar in action to STa by being functionally similar to guanylin.

Other Enteric Toxins. Escherichia coli produces other proteins that affect the cells of the intestinal tract. Though these products have "enterotoxic" activity, the term "enterotoxin" is reserved for LT, ST, and EAST1 as discussed above. The other enteric toxins include shiga and shiga-like toxins, cytotoxic necrotizing factor, a plasmid encoded toxin, and a cytolethal-distending toxin:

1. SLT (for *S*higa and shiga-*l*ike *t*oxin). SLTs (also known as Vero tissue culture toxins because of their characteristic effects on Vero cells) are protein toxins similar to shiga toxin produced by *Shigella* (see Chapter 11). These toxins are composed of an A subunit and a B subunit. The B subunit is responsible for binding of the toxin to endothelial cells. The A subunit inhibits protein synthesis of the target cell (an endothelial cell) following interaction with the 60S ribosomal subunit. There are two types of shiga-like toxins, SLT-I and SLT-II. SLT-I is neutralized by antibody specific for the shiga toxin produced by *Shigella* spp.; SLT-II is not. SLT-I is probably identical to shiga toxin, whereas SLT-II is a variant. A family of bacteriophages has been shown to encode the shiga and shiga-like toxins. A variant of SLT-II, called SLT-IIe, is responsible for the vascular damage characteristic of edema disease of swine. The genes encoding SLT-IIe do not appear to be bacteriophage-associated.

2. CNF (for *c*ytotoxic *n*ecrotizing *f*actor). CNFs are proteins that interact with epithelial cell small GTP-binding protein Rho, resulting in membrane "ruffles." There are two types of CNF, CNF1 and CNF2, which are immunologically related and similar in size. The gene encoding CNF1 is located on the chromosome in a Pathogenicity Island (a cluster of genes encoding virulence determinant[s], an integrase protein, a specific insertion site, and mobility). The Pathogenicity Island that contains the gene encoding CNF1 also contains the genes encoding a number of other chromosomally encoded virulence traits, e.g., hemolysin, serum resistance, and the adherence protein Pap, needed by some strains of *E. coli* to adhere to urinary tract epithelium antecedent to urinary tract disease. The gene encoding CNF2 is plasmid-based.

3. Pet (for *p*lasmid-*e*ncoded *t*oxin). Pet is a serine protease enteric-acting toxin that affects the cellular cytoskeleton of affected intestinal epithelial cells, resulting in damage to the cell and stimulating an inflammatory response. Diarrhea is thought to result from prostaglandin synthesis by the recruited PMNs and affected epithelial cells, as well as activation of various inositol-signaling pathways within affected host cells. The net result is the secretion of chloride ions and water.

4. Cdt (for *c*ytolethal *d*istending *t*oxin). Cdts are a family of related toxins that affect the mammalian cell cycle. A role in pathogenicity has not been provided.

Hemolysins. Escherichia coli produce at least three hemolysins: alpha hemolysin, enterohemolysin (Ehx for *en*tero*h*emorrhagic *E. coli* toxin), and cytolysin A (Cly):

1. Alpha hemolysin. Alpha hemolysin (Hly) as well as enterohemolysin (see below) belongs to the RTX (*r*epeats in *t*oxin, so called because of the common feature of repeats in glycine-rich sequences within the protein) family of toxins (see also *Pasteurella/Mannheimia* leukotoxin in Chapter 12, *Actinobacillus* haemolysin in Chapter 13, adenylyl cyclase toxin of *Bordetella* in Chapter 15, *Moraxella* cytotoxin in Chapter 19). Hly is secreted by many virulent strains of *E. coli*. Loss or gain of *hly* by genetic manipulation produces corresponding changes in virulence of *E. coli* strains. Hly damages cell membranes, and is detected by growth in vitro on a medium containing red blood cells.

2. Enterohemolysin. Enterohemolysin (Ehx, for *en*tero*h*emorrhagic *E. coli* toxin) as well as Hly (see above) belongs to the RTX (*r*epeats in *t*oxin, so called because of the common feature of repeats in glycine-rich sequences within the protein) family of toxins (see also *Pasteurella/Mannheimia* leukotoxin in Chapter 12, *Actinobacillus* haemolysin in Chapter 13, adenylate cyclase toxin of *Bordetella* in Chapter 15, *Moraxella* cytotoxin in Chapter 19). Evidence suggests that Ehx may be the result of a defect in the secretion system for Hly. Ehx is secreted by many virulent strains of *E. coli* (especially those that produce SLT, see above) and is detected on media that contains red blood cells and added calcium.

3. Cytolysin A. The gene encoding cytolysin A commonly occurs among strains of *E. coli*. Expression of cytolysin A (Cly) occurs following infection of the bacterial cells with the temperate bacteriophages Ehy1 and 2 (incorrectly termed "*en*tero*h*emol*y*sins 1 and 2").

Iron Acquisition. Iron is an absolute growth requirement for most, if not all, living things. Siderophores (e.g., aerobactin) that remove iron from host iron-binding proteins are necessary if a microbe is to have invasive capabilities.

Miscellaneous Products. Miscellaneous cellular products include the following:

1. Acid tolerance. RNA polymerase containing RpoS (the sigma factor associated with stationary phase) preferentially transcribes genes responsible for acid tolerance (survival at pH, 5), allowing safe transit through the stomach.
2. Intimin. Intimin is a protein encoded by *eae* (for *E. coli a*ttaching *e*ffacing) located within a Pathogenicity Island (a cluster of genes encoding virulence determinant(s), an integrase protein, a specific insertion site, and mobility) called LEE (*l*ocus *e*ffacing *E. coli*). Intimin attaches to another secreted bacterial protein, Tir (*t*ranslocated *i*ntimin *r*eceptor) inserted into the host cell membrane.

3. Type III secretion system. The genes encoding a Type III secretion system (an assemblage of proteins—more than 20—that form a hollow tube-like structure through which effector proteins are "injected" into host "target" cells) also located within LEE (see above).

4. Esp. The genes encoding Esp (for *EP*EC *s*ignaling *p*rotein, also located within LEE, see above) activates a tyrosine phosphokinase in the affected cell resulting in cytoskeletal rearrangements leading to "collapse" of the microvilli (effacement). Diarrhea occurs secondary to increases in intracellular calcium ions and activation of protein kinase C. Protein kinase C is responsible for phosphorylation of proteins composing the chloride channels resulting in loss of chloride and water into the intestinal lumen, as well as the phosphorylation of the membrane associated ion transport proteins resulting in blockage of absorption of NaCl.

Variability

The variability of *E. coli* resides in the antigenic makeup of the O-repeat units (type of sugar subunits, how the subunits are hooked together, and the length of the chain), the composition of the flagellar protein (flagellin), and the composition of the capsule. There are at least 80 distinct K-antigens, approximately 165 serologically distinct O-groups, and at least 50 serologically different flagellar (H) antigens. The O-, H-, and K-antigens are used in serotyping a particular isolate. For example, O141:K85:H3 describes an isolate with antigens of the 141 serogroup, capsular antigen number 85, and flagellar antigen number 3.

Ecology

Reservoir and Transmission

Strains of *E. coli* capable of producing disease reside in the lower gastrointestinal tract and are abundant in environments inhabited by animals. Transmission is through the fecal-oral route.

Pathogenesis

Mechanisms and Disease Patterns. It is very difficult for most strains of *E coli* to produce disease because they do not have the necessary genes encoding the proteins needed to do so. If the genes are acquired (by transduction, conjugation, or transformation), the nonpathogenic strain may be changed to one with pathogenic potential. The type of disease produced would depend upon the genes acquired.

Enterotoxigenic Diarrhea. This disease occurs in neonatal pigs, calves, and lambs, and in weanling pigs. It has been reported in dogs and horses.

Enterotoxigenic diarrhea is caused by strains of *E. coli* that produce adhesins that promote attachment to glycoproteins on the surface of epithelial cells of the jejunum and ileum, and an enterotoxin(s) that affects the epithelial cell (to which the enterotoxigenic strain of E. coli is adhered), resulting in fluid secretion and diarrhea. Both traits are necessary for disease to result, since unless the ingested strain adheres to these cells, peristalsis will move it into the large bowel. The cells of the jejunum and the ileum are susceptible to the action of enterotoxin; the cells of the large bowel are not.

At least four adhesins may be found on enterotoxigenic E. coli, F4, F5, F6, and F41. They possess some host species specificity: F4 and F6 are almost always associated with isolates from swine; F5 with isolates from cattle, sheep, and swine; and F41 with those from cattle. The epithelial cell receptors for these adhesins regulate the age incidence of this disease as well. In calves and lambs, the receptors appear transiently during the first week or so of life. Analogous receptors are present in pigs throughout the first six weeks of life. There are many uncharacterized adhesins that probably play a role.

Aside from the adhesins outlined above, some enterotoxigenic strains of E. coli express curli. So, in addition to adherence to glycoproteins on the surface of epithelial cells, some strains adhere to extracellular matrix proteins. The presence of curli may explain the increase in the window of age susceptibility to enterotoxigenic disease in animals concurrently infected with rotavirus or cryptosporidia, two agents that may cause enough tissue damage to lead to exposure of extracellular matrix proteins.

In addition to adherence to the target tissues of the small intestine, enterotoxigenic strains must have the genetic capability of synthesizing enterotoxin. Strains producing only ST are the most common, followed by those secreting both ST and LT, and then by those secreting LT only.

Some of the adhesins and enterotoxins are encoded on plasmid DNA. As a consequence, it is difficult to predict which strain of E. coli possesses the genetic information necessary to produce disease. Some adhesins prefer to be associated with certain serotypes. In particular, the genes encoding the protein for the F41 adhesin are almost always found within strains of E. coli of the O9 and the O101 serogroups. As might be expected, the genes encoding the proteins for F41 adhesin are located on chromosomal DNA.

Following ingestion by the host, enterotoxigenic strains of E. coli adhere to target cells, multiply, and secrete enterotoxin. Fluid and electrolytes accumulate in the lumen of the intestine, resulting in diarrhea, dehydration, and electrolyte imbalances. In time, the infecting strain is moved distally away from the target cell and the disease process stops, due probably in part to the cessation of expression of the adhesin along with a decrease in available substrate following the almost explosive multiplication of the strain in the small intestine. Unless steps are taken to correct the fluid and electrolyte imbalances, the disease has high mortality.

The diarrhea produced is watery and nonbloody. There are minimal, if any inflammatory changes in the small intestine. Bacteria will be observed histologically coating the villi of the mid to distal portions of the small intestine.

Enteroaggregative Diarrheal Disease. Enteroaggregative strains of E. coli (EAggEC) associated with this disease are isolated from weaned pigs and calves with diarrhea. EAggEC adhere to cells lining the small intestine by way of the AAF adhesin. Following adhesion, EAggEC secrete a protein (encoded by a gene termed *agg* for aggregation) that promotes the formation of a sheet of microorganisms strongly adherent one to another (some have referred to this as a "biofilm"), thus the description, "enteroaggregative." EAggEC produce EAST1 and Pet, both potential causes of diarrhea.

The diarrhea is usually watery (though blood and leukocytes may be observed in some cases). Histologically, sheets of bacteria (entrapped in mucus) will be seen covering the small intestinal epithelia.

Invasive Disease. Association of susceptible animals (usually a neonate that has received inadequate amounts of colostrum or colostrum of inadequate quality) with invasive strains of E. coli may occur by way of the conjunctivae, inadequately treated umbilicus, or ingestion. If the invasive strain associates via ingestion, it first adheres to target cells in the distal small bowel. Adherence is probably related to expression of any number of adhesins, but CS31A is one that is commonly associated with invasive E. coli. Likewise, the adhesin F17 originally described on a plasmid termed *Vir* (so-called because of its association with virulent or invasive E. coli) is prevalent on invasive E. coli. Following adherence, invasive strains "induce" their own uptake by expression of either CNF1 or CNF2, resulting in the formation of "ruffles" that entrap adhering bacteria and "pull" them into the intestinal epithelial cell. Entry into the lymphatics and subsequently the bloodstream follows. Extensive multiplication within the intestinal epithelial cell probably does not occur. The mechanism by which the invasive strain gains access to lymphatics after uptake by the epithelial cell is unknown. Likewise, the mechanism of entry into lymphatics after association with conjunctivae or the umbilicus is unknown. Once the epithelial surface is traversed, expression of adhesins is repressed (otherwise adhesin-expressing bacteria could adhere to host phagocytic cells with disastrous consequences for the bacterium).

The infecting strain multiplies in the lymphatics and bloodstream and endotoxemia develops (Fig 8.1). Death of the host occurs if antibacterial therapy, the immune system, or both do not remove the microorganism.

Invasive strains have special qualities, e.g., they must escape phagocytosis, complement-mediated lysis, and have a mechanism to acquire iron. Capsule and various outer membrane proteins confer resistance to complement-mediated lysis (serum resistance). How capsules protect the outer membrane from insertion of the membrane attack complex is not known. Certain capsules (such as K1) are chemically similar to the surface of host cells in that they are composed mainly of sialic acid. Complement components associating with surfaces composed of sialic acid are shunted to degradative pathways rather than amplification and formation of membrane attack complexes.

Escape from phagocytosis is also related to capsule and certain outer membrane proteins. How outer membrane proteins function as antiphagocytic factors is not known.

The genes encoding the adhesin (e.g., CS31A, F17) and

FIGURE 8.1. *Cascade of biologically active mediators following interaction of lipopolysaccharide (LPS) with the body. When gram-negative microorganisms grow in the body, LPS is released (not on purpose, but when a bacterial cell makes LPS, some of it escapes). If LPS is in the bloodstream (endotoxemia), then a generalized cytokine "storm" plus activation of some of the enzyme cascades (complement is one) results in intravascular clotting, and increased vascular permeability, which leads to decreased organ perfusion and multiple organ failure, and very serious pH problems. This "state" is called "septic shock." The same occurs in a limited area if LPS is liberated "locally" (as might occur when a gram-negative bacteria grows in tissue). (*IL-8 attracts PMNs, and MCAF [macrophage chemotactic factor] attracts macrophages.)*

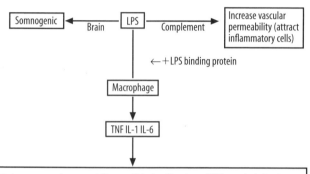

1. Increase vascular permeability–arachidonic acid pathway (TNF on endothelium)
2. Increase intravascular clotting–arachidonic acid pathway (TNF on endothelium)
3. Attract inflammatory cells–(TNF/IL-1 induce endothelium to produce IL-8 and MCAF)*
4. Release of acute phase proteins (liver) (IL-6)
5. Endogenous pyrogen (TNF, IL-1, IL-6) (brain)
6. Somnogenic (TNF, IL-1) (brain)

FIGURE 8.2. *Electron photomicrograph of an enteropathogenic strain of* Escherichia coli *(EPEC) showing (a) bundle forming pili, (b) the attaching and effacing lesion produced by this strain, and (c) a diagrammatic depiction of the generation of this lesion. See text for explanation of Tir and intimin. WASP: Wiskett-Aldrich syndrome protein; Arp2/3: nucleation site protein. (Reproduced with permission of Donnenberg MS, Whittam TS. Pathogenesis and evolution of virulence in enteropathogenic and enterohemorragic* Escherichia coli. Journal of Clinical Investigation *2001;107:539.)*

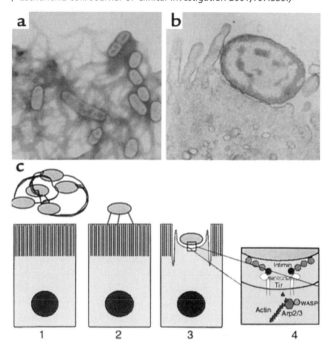

those responsible for siderophore production reside on plasmids. As mentioned above, the genes encoding F17 have been associated with the plasmid Vir, as has the gene encoding CNF2; those responsible for siderophore production have been associated with the plasmid pColV. In the latter instance, the siderophore genes are linked closely with the genes for the production of colicine V. The siderophore, aerobactin, has a high affinity for iron.

Many of the strains with invasive capability, except those from foals, produce a hemolysin (Hly) and are hemolytic on blood agar.

Histopathologically there are inflammatory changes in liver, spleen, joints, and meninges. There may be hemorrhages on pericardium, peritoneal surfaces, and adrenal cortices.

Nonenterotoxigenic Diarrheas. Enteropathogenic strains of *E. coli* (EPEC) produce diarrhea in all animal species, including human beings. EPEC do not produce ST, LT, or any other diarrhea associated toxin. They do, however, produce a characteristic lesion in the intestinal tract that is described as an *attaching and effacing* lesion. The characteristic lesion occurs because of the "collapse" of the microvilli of the affected cell giving the histopathologic appearance of "effacement" (Fig 8.2). The location in the tract is the distal small intestine, and upper large.

EPEC have a number of attributes that are involved in pathogenesis. The first is the production of the adhesin

Bfp. Bfp is responsible for "targeting" the particular intestinal epithelial cell that will become involved in the process. After association with an intestinal epithelial cell, a more intimate attachment occurs by way of intimin, which binds to the protein Tir that has been inserted into the "targeted" cell. Esp proteins are produced and are "injected" into the target cell by way of the Type III secretion system. The Esp proteins produce the effacement lesion, and diarrhea. Many EPEC also produce enterohemolysin (Ehx). It is unclear what role Ehx plays in enteropathogenic disease.

Some attaching and effacing strains of *E. coli* are lysogenized with the bacteriophage(s) that encode the shiga-like toxins SLT-I and/or SLT-II. These strains are termed *enterohemorragic E. coli* (EHEC) because, in addition to producing attaching and effacing lesions, they also produce hemorrhagic diarrhea. However, the target cells are those of the large intestine. Thus, the Bfp adhesin is not involved, and evidence strongly suggests that it is OmpA. The prototype EHEC is a strain of *E. coli* of the serotype O157:H7 that produces disease in human beings, and calves given the strain experimentally. Following attachment (the large intestine via OmpA), an attaching and effacing lesion is produced (the intimin produced by EHEC strains is slightly different from that produced by EPEC, reflecting the different target cell), and SLT is produced. The SLTs affect endothelial cells, leading to their injury and loss of integrity. The effects of

SLTs are local, i.e., the endothelial cell under the cell to which EHEC is attached, and systemic, i.e., the endothelial cells elsewhere in the body but mainly in the kidney and brain. The local effect is hemorrhage. The systemic effects of SLT, at least in humans, result in a syndrome called the *hemolytic uremic syndrome* (HUS), characterized by microangiopathic hemolytic anemia, glomerulonephritis, and thrombocytopenia. How SLT is absorbed locally or systemically is not understood. HUS does not appear to be a significant sequela of EHEC-based disease in nonhuman animals. Approximately 5% to 10% of human patients affected with EHEC (almost all are O157:H7) will develop HUS. Virtually all strains of O157:H7 produce Ehx.

All affected animals acquire EPEC/EHEC by way of the oral route. It is not clear whether EPEC have zoonotic potential, but animals (including humans) probably acquire the infecting strain by the fecal-oral route. Strain O157:H7 is a part of the normal flora of nonhuman animals, especially bovines. Human beings become infected following ingestion of contaminated food, mainly beef. At slaughter, the surface of the carcass becomes contaminated with fecal microorganisms. The surfaces of cuts of meat derived from an infected carcass are readily sterilized by cooking. When the meat is ground, the microorganisms on the surface become mixed throughout. Though improper cooking will readily kill surface microorganisms, including O157:H7, those inside may not be killed.

Diarrhea associated with EPEC will be watery, usually without blood and inflammatory cells. The characteristic histopathologic lesion is an "attaching and effacing" one affecting cells of the small intestine. Attachment is localized. Diarrhea associated with EHEC will be hemorrhagic. The characteristic histopathologic lesion will also be an "attaching and effacing" one, but affecting the large intestine.

Edema Disease. Edema disease is an acute, often fatal "enterotoxemia" of weaned pigs. The disease is characterized by subcutaneous and subserosal edema, caused by absorption of SLT-IIe produced by certain serotypes of *E. coli* (e.g., O141:K85, O138:K81, and O139:K82). The toxin attaches to and affects endothelial cells throughout the pig, resulting in extensive edema. The toxigenic strains inhabit the large bowel of normal pigs, and these strains are thought to increase in numbers during nutritional, social, or physical stress.

The typical lesion is generalized edema of various organs and tissues (e.g., head, neck, colon, stomach, intestine, brain).

Colibacillosis of Fowl. Colibacillosis of fowl is an economically important disease caused by invasive strains of *E. coli.* The disease takes many forms in fowl, depending upon the age of the host and mode of infection.

The egg surface can be contaminated with potentially pathogenic strains at the time of laying. The bacteria penetrate the shell and infect the yolk sac. If the bacteria grow, the embryo dies, usually late in incubation. Embryos that survive may die shortly after, with losses occurring as late as 3 weeks after hatching.

Fowl may also be infected by the respiratory tract and develop respiratory or septicemic disease. The course may be rapidly fatal or chronic, manifested by debilitation, diarrhea, and respiratory distress.

Other clinical syndromes seemingly caused by *E. coli* include cellulitis, synovitis, pericarditis, salpingitis, and panophthalmitis.

The *E. coli* responsible for this disease have been shown to possess some of the same virulence determinants as those isolated from mammals, most notably adhesins, production of aerobactin and associated iron-regulated outer membrane proteins.

Immunologic Aspects

Immunologic defense against diseases produced by pathogenic *E. coli* occurs at two levels: at the site of attachment to the target cell and through destruction of the bacteria or neutralization of its products.

Enterotoxigenic Diarrhea. Specific anti-adhesin antibody (sIgA and sIgm) found in colostrum and milk, prevent attachment to "target cells." Likewise, specific anti-LT neutralizes LT enterotoxin.

Enteroaggregative Diarrhea. Specific anti-AAF (adhesin) antibody (sIgA and sIgM) found in colostrum and milk prevents attachment to "target cells."

Invasive Disease. The neonate acquires immunity from the dam and, depending upon the isotype of the immunoglobulin (IgA, IgG, or IgM) the type of protection differs. For the first 36 hours or so of life, ingested IgG and IgM attach to receptors on the surface of epithelial cells of the small intestine. Transfer across the cell into the systemic circulation follows attachment. If the antibodies are specific for a virulence determinant, then disease may not result if the neonate encounters a pathogenic strain expressing that virulence determinant. For example, anticapsular antibodies acquired from the dam will protect the newborn from fatal invasive disease by strains of *E. coli* possessing that particular capsule.

Nonenterotoxigenic Diarrhea. Specific anti-Bfp antibody (sIgA and sIgM) found in colostrum and milk prevents attachment to "target cells." Antibody specific for SLT will neutralize this toxin, preventing its activity on endothelial cells.

Edema Disease. Antibody specific for SLT IIe will prevent the edema associated with this condition.

It is imperative, therefore, that the dam be exposed either naturally or artificially to the microorganism and its virulence determinants before parturition. Such exposure allows for antibodies to be made for secretion into colostrum and milk.

Laboratory Diagnosis

Demonstration of Enterotoxigenic Strains of *Escherichia coli*

Enterotoxigenic strains multiply to numbers approaching 10^8 to 10^9/ml of luminal contents. If the animal survives the fluid and electrolyte imbalances, large numbers are shed into the environment. Diagnosis is based on the suspicion that the disease is due to enterotoxigenic *E. coli.* The least troublesome and least invasive procedure (and also the least reliable) for verification of this suspicion is to demonstrate large numbers of specific adhesin-expressing *E. coli* in the feces. Demonstration entails plating a portion of a fecal sample onto a selective medium (MacConkey agar, for example). As adhesins are expressed poorly on selective media, a number of colonies are subcultured onto media that will promote the expression of the various adhesins: for F4, E medium; for F5 and F6, Minca medium; and for F41, E or Minca medium. Slide agglutination tests are run on each colony using antiserum specific for the various adhesins. An enzyme-linked immunosorbent assay has been developed to measure directly the presence of F4 and F5 adhesin-expressing bacteria in feces. Such a method eliminates many of the problems inherent in the analysis of feces for fimbriated bacteria. Gene-specific primers have been developed so that demonstration of appropriate genes in isolated colonies can be made by use of the polymerase chain reaction.

A more reliable method to verify the clinical diagnosis of enterotoxigenic *E. coli*-induced diarrhea is to quantitate the number of *E. coli* in the small intestine. Normally, there should be very few *E. coli* in such sites, especially in the jejunum, and the presence of large numbers of bacteria in these locations is highly suggestive of enterotoxigenic *E. coli* disease. Samples are plated onto different media chosen to promote the expression of the various adhesins, and colonies are picked and tested with the monospecific anti-adhesin sera. Examination of stained smears of the contents of the small intestine is another method based upon the increased numbers of enterotoxigenic *E. coli* in this location; finding >100 per oil immersion field implies >10^6/ml of contents. Although this method lacks specificity, it strengthens the diagnosis.

Fluorescent-labeled antibody techniques provide the easiest method and are probably the most reliable except for demonstration of the toxin. Smears of scrapings taken from the small intestine are flooded with antisera that are specific for the various adhesins. After treatment with fluorescent-labeled secondary antiserum, preparations are examined for labeled bacteria adhering to the epithelial cells.

Enterotoxin production by isolated strains of *E. coli* is best detected by utilizing an ELISA test specific for ST and LT. This test is reputed to detect 140pg/ml of ST (>100 times more sensitive than the suckling mouse assay) and 290 pg/ml of LT.

E. coli containing the genes encoding the various adhesins, as well as the enterotoxins can be detected by using DNA probes or polymerase chain reaction (PCR) primers specific for the corresponding base sequences encoding a specific trait (e.g., an adhesin or an enterotoxin). Such probes or primers have been used to detect the genes (in bacteria) in feces as well as in culture.

Demonstration of Strains Producing Enteroaggregative Disease

Isolates suspected as being capable of producing enteroaggregative diarrheal disease, can be tested for their ability to associate with HEp-2 tissue culture cells in aggregative pattern (the "gold standard"). However, demonstration of the presence of DNA associated with the genes encoding EAST1 and/or AAF is certainly easier and more cost effec-

tive. Histopathologically, a diagnosis of enteroaggregative disease is supported by the presence of sheets of bacteria associated with the intestinal epithelium.

Demonstration of Strains Producing Invasive Disease

The microbiological diagnosis of invasive disease is based upon the demonstration of *E. coli* in normally sterile sites or locations (joint, bone marrow, spleen, or blood). In fowl, the same sites are cultured, plus those grossly affected (lung, air sac). Dead in-shell embryos are cultured. Culture of the liver is to be avoided even though the Kupffer cells remove bacteria from the blood, because retrograde movement of enteric bacteria during the agonal stages of the disease complicates the microbiologic findings.

Demonstration of EPEC/EHEC Strains

The presence of genes encoding shiga-like toxins can be determined by specific DNA probes or by PCR. More cumbersome is the demonstration of cytotoxin activity for tissue culture cells (vero cells).

The demonstration of attaching and effacing strains as the cause of disease in the live animal is more difficult. Aside from biopsy of intestinal mucosa and the finding of attaching and effacing lesions, detection of genes associated with EPEC/EHEC, *eaeA*, *bfp*, or *slt* have been used (specific DNA probes or polymerase chain reaction with sequence-specific primers), or function assays testing for SLT activity for tissue culture cells. Fecal isolates obtained from a selective medium (e.g., MacConkey agar) can be tested for the genes or production of shiga-like toxin in culture supernatants that are tested for cytotoxicity for tissue culture cells. Most of these isolates have been shown to produce urease, an uncommon trait for *E. coli*. *Escherichia coli* O157:H7 does not ferment sorbitol. MacConkey agar containing this sugar instead of lactose is used to examine feces for the presence of sorbitol negative isolates, which are then tested for antiserum specific for O157 and/or H7. Since Ehx production is found with considerable number of SLT-producing strains of *E. coli*, demonstration of these strains can be made on blood agar plates supplemented with calcium.

Demonstration of Strains Producing Edema Disease

The microbiological diagnosis of edema disease depends upon the isolation and demonstration of certain serotypes that have been shown to play a role in this disease. The characteristic gross and microscopic tissue changes make this disease relatively easier to diagnose pathologically than microbiologically.

Treatment, Control, and Prevention

Treatment of an animal that has diarrhea due to an infectious cause centers on correcting fluid and electrolyte imbalances. If the animal is in shock due to cardiovascular collapse, then the fluid and electrolytes (sodium bicarbonate, KCl) are given IV; if not, oral electrolyte solutions are given. Since the animals are acidotic, sodium bicarbonate is included. Adding glucose to oral electrolytes will enhance the absorption of the sodium ions being excreted. The use of antimicrobials is controversial. Because the concentration of antimicrobic achievable (and available) in the lumen of the bowel is not known, the results of in vitro susceptibility tests to guide therapy are of doubtful reliability. Administration of nonabsorbable antimicrobics (such as neomycin) will sufficiently reduce the numbers of *E. coli* in the upper small bowel to allow correction of fluid and electrolyte imbalances. Such reduction occurs even though in vitro tests show that strains of *E. coli* commonly test "resistant" to neomycin. The fact that in vitro tests measure susceptibility to microgram amounts whereas milligram amounts may be available locally accounts for the discrepancy.

Antimicrobial agents, fluid, and electrolyte augmentation are necessary to successfully treat septicemic disease produced by invasive strains of *E. coli*. Invasive disease results in an endotoxemia progressing to a lactic acidosis because of decreased organ perfusion secondary to hypotension and disseminated intravascular coagulation. This should be taken into account when the electrolyte replacement is chosen. Antimicrobial agents should be chosen according to susceptibility trends in the practice area. Usually *E. coli* isolated from farm animals are susceptible to gentamicin or amikacin, trimethoprim-sulfonamides, and ceftiofur. They are usually resistant to tetracyclines, streptomycin, sulfonamides, ampicillin, and kanamycin. The severity of the signs of endotoxemia has been reduced experimentally by administering antibodies to the lipid A portion of the LPS.

Prevention and control of the enteric diseases produced by pathogenic strains of *E. coli* are one and the same. The key is sound husbandry practices. It is important that the dam be exposed to the antigenic determinants of the various virulence factors expressed on or by the infecting strains. Exposure can be provided naturally by placing the dam into the environment in which parturition will take place or artificially by vaccinating the dam with preparations containing the antigenic determinants perceived to be a threat to the newborn. Commercially produced preparations containing monoclonal antibodies to the adhesins (for ETEC) can be given orally to the neonatal animal. Although this practice will not significantly reduce the incidence of diarrhea, it will reduce the severity and mortality.

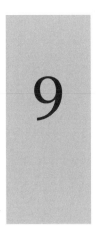

9

Enterobacteriaceae: Salmonella

Dwight C. Hirsh

The genus *Salmonella* is a member of the family *Enterobacteriaceae*, and is composed of two species, *S. bongori* and *S. enterica*. There are six subspecies within *S. enterica, enterica* (sometimes designated as subspecies I), *salamae* (subspecies II), *arizonae* (supspecies IIIa), *diarizonae* (subspecies IIIb), *houtenae* (subspecies IV and VII), and *indica* (subspecies VI) (those belonging to subspecies V were placed into *S. bongori*). There are numerous serotypes (serovars), more than 2000, within *S. bongori*, and the subspecies of *S. enterica*. The majority of these serovars have been given names that are capitalized and depicted in roman print. Others are merely denoted by antigenic formulae. Those belonging to *S. bongori* and *S. enterica* subspecies II through VII are mainly associated with cold-blooded vertebrates, while those belonging to *S. enterica* subspecies I are more commonly found in mammals and birds. However, each serovar is capable of producing disease regardless of the host.

In this chapter, the subspecies designation will not be used unless important to the discussion. For example, *Salmonella enterica* subspecies *enterica* serotype Typhimurium will first be denoted as *Salmonella enterica* serotype Typhimurium, and then, simply *S.* Typhimurium.

Descriptive Features

Cellular Anatomy and Composition

There is one capsular type, Vi (for virulence), though most members of the genus do not produce one. The cell wall is typical of gram-negative bacteria, composed of lipopolysaccharide (LPS), and protein. The antigenic composition of the polysaccharide portion of the LPS in part determines the serotype. The kind and number of sugars together with the linkage between them determine the antigenic determinants comprising the O-antigens of the particular isolate. The O-antigens, together with the antigenic determinants on the surface of the flagella (H-antigens), which are possessed by most salmonellae, help to define an isolate serologically (Table 9.1). This classification scheme is called the *Kauffman-White* schema.

Cellular Products of Medical Interest

Adhesins. Adhesins (also known as *fimbria* or *pili*) mediate adherence to target cells in the gastrointestinal tract and to cells comprising the niche for the strain. Because of their relative hydrophobicity, adhesins may also promote association with the membrane of phagocytic cells. Adhesins are important virulence factors only when the microbe is on mucosal surfaces. There are at least three different adhesins implicated in the interaction between salmonellae and target cells (M cells, intestinal epithelial cells) of the host—Pef, Agf, and Lpf:

1. Pef (*p*lasmid *e*ncoded *f*imbriae) are responsible for attachment to small intestinal epithelial cells.
2. Agf (thin *ag*gregative *f*imbriae, or curli) are responsible for attachment to small intestinal epithelial cells.
3. Lpf (*l*ong *p*olar *f*imbriae) are responsible for attachment to M cells.

Capsule. The role of the capsule (Vi) is unclear. Since salmonellae are primarily intracellular parasites, possession of a capsule does not seem to be a strategy that is consistent with the role this structure has in other microorganisms (i.e., antiphagocytic). However, Vi protects the outer membrane from effective interactions with membrane attack complexes generated by the complement system. This is useful in protecting salmonellae when extracellular.

Cell Wall. The lipopolysaccharide (LPS) in the outer membrane is an important virulence determinant. Not only is the lipid A component toxic (endotoxin), but the length of the side chain in the O-repeat unit hinders the attachment of the membrane attack complex of the complement system to the outer membrane. LPS binds to lipopolysaccharide-binding protein (a serum protein), which in turn transfers it to the blood phase of CD14. The CD14-LPS complex binds to Toll-like receptor proteins (see Chapter 2) on the surface of macrophage cells triggering the release of proinflammatory cytokines.

Effector (Toxin) Proteins. Several of the genes responsible for *Salmonella* virulence are located in clusters, called Pathogenicity Islands, a cluster of genes encoding virulence determinant(s), an integrase protein, a specific insertion site, and mobility. There are at least five Salmonella Pathogenicity Islands (SPIs). While SPI-1 is found in both species of *Salmonella*, SPI-2 (and presumably SPI-3 through 5) is found only in *S. enterica*. All five SPIs contain genes encoding the proteins necessary for the Type III secretion system (though the genes and their products are different

Table 9.1.   Representative Antigenic Formulas for Salmonellae

O-group	Serovariety	Antigenic Formula[a]
B	*Salmonella* Typhimurium	**1,4,5,12**:i:1,2
B	*Salmonella* Agona	**4,12**:f,g,s:-
D	*Salmonella* Dublin	**1,9,12**:g,p:-
E	*Salmonella* Anatum	**3,10**:e,h:1,6
G	*Salmonella* Worthington	**1,13,23**:z:1,w

[a] O-antigens: boldface numerals. Phase 1 H-antigen: lowercase letter. Phase 2 H-antigen: numeral (or lowercase letter).

for each island), and may or may not contain the effector proteins (those proteins that interact with the host "target" cell). The Type III secretion system consists of an assemblage of proteins (more than 20) that form a hollow tube-like structure through which effector proteins are "injected" into host "target" cells.

The effector proteins associated with SPI-1 include Ssps (*Salmonella* secreted proteins, encoded by a number of *ssp* genes located within SPI-1), and Sops (*Salmonella* outer protein, encoded by a number of *sop* genes, located outside of SPI-1). Ssps and Sops are involved with uptake of salmonellae by the target cell(s) by inducing membrane "ruffles" that follow the rearrangement of the actin cytoskeleton following the activation of the small GTP-binding proteins, CDC42 and Rac. In addition, Ssps also interacts with caspase-1 causing the death of activated macrophages.

The effector proteins associated with SPI-2 include Sses (secretion system effectors, encoded by a number of *sse* genes located within SPI-2), Ssas (secretion system apparatus, encoded by a number of ssa genes, located within SPI-2). Both Sses and Ssas are induced by low pH (stomach, phagosome), and interfere with macrophage function.

The effector proteins associated with SPI-3 include Mgts (*magnesium transport system*, encoded by a number of *mgt* genes located within SPI-3). These genes are induced by low concentration of magnesium ions (as occurs within macrophages), and the encoded proteins appear to be important for survival inside of macrophages.

The effector proteins associated with SPI-4 and SPI-5 are associated with intracellular survival, and as yet are not clearly defined.

Enterotoxin. Members of the genus *Salmonella* secrete an enterotoxin, Stn (*Salmonella* enterotoxin) associated with water and electrolyte secretion by host target cells. Stn differs from cholera toxin and LT of *Escherichia coli* (see Chapter 8) by being a peptide rather than being composed of subunits. The role (if any) of Stn in the production of diarrhea is unclear.

Iron Acquisition. Salmonellae produce siderophores (enterobactin) when growing in iron-limiting conditions.

Stress Proteins. Stress proteins are defined as proteins made when the microorganism is placed under conditions of stress (e.g., heat, cold, low pH, high pH). RNA polymerase containing RpoS preferentially transcribes genes responsible for acid tolerance (survival at pH 5) and regulates genes found on Spv plasmids (see below). RNA poly-

merase containing RpoE is involved with survival within phagocytic cells.

Virulence Plasmids. Salmonellae possess plasmids of various sizes, some of which have been associated with virulence. The most notable is a family of large (approximately 50 to 100 kilobases [kb]) plasmids, termed "*Salmonella* virulence plasmids" (Spv plasmids) that are found within those species of salmonellae with potential to produce disseminated disease. Some of the genes (*spv* genes) carried by these plasmids are necessary for intracellular growth and are regulated in part by RNA polymerase containing the stationary phase sigma factor, RpoS (see "Stress Proteins," above). Other genes on these plasmids are responsible for serum resistance and may be involved with adherence and invasion of the cellular target.

Miscellaneous Products. The transcriptional regulator, SlyA (for salmolysin), is in part responsible for survival of salmonellae within macrophages, perhaps affording protection from the toxic products generated by oxygen-dependent pathways. The products of the *phoP/phoQ* operon are responsible for resistance of salmonellae to defensins found in the lysosomal granules of phagocytic cells (by directing the remodeling of the salmonella outer membrane). The product of the *shdA* (for shedding) gene governs fecal shedding of salmonellae by an infected host. This gene is restricted to serotypes of *S. enterica* subspecies *enterica*. Arc (for *aerobic regulation control*), is a two-component global regulator system involved with intracellular survival.

Ecology

Reservoir

The reservoir for members of the genus *Salmonella* is the gastrointestinal tract of warm- and cold-blooded animals. Sources of infection include contaminated soil, vegetation, water, and components of animal feeds (such as bone, meat, and fish meal), particularly those containing milk-, meat-, or egg-derived constituents, and the feces of infected individuals. Lizards and snakes (usually asymptomatic) are commonly infected, sometimes with several serotypes. *Salmonella enterica* subspecies *enterica* are almost exclusively found in warm-blooded mammals and birds (evidence suggests that the possession of the *shdA* gene product is responsible).

Transmission

Infection occurs following the ingestion of salmonellae. The outcome of the interaction between host and *Salmonella* depends upon the state of the colonization resistance of the host (a measure of the "barrier" produced by the normal flora), the infectious dose, and the particular species of *Salmonella*. Disease may or may not occur following ingestion. If it occurs, it may do so immediately, or at some later date. In the later instance, the initial interaction may result in the colonization (without disease) of the host, but with a change in the intestinal environment, brought on, for example, by stress or antibiotics (activities that affect the normal flora), and disease may follow.

Pathogenesis

Mechanisms. The most common clinical manifestation of salmonellosis is diarrhea. In certain instances (defined by host factors, the strain of *Salmonella*, and dose) septicemia occurs. Host factors include age, immune status, concurrent disease, and "health" of the normal flora (colonization resistance).

Stationary phase salmonellae appear best suited to initiate disease, because under these conditions, RNA polymerase containing the alternative sigma factor, RpoS, initiates transcription of genes responsible for acid tolerance and subsequent survival through the stomach. Also, RNA polymerase containing RpoS is a positive regulator for the genes found on the Spv plasmids.

The target cells are the M cells atop the lymphoid nodules and the epithelial cells of the distal small intestine and the upper large bowel. If the target cell is "vacant" relative to the numbers of salmonellae (a reflection of the colonization resistance), disease may result. Vacancy of the target cell depends upon the status of the normal flora. If the flora is disrupted (stress, antibiotics), then the infectious dose does not have to be as high for salmonellae to gain access to the target cell. It appears that the M cell is the preferred target, and it is this cell that is affected first. Adhesion is the first step in the disease process, mediated by one or more of the adhesins Agf, Pef, Lpf, or by others yet to be determined. Following adhesion, salmonellae are internalized following the induction of membrane ruffles in the target cells triggered by Ssps and Sops subsequent to their "injection" by the Type III secretion system. The target cell is irreversibly damaged by this interaction, undergoing apoptosis. Salmonellae are now found within the target cells, the lymph nodule, and submucosal tissue. An inflammatory response is initiated by release of various chemokines from affected host cells, as well as release of proinflammatory cytokines following host interaction with cell wall LPS—activities that result in an influx of polymorphonuclear neutrophil leukocytes (PMNs) and macrophages. The influx of PMNs may be reflected in a transient peripheral neutropenia. PMNs are highly efficient in phagocytosing and destroying salmonellae, the macrophage less so. If the immune status of the host and the characteristics of the salmonellae are such, the infectious process is arrested at this stage. Diarrhea is thought to result from prostaglandin synthesis by the recruited PMNs (and perhaps by the affected host cells), as well as activation of various inositol-signaling pathways within affected host cells. The net result is the secretion of chloride ions and water. The role of Stn in the production of diarrhea is unclear.

If the infecting strain of *Salmonella* has properties that allow dissemination (possession of SPI-2, 3, 4, and 5—associated gene products that allow growth within macrophages; Spv plasmid encoding ability to grow intracellularly and serum resistance; PhoQ/PhoP system allowing resistance to defensins; SlyA allowing resistance to oxygen-dependent by-products; *arcA*), septicemia may result. The likelihood of this occurring is increased if immune status of the host is diminished. Salmonellae disseminate and multiply within phagocytic cells (macrophages mainly) within phagosomes. Not only are the invasive strains better able to withstand the action of lysosomal contents, some "sort" to phagosomes that do not fuse with lysosomes. The presenting signs are usually, but not always, septicemia and shock (see Fig 8.1). Strains producing this form of disease escape destruction by the host and multiply within macrophages of the liver and spleen, as well as intravascularly. During the dissemination process, salmonellae are occasionally outside of the intracellular environment and therefore at risk from the formation of complement membrane attack complexes on their surfaces. This occurrence is discouraged by at least two mechanisms: a product of the Spv plasmid and the length of the O-repeat unit of the LPS (there is a direct correlation between O-repeat length and virulence).

Invasive salmonellae are capable of secreting a siderophore, enterobactin that removes iron from the iron-binding proteins of the host, although it is doubtful whether this is needed within the cells of the host.

Multiplication of the organism results in endotoxemia (see Fig 8.1), which accounts for most signs and the course of illness.

Pathology. If the infectious process is limited to the intestinal tract, the lesions will consist of a hemorrhagic inflammation of the distal small intestine and large bowel. There may be superficial necrosis. In the septicemic form of the disease, there are inflammatory changes in liver, spleen, and intestinal tissue. There may be hemorrhages on pericardium, peritoneal surfaces, and adrenal cortices.

Disease Patterns

Ruminants. Salmonellosis is a significant disease of ruminants, mainly cattle. The disease affects young (usually 4 to 6 weeks of age) as well as adult animals. Animals in feedlots are commonly affected. The disease may be a septicemia or be limited to the enteric tract. Pneumonia, hematogenously acquired, is a common presenting sign in calves with septicemia due to *S. enterica* serotype Dublin (*S.* Dublin). Abortion may follow septicemia. *S. enterica* serotype Typhimurium, *S.* Dublin, and *S. enterica* serotype Newport are the serotypes commonly isolated from cattle, *S.* Typhimurium the serotype from sheep.

Swine. Salmonellosis in swine can present as an acute, fulminating septicemia or as a chronic debilitating intestinal disease. The form depends upon the strain of *Salmonella*, the dose, and the colonization resistance of the infected animal. The disease is seen most often in pigs that have been stressed. Such conditions occur often in feeder pigs, an age group in which salmonellosis commonly occurs. *S.* Typhimurium and *S. enterica* serotype Cholerae-suis are the predominant serotypes.

Horses. Adult horses are commonly affected with *Salmonella*. The pattern is diarrhea, though septicemia is seen occasionally. Colic, gastrointestinal surgery, and antimicrobial agents predispose the horse to the development of clinical signs. The agent is either carried normally (as in approximately 3% of clinically normal horses) or acquired from other sources (e.g., a veterinary hospital). *S.*

Typhimurium and *S. enterica* serotype Anatum are most commonly isolated.

Dogs and Cats. Salmonellosis is uncommon in dogs and cats, although carriage is reportedly high in clinically normal pound dogs (upwards of 35%). When outbreaks occur they are usually associated with a common source, such as contaminated dog food or "treats" (e.g., dried pig's ears). *Salmonella* should be high on the microbiological differential list for cats with signs of septicemia.

Poultry. See "Salmonellosis of Poultry."

Epidemiology

Salmonella spp. are ubiquitous geographically and zoologically. Some serotypes are relatively host-specific (*S.* Dublin—cattle; *S. enterica* serotype Typhisuis—swine; *S. enterica* serotype Pullorum—fowl), while others, notably *S.* Typhimurium, *S.* Anatum, and *S.* Newport, affect a wide host range among which feral birds and rodents play important roles in interspecific dissemination of infection. Long periods of asymptomatic and convalescent shedding ensure widespread, unchecked distribution of the organisms.

Clinical outbreaks are correlated with depressed immune states, as in newborn animals (calves, foals) and stressed adults, parturient cows, equine surgical patients, and swine with systemic viral diseases. All animals are at increased risk of developing disease if their normal flora is disrupted (stress, antibiotics). These circumstances render animals susceptible to exogenous exposure or activation of silent infections.

Humans appear to be susceptible to all *Salmonella* serotypes, the most important source for which are animals and their by-products. Poultry and poultry products (eggs) are a major source of *Salmonella* in humans. *Salmonella enterica* serotype Enteriditis (e.g., phage type 4) is especially adapted for egg transmission. Whether a person develops disease following ingestion of salmonellae from the environment depends upon the dose of organisms, the serotype of *Salmonella*, and the colonization resistance of the infected individual. *Salmonella* Typhimurium is most common, usually producing gastroenteritis. Some serotypes have greater invasion potential, for example, *S.* Cholerae-suis (from swine), and *S.* Dublin (infected milk). Though *S.* Typhimurium DT104 (the *Definitive Type* designation specifies a particular phage type), which is acquired from cattle, appears more prone to systemic disease, though this has been difficult to prove experimentally. Asymptomatic reptiles have become an important source of *Salmonella* in humans.

Immunologic Aspects

Protection depends upon specific and nonspecific immunological factors and microbiological defense mechanisms. Disease may be prevented by an intact colonization resistance at the level of the target cell (see Chapter 2). Whether infection can be prevented is not known.

Antibodies specific for surface structures of *Salmonella*, possibly adhesins, prevent adherence to target cells. The newborn is protected passively by ingesting specific sIgA or IgG$_1$ (bovine). The immunologically mature animal is protected by exudation of specific immunoglobulins (IgM and IgG) at the site of invasion or by the production of secretory immunoglobulins.

Another, more novel approach has been to feed animals microorganisms that out-compete salmonellae for niches along the gastrointestinal tract. *Competitive exclusion*, as this phenomenon is called, may be quite useful because, theoretically, salmonellae of any serotype would be excluded as long as they shared the same niche as the competing strain.

Antibodies in the circulation act as opsonins and promote the phagocytosis of the organism. Destruction of the salmonellae that have been phagocytosed follows the immunological activation of the macrophages by specifically stimulated lymphocytes (T cells), though activated macrophages are damaged or killed by Ssps. NK cells lyse *Salmonella*-infected cells.

Acquired immunity revolves around activation of macrophages, which takes place as follows. After initial interaction between salmonella and macrophage, IL-12 is released by the affected macrophage. IL-12 activates the T$_{H1}$ subset of T helper cells (see Chapter 2). This subset secretes, among other cytokines, interferon gamma, which activates macrophages. Activated macrophages are efficient killers of intracellular salmonellae.

Artificial immunization against salmonellae is difficult. Bacterins have had limited success. Apparently, they do not stimulate strong cellular immunity, even though abundant antibody is produced. Antibodies that are produced locally or passed in colostrum or milk interfere with adsorption to the target cell and protect against disease in this location. Macrophages can be activated and antibody production stimulated in response to modified live vaccines. If given orally, these vaccines stimulate local secretory immunity and cell-mediated activation of phagocytic cells. Aromatic-dependent mutants of *Salmonella* show promise as effective modified live vaccines, especially for calves. *aroA* mutants of *Salmonella* cannot multiply within the host since vertebrate tissue does not contain the needed precursors for aromatic acid synthesis.

Laboratory Diagnosis

In cases of intestinal infection, fecal samples are collected; in systemic disease, a blood sample is collected for standard blood culture. Spleen and bone marrow are cultured for the salmonellae when postmortem diagnosis of systemic salmonellosis is required.

Fresh fecal samples are placed onto one or more selective media, including MacConkey agar, XLD agar, Hektoen enteric medium, and brilliant green agar. For enrichment, Selenite F, tetrathionate, or gram-negative broth (GN) is recommended.

Salmonellae appear as lactose-nonfermenting colonies on lactose-containing media (lactose-fermenting strains of *Salmonella* have been reported, but these are rarely encountered). Since most serotypes of salmonellae produce H_2S, colonies on iron-containing media (e.g., XLD agar), they will have a black center. Suspicious colonies can be tested directly with polyvalent anti-*Salmonella* antiserum or inoculated into differential media and then tested with antisera.

To cultivate salmonellae from tissue, blood agar can be used.

Definitive identification involves determination of somatic and flagellar antigens and possibly bacteriophage type.

Various *Salmonella*-specific DNA probes and primers for the polymerase chain reaction have been developed for identification as well as detection in samples (food, feces, water) containing other microorganisms.

A multiplex polymerase chain reaction (PCR) assay using primers designed to detect the common diarrhea-associated microorganisms of swine (*Brachyspira hyodysenteriae*, *Lawsonia intracellularis*, and *Salmonella*) has been described.

Treatment, Control, and Prevention

Nursing care is the principal treatment for the enteric form of salmonellosis. The use of antimicrobial agents is controversial. Some studies show that antibiotics do not alter the course of the disease. In addition, there is evidence that antibiotics promote the carrier state and select for resistant strains. Proponents of antibiotic usage recommend a member of the fluoroquinolone class of drug (e.g., enrofloxacin or ciprofloxacin).

Treatment of the systemic form of salmonellosis includes nursing care and appropriate antimicrobial therapy as determined by retrospectively acquired susceptibility data. Since salmonellae survive in the phagocytic cell, the antimicrobial drug should be one that penetrates the cell. Examples of those that distribute in this manner include ampicillin, enrofloxacin, trimethoprim-sulfonamides, and chloramphenicol/florfenicol. Treatment options may be compromised due to acquisition of R plasmids or integrons encoding resistance to multiple antibiotics. A serious global epidemic of S. Typhimurium DT104 (the *Definitive Type* designation specifies a particular phage type), a type of salmonella that affects humans and other animals worldwide, contains a "cluster" of antibiotic resistance-encoding genes within its chromosome. This "cluster," called "Salmonella genomic island 1" (SGI1), contains the genes for resistance to ampicillin, chloramphenicol/florfenicol, streptomycin/spectinomycin, sulfonamides, and tetracyclines bounded by two integrons. SGI1 has moved into *S. enterica* serotype Albany (fish in Southeast Asia) and *S. enterica* serotype Paratyphi B (tropical fish in Singapore).

Salmonellosis is controlled through strict attention to protocols designed to curtail the spread to susceptible animals of any contagious agent found in feces. Artificial immunization with modified live products has shown promise (e.g., *aroA* mutants, see above). Attempts have been made to treat and prevent the endotoxemia produced by the systemic form of the disease by administering serum containing antibodies to the core LPS. Likewise, the ad-

ministration of J5, a rough variant of *E. coli*, has been shown to stimulate the production of antibody to the core LPS. Both methods appear to prevent and control the signs of disease produced by systemic salmonellosis.

Salmonellosis of Poultry

Paratyphoid

"Paratyphoid" is salmonellosis produced by any of the motile strains of *Salmonella* (all but *S. enterica* serotype Pullorum and *S. enterica* serotype Gallinarum are motile). The disease produces its highest losses in the first 2 weeks of life as a septicemic disease. Survivors become asymptomatic excretors.

Infection is through ingestion. The source is usually feces or fecally contaminated materials (litter, fluff, water).

Diagnosis is made by culturing the organism from affected tissue (spleen, joints) from birds that had been showing clinical signs of disease. It is more difficult to detect an asymptomatic carrier because such carriers only periodically shed the organism in feces. Some have suggested that culture of fluff and litter could be used to detect carrier flocks.

Treatment does not eliminate carriers, although it does control mortality. Treatment regimens have included avoparcin, lincomycin, furazolidone, streptomycin, and gentamicin. Exclusion of salmonellae by feeding "cocktails" of normal flora has been used with some success to reduce the number of salmonellae shed by carrier birds (competitive exclusion).

Pullorum Disease

Pullorum disease, caused by *S*. Pullorum, is rare in North America but not in the rest of the world. The disease has almost been eliminated in the United States due to a breeding flock testing program.

Salmonella Pullorum infects the ova of turkeys and chickens (see Fig 74.7). Thus, the embryo is already infected when the egg is hatched. The hatchery environment is contaminated following hatching of an infected egg, leading to infection of other chicks and poults. Mortality is due to septicemia and is greatest in the second to third week of life. Surviving birds carry the bacterium and may pass it to their offspring. It is difficult to detect infected breeding hens by bacteriologic means. Agglutination titers, produced 3 to 10 days after infection, are used to detect carrier birds.

Eliminating infected breeding birds detected serologically controls this disease. Treatment with antimicrobial agents (mainly sulfonamides) reduces mortality in infected flocks.

Fowl Typhoid

Fowl typhoid, caused by *S*. Gallinarum, is an acute septicemic or chronic disease of domesticated adult birds, mainly chickens. Fowl typhoid is rare now in the United States due to control programs.

The disease is diagnosed by culturing the organism from liver or spleen. It is treated with antimicrobial agents, mainly sulfonamides (sulfaquinoxaline) and nitrofurans. Fowl typhoid is controlled by management and eliminating infected birds. A bacterin made from a rough variant of *S.* Gallinarum, 9R, has been shown to decrease mortality.

Avian Arizonosis

Salmonella enterica subspecies *arizonae* and *S. enterica* subspecies *diarizoniae* (*Arizona hinshawii*) are most often isolated from reptiles and fowl, although these species can be isolated from any animal. Turkeys are most commonly affected. There are 55 serologic types affecting fowl, with type 7:1,7,8 most commonly isolated in the United States.

Salmonella enterica subspecies *arizonae* and *S. enterica* subspecies *diarizoniae* are maintained in turkey flocks via hatching eggs, which become infected following ingestion by the hen. Feces also spread it.

Diagnosis is made by culturing salmonellae from the liver, spleen, blood, lungs, or kidneys of affected birds, or from dead poults and hatch debris.

Most serotypes of *Salmonella enterica* subspecies *arizonae* and *S. enterica* subspecies *diarizoniae* possess R plasmids, which sometimes makes it difficult to prevent and treat this disease. Various antimicrobial agents such as furazolidone and sulfamerazine added to feed have shown some success in lowering mortality. Injection of day-old poults with gentamicin or spectinomycin decreases mortality, but survivors still harbor (and shed) the organism.

Control measures should be aimed at prevention rather than treatment. Because of the multiplicity of serotypes, no effective vaccine is available.

10 *Enterobacteriaceae: Yersinia*

Dwight C. Hirsh

The genus *Yersinia* is included in the family *Enterobacteriaceae*. There are 11 species, one of which, *Y. ruckeri*, affects only fish. *Yersinia enterocolitica* and *Y. pseudotuberculosis* are associated with mesenteric lymphadenitis, terminal ileitis, acute gastroenteritis, and septicemia. While *Y. enterocolitica* affects mainly domestic animals and primates, *Y. pseudotuberculosis* affects largely birds and rodents, and only occasionally domestic animals and primates. Plague, caused by *Y. pestis*, is a rodent-based zoonosis. The zoonotic aspects of *Y. enterocolitica, Y. intermedia, Y. frederiksenii,* and *Y. kristensenii* are uncertain. *Yersinia aldovae, Y. rohdei, Y. mollaretii,* and *Y. bercovieri* are without known pathogenic potential.

Descriptive Features

Morphology and Staining

Members of the genus *Yersinia* are gram-negative coccobacilli. Bipolarity is common in tissue smears. Most species are flagellated at ambient temperatures.

Growth Characteristics

Yersiniae grow on ordinary laboratory media, including MacConkey agar, although they grow slower than most other members of the family *Enterobacteriaceae*. Colony diameters range from under 1 mm (*Y. pestis*) up to 1.5 mm for most other yersiniae. They are not hemolytic when grown on blood agar.

In biochemical activities and resistance, yersiniae resemble other members of the family *Enterobacteriaceae*.

YERSINIA PESTIS (PLAGUE BACILLUS)

Yersinia pestis is the cause of the rodent-based zoonotic disease called *plague*. In human patients, and susceptible domestic animal species (mainly cats), plague is manifest as a local lymphadenitis (bubonic plague), pneumonia (pneumonic plague), or septicemia (septicemic plague). Analysis of DNA sequences of the genes encoding the 16S ribosomal RNA indicates that *Y. pestis* is a subspecies of *Yersinia pseudotuberculosis*.

Descriptive Features

Cellular Composition and Products of Medical Importance

Yersinia pestis contains the plasmids pYV (encoding the Type III secretion system, Yops, and LcrV), pMT1 (encoding the capsule, and Ymt), and pPCP1 (encoding pesticin, coagulase, and plasminogen activator). A chromosomal locus called the *High Pathogenicity Island* contains the genes encoding iron uptake, and the Hms phenotype. Also located on the chromosome are the genes encoding the protein Gsr.

Capsule. The capsule plays many roles, the most important of which are interference with phagocytosis (antiphagocytic), and the protection of the outer membrane from the deposition of membrane attack complexes generated by activation of the complement system. The capsule of *Y. pestis* is called Caf1 (for *c*apsular *a*ntigen *f*raction 1), and is encoded by genes that reside on plasmid pMT1 (which also carries the genes encoding the toxin Ymt, see below).

Cell Wall. The cell wall of *Y. pestis* does not have O-antigen (rough phenotype). The lipopolysaccharide (LPS) in the outer membrane is an important virulence determinant. LPS binds to lipopolysaccharide-binding protein (a serum protein), which in turn transfers it to the blood phase of CD14. The CD14-LPS complex binds to Toll-like receptor proteins (see Chapter 2) on the surface of macrophage cells triggering the release of proinflammatory cytokines

High Pathogenicity Island. High Pathogenicity Island (HPI), so-called because its presence is related to increased virulence as compared to strains that do not contain it, is a cluster of chromosomal genes involved with iron acquisition (see below, "Iron Acquisition").

Hms Phenotype. The Hms (for *hem*in storage) phenotype is associated with iron acquisition and colonization of fleas (see below, "Iron Acquisition").

Iron Acquisition. Iron is an absolute growth requirement and must be removed from iron-binding proteins of the host. The genes encoding products involved with iron acquisition reside on a chromosomal pathogenicity island HPI (a cluster of genes encoding virulence determinant(s), an integrase protein, a specific insertion site, and mobility.) The HPI of *Y. pestis* encodes the genes for the iron-acquiring siderophore yersiniabactin, and the Hms (for hemin storage) phenotype. Colonies growing on the surface of blood agar plates that display the Hms phenotype appear pigmented (they are not) due to the binding of hemoglobin (or Congo Red if present). It is probable that bound hemoglobin is used as a source of iron. The genes responsible are encoded by the *pgm* (for *pigment*) locus. In addition to playing a role in iron acquisition, the Hms phenotype is somehow involved with colonization and blockage of the proventriculus of fleas.

Type III Secretion System. The Type III secretion system consists of an assemblage of proteins (more than 20) that form a hollow tube-like structure through which effector proteins (Yops, LcrV) are "injected" into host "target" cells. The genes encoding the proteins needed by the Type III secretion system reside on plasmid pYV (along with the genes encoding Yops and LcrV, see below).

Toxins. Yersinia pestis produces a number of toxins that are secreted by way of a Type III secretion system (see above):

1. Yops. Following their "injection" into macrophages, Yops (for *Yersinia outer protein*) interfere with the actin cytoskeleton, thereby blocking phagocytosis, and down regulating the inflammatory responses by the inhibition of NF-κB. "Injection" into neutrophils, results in a decrease in the expression of endothelial cell-adhesion proteins, thereby reducing effective inflammatory responses. The genes encoding Yops reside on the plasmid pYV (also known as pCD1). The genes residing on this plasmid encode Yops, LcrV, and the Type III secretion system. They are down regulated at 26°C, and up regulated at 37°C and low calcium.

2. LcrV. LcrV (for *low calcium response virulence*, also known as Factor V) is a protein located on the surface of *Y. pestis*. LcrV has several roles: it aids in the "injection" of effector proteins (e.g., Yops) into target cells; after "injection" into phagocytic cells, it reduces the excretion of proinflammatory cytokines and inhibits neutrophil chemotaxis. The genes encoding LcrV reside on the plasmid PYV (also known as pCD1). The genes residing on this plasmid encode Yops, LcrV, and the Type III secretion system. They are down regulated at 26°C, and up regulated at 37°C and low calcium.

3. Ymt. The genes encoding Ymt (for *Yersinia mouse toxin*) reside on the plasmid pMT (which also contains the genes for the capsule, see above). Ymt is a phospholipase D that is expressed at 25°C (and poorly at 37°C), and plays a role in protecting *Y. pestis* from the digestive enzymes within the midgut of fleas.

4. Pesticin. Pesticin is a bacteriocin produced by *Y. pestis* with an uncertain role in the production of disease. Genes on plasmid pPCP1 encode Pesticin (along with Plasminogen Activator).

5. Plasminogen Activator. Plasminogen Activator is responsible for the coagulase, fibrinolytic, and C3 degradative activity of *Y. pestis* at 37°C. Genes on plasmid pPCP1 encode Plasminogen Activator (along with Pesticin).

6. Coagulase. See "Plasminogen Activator," above.

7. Gsr. Gsr (for *global stress requirement*) is expressed at 37°C while *Y. pestis* is within the macrophage phagolysosome. The Gsr protein is responsible for the survival of *Y. pestis* within this environment.

Variability

Yersinia pestis is serologically uniform. There are three biotypes (based on carbohydrate fermentation and ability to reduce nitrate): Antiqua, Medievalis, and Orientalis.

Ecology

Reservoir

Tolerant rodents in endemic areas (see below) constitute the plague reservoir. They rarely develop fatal disease and are called *maintenance* or *enzootic* hosts. In North America along the coastal regions of California, the meadow mouse *Microtus californicus* is such a host.

Transmission

Transmission is by fleas. They may carry *Y. pestis* to more susceptible, epizootic, or amplification hosts, such as ground squirrels or rats. When these die, still other hosts, such as humans, are attacked. Infected mammals may spread plague by the airborne route. Oral acquisition is by predation, cannibalism, and scavenging.

Pathogenesis

Fleas feed on an infected host. *Yersinia pestis* inside fleas proliferate until they block (obstruct) the flea's proventriculus (function of Ymt and Hms). "Blocked" fleas infest a new host and contaminate the feeding site with *Y. pestis* when attempting to feed. At flea temperature, the Type III secretion system, Yops, LcrV, Caf1, and Gsr are not produced. The bacteria, thus introduced into a vertebrate host, lack defense against the host's innate immune system, and are killed when ingested by neutrophils (an inflammatory response is generated due to products of the flea bite along with the gram-negative cell wall components of *Y. pestis*). In mononuclear phagocytes, at mammalian temperatures, and low-calcium ion concentrations, and while protected by Gsr, *Y. pestis* activates the Type III secretion system; produces Yops, LcrV, and Caf1; and is released from the phagocytic cell following initiation of apoptosis. Yersiniae acquire resistance to further phagocytosis and intracellular killing by neutrophil and mononuclear phagocytes (LcrV reduces the excretion of proinflammatory cytokines, and inhibits neutrophil chemotaxis; "injected" Yops prevent phagocytosis; Caf1 prevents phagocytosis and promotes serum resistance). Thus, early in the disease process, *Y. pestis* is an intracellular parasite, and later, an extracellular one.

Extracellular multiplication made possible by iron acquisition systems and capsule production elicits a hemorrhagic inflammatory lesion, followed by local lymph node involvement (bubo). This form is called *bubonic plague.*

The infection commonly becomes septicemic and, if untreated, terminates fatally (an endotoxemia aided by the function of Plasminogen Activator, which accelerates initiation of disseminated intravascular coagulation, see Fig 8.1). Some individuals develop plague pneumonia and shed *Y. pestis* in sputum and droplet nuclei. Others contract primary pneumonic plague from this source and transmit it by the same route. Under epidemic conditions this form is nearly always fatal.

Among domestic animals, cats acquire natural clinical infection, often by ingestion of infected prey. Signs include regional (particularly mandibular) lymphadenitis, fever, depression, anorexia, sneezing, coughing, and occasionally central nervous system disturbances. Most cases end fatally. Lesions, mainly in the respiratory and alimentary tracts, include lymphadenitis, tonsillitis, cranial and cervical edema, and pneumonia.

Human plague has been traced to feline infections. Suspected inoculation routes are via cuts, bites, scratches, and airborne and flea-borne pathways, although the latter is unlikely since the cat flea (*Ctenocephalides felis*) does not become blocked.

Epidemiology

Plague is concentrated in certain endemic areas in southern and southeastern Asia, southern and west central Africa, western North America, and north central South America. Endemicity largely parallels presence of enzootic and epizootic rodent hosts. Human plague epidemics have historically been precipitated by importation of infected rats on board ships coming from endemic regions. Today, most human cases result from infection following contact with rural wild animals (sylvatic plague).

Plague is a disease of rodents. The organism is maintained in endemic hosts (certain species of *Microtus* and *Peromyscus*, i.e., voles and meadow mice). Endemic hosts are infected following the bite of infected fleas. Though endemic hosts are fairly resistant to development of serious disease, when their populations rapidly increase and spread of *Y. pestis* is rapid, die off of endemic hosts occurs. Infected fleas, having a shortage of preferred hosts, feed on epidemic, highly susceptible species such as prairie dogs, rats, mice, and ground squirrels. What constitutes an endemic host and an epidemic host is somewhat clouded since there is considerable overlap between the two.

In endemic areas, infections are clustered during the warm months. "Off-season" plague affects mostly persons handling infected rabbits, bobcats, and occasionally house cats. Carnivores such as canids (wild and domestic), bears, raccoons, and skunks, as well as raptors, seroconvert following infection (ingestion, flea bite), but rarely develop clinical disease. Cat fleas and dog fleas, *Ctenocephalides felis* and *C. canis*, respectively, do not transmit *Y. pestis* efficiently because neither flea becomes "blocked." Thus, infection of humans from an infected cat (rarely dog) occurs from infections of scratches or bites with infected saliva or from inhalation of infected droplets.

Immunologic Aspects

Specific resistance to plague probably requires antibody and cell-mediated responses. Capsular antigens (F1 antigen) evoke opsonin formation. Antibody to the LcrV antigen is protective. Disposal of intracellular organisms depends on activated macrophages. Immunity following recovery is good, but temporary. Detection of antibodies to *Y. pestis* in resistant species (e.g., canids) is a way of determining the presence of the organism in a particular environment.

Laboratory Diagnosis

Diagnostic attempts should be supervised by qualified public health personnel (see below). Samples from affected sites (i.e., edematous tissues, lymph nodes, and nasopharynx), transtracheal aspirates, cerebrospinal fluid, and blood (for culture and serology) are collected.

Direct smears are examined following immunofluorescent, Wayson's staining, or Gram staining. Culture is done on blood or infusion agar. Identification is confirmed by immunofluorescence or bacteriophage susceptibility. Mice or guinea pigs injected subcutaneously with *Y. pestis* die within 3 to 8 days. DNA techniques utilizing molecular probes or the amplification of specific DNA sequences by the polymerase chain reaction are available.

Serologic tests (hemagglutination, hemagglutination-inhibition, enzyme-linked immunosorbent assay [ELISA]) are useful for retrospective studies.

Treatment and Control

If plague is suspected in domestic cats, the following recommendations from the Centers for Disease Control apply:

1. Arrange immediately with local and state public health officials for laboratory diagnostic assistance and steps to prevent spread and contamination.
2. Place all suspect cats in strict isolation.
3. When handling such cats, wear gown, mask, and gloves.
4. Treat every suspect for fleas (5% carbaryl dust for residual effect).

Flea elimination should precede rodent control.

Aminoglycosides, chloramphenicol, fluoroquinolones, and tetracycline are effective antimicrobics.

No vaccines for animals are available. Protection of humans by bacterins is transient.

YERSINIA PSEUDOTUBERCULOSIS

Yersinia pseudotuberculosis is associated with mesenteric lymphadenitis, terminal ileitis, acute gastroenteritis, and septicemia, affecting mainly birds and rodents, and only occasionally domestic animals and primates. *Yersinia pseu-*

dotuberculosis is closely related to *Y. pestis,* and many consider *Y. pestis* to be a subspecies.

Descriptive Features

Cellular Composition and Products of Medical Importance

Yersinia pseudotuberculosis contains the plasmid pYV (encodes the Type III secretion system, Yops, and LcrV). A chromosomal locus called the *High Pathogenicity Island* contains the genes for iron uptake. Also located on the chromosome are the genes encoding the proteins Ail, Inv, YadA, and Gsr.

Adhesins. Yersinia pseudotuberculosis produces three adhesins that are responsible for adherence to ß integrins on the luminal surface of M cells and the basolateral surface of ileal epithelial cells —Ail, Inv, and Yad:

1. Ail (for *a*ttachment *i*nvasion *l*ocus) adheres to receptors on the surface of M cells. Ail also protects the outer membrane from insertion of the membrane attack complexes generated by activation of the complement system.
2. Inv (for *inv*asin) adheres to receptors on the surface of M cells and the basolateral surface of ileal epithelial cells.
3. Yad (for *y*ersinia *ad*hesin) adheres to receptors on the surface of M cells and the basolateral surface of ileal epithelial cells. Yad also protects the outer membrane from insertion of the membrane attack complexes generated by activation of the complement system.

Cell Wall. The cell wall of *Y. pseudotuberculosis* has O-antigens (smooth phenotype). The cell wall of the members of this genus is one typical of gram negatives. The lipopolysaccharide (LPS) in the outer membrane is an important virulence determinant. Not only is the lipid A component toxic (endotoxin), but the length of the side chain in the O-repeat unit hinders the attachment of the membrane attack complex of the complement system to the outer membrane. LPS binds to lipopolysaccharide-binding protein (a serum protein), which in turn transfers it to the blood phase of CD14. The CD14-LPS complex binds to Toll-like receptor proteins (see Chapter 2) on the surface of macrophage cells triggering the release of proinflammatory cytokines

High Pathogenicity Island. See above, *"Yersinia pestis,* Cellular Composition and Products of Medical Importance.".

Iron Acquisition. Iron is an absolute growth requirement, and must be removed from iron-binding proteins of the host. The genes encoding products involved with iron acquisition reside on a chromosomal pathogenicity island. The HPI of *Y. pseudotuberculosis* encodes the genes for the iron-acquiring siderophore yersiniabactin.

Type III Secretion System. See above, *"Yersinia pestis,* Cellular Composition and Products of Medical Importance."

Gsr (Global Stress Requirement). See above, *"Yersinia pestis,* Cellular Composition and Products of Medical Importance."

Toxins. Yersinia pseudotuberculosis produces toxins that are involved with pathogenicity:

1. Yops—See above, *"Yersinia pestis,* Cellular Composition and Products of Medical Importance."
2. LcrV—See above, *"Yersinia pestis,* Cellular Composition and Products of Medical Importance."

Variability

There are approximately 21 serotypes based on variability of the somatic (O) antigens.

Ecology

Reservoir

Yersinia pseudotuberculosis is a parasite of wild rodents, lagomorphs, and birds, but it infects other mammals and reptiles and persists in the environment. The cat is the most commonly infected domestic mammal. Minor epidemics occur among sheep, pigs, nonhuman primates, fowl, and pet birds.

Transmission

Exposure is primarily through ingestion.

Pathogenesis

Yersinia pseudotuberculosis attaches to M cells of lymphoid nodules of the distal small intestine following expression of the cell surface proteins Inv, Ail, and YadA. Attachment triggers actin cytoskeletal changes resulting in a "zippering" phenomenon that leads to the enclosure of the cell membrane around the attached yersiniae, resulting in their internalization. Internalized microorganisms pass through to the lymphoid nodule where they are phagocytosed by macrophages within the nodule. Expression of Gsr permits intracellular survival. Within macrophages (37°C, low calcium), the Type III secretion apparatus is activated, Yops and LcrV produced. Ingested yersinae are released after initiation of apoptosis of the macrophage. Now extracellular, yersiniae interfere with further phagocytosis. Invasion of the basolateral surface of ileal epithelial cells occurs following attachment of YadA and Inv, and internalization follows. Inflammation induced by extracellular yersiniae (lps), together with interferon secretion by natural killer cells and gamma delta T cell-recognition of infected epithelial cells (as well as lipopolysaccharide), results in an influx of polymorphonuclear neutrophil leukocytes (PMNs). Extracellular yersiniae avoid phagocytosis (Yops), and destruction by complement-mediated mechanisms by expression of Ail and YadA, both of which impart complement resistance. *Yersinia pseudotuberculosis* acquires iron from iron-binding proteins of the host following secretion of yersiniabactin (encoded within the HPI). Diarrhea is thought to result from prostaglandin synthesis by the recruited PMNs (and perhaps by the affected host cells), as well as activation of various inositol-signaling pathways within affected host cells. The net result is the secretion of chloride ions and water. Septicemia results from the host's inability to "clear" yersiniae from infected sites (serum resistance, antiphagocytic traits, and iron scavenging). The result is enteritis and septicemia.

Yersinia pseudotuberculosis causes intestinal infections with formation of necrotic foci in the intestinal wall, abdominal lymph nodes, and viscera, particularly liver and spleen. There may be vomiting, diarrhea, or constipation, and weight loss, pale to subicteric mucous membranes, and depression. Fever is inconsistent. Few cases are diagnosed clinically antemortem. Mastitis is seen in cattle and abortion in ruminants and monkeys. In immunocompetent humans, the disease is generally an enteritis and abdominal lymphadenitis that is self-limiting or responsive to treatment.

Epidemiology

Pseudotuberculosis occurs worldwide. Cases tend to cluster in the cold months. In cats, prevalence is biased toward adult, rural, outdoor cats.

Immunologic Aspects

Natural infection leaves surviving individuals immune. Avirulent live vaccine protects against homologous challenge. It is not available commercially.

Laboratory Diagnosis

Diagnosis involves isolation of the agent antemortem from feces or lymph node aspirates. Isolation, particularly from mixed sources, is enhanced by cold enrichment, that is, incubation of a 10% mixture of inoculum in a minimal medium for several weeks at 4°C. DNA techniques utilizing molecular probes or the amplification of specific DNA sequences by the polymerase chain reaction are available.

Treatment and Control

Pseudotuberculosis responds to the same antimicrobics as plague.

YERSINIA ENTEROCOLITICA

Yersinia enterocolitica is associated with mesenteric lymphadenitis, terminal ileitis, acute gastroenteritis, and septicemia in domestic animals and primates.

Descriptive Features

Cellular Composition and Products of Medical Importance

Yersinia enterocolitica contains the plasmid pYV (encodes the Type III secretion system, Yops, and LcrV). A chromo-

somal locus called the *High Pathogenicity Island* contains the genes for iron uptake. Also located on the chromosome are the genes encoding the proteins Ail, Inv, YadA, Gsr, and Yst.

Adhesins. See above, "*Yersinia pseudotuberculosis*, Cellular Composition and Products of Medical Importance."

Cell Wall. See above, "*Yersinia pseudotuberculosis*, Cellular Composition and Products of Medical Importance."

Gsr (Global Stress Requirement). See above, "*Yersinia pestis*, Cellular Composition and Products of Medical Importance."

High Pathogenicity Island. See above, "*Yersinia pestis*, Cellular Composition and Products of Medical Importance."

Iron Acquisition. See above, "*Yersinia pseudotuberculosis*, Cellular Composition and Products of Medical Importance."

Type III Secretion System. See above, "*Yersinia pestis*, Cellular Composition and Products of Medical Importance."

Toxins. *Yersinia enterocolitica* produces a number of toxins that are involved with pathogenicity:

1. Yops—See above, "*Yersinia pestis*, Cellular Composition and Products of Medical Importance."
2. LcrV—See above, "*Yersinia pestis*, Cellular Composition and Products of Medical Importance."
3. Yst (for *Yersinia stable toxin*)—Yst is a chromosomally encoded enterotoxin unique to *Y. enterocolitica*. Yst affects the guanylyl cyclase system by deregulating cGMP synthesis (increases in intracellular cGMP leads to the opening of chloride channels with the resultant flow of chloride and water into the intestinal lumen), resulting in fluid and electrolyte accumulation in the bowel lumen subsequent to blockage of sodium and chloride ion (and thus water) absorption (tip cells) and loss of chloride ions (crypt cells) (see also, ST enterotoxin of *Escherichia coli*, Chapter 8).

Variability

There are approximately 34 O-antigen and 20 H-antigen serogroups. O groups 3, 5, 27, 8, and 9 are associated with classical disease of the gastrointestinal tract. There are five biotypes.

Ecology

Reservoir and Transmission

Water, food, soil, fruits, vegetables, and asymptomatic individuals from humans to mollusks have been proposed as reservoirs for *Y. enterocolitica*. Expression of certain virulence determinants at 22°C to 25°C suggests that mammals acquire *Y. enterocolitica* from a "cold" source (water and food, for example) rather than a warm-blooded animal. Infection follows ingestion of organisms expressing the adhesin.

Transmission

Exposure is primarily through ingestion.

Pathogenesis

The pathogenesis of disease produced by *Y. enterocolitica* is the same as *Y. pseudotuberculosis* (see above). In addition to diarrhea associated with invasion of epithelial cells and inflammation (as with *Y. pseudotuberculosis*), *Y. enterocolitica* produces Yst.

Epidemiology

Certain serotypes are geographically restricted. O:8 is indigenous to the United States but not the rest of the world. O:3 until recently was rarely isolated in the United States but is common in the rest of the world, and is becoming more so in the United States. O:9 has not been reported outside of Europe.

The chief interest in animal yersiniosis derives from its possible epidemiologic relation to human yersinial infections. Outbreaks linked to animals and animal products have been rare. Serotyping and biotyping suggest that there is little relationship between animal strains and human disease isolates.

Immunologic Aspects

Yersinia enterocolitica is an extracellular microorganism. Phagocytic cells readily destroy it, even though the microorganism excretes proteins (Yops) that interfere with this process. Most often, *Y. enterocolitica* disease is self-limiting due to the innate immune response: phagocytosis, lysis of infected epithelial cells, iron sequestration, and complement proteins.

A serologic relationship between O:9 serotype, common in swine, and *Brucella* spp. has complicated swine brucellosis eradication programs.

Laboratory Diagnosis

Samples of feces, lymph node biopsy, and biopsy from affected tissues are examined microbiologically. Selective media containing bile salts are somewhat inhibitory to *Y. enterocolitica*; especially at 37°C. MacConkey agar is least inhibitory. There are special media designed for the isolation of *Y. enterocolitica* (e.g., CIN medium). Cold enrichment of the sample at 4°C aids in attempts to isolate small numbers of *Y. enterocolitica* from a contaminated environment. Isolation from tissue necessitates the use of blood agar plates incubated at 37°C. DNA techniques utilizing molecular probes or the amplification of specific DNA sequences by the polymerase chain reaction are available.

Treatment and Control

Antimicrobial agents useful for treating disease produced by *Y. enterocolitica* are the fluoroquinolones, tetracycline, trimethoprim-sulfonamides, and chloramphenicol. R plasmids are common in *Y. enterocolitica*, and genes encoding resistance to tetracycline and streptomycin are most commonly found.

YERSINIA RUCKERI

"Enteric redmouth" is a hemorrhagic inflammation of the perioral subcutis of freshwater fish, particularly rainbow trout. Infection is systemic and causes significant mortality in hatcheries of North America, Australia, and Europe. The agent is disseminated by asymptomatic carrier fish and possibly riparian mammals (muskrats). Outbreaks appear to be related to massive exposure.

The pathogenesis of this disease has not been described. A protease, Yrp (*Yersinia ruckeri* protease) appears to play an important role since inactivation of the encoding gene significantly reduces virulence.

Outbreaks are brought under control with antimicrobics (e.g., sulfonamides, tetracycline, trimethoprim-sulfonamide), and bacterins have been successful in lowering mortality.

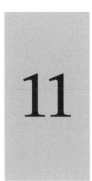

11   *Enterobacteriaceae: Shigella*

Dwight C. Hirsh

Members of the genus *Shigella* belong to the family *Enterobacteriaceae*, and cause bacillary dysentery in primates. The discussion that follows is limited to the disease in nonhuman primates. The disease occurs almost exclusively in captive primates and appears to be related to stressful situations (e.g., transportation, crowding) or immunological dysfunctions (e.g., simian acquired immunodeficiency syndrome). Humans may be affected by all four species of shigellae, *S. dysenteriae*, *S. flexneri*, *S. boydii*, and *S. sonnei*, whereas nonhuman primates are affected by *S. flexneri*, *S. boydii*, and *S. sonnei*.

Descriptive Features

Cellular Anatomy and Composition

The anatomy of the members of the genus *Shigella* is typical for the family *Enterobacteriaceae*. However, they possess neither capsules (K antigens) nor flagella (H antigens). All express adhesins (IpaD) and a typical gram-negative cell wall composed of lipopolysaccharides (O-antigen) and proteins.

There are four serotypes, identification of which is dependent upon the composition of the O-repeat units of the lipopolysaccharide (LPS). Each of the four serotypes has been given species designation. Within each species there are a number of serotypes (Table 11.1). Conversion of one serotype to another is under the regulation of the genes contained within a Pathogenicity Island (Shi-0 for *Shi*gella *I*sland) a cluster of genes encoding virulence determinant(s), an integrase protein, a specific insertion site, and mobility. In the case of Shi-0, the genes are contained within a defective (immobile) lysogenic bacteriophage, so the serological traits are stable.

Cellular Products of Medical Interest

Adhesins. A surface protein, IpaD (for *i*nvasion *p*rotein *a*ntigen) is responsible for adherence of shigellae to ß integrins on the surface of M cells, and the basolateral surface of large intestinal epithelial cells.

Cell Wall. The cell wall of the members of this genus is one typical of gram negatives. The lipopolysaccharide (LPS) in the outer membrane is an important virulence determinant. Not only is the lipid A component toxic (endotoxin), but the length of the side chain in the O-repeat unit hinders the attachment of the membrane attack complex of the complement system to the outer membrane.

LPS binds to lipopolysaccharide-binding protein (a serum protein), which in turn transfers it to the blood phase of CD14. The CD14-LPS complex binds to Toll-like receptor proteins (see Chapter 2) on the surface of macrophage cells triggering the release of proinflammatory cytokines

"Invasion" Proteins. Virulence factors (invasion proteins) produced by members of this genus are mainly encoded on large plasmids (termed *invasion plasmids*). These genes, for the most part, are regulated by at least six chromosomal genes. The plasmid gene products encode proteins that are responsible for a Type III excretion apparatus whereby some invasion proteins (Ipa for *i*nvasion *p*lasmid *a*ntigen) are "injected" into host cells, namely IpaB,C. The Type III secretion system consists of an assemblage of proteins (more than 20) that form a hollow tube-like structure through which effector proteins are "injected" into host "target" cells:

1. IpaB. "Injection" of IpaB (like IpaC) into the host target cell leads to activation of small GTP-binding proteins of the Rho family resulting in cytoskeletal changes and the formation of "ruffles." IpaB also is responsible for lysis of the membrane of the phagosome containing entrapped shigellae. Within macrophages, IpaB activates caspase-1 resulting in apoptosis.
2. IpaC. "Injection" of IpaC (like IpaB) leads to activation of small GTP-binding proteins of the Rho family resulting in cytoskeletal changes and the formation of "ruffles."
3. IcsA. The surface protein IcsA (for *i*ntra*c*ellular *s*pread) is required for intracellular spread. IcsA is required and is sufficient for actin deposition and motility when shigellae are within host epithelial cells.
4. IcsB. The surface protein IcsB (for *i*nter*c*ellular *s*pread) is for intercellular spread.

Enterotoxins. Two enterotoxins have been described, ShET1 (*Sh*igella *e*nterotoxin, encoded within the chromosomal Pathogenicity Island, Shi-1—a cluster of genes encoding virulence determinant(s), an integrase protein, a specific insertion site, and mobility) and a 63kDa product of the *sen* gene (*S*higella *en*terotoxin, encoded on the invasion plasmid). How these proteins elicit fluid secretion is not known.

Exotoxins. Shigella dysenteriae is the only member of the group that has the genes necessary for production of shiga toxin. Shiga toxin is chromosomally encoded. The toxin is

Table 11.1. Species of *Shigella*

Species	Group (Types)
S. dysenteriae	A (1–10)
S. flexneri	B (1–6)
S. boydii	C (1–15)
S. sonnei	D (1)

a protein of 70,000MW composed of an A subunit (32,000MW) and five identical B subunits (each about 7700MW). The target cells for the toxin are the endothelial cells that line blood vessels. Receptors on these cells are recognized by the B subunit. The toxin, by way of the A subunit, inhibits peptide chain elongation at the level of the ribosome by affecting elongation factor 1-dependent processes. This action results in the death of the cell. The production of toxin is iron-regulated (by way of *Fur*, see below), more being produced in conditions of low iron concentration. The virulence of a particular strain or isolate is directly related to the amount of toxin produced.

Other Exotoxins. Shigellae produce at least two other exotoxins that, at least theoretically, play a role in pathogenesis. These two proteins are SigA and Pic:

1. SigA (for *Shigella IgA* protease). SigA is postulated to play a role by inactivating *Shigella*-specific IgA in the intestinal tract, thereby allowing the disease process to progress. SigA is encoded within the chromosomal Pathogenicity Island, Shi-1.
2. Pic (for *p*rotein involved in *i*ntestinal *c*olonization). Pic is a serine protease, which is thought to digest intestinal mucus that overlays the intestinal epithelial cells so that shigellae have access to host "target" cells. The genes encoding Pic are within the chromosomal Pathogenicity Island, Shi-1.

Regulatory Genes. Shigellae possess a number of genes whose activation results from certain environmental cues. These include Fur and an RNA polymerase containing RpoS:

1. Fur (*f*erric *u*tilization *r*esponse-iron levels). The Fur system "senses" available iron concentration, and when low (as would be inside the host, since most iron is bound to host iron-binding proteins), activates the synthesis and secretion of the siderophore, aerobactin, and shiga toxin (see above). Genes within the Pathogenicity Island Shi-2 encode Fur.
2. RNA polymerase. RNA polymerase containing RpoS preferentially transcribes genes responsible for acid tolerance (survival at pH 5), permitting safe transit through the stomach.

Variability

Shigellae are "typed" based upon the makeup of the O-antigen (species designation). Within each species, there are a number of serotypes (see Table 11.1).

Ecology

Reservoir

The reservoir for members of the genus *Shigella* is the large bowel of clinically ill, recovered, or asymptomatic primates

Transmission

The disease is transmitted by the fecal-oral route, but the infective dose is so small that fomites may also play a role. Members of the genus *Shigella* are greatly influenced by the colonization resistance (a measurement of the "barrier" effect the normal flora has in excluding "foreign" microorganisms from the tract) in the large bowel. Antimicrobial drugs, stress, or dietary changes promote risk by reducing colonization resistance (by decreasing the numbers of the normal flora resulting in a reduction of the "barrier"), which may lead to disease in asymptomatic carrier animals or by lowering the oral dose needed for infection and subsequent disease.

The mode of transmission of *S. flexneri* 4 associated with periodontal disease of nonhuman primates is unknown, but it is assumed to be feces.

Pathogenesis

Environmental cues trigger the expression and excretion of virulence proteins. Ingested shigellae safely traverse the stomach (RpoS directed acid tolerance response). The target cells are the apical surface of M cells in the large intestine to which shigellae attach by way of IpaD after digestion of the overlying mucus layer (Pic). Cell-associated bacteria are trapped in the "ruffles" formed following the "injection" of IpaB,C by way of the Type III secretion system. Some of the shigellae within the vacuole are transported into the nodule, where the uptake is again triggered, but by macrophages within the nodule. Ingested shigellae may initiate apoptosis of the macrophage (IpaB) and/or other abnormalities reflected in a drop in concentration of intracellular adenosine triphosphate (ATP). Either effect results in the death of the macrophage. The liberated shigellae adhere to the basolateral surface of the colonic epithelial cell (IpaD) and induce their own uptake as before. Shigellae escape the vacuole by secretion of IpaB resulting in the deposition of the microorganism into the cytoplasm of the epithelial cell. Expression of Ics and formation of actin at one pole of the bacterium results in intracellular movement. Movement appears to be more concentrated along actin "stress fibers" and shigellae with their actin "tails" move toward cadherin proteins marking intercellular bridges. Thus, shigellae move laterally. IcsB lyses the double membrane resulting from movement between cells. Affected host cells together with dead and dying macrophages secrete various chemokines (including IL-1 and IL-18), which results in an intense inflammatory response. Likewise, extracellular shigellae also initiate inflammation (by virtue of their LPS). Transepithelial migration of polymorphonuclear neutrophil leukocytes (PMNs) is stimulated by LPS. Natural Killer cells have been implicated in lysis of infected epithelial cells, another inflammation-inducing process. Tissue destruction with numerous PMNs is the hallmark of dysentery caused by shigellae. The origin of hemorrhage produced by non-shiga toxin-producing shigellae is not known, but the tissue destruction, which includes endothelial cell damage, is probably responsible. PMNs phagocytose and destroy shigellae, limiting the process to the intestinal tract.

Diarrhea is brought about by the activation of phospholipase C (perhaps due to "ruffle" formation) leading to increases in intracellular calcium ions, activation of protein kinase C and subsequent phosphorylation of proteins of the chloride ion channels and those of the membrane-associated ion transport proteins involved in NaCl absorption. These activities lead to diarrhea.

The role of enterotoxin in this disease is unclear. The diarrhea, sometimes watery, may be caused by interactions of enterotoxin with small intestinal epithelial cells and in part be due to changes in the colonic epithelium brought about by the invasion/inflammatory process.

Shigella dysenteriae produces shiga toxin. This toxin damages submucosal endothelial cells (hemorrhage) and may cause the development of hemolytic uremic syndrome (HUS) (see Chapter 8).

Shigella flexneri 4 has been encountered in periodontal disease of monkeys. A causal role is suspected but undefined.

Epidemiology

The disease is seen almost exclusively in captive primates.

Immunologic Aspects

Protection from bacillary dysentery is by specific secretory immunoglobulin found on the luminal side of the intestinal canal. These antibodies prevent adherence and subsequent uptake. Shigellae are serum-sensitive (i.e., they are quickly destroyed by complement-generated membrane attack complexes), and PMNs deal with them effectively. As a result, extracellular shigellae (those outside of the M cell, macrophage, and colonic epithelial cell) are dealt with effectively by complement proteins in tissue fluids, and the constituents of the inflammatory exudate (complement proteins and PMNs).

Whether nonhuman primates after infection and disease are resistant to reinfection (exacerbation) is not known. Reinfection or exacerbation occurs in human beings in stressful situations such as in prisoner-of-war camps. Bacterins given orally or parenterally have been ineffective. Some protection has been demonstrated following vaccination with avirulent, live oral vaccines. These are not universally available.

Laboratory Diagnosis

Rectal swabs or samples of feces obtained from the rectum are collected for laboratory diagnosis. Direct examination of stained smears of fecal material will reveal the presence of inflammatory cells, cellular debris, and red blood cells (RBCs). Such a finding is not diagnostic, however, since enteritis produced by *Campylobacter* results in the same signs. The presence of curved rods in the direct smear suggests that *Campylobacter* is the cause of the disease.

The sample is plated onto a selective medium that is less inhibitory than media for isolation of salmonellae. Suitable media include MacConkey agar, XLD agar, and Hektoen Enteric medium. SS agar is often too inhibitory for some strains of shigellae, and brilliant green does not work at all. For enrichment, GN broth is preferred. Selenite or tetrathionate broths do not enrich for shigellae.

Shigellae appear as lactose-nonfermenting colonies on lactose-containing media. Although some species (*S. sonnei* and *S. boydii* 9) ferment this sugar, not enough is fermented within the 24- to 48-hour incubation period to affect the selection of appropriate colonies for further testing. Suspicious colonies are tested directly with shigellae-specific antisera or inoculated into differential media and then tested with antisera.

Primers have been designed to amplify (by the polymerase chain reaction) DNA specific for shigellae. This assay has been used to detect and identify members of this genus.

Treatment, Control, and Prevention

Treatment of shigellosis involves nursing and supporting care. Antimicrobics are indicated in serious cases but not routinely since their use in an animal facility selects for resistant strains. Trimethoprim-sulfonamide, or a fluoroquinolone, is effective against most strains and these drugs do not disrupt the normal flora (colonization resistance) as much as other antimicrobials. The yeast *Saccharomyces boulardii* has been shown to reduce susceptibility of experimental animals to challenge by *Shigella flexneri*, supposedly by interfering with attachment of shigellae to host target cells.

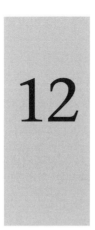

12

Pasteurellaceae: Pasteurella, Mannheimia

Dwight C. Hirsh   Ernst L. Biberstein

The family *Pasteurellaceae* contains the genera *Actinobacillus, Gallibacterium, Haemophilus, Histophilus, Lonepinella, Mannheimia, Pasteurella,* and *Phocoenobacter*. All but *Lonepinella* (*L. koalarum*—a tannin degrading bacterium isolated from normal Koala feces) and *Gallibacterium* (*G. anatis*—isolated from the intestine of normal ducks) contain species that are of medical importance.

All the members of the family *Pasteurellaceae* are gramnegative coccobacilli. They are facultative anaerobes, and typically oxidase-positive (which sets them apart from members of the family *Enterobacteriaceae*). Most are commensal parasites of animals.

The genus *Pasteurella*, particularly *P. haemolytica*, has undergone extensive taxonomic changes over the past several years. *Pasteurella haemolytica* at one time contained 17 capsular types, and 2 biotypes (A for arabinose fermentation, and T for trehalose fermentation). Thus, each strain of *P. haemolytica* was identified by a letter (either an A or T) designating the biotype, and a number (1–17) designating the capsular type. For example, *P. haemolytica* of the A biotype possessing a type 1 capsule was designated as *P. haemolytica* A1. Genetic analysis showed that all of the A biotypes comprised a new and separate genus, designated as *Mannheimia*. Thus, all but one of the *P haemolytica* A biotypes became *Mannheimia haemolytica*. The one exception, *P. haemolytica* A11, became a different species, *M. glucosida*. All of the T biotypes were placed into a new species, *P. trehalosi*. Consequently, "*Pasteurella haemolytica*" is obsolete.

Discussed in this chapter are the genera *Pasteurella* and *Mannheimia*, whose members play an important role in diseases of several animal species (Table 12.1). *Photobacterium damsela* (previously *Pasteurella piscicida*) and *Riemerella anatipestifer* (previously *Pasteurella anatipestifer*) will be discussed briefly, as will Eugonic fermentor 4 (EF-4) a bacterium that resembles *Pasteurella*.

Descriptive Features

Morphology and Staining

Members of the genera *Pasteurella* and *Mannheimia* are gram-negative coccobacilli measuring 0.2 µm by up to 2.0 µm. Bipolarity, that is, the staining of only the tips of cells, is demonstrable with polychrome stains (e.g., Wright's stain).

Structure and Composition

Capsules contain acidic polysaccharides. The capsule of *P. multocida* type A is made of hyaluronic acid, the capsule of type D is made of heparin, and the capsule of type F is made of chondroitin (see below, "Variability," for discussion of *P. multocida* capsule nomenclature). Some *P. multocida* and *M. haemolytica* strains express adhesins.

Cell walls are typical of gram-negative microorganisms consisting mainly of lipopolysaccharides and proteins. Some of the latter are iron-regulated (i.e., they are expressed under iron-poor conditions).

Cellular Products of Medical Interest

Adhesins. Some, and probably all members of the family *Pasteurellaceae* produce adhesins (and possibly more than one kind). A type 4 fimbria (adhesin) has been described for avian strains of *P. multocida*, and an *adh*esin (termed Adh1) is expressed by *M. haemolytica*. As with other microorganisms, the expression of adhesins probably depends upon environmental cues. That is, adhesins are expressed while the microorganism inhabits an epithelial surface, but repressed when the microorganism is inside the host where adherence to a phagocytic cell could be disastrous. *Mannheimia haemolytica* and *P. trehalosi* produce fibrinogen-binding proteins. The role of these proteins is unclear at present, but in the streptococci (see Chapter 28) fibrinogen-binding proteins impart an antiphagocytic property to the streptococcal particle by "coating" the bacterial cell, thereby "covering" sites for complement activation (and thus decrease opsonization, and the generation of functional membrane attack complexes) as well as those recognized by serum proteins (collectins/ficollins) that opsonize foreign particles. The hyaluronic acid capsule of type A strains *P. multocida* serves as an adhesin probably similar to hyaluronic acid encapsulated *Streptococcus pyogenes* (Chapter 28), which binds to human epithelial cells via CD44, a hyaluronic acid–binding glycoprotein.

Capsule. The capsule plays many roles, the most important of which are interference with phagocytosis (antiphagocytic) and the protection of the outer membrane from the deposition of membrane attack complexes generated by activation of the complement system. The amount of capsule produced is inversely proportional to the amount of available iron. In vivo, where the amount of

Table 12.1.   Members of the Genera *Pasteurella, Mannheimia, Gallibacterium*, and *Phocoenobacter* and Their Usual Source or Associated Condition

Species	Usual Source or Associated Condition
Pasteurella aerogenes	Associated with gastroenteritis in swine; abortion in swine; fowl
P. avium	Respiratory tract of fowl
P. bettyae (CDC Group HB-5)	Human Bartholin gland abscess; septicemia in immunocompromised patients; periparturient septicemia in human infants
P. caballi	Pneumonia and associated conditions in horses
P. canis	Pneumonia in dogs; other "mouth" related conditions in dogs
P. dagmatis	Respiratory tract of dogs; respiratory tract of fowl
P. gallinarum	Respiratory tract of fowl
P. langaa	Respiratory tract of fowl
P. lymphangitis	Bovine lymphangitis
P. mairi	Abortion in swine; septicemia in piglets
P. multocida	Pneumonia and respiratory conditions in ruminants, swine, dogs, and cats; other "mouth" related conditions of dogs and cats; septicemia in ruminants; septicemia in fowl; abscesses and pneumonia in rabbits
P. pneumotropica	Pneumonia in rodents
P. stomatis	Pneumonia in dogs; other "mouth" related conditions in dogs
P. skyensis	Septicemia in farmed Atlantic salmon
P. testudinis	Respiratory tracts of desert tortoise and box turtles
P. trehalosi (*P. haemolytica* T-strains)	Pneumonia and septicemia in ruminants
P. volantium	Wattles of fowl
Mannheimia haemolytica (*Pasteurella haemolytica*)	Pneumonia and respiratory conditions in ruminants
M. granulomatis	Panniculitis in ruminants; respiratory conditions in ruminants, deer, and hares
M. glucosida	Respiratory conditions of ruminants
M. ruminalis	Normal flora of rumen
M. varigena	Respiratory tract conditions of ruminants and swine; septicemia in ruminants and swine; mastitis in cattle
Gallibacterium anatis (*Pasteurella anatis*)	Intestinal contents of normal ducks
Phocoenobacter uteri	Uterus of harbor porpoise

available iron is low, the amount of capsule formed is less (but sufficient to protect the microorganism from phagocytosis and complement-mediated lysis). *Pasteurella multocida* type A capsules are made of hyaluronic acid, type D capsules are made of heparin, and type F capsules are made of chondroitin (see below, "Variability," for discussion of *P. multocida* capsule nomenclature). These substances are similar (if not identical) to host tissue components, and are thus poorly antigenic, as well as binding complement components poorly (and are therefore, antiphagocytic). The hyaluronic acid capsule also serves as an adhesin for respiratory tract epithelial cells as in the case of capsule type A strains of *P. multocida* (see above).

Cell Wall. Lipopolysaccharide (LPS) elicits an inflammatory response following binding to lipopolysaccharide-binding protein (a serum protein), which in turn transfers it to the blood phase of CD14. The CD14-LPS complex binds to Toll-like receptor proteins (see Chapter 2) on the surface of macrophage cells triggering the release of proinflammatory cytokines. In addition, LPS is not only directly toxic to respiratory tract epithelial cells, but also acts synergistically with the *M. haemolytica* leukotoxin that affects alveolar macrophages (see below).

Toxins. Mannheimia and *Pasteurella* produce a number of proteins with toxic activity. At least two of these are important in the pathogenesis of disease (i.e., reduction of virulence results from inability to produce these toxins): an RTX, and a Rho activating toxin:

1. RTX toxin. The RTX (repeats in *toxin*, so called because of the common feature of repeats in glycine-rich sequences within the protein) type of toxin is a leukotoxin (Lkt) produced by *M. haemolytica, P. trehalosi*, and *P. glucosida* (a comparable toxin is produced by *P. aerogenes, P. mairi*, and *M. varigena*). Though similar in amino acid sequence to other members of the RTX family (see also *Escherichia* hemolysins in Chapter 8, *Actinobacillus* haemolysin in Chapter 13, adenylyl cyclase toxin of *Bordetella* in Chapter 15, *Moraxella* cytotoxin in Chapter 19), Lkt specifically affects bovine leukocytes, and erythrocytes. The effect on erythrocytes probably has little importance in vivo, but is responsible for the hemolysis observed when *M. haemolytica, P. trehalosi*, and *P. glucosida* are grown on blood agar plates. Lkt binds to CD18 (a β_2 integrin), which is expressed on

the surface of bovine leukocytes (neutrophils, macrophages, platelets, and lymphocytes). At low concentrations, Lkt causes target cell activation, at higher concentrations, apoptosis is initiated, and at very high concentrations, necrosis is produced (due to production of transmembrane pores). Upon contact with Lkt, neutrophils degranulate releasing potent enzymes that produce as well as aggravate inflammation, macrophages release proinflammatory cytokines (magnified in the presence of LPS), lymphocytes undergo apoptosis and necrosis, and platelets respond by increased adhesion. In addition, tissue mast cells degranulate releasing vasoactive amines. In summary, LKT drives a tissue-destroying inflammatory response.

2. Rho activating toxin. The Rho activating toxin is produced by *P. multocida* capsule type D, (see below, "Variability," for discussion of *P. multocida* capsule nomenclature) associated with Atrophic Rhinitis of swine. The toxin, Pmt (*P. multocida* toxin), stimulates two different signaling proteins: the small GTPase Rho, and heterodimeric G proteins. Unlike similar toxins (CNF produced by *Escherichia coli*, see Chapter 8, and dermonecrotic toxin produced by *Bordetella bronchiseptica*, see Chapter 15), Pmt does not enzymatically affect either of these regulatory proteins. However, the interaction of Pmt with either results in toxicity mediated by increases in intracellular calcium. In addition, Pmt binds to vimentin, an intracellular intermediate filament responsible for providing mechanical strength to the cell.

3. Miscellaneous toxins. Some strains of *P. multocida* produce hyaluronidase and neuraminidase. The role played by these enzymes in the pathogenesis of disease is unclear. It is tempting to speculate that hyaluronidase is active in vivo and may be responsible for the microorganism's ability to "spread" through tissue. Neuraminidase has been postulated to play a role in the colonization of epithelial surfaces by removing terminal sialic acid residues from mucin, thereby modifying normal host innate immunity.

Iron Acquisition. Because iron is an absolute growth requirement, microorganisms must acquire this substance if they are to exist within the host. Some avian strains of *P. multocida* produce a siderophore, multicidin, which is neither a phenolate nor hydroxynate type siderophore. Siderophores have not been demonstrated in *Pasteurella* or *Mannheimia* from other sources or species. However, *Pasteurella* and *Mannheimia* bind transferrin-iron complexes by virtue of iron-regulated outer membrane proteins expressed under iron-poor conditions (so-called *transferrin-binding proteins*, or Tbps). Iron is acquired from the transferrin-iron complexes that bind to the surface of the microorganism. *Pasteurella multocida* also binds heme and hemoglobin, which are other possible sources of iron.

Miscellaneous Products. Some avian strains of *P. multocida* express an outer-membrane protein that is toxic to phagocytic cells. It is unclear what role this protein might play in the pathogenesis of disease. If capsule formation is down regulated in vivo due to low available iron concentrations, then the toxic outer membrane protein might serve to protect the microorganism from phagocytosis.

Growth Characteristics

Pasteurella and *Mannheimia* grow best in the presence of serum or blood. After overnight incubation (35–37°C), colonies are about 1mm in diameter, clear, and smooth or mucoid. *Mannheimia haemolytica*, *P. trehalosi*, and *P. glucosida* produce hemolysis on ruminant blood agar. All are gram-negative, nonmotile coccobacilli. They are facultative anaerobes, typically oxidase-positive, reduce nitrates, and attack carbohydrates fermentatively.

Resistance

Cultures die within 1 or 2 weeks. Disinfectants, heat (50°C for 30 minutes), and ultraviolet light are promptly lethal. *Pasteurella multocida* survives for months in bird carcasses.

Pasteurella and *Mannheimia*, especially from food animals, have become increasingly resistant to penicillins, tetracyclines, and sulfonamides, to which they were originally susceptible. The gene encoding tetracycline resistance is unique to *Pasteurella* and *Mannheimia*. Resistance encoding genes are frequently associated with R plasmids.

Variability

Pasteurella multocida consists of five capsular (A, B, D, E, F) and 11 somatic (1–11) serotypes occurring in 20 different combinations. Serotypes are often related to host specificity and pathogenicity. The serotype is designated with a letter designating the capsule type and a number designating the somatic type, e.g., A:1.

Mannheimia haemolytica consists of 12 capsular types (1, 2, 5-9, 12–14, 16, 17), *P. trehalosi*, four. (3, 4, 10, 15).

Ecology

Reservoir

Pasteurella and *Mannheimia* are carried on mucous membranes (most commonly in the oropharyngeal region) of susceptible host species (adherence to these surfaces is due to adhesins). Carriage may be widespread, as with *P. multocida* in carnivores, or exceptional, as with avian cholera-producing strains in birds or hemorrhagic septicemia-producing strains in ruminants. In avian cholera, one host species may serve as reservoir for another.

Transmission

Infection is by inhalation, ingestion, or bites and scratch wounds. Many infections are probably endogenous. In bovine hemorrhagic septicemia and avian cholera, environmental contamination contributes to indirect transmission.

Pathogenesis

Mechanisms. In general, there are three manifestations of *Pasteurella/Mannheimia*-induced disease: respiratory tract involvement, septicemia, and trauma-associated conditions:

1. Respiratory tract involvement is either pneumonia or upper tract disease (Atrophic Rhinitis in swine). Pneumonia is seen most frequently in ruminants and is usually associated with *M. haemolytica*, *P. multocida*, or *P. trehalosi*. Environmental stress (e.g., shipping, weaning), virus infection, or other bacterial infections (e.g., *Mycoplasma*) usually precede pneumonia, and are thought to decrease host defenses of the tract allowing commensal bacteria living in the upper tract (most commonly *M. haemolytica*, *P. multocida*, or *P. trehalosi*) to infect the lung (Table 12.2). *Mannheimia haemolytica/P. trehalosi* from the upper respiratory tract is deposited in the lung, and secrete Lkt and, along with LPS from their cell walls, initiate an intense inflammatory response with fibrin deposition. Though *P. multocida* has not been shown to produce Lkt, its deposition in the lung initiates an inflammatory response by virtue of having LPS. Capsule, iron-scavenging abilities, and perhaps binding of fibrinogen enhance survival of the bacteria within the lesion.

    Upper tract disease is limited to Atrophic Rhinitis of swine. The serious (or progressive) form of this disease is one in which *Bordetella bronchiseptica* (see Chapter 15) first adheres to the nasal mucosa, and secretes a toxin, called dermonecrotic toxin, which mildly damages the epithelium. Capsule type D strains of *P. multocida* adhere to this mildly damaged epithelium and secrete Pmt (these strains do not readily adhere to a normal epithelium). It is Pmt that is responsible for the destruction of the nasal turbinates. The action of *B. bronchiseptica* toxin alone, without the participation of *P. multocida*, results in a mild, nonprogressive turbinate hypoplasia.

2. Septicemic disease produced by members of the family *Pasteurellaceae* is almost exclusively caused by *Pasteurella* in ruminants (hemorrhagic septicemia in cattle; septicemia in sheep) or in avian species (avian cholera). Why these strains produce septicemia is not understood. However, capsule and iron scavenging are crucial for survival of the organisms within the host. Outer membrane proteins on avian strains of *P. multocida* appear to play some role by decreasing phagocytosis. Signs and outcome of this disease are attributable to endotoxemia (see Fig 8.1).

3. Trauma-related conditions are those in which "mouth" microorganisms (*Pasteurella* is the most common) are inoculated into the site of infection. Examples include bite wounds, licking compromised sites (e.g., a surgical wound).

Pathology. Lesions vary with site of infection, virulence of strains, and host resistance. In septicemias, vascular damage results in hemorrhage and fluid loss but little cellular inflammatory response. Focal necrosis in parenchymatous organs or ulcerations of mucous membranes may occur. Mammals develop generalized hemorrhagic lymphadenopathy.

In most pneumonias, inflammatory cells are prominent, with erythrocytes, neutrophils, and mononuclear cells appearing and predominating successively. The tissue appearance changes accordingly from reddish-black to red, pink, and gray. Necrosis, abscess formation, and fibrin deposition vary in severity. In chronic fowl cholera, caseopurulent inflammation occurs in joints, middle ear, ovaries, or wattles.

Atrophic rhinitis of pigs (see also under *Bordetella bronchiseptica*, Chapter 15) is a chronic rhinitis accompanying disturbed osteogenesis adjacent to the inflamed areas. Increased osteoclastic and diminished osteoblastic activity destroys the turbinates and bones of the snout, resulting in distortions of facial structures (see Fig 73.1). Histologically, fibrous tissue replaces osseous tissue. Bone atrophy is accompanied by inflammation of varying acuteness.

The pathology of lesions that are "mouth" related is unremarkable with neutrophils predominating.

Disease Patterns

Cattle. *Pneumonia.* The most common form of bovine "pasteurellosis," involving *M. haemolytica*, *P. multocida*, or *P. trehalosi*, is shipping fever, a fibrinous pleuropneumonia or bronchopneumonia seen wherever cattle, especially calves, are transported, assembled, and handled under stressful conditions (see Figs 73.6 and 73.7). While the ultimate cause is uncertain (see Table 12.2), the agents pro-

Table 12.2. Etiologic and Possible Contributory Factors in Bovine Shipping Fever (after C.A. Hjerpe)[c]

Bacteria[a]	Mycoplasmas	Viruses[b]	Environmental Stress
Mannheimia haemolytica	Mycoplasma bovis	Infectious bovine rhinotracheitis virus)	Exhaustion, starvation, dehydration, weaning, ration changes,
Pasteurella multocida	Mycoplasma dispar	Parainfluenza-3	overcrowding, chilling, overheating, excess or irregular
Histophilus somni	Ureaplasma	Bovine respiratory syncytial virus	high-energy feed, poor ventilation, excess humidity, non-
			respiratory disease, castration, dehorning, social maladjustment

[a] Other bacteria uncommonly associated: *Salmonella, Streptococcus, Staphylococcus aureus, Escherichia. coli, Arcanobacterium. pyogenes,* obligate anaerobes, *Chlamydia.*
[b] Other viruses uncommonly associated: bovine virus diarrhea virus, adenovirus, rhinovirus, reovirus, herpesvirus, enterovirus, calicivirus, and coronavirus.
[c] Hjerpe, CA. Bovine respiratory disease complex. Curr Vet Ther 1986;2:670.

ducing severe illness and death are bacteria, most commonly and acutely *M. haemolytica* capsule type 1.

The onset, 1 to 2 weeks after stress, is marked by fever, inappetence, and listlessness. Respiratory signs (nasal discharge, cough) are few and variable. At more advanced stages, the fever may drop but respiratory distress will be obvious. Abnormal lung sounds can be detected, especially over the apical lobes, which are first and most severely affected.

Hemorrhagic Septicemia. Hemorrhagic septicemia is an acute systemic infection with *P. multocida*, serotype B:2 (Southern and Southeast Asia) or E:2 (Africa), occurring in tropical areas as seasonal epidemics with high morbidity and mortality. Signs include high fever, depression, subcutaneous edema, hypersalivation and diarrhea, or sudden death. All excretions and secretions are highly infectious.

Mastitis. *Mannheimia haemolytica* may cause mastitis with much tissue destruction, hemorrhage, and systemic toxic complications, which are often fatal. A somewhat less severe form is caused by *P. multocida*.

Sheep and Goats.   *Septicemia.* Septicemic pasteurellosis, usually due to *P. trehalosi* in feeder lambs and *M. haemolytica* in nursing lambs, resembles bovine hemorrhagic septicemia, although intestinal involvement is often absent and the morbidity rate is much lower.

Enzootic Pneumonia. Enzootic pneumonia of sheep is the ovine equivalent of bovine shipping fever. *Mannheimia haemolytica* is most often involved.

Mastitis. Gangrenous mastitis due to *M. haemolytica* (usual) or *P. trehalosi* occurs late in lactation, when large lambs bruise the udder and provide the inoculum from their oropharyngeal flora. Acute systemic reactions accompany disease of the udder, parts of which undergo necrosis ("blue bag") and may slough.

Swine.   *Atrophic Rhinitis.* Atrophic rhinitis of young pigs (3 weeks to 7 months) leading to turbinate destruction and secondary complications results from synergistic nasal infection by *P. multocida* (usually capsule type D) and *Bordetella bronchiseptica*. In addition, ammonia (in concentrations sometimes found in swine-rearing houses) acts synergistically with Pmt.

Signs include sneezing, epistaxis, and staining of the face due to tear-duct obstruction. Skeletal abnormalities produce lateral deviation of the snout or wrinkling due to rostrocaudal compression. Secondary pneumonia is due in part to the elimination of the turbinates as defenses of the respiratory tract (see Fig 73.1).

Pneumonia. A fibrinous pneumonia, associated with *P. multocida*, often follows viral infections.

Rabbits.   *Respiratory Tract Conditions.* "Snuffles," a mucopurulent rhinosinusitis of rabbits due to *P. multocida*, develops under stress of pregnancy, lactation, or mismanagement. Complications include bronchopneumonia, middle and inner ear infection, conjunctivitis, and septicemia.

Genital Tract Disease. In the genital tract, *P. multocida* may cause orchitis, balanoposthitis, and pyometra.

Avian Species.   *Avian Cholera.* Avian cholera, a systemic infection due to *P. multocida* (most commonly capsule type A), is acquired by ingestion or inhalation and affects mainly turkeys, waterfowl, and chickens. The peracute form kills about 60% of infected birds without preceding signs of illness. The acute type, marked by listlessness, anorexia, diarrhea, and nasal and ocular discharges, may last several days and be about 30% lethal. The subacute form is mostly respiratory and is manifested by rales and mucopurulent nasal discharges. In chronic fowl cholera, there is localization of caseous lesions. *Pasteurella gallinarum* is sometimes isolated from chronic cases.

Dogs and Cats.   *Mouth Related Conditions. Pasteurella multocida* (cats) and *P. canis* (dogs) are found alongside predominantly anaerobic flora in wound infections, serositides (e.g., feline pyothorax), and foreign body lesions.

Equine.   *Respiratory Tract Conditions. Pasteurella caballi* occurs in equine respiratory disease, usually in association with *Streptococcus equi* subspecies *zooepidemicus*.

Laboratory Rodents.   *Pasteurella pneumotropica*, a common commensal, may contribute to opportunistic infections such as pneumonia. Phenotypically similar organisms in other hosts probably belong to different species (e.g., *P. dagmatis*).

Human Beings.   *Pasteurella multocida* (and rarely other pasteurellae) causes wound infections in humans resulting from animal bites or scratches. A second form, especially in the respiratory tract, is usually not directly traceable to animal sources.

Epidemiology

Table 12.3 shows the relative roles of exogenous reservoir, dissemination, and stress in various conditions associated with *Pasteurella* and *Mannheimia*. In avian cholera, feral sources are sometimes implicated.

Immunologic Aspects

Basis of Immunity

Circulating antibody is significant in protection against hemorrhagic septicemia and fowl cholera. The type-specific capsular antigens are essential immunogens in hemorrhagic septicemia. With other forms of disease associated with *Pasteurella* and *Mannheimia*, the picture is less clear. Both antitoxic and antibacterial antibodies are important in protection.

Artificial Immunization

Pasteurella adjuvant bacterins are effective in preventing bovine hemorrhagic septicemia, conferring protection for up to 2 years. Antiserum is useful for short-term protection.

The essential attributes of an effective avian cholera vaccine are not known. Field performance of bacterins has

Table 12.3. The Relative Roles of Stress, Agent Introduction, and Agent Dissemination in Various Types of *Pasteurella* Infections

	Importance of:		
	Introduction of Agent into Population	Dissemination of Agent Within Population	Environmental or Individual Stress or Injury
Avian cholera	+++	++++	?
Bovine hemorrhagic septicemia	+++	++++	+
Bovine shipping fever, ovine enzootic pneumonia, ovine septicemic pasteurellosis, rabbit pasteurellosis	+	++	+++
Human pasteurellosis	+?	–	++++
Sporadic pneumonia in ruminants, *Pasteurella* infection in dogs and cats	–	–	++++

Legend: - = irrelevant; + = contributory; ++ = significant; +++ = critical; ++++ = paramount.

been inconsistent, even with autogenous preparations. Most promising have been live vaccines containing attenuated organisms (e.g., CU or M-9). Attenuation appears inversely related to immunogenicity.

Most shipping fever vaccines are bacterins of mixtures of *M. haemolytica*, *P. multocida*, and *P. trehalosi* combined with suspect viruses and other bovine bacterial pathogens. Benefits are inconsistent. Vaccination of calves with bacterins prepared from *M. haemolytica* reduces the degree of colonization of the upper respiratory tract by this organism. The effectiveness of modified live vaccines awaits field confirmation. Recombinant Lkt alone does not protect cattle from *M. haemolytica*-induced pneumonia. The gene encoding Lkt has been cloned into the genome of—and subsequently expressed by—white clover, the strategy being to immunize by feeding. No data are available on the usefulness of this method.

Pasteurella multocida and *B. bronchiseptica* bacterins with toxoid are valuable in the control of atrophic rhinitis.

Laboratory Diagnosis

Direct Examination

Exudate, tissue impressions, sediments of transtracheal aspirates, and, in birds, blood smears can be stained with a polychrome stain (e.g., Giemsa, Wright's, Wayson's) and examined for bipolar staining microorganisms. Their presence is suggestive but not unique to *Pasteurella/ Mannheimia*. On Gram stain, *Pasteurella/Mannheimia* do not look distinctive.

Isolation and Identification

Pasteurella/Mannheimia grow overnight (35–37°C) on bovine or sheep blood agar and are identified using differential tests. Capsule and somatic typing are done in a reference laboratory. DNA probes and primers designed to

amplify specific regions of the bacterial chromosome by the polymerase chain reaction are available for demonstration and identification of *Pasteurella/Mannheimia*.

Treatment and Control

Diseases produced by *Pasteurella/Mannheimia* respond to timely antimicrobial therapy. Strains from carnivores and humans are generally susceptible to almost all antimicrobials. Most *Pasteurella/Mannheimia* show moderate resistance to aminoglycosides, which is probably not significant clinically. Those from food-producing animals vary. In these species, cost and withdrawal requirements before slaughter are additional considerations. Consequently, sulfonamides, penicillin G, ceftiofur, tilmicosin, florfenicol, and tetracyclines are preferred. Their appropriateness should be confirmed by susceptibility tests. Sulfonamides, penicillin G, fluoroquinolones, and tetracycline are used to treat avian cholera.

Sulfonamides, penicillin G, and tetracyclines in swine and poultry, are suitable for mass medication via feed or water, therapeutically or prophylactically.

Management practices directed at reducing stress are important in preventing *Pasteurella/Mannheimia*-associated disease in livestock.

Immunization has been dependable only in bovine hemorrhagic septicemia and atrophic rhinitis control.

RIEMERELLA ANATIPESTIFER

Riemerella anatipestifer, the agent of "new duck disease," produces a severe polyserositic disease especially of ducklings (duck septicemia, infectious serositis of ducks). At various times in the past, this microorganism has been called *Pasteurella anatipestifer* or *Moraxella anatipestifer*.

Descriptive Features

Riemerella anatipestifer is a gram-negative, nonmotile, encapsulated, occasionally bipolar coccobacillus. It grows best under increased carbon dioxide tension on blood or chocolate agar (see Chapter 14 for a description of this agar). Colonies are nonhemolytic, transparent, and may exceed 1 mm in diameter after 24 hours of incubation. The organism is oxidase and catalase-positive, proteolytic, ferments no carbohydrates, and survives for weeks in litter. There are 21 serotypes (1–21) occurring in several combinations.

Ecology

Reservoir

The agent occurs in ducks and other fowl. Carrier birds constitute the reservoir.

Transmission

Infection occurs via respiratory, percutaneous, and possibly other routes.

Pathogenesis

Riemerella anatipestifer septicemia causes sudden mortality, or, less acutely, respiratory signs with sneezing, coughing, and discharges from nose and eyes. Central nervous involvement produces head tremors, torticollis, and ataxia. Diarrhea is also seen.

Fibrinous polyserositis is observed in the acute disease. The exudate is mostly mononuclear. In protracted cases, fibroblasts and giant cells are seen.

Mortality rates vary from 5% to 75%; duration is from one day to several weeks.

Epidemiology

Only ducks are consistently at risk. Stress factors play a significant predisposing role. Young birds are most susceptible.

Immunologic Aspects

Recovered birds are resistant following re-exposure to the bacterium. Immunity is serotype-specific and may be induced by bacterins.

Laboratory Diagnosis

Isolation and identification of the agent are mandatory for diagnosis. Organisms may be demonstrated in organs and fluids by Gram stain or immunofluorescence.

Culture plates are incubated under increased carbon dioxide tension.

Treatment and Control

Sulfonamides (sulfamethazine, sulfadimethoxine, sulfaquinoxaline) may be given prophylactically in feed or water. Penicillin G, tetracycline, erythromycin, and novobiocin are used therapeutically. Corticosteroids administered along with antibiotics (penicillin G) do not influence resolution of lesions.

Vaccination with killed or live avirulent bacteria of appropriate serotypes is beneficial.

PHOTOBACTERIUM DAMSELA

Photobacterium damsela contains two subspecies, *piscicida* and *damselae*. *Photobacterium damsela* ssp. *piscicida* (previously classified as *Pasteurella piscicida*) is the agent of fish pasteurellosis. *Photobacterium damsela* ssp. *damselae* was previously classified as *Vibrio damsela*. Both subspecies produce septicemic disease in farmed marine fish of a variety of species. *Photobacterium damsela* ssp. *damselae* is capable of producing septicemia in mammals (dolphins and humans).

Photobacterium damsela is a gram-negative, oxidase-positive, halophilic rod. Differentiation of the subspecies is done using traditional biochemical tests, or by determination of DNA sequences of the gene encoding the 16S rRNA (subspecies-specific primers are available and the test is done by using the polymerase chain reaction).

Both subspecies are susceptible to a variety of antimicrobials, including tetracyclines and beta lactams. R plasmid-mediated resistance has made treatment difficult in some outbreaks.

Group EF-4 (Eugonic Fermentor)

A gram-negative nonmotile bacterium, superficially resembling *Pasteurella* spp., occurs in the mouth of carnivores and sporadically causes apparently endogenous fatal, acute focal, pyogranulomatous pneumonias. In humans it is implicated in animal bite wound infections.

It is oxidase, catalase, and nitrate-positive; it ferments glucose slowly and has no other diagnostically dependable characteristics.

Isolates from humans stemming from animal bites test susceptible to the macrolides (erythromycin, clarithromycin, azithromycin), cephalosporins, ampicillin, tetracycline, aminoglycosides, and fluoroquinolones.

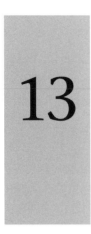

13

Pasteurellaceae: Actinobacillus

Dwight C. Hirsh   Ernst L. Biberstein

The family *Pasteurellaceae* contains the genera *Actinobacillus, Gallibacterium, Haemophilus, Histophilus, Lonepinella, Mannheimia, Pasteurella,* and *Phocoenobacter.* All but *Lonepinella* (*L. koalarum*—a tannin degrading bacterium isolated from normal Koala feces) and *Gallibacterium* (*G. anatis*—isolated from the intestine of normal ducks) contain species that are of medical importance.

Although they are genetically distinct, the genera *Actinobacillus* and *Pasteurella* overlap phenotypically. As is the case with the genus *Pasteurella,* the genus *Actinobacillus* is undergoing a considerable amount of taxonomic change. As of this writing, the genus *Actinobacillus* contains 20 species, many of which are associated with disease in several animal species (Table 13.1). Discussed in this chapter are *A. equuli* subspecies *equuli* (previously *A. equuli,* the cause of neonatal septicemia of foals), *A. equuli* subspecies *haemolytica* (previously *A. suis*-like, and occurs mainly in respiratory tract disease of horses), *A. lignieresii* (the agent of pyogranulomatous processes, primarily of ruminants), *A. suis* (associated with respiratory, septicemic, and localized infections of swine), and *A. pleuropneumoniae* (the agent of porcine pleuropneumonia).

All the members of the family *Pasteurellaceae* are gram-negative coccobacilli. They are facultative anaerobes, and typically oxidase-positive (setting them apart from members of the family *Enterobacteriaceae*). Most are commensal parasites of animals.

Descriptive Features

Morphology and Staining

Members of the genus *Actinobacillus* are gram-negative coccobacilli, approximately 0.5 μm wide and variable in length.

Structure and Composition

Capsules are polysaccharide. The cell wall is typical of gram-negative microorganisms consisting mainly of lipopolysaccharides and proteins. Some of the latter are iron-regulated (i.e., they are expressed under iron-poor conditions).

Cell Products of Medical Interest

Adhesins. The role of adhesins, as in other microorganisms, is to allow the bacterium expressing them to adhere to cells lining a particular niche, as well as to the surface of so-called "target" cells prior to the initiation of disease (in some cases, niche and target cells may be the same). The expression of adhesins depends upon various environmental cues. Some, and probably all, members of the family *Pasteurellaceae* express adhesins (and possibly more than one kind).

Except for *A. pleuropneumoniae,* virtually nothing is known about the adhesins of the other actinobacilli associated with diseases of animals of veterinary importance. *Actinobacillus pleuropneumoniae* adheres to two different cell types, those lining the nasal cavity and tonsilar crypts (as is the case with carrier animals), and the cells of the terminal bronchioli and alveoli (antecedent to disease). *Actinobacillus pleuropneumoniae* produces two structures that function as adhesins. The first is an adhesin in the classic sense, i.e., a structure composed of protein subunits whose main function is to bind to the surface of host cells. These adhesins are type 4 fimbria, and it is unknown to which cell type they adhere. The other, cell wall lipopolysaccharide, is not usually considered an adhesin. Nevertheless, the lipopolysaccharide (in particular the core portion) of *A. pleuropneumoniae* is responsible for the adherence of this microorganism to cells of the lower respiratory tract of swine.

Capsules. The capsule plays many roles, the most important of which are interference with phagocytosis (antiphagocytic) and protection of the outer membrane from the deposition of membrane attack complexes generated by activation of the complement system. The amount of capsule produced is inversely proportional to the amount of available iron. In vivo, where the amount of available iron is low, the amount of capsule formed is less (but sufficient to protect the microorganism from phagocytosis and complement-mediated lysis). It is difficult to reconcile capsule expression and lipopolysaccharide as an adhesin in adherence in *A. pleuropneumoniae.*

Cell Wall. Lipopolysaccharide elicits an inflammatory response following association with lipopolysaccharide-binding protein (a serum protein), which in turn transfers it to the blood phase of CD14. The CD14-LPS complex binds to Toll-like receptor proteins (see Chapter 2) on the

Table 13.1.   Members of the Genus *Actinobacillus* and Their Usual Source or Associated Condition

Species	Usual Source or Associated Condition
A. actinomycetemcomitans	Oral cavity, periodontal disease in primates; endocarditis in primates
A. arthritidis	Septicemia of foals and horses; normal flora of oral cavity of horses
A. capsulatus	Arthritis of rabbits
A. delphinicola	Septicemia in sea mammals
A. equuli ssp. equuli (A. equuli)	Septicemia in neonatal foals
A. equuli ssp. haemolytica (A. suis-like)	Respiratory tract conditions in horses
A. hominis	Respiratory tract conditions in humans
"A. indolicus"	Pleuropneumonia and pneumonia in swine
A. lignieresii	Chronic granulomatosis in ruminants ("Wooden Tongue")
"A. minor"	Pleuropneumonia and pneumonia in swine
A muris	Respiratory tract conditions of rodents
A. pleuropneumonieae	Pleuropneumonia in swine
"A. porcinus"	Pleuropneumonia and pneumonia in swine
A. rossii	Reproductive tract of sows
"A. salpingitidis" (will become Gallibacterium sp)	Conditions of the respiratory and reproductive tracts of chickens
A. scotiae	Septicemia in harbor porpoises
A. seminis	Reproductive conditions of sheep (epididymitis in lambs); normal flora of genital tract of sheep
A. succinogenes	Bovine rumen
A. suis	Respiratory tract conditions, and septicemia in swine
A. ureae	Respiratory tract conditions in humans

surface of macrophage cells triggering the release of proinflammatory cytokines

Toxins. Members of the genus *Actinobacillus* produce at least two products that have toxic activity. The most important is an RTX type of toxin, and the other is the enzyme urease:

1. RTX type toxin. The RTX (repeats in *to*xin, so called because of the common feature of repeats in glycine-rich sequences within the protein, see also *Escherichia coli* hemolysin in Chapter 8, *Pasteurella/ Mannheimia* leukotoxin in Chapter 12, adenylyl cyclase toxin of *Bordetella* in Chapter 15, *Moraxella* cytotoxin in Chapter 19) type of toxin is produced by *A. pleuropneumoniae*, *A. suis*, and *A. rossii*. The toxin is termed Apx (for *A. p*leuropneumoniae to*x*in). *Actinobacillus equuli* ssp. *haemolytica* produces a very similar toxin, Aqx (for *A. e*quuli to*x*in). Even though *A. lignieresii* contains the genes encoding Apx, it does not express them (lacks a functioning promoter). As with other RTX type toxins, there is a dose effect. At low concentrations these toxins interfere with macrophage and neutrophil function by triggering degranulation, and at higher concentrations they are cytolytic for macrophages, neutrophils, and alveolar epithelial cells. In addition, the RTX toxins lyse erythrocytes (explaining the hemolytic phenotype of actinobacilli expressing them when grown on blood agar), and are responsible for

a CAMP reaction when cross-streaked with a beta toxin–producing strain of *Staphylococcus* (see Chapter 28). The effect on erythrocytes probably plays little if any role in disease production. There are four types of Apx toxin (ApxI, ApxII, ApxIII, ApxIV), each with a different degree of cytotoxicity (ApxI is the most potent of the four, followed by ApxIII, and then ApxII—the potency of ApxIV is unknown). Actinobacilli may contain the genes encoding any combination of the four toxins. In the case of *A. pleuropneumoniae*, serotypes (see "Variability," below) 1, 5, 9, 10, and 11 produce ApxI, all the serotypes (except serotype 10) produce ApxII, serotypes 2, 3, 4, 6, and 8 produce ApxIII, and all of the serotypes produce ApxIV. *Actinobacillus rossii* produces ApxII and ApxIII, whereas *A. suis* produces ApxI and ApxII.

2. Urease. Urease produced by *A. pleuropneumoniae*, has been shown to be important in disease produced by this microorganism (it is unknown whether this enzyme plays a role in the diseases produced by the other urease-positive species of actinobacilli). Urease is responsible for the liberation of ammonia from urea (the association constant of *A pleuropneumoniae* urease is extremely high allowing effective association with the very low concentrations of urea found in blood and tissue fluids). In addition to attracting and activating neutrophils and macrophages, ammonia inhibits phagolysosome

fusion and increases the pH within phagolyso-somes, thereby reducing the effectiveness of various acid hydrolases. These effects result not only in a decrease in the host's ability to clear the microorganism from the lung, but also to assure effective colonization of the upper respiratory tract, thereby promoting the carrier state (mutants unable to produce urease are cleared rapidly from the respiratory tract).

Iron Acquisition. Because iron is an absolute growth requirement, microorganisms must acquire this substance if they are to exist within the host. Actinobacilli bind transferrin-iron complexes by virtue of iron-regulated outer membrane proteins expressed under iron-poor conditions (so-called *transferrin-binding proteins*, or Tbps). Iron is acquired from the transferrin-iron complexes that bind to the surface of the microorganism. In addition to acquiring iron by way of Tbps, *Actinobacillus pleuropneumoniae* also utilizes siderophores (both hydroxamates and catechols) produced by other species of bacteria even though it does not produce them itself.

Miscellaneous Products. Other products produced by actinobacilli (specifically *A. pleuropneumoniae*) that may play a role in disease production include IgA and IgG proteases (prevent adherence, and opsonization, respectively), and periplasmic superoxide dismutase (suggested as a strategy to prevent digestion within the phagolysosome by inactivating superoxide molecules).

Growth Characteristics

Actinobacilli grow on blood and serum-containing media at 20°C to 42°C. Colony sizes at 24 hours reach 1–2 mm. Some actinobacilli (*A. indolicus*, *A. minor*, *A. pleuropneumoniae* biotype 1, and *A. porcinus*) require nicotinamide adenine dinucleotide (NAD) for growth, while *A. pleuropneumoniae* biotype 2 does not. Hemolysis depends upon expression of ApxI, ApxII, or Aqx (toxins with hemolytic activity).

Carbohydrates are fermented without gas production. Urease, orthonitrophenyl-beta-d-galactopyranosidase (ONPGase, "beta-galactosidase"), and nitratase are typically present. No indole is produced, and most strains grow on MacConkey agar (but poorly). Cultures die within a week. They are facultative anaerobes, and typically oxidase-positive.

Resistance

Actinobacillus pleuropneumoniae contains R plasmids encoding resistance to sulfonamides, tetracycline, and penicillin G.

Variability

Actinobacillus lignieresii and *A. equuli* are antigenically diverse. The six somatic types of *A. lignieresii* have some relation to geographic and host species predilection. There are 15 somatic serotypes of *A. pleuropneumoniae* (1–15), and two biotypes (biotype 1 requires NAD for growth, biotype 2 does not). *Actinobacillus suis* has at least two somatic serotypes (O1 and O2).

Ecology

Reservoir

Actinobacilli (except possibly *A. capsulatus*) are commensal parasites on mucous membranes. *Actinobacillus pleuropneumoniae* are more closely associated with the respiratory tracts of sick or recovered animals.

Transmission

Except in neonates, most actinobacilloses are probably endogenous infections. Neonatal foals acquire *A. equuli* ssp. *equuli* before, at, or shortly after birth from their dams, commonly via the umbilicus.

Pathogenesis

Mechanisms. Most disease produced by members of the genus *Actinobacillus* result from "contamination" (infection) of a normally sterile, compromised site by microorganisms living on a contiguous site (niche). Common compromises are viral infections, trauma, or stress. Sometimes it is difficult to determine the nature of the antecedent event (especially true for neonates with septicemia). Deposition of actinobacilli into a normally sterile site results in initiation of an inflammatory response due to the lipopolysaccharide of the cell wall, and urease if the infecting strain produces this enzyme. The capsule interferes with phagocytosis (antiphagocytic) and protects the outer membrane from the deposition of membrane attack complexes generated by activation of the complement system. Transferrin-binding proteins participate in iron acquisition. The RTX toxins (Apx, Aqx) intensify the inflammatory response by activating and damaging neutrophils and macrophages. If the infectious process involves the lungs, alveolar epithelial cells are also damaged. Urease-producing actinobacilli that are phagocytosed resist destruction by generating ammonia, and perhaps superoxide dismutase. Opsonization is reduced by the production of IgG protease.

In the case of neonatal septicemias (*A. equuli* ssp. *equuli*, in particular), actinobacilli gain access to the systemic circulation. Capsule and Tbps permit multiplication within the bloodstream resulting in an endotoxemia (see Fig 8.1).

Pathology. Lung lesions (usually produced by *A. equuli* ssp. *haemolytica*, *A. pleuropneumoniae*, and *A. suis*) are suppurative. Inflammatory cells are prominent, with erythrocytes, neutrophils, and mononuclear cells appearing and predominating successively. The tissue appearance changes accordingly from reddish-black to red, pink, and gray.

A soft tissue process, mainly produced by *A. lignieresii*, is a chronic granuloma in the ruminant tongue. At its center is a colony of *A. lignieresii*, ringed by eosinophilic, club-like processes forming a "rosette." The complex is surrounded by neutrophils and granulation tissue containing macrophages, plasma cells, lymphocytes, giant cells, and fibroblasts. Plant fibers are often present. Through coalescence, larger granulomas (1 cm or more in diameter) may be formed. Infection spreads to lymph nodes, producing granulomas along the way. The proliferative tissue reaction causes the tongue to protrude from the mouth. Other tissues in the vicinity, and occasionally along the gastrointestinal tract, may be involved, along with adjacent lymph nodes. Superficial lesions often ulcerate. In sheep, suppurative infections occur around the head and neck and in the skin and mammary gland. Tongue involvement is not typical.

Disease Patterns

Ruminants.   "Actinobacillosis" or "Wooden Tongue" involving *A. lignieresii* occurs in ruminants and, rarely, dogs and horses. In ruminants, the agent (normal inhabitant of the nasopharynx) is probably inoculated by trauma (plant fibers), initiating the process described. The course is protracted and healing slow. Interference with feed intake causes weight loss and dehydration.

Swine.   *Pneumonia. Actinobacillus pleuropneumoniae* (serotypes 1 and 5 are more common in North America; serotype 2 is more common in Europe) causes a primary pneumonia of swine, particularly young pigs 2 to 6 months old. Spread is favored by crowding and poor ventilation. Early signs include fever and reduced appetite, followed within a day by acute respiratory distress. Animals may die within 24 hours. Morbidity may reach 40%, with mortality up to 24%. Survivors show intermittent cough and unsatisfactory weight gains. Chronic infections, often without preceding acute episodes, are the source of persistent herd problems. Lesions consist of fibrinous pneumonia and pleuritis. Arthritis, meningitis, and abortion occur as complications. Pneumonia in older animals may be caused by *A. suis.*

Septicemia. Septicemia of young pigs and arthritis, endocarditis is sometimes associated with *A. suis.*

Horses.   *Pneumonia.* Bacterial pneumonia in horses (of any age) is usually associated with a mixture of beta hemolytic streptococcus (usually *S. equi* subspecies *zooepidemicus*) and a gram-negative microorganism (commonly *A. equuli* ssp. *haemolytica*).

Septicemia. Foal septicemia due to *A. equuli* ssp. *equuli* ("sleepy foal disease") occurs within a few days of birth and is marked by fever, inappetence, prostration, and diarrhea (see Fig 74.1). Animals surviving the first day typically develop lameness due to (poly)arthritis. Some foals develop umbilical infections with this microorganism ("navel ill").

Epidemiology

Actinobacilli are opportunistic pathogens producing disease when their host's integrity is compromised, as by trauma, immaturity, or other stress. Trauma to mucous membranes of ruminants by rough feed may cause herd outbreaks suggestive of transmissible diseases.

In the case of Porcine Pleuropneumonia, chronic asymptomatic carriers are the apparent reservoirs. Disease occurs when nonimmune animals are exposed to subclinically infected individuals. That prevalence is highest in the colder months is due probably more to management (i.e., the mixing of individuals with different exposure histories) than climatic factors.

Immunologic Aspects

The pathology of "Wooden Tongue" suggests a cell-mediated hypersensitivity. Antibodies of no known protective function appear during infection. The benefits of bacterins have not been established. Antibody to *A. pleuropneumoniae* is opsonizing and colostrum protects piglets. Antibody to RTX-type toxin is protective.

Laboratory Diagnosis

Actinobacilli can often be demonstrated in gram-stained exudates. They grow best on blood agar under increased amounts of carbon dioxide (35–37°C). Colonies are often sticky. Speciation is accomplished by cultural and biochemical tests. DNA primers have been developed to aid in identification by means of the polymerase chain reaction.

Treatment and Control

Porcine pleuropneumonia is controlled and treated by a combination of management practices, immunoprophylaxis, and antimicrobial therapy. Management practices include minimizing contact of piglets with mature (carrier) animals (e.g., "all in, all out" rearing practices; identification and elimination of carrier sows by serological testing, culture, and/or by polymerase chain reaction using primers designed to detect the genes encoding one of the *apx* genes—*apxIV* appears to be the most useful since it is unique and in all serotypes). Vaccination strategies include bacterins (these are serotype-specific and do not prevent carrier states) and modified live vaccines (*A. pleuropneumoniae* with Apx and urease deletion mutants). Potentially useful antimicrobial agents include penicillin G, tetracycline, gentamicin, kanamycin, cephalosporins, tilmicosin, tiamulin, florphenicol, ceftiofur, enrofloxacin, and trimethoprim-sulfas.

In "Wooden Tongue" iodides given orally or intravenously promptly reduce the inflammatory swelling, which is the main clinical problem. Avoidance of harsh, dry feed reduces the likelihood of development of this condition.

Good foaling hygiene, including navel disinfection, reduces the likelihood of foal septicemia. Potential effective antimicrobials for treatment of septicemia produced by *A. equuli* ssp. *equuli* include penicillin G, ceftiofur, and gentamicin.

Actinobacillus equuli ssp. *haemolytica* responds to most antimicrobics.

14

Pasteurellaceae: Haemophilus and Histophilus

Dwight C. Hirsh   Ernst L. Biberstein

The family *Pasteurellaceae* contains the genera *Actinobacillus*, *Gallibacterium*, *Haemophilus*, *Histophilus*, *Lonepinella*, *Mannheimia*, *Pasteurella*, and *Phocoenobacter*. All but *Lonepinella* and *Gallibacterium* contain species that are of medical importance.

Members of the genus *Haemophilus*, beyond sharing the family traits of the family *Pasteurellaceae*, require for propagation one or both of two growth factors: porphyrins (heme) or nicotinamide adenine dinucleotide (NAD, NADP), originally called X (heat-stable), and V (heat-labile) factor, respectively. Some members of the family *Pasteurellaceae* showing these needs are genetically unrelated to the type species *H. influenzae* (associated with oropharyngeal, middle ear, and respiratory tract conditions in human patients).

Discussed in this chapter are *Haemophilus paragallinarum* (the cause of infectious coryza in chickens), *H. parasuis*, (the cause of a septicemic disease called Glässer's disease or polyserositis, and secondary respiratory disease of swine), and *Histophilus somni* (the cause of septicemic, respiratory, and genital tract disease in cattle and sheep). *Histophilus somni* is the name now given to those microorganisms previously denoted as "*Haemophilus somnus*," "*Haemophilus agni*," "*Histophilus ovis*." Briefly discussed is *Ornithobacterium rhinotracheale*, a bacterium that is not a member of the family *Pasteurellaceae*, but phenotypically (and clinically) resembles some strains of *H. paragallinarum*.

All the members of the family *Pasteurellaceae* are gram-negative coccobacilli. They are facultative anaerobes, and typically oxidase-positive (setting them apart from members of the family *Enterobacteriaceae*). Most are commensal parasites of animals.

Descriptive Features

Morphology and Staining

Members of the genera *Haemophilus* and *Histophilus* are gram-negative rods, less than a micrometer wide and 1 to 3 μm long, but sometimes form longer filaments. Some species (*H. paragallinarum* and *H. influenzae*) are encapsulated.

Cellular Constituents and Products

Capsules are polysaccharide. The cell wall is typical of gram-negative microorganisms consisting mainly of lipopolysaccharides and proteins. Some of the latter are iron-regulated (i.e., they are expressed under iron-poor conditions).

Cellular Products of Medical Interest

Adhesins. The role of adhesins, as in other microorganisms, is to allow the bacterium expressing them to adhere to cells lining a particular niche, as well as to the surface of so-called "target" cells prior to the initiation of disease (in some cases, niche and target cells may be the same). The expression of adhesins depends upon various environmental cues. Some, and probably all members of the family *Pasteurellaceae* express adhesins (and possibly more than one kind).

Histophilus somni also produces a particular surface protein, appearing as fibrils when viewed with an electron microscope. These structures are responsible for the binding of the microorganism to endothelial cells (in which apoptosis is triggered with subsequent fibrin deposition, see below, "Mechanisms"). The protein comprising this fibrillar network is one of two immunoglobulin-binding proteins (IgBPs) produced by *Histophilus somni*—in particular, the so-called high molecular weight IgBP (see below).

Little else is known about the adhesins of the haemophili and *Histophilus*, except for the human pathogen *H. influenzae*, which produces several (also called *fimbriae* or *pili*) that are responsible for adherence to human upper respiratory tract epithelium.

Capsules. The capsule plays many roles, the most important of which are interference with phagocytosis (antiphagocytic) and the protection of the outer membrane from the deposition of membrane attack complexes generated by activation of the complement system. *Haemophilus influenzae* and *H. paragallinarum* produce capsules.

Cell Wall. Lipopolysaccharide (LPS) elicits an inflammatory response following binding to lipopolysaccharide-binding protein (a serum protein), which in turn transfers it to the blood phase of CD14. The CD14-LPS complex binds to Toll-like receptor proteins (see Chapter 2) on the surface of macrophage cells triggering the release of proinflammatory cytokines

The cell wall lipopolysaccharide of *Histophilus somni* is termed lipooligosaccharide (LOS). LOS, under the direction of the gene *lob* (for *LOS b*iosynthesis), undergoes phase variation resulting in different epitope expression subsequent to changes in the carbohydrate portions of the LOS. *Histophilus somni* that phase vary are more virulent. Explanations for this include immune evasion, and phase varying isolates are more serum resistant (an in vitro measure of resistance to complement mediated lysis) than those that do not phase vary. Clinical isolates (from central nervous system, lungs, joints, and aborted fetuses) phase vary, most isolates from carrier sites (prepuce, vagina), do not (or cannot).

There are two different immunoglobulin-binding proteins (IgBPs) expressed on the surface of *Histophilus somni*, a 41 kDa protein, and a high molecular weight protein (100–350 kDa). Both IgBPs bind immunoglobulin, but the high molecular weight protein preferentially binds IgG_2. Immunoglobulin molecules bind to IgBPs by way of the Fc portion rendering the antibody ineffectual in opsonization or triggering complement activation. In addition, the high molecular weight IgBP serves as an adhesin (see above).

Iron Acquisition. Because iron is an absolute growth requirement, microorganisms must acquire this substance if they are to exist within the host. Haemophili and *Histophilus* bind transferrin-iron complexes by virtue of iron-regulated outer membrane proteins expressed under iron-poor conditions (so-called *t*ransferrin *b*inding *p*roteins, or Tbps). Iron is acquired from the transferrin-iron complexes that bind to the surface of the microorganism.

Growth Characteristics

Members of the genera *Haemophilus* and *Histophilus* are facultative anaerobes, typically oxidase-positive, and attack carbohydrates fermentatively. Carbon dioxide enhances growth of some strains. On adequate media members of this genus produce within 24 to 48 hours turbidity in broth and colonies 1 mm in diameter on agar (35–37°C). Growth factors may be supplied as hemin (X factor) and NAD (V factor). A medium naturally containing them is chocolate agar, a blood agar prepared by addition of blood when the melted agar is at 75–80°C (rather than 50°C when making regular blood agar). This procedure liberates NAD from cells and inactivates enzymes destructive to NAD.

Alternatively, a "feeder" bacterium (e.g., *Staphylococcus*) may be inoculated across plates where *Haemophilus* has been streaked. On otherwise inadequate media, growth occurs only near the feeder streak, a phenomenon called *satellitism* (Fig 14.1). It may be duplicated by commercially prepared X and V factor-impregnated filter papers placed on the inoculated area (Fig 14.2). For the X and V factor requirements, see Table 14.1.

Biochemical Activities

Haemophilus and *Histophilus* of animals are oxidase and nitratase-positive and ferment carbohydrates.

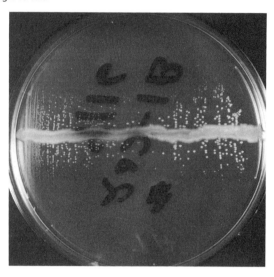

FIGURE 14.1. *Satellitic growth of* Haemophilus *on a feeder streak of* Staphylococcus. Haemophilus *was inoculated evenly over the entire surface. The staphylococcus was then inoculated in a single streak.*

Resistance

Haemophilus and *Histophilus* are readily killed by heat and die rapidly in culture and storage unless freeze dried or stored at minus 70°C. At cool temperatures, *H. paragallinarum* survives in exudates for several days.

Variability

Serotypes may differ in pathogenicity and geographic prevalence, and determine the specificity of bacterin-induced immunity. There are three serotypes (A–C in the so-called Page scheme, or I–III in the Kume scheme) of *H. paragallinarum* and at least seven of *H. parasuis*. NAD independent strains of *H. paragallinarum* have been isolated from South Africa. Since NAD-dependency is used in the cultural diagnosis of Infectious Coryza, this has become a serious issue.

Ecology

Reservoir

Members of the genera *Haemophilus* and *Histophilus* live in the upper respiratory tract, or in the lower genital tract. *Haemophilus parasuis* lives in the nasopharynx of normal swine, while *H. paragallinarum* is more closely associated with the respiratory tracts of sick or recovered poultry. *Histophilus somni* is found in normal cattle both in the lower genital tract (prepuce, vagina) as well as in the upper respiratory tract. Oddly, isolates from these sites do not seem to phase vary their LOS (and are thus relatively avirulent). *Histophilus somni* also inhabits the lower genital tract of normal sheep.

FIGURE 14.2.   *Determination of cofactor needs with (left to right) XV, V, and X factor-impregnated filter paper discs. Growth has occurred around the XV and X discs (lower left and right), but not the V disc (top center). The organism accordingly was identified as* Haemophilus haemoglobinophilus, *which requires X but not V factor.*

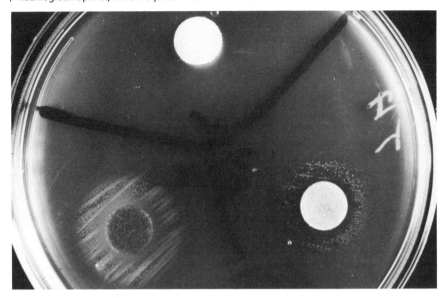

Table 14.1.   Pathogenic and Common Species of *Haemophilus* and *Histophilus*

	X	V	Host	Clinical Significance
Haemophilus influenzae	+	+	Human	Meningitis, septicemia, otitis, epiglottitis, conjunctivitis, bronchopneumonia
H. paragallinarum	–	+	Fowl	Infectious coryza of fowl
H. parasuis	–	+	Swine	Secondary pneumonia, Glässer's disease
Histophilus somni	–*	–*	Cattle, sheep	Septicemia, meningoencephalitis, pneumonia, abortion, epididymitis
H. felis	–	+	Cat	Conjunctivitis of cats
H. haemoglobinophilus	+	-	Dog	None (opportunistic)

*Requires cyst(e)ine, is stimulated by thiamine pyrophosphate.

Transmission

Transmission of haemophili and *Histophilus* is probably airborne or by close contact. Indirect transmission is likely during epidemics.

Pathogenesis

Mechanisms. Disease is usually produced when haemophili and *Histophilus* find their way to a normally sterile site (a possible exception is *H. paragallinarum*). Whether an invasive phenotype is triggered by as yet some undefined event (*Histophilus somni* septicemia, for example), or whether it is just happenstance "contamination" of a previously compromised site (e.g., *H. parasuis* pneumonia following stress), or both is not known.

In septicemic disease produced by *Histophilus somni*, the microorganism is resistant to complement-mediated lysis (LOS phase variation) and survives within phagocytic cells by an unknown mechanism. Iron is acquired by removal from transferrins of the host. Effective immune responses are evaded by means of phase variation of the outer surface (LOS). In addition, antibody (especially that belonging to the IgG$_2$ isotype) binds to IgBPs by their Fc portion (antibody bound in such fashion does not trigger complement activation, nor does it serve as an opsonin). *Histophilus somni* adheres to endothelial cells by way of the high molecular weight IgBPs, and triggers apoptosis of this cell. Thrombosis occurs upon the surface of the damaged endothelial cell. Intravascular multiplication brings about endotoxemia (see Fig 8.1).

Deposition of *Histophilus somni* or *H. parasuis* into the lower respiratory tract stimulates an inflammatory response by virtue of their cell wall lipopolysaccharide (also known as lipooligosaccharide, or LOS). Iron is acquired from transferrin. Immune evasion occurs because of LOS phase variation, as well as IgBPs sidetracking antibody mediated opsonization, and complement activation. *Histophilus somni* survives intracellularly within phagocytic cells (*H. parasuis* does not have this property).

Haemophilus paragallinarum is resistant to complement mediated lysis and phagocytosis because of its capsule. Though little is known regarding the production of disease by this microorganism, the lipopolysaccharide component of the cell wall triggers an inflammatory response.

Pathology. All infections have suppurative components brought about by the chemistry of the gram-negative cell wall, which triggers the release of proinflammatory cytokines from macrophages. Infection of lungs, body cavities, and joints tends to be serofibrinous to fibrinopurulent. Bacterial colonization of the meningeal vessels produces a thrombotic vasculitis leading to encephalitis and meningitis. Hemorrhagic necrotizing processes are caused by *Histophilus somni*.

Fowl coryza is marked by catarrhal inflammation with heterophil exudates.

Disease Patterns

Cattle. *Thromboembolic Meningoencephalitis.* TEME (Thromboembolic *m*eningoencephalitis) is a consequence of septicemia produced by *Histophilus somni* leading to thrombotic meningoencephalitis and infarcts in brain and cerebellum. The preencephalitic stage is marked by high fever. With central nervous system (CNS) involvement, motor and behavioral abnormalities develop.

Pneumonia. *Histophilus somni* occurs in pneumonic processes, usually with other agents, for example, *Pasteurella/ Mannheimia* spp., as part of the shipping fever complex.

Septicemic Disease. *Histophilus somni* may produce septicemia (manifesting as an endotoxemia), sometimes resulting in arthritis, mycoarditis, or abortion.

Abortion. Abortion due to *Histophilus somni* sometimes occurs. Whether this is secondary to septicemia, or to genital tract disease (initiated by an ascending route) is unknown.

Swine. *Pneumonia.* *Haemophilus parasuis* can cause bronchopneumonia secondary to virus infections (e.g., swine influenza). Other bacteria (e.g., *Pasteurella* spp. and *Mycoplasma* spp.) may also participate.

Septicemic Disease. In young weaned pigs, *H. parasuis* also causes Glässer's disease (polyserositis), an acute inflammation affecting pleura, peritoneum, mediastinum, pericardium, joints, and meninges. Weaning, transport, and management stress are predisposing causes. The disease strikes sporadically within days of the stressing event. Morbidity and mortality are often low because of widespread acquired resistance, but they may be high in previously unexposed herds (e.g., specific pathogen-free herds). Disease manifestations include fever and general malaise, respiratory and abdominal distress, lameness, and paralytic or convulsive signs. Recovery begins in 1 to 2 weeks. Similar syndromes are due to *Mycoplasma hyorhinis*.

Poultry. *Infectious Coryza.* Infectious coryza (caused by *H. paragallinarum*) is an acute contagious upper-respiratory infection of chickens. It affects birds of practically all ages. The signs include nasal discharge, swelling of sinuses, facial edema, and conjunctivitis. With air sac and lung involvement, rales may be detected. In the uncomplicated infection, mortality is low. Loss of productivity is the most damaging aspect. Superimposed infections with mycoplasmas and helminth parasites exacerbate and prolong outbreaks. Of other species, only Japanese quail are highly susceptible.

Sheep. *Histophilus somni* causes respiratory and mammary infections, epididymitis of immature rams, and occasionally septicemias (see Fig 74.6).

Dogs and Cats. *Dogs. Haemophilus haemoglobinophilus*, a commensal of the canine lower genital tract, sometimes causes cystitis and neonatal infections. Its role in balanoposthitis and vaginitis, where it is frequently found, is uncertain.

Cats. Haemophilus felis is associated with conjunctivitis (following *Chlamydophila felis* and *Mycoplasma* spp. in prevalence).

Epidemiology

All the agents named, except for *H. paragallinarum*, inhabit normal mucous membranes of the respiratory or genital tract. Sources of infection are therefore often endogenous to herds or individuals. Colonization of pigs with *H. parasuis* probably occurs while animals are shielded by maternal immunity. Glässer's disease in pigs of all ages occurs in previously *H. parasuis*-free, stressed populations.

Respiratory and septicemic diseases produced by *Histophilus somni* are similarly related to stress factors, as their predilection for feedlots and the fall and winter months suggests.

Haemophilus and *Histophilus* are generally host-specific.

Immunologic Aspects

Circulating antibody develops in infected individuals and has a protective function, at least in mammals. Presence of serum antibody correlates well with resistance to *Histophilus somni* infection. The role of cell-mediated immunity is unknown.

Immunity develops after infection. Following infectious coryza, it extends to heterologous serotypes.

Immunoprophylaxis is used to control infectious coryza, polyserositis (Glässer's disease), and TEME. Bacterins prevent serious disease but not infection owing to homologous serotypes.

Laboratory Diagnosis

Recovery of the organism from infected tissues or fluids is usually required to establish a diagnosis, though detection of genus and species-specific DNA makes this considerably easier (however, diagnosis made in this manner is without an isolate, making type and susceptibility testing difficult, if not impossible). Observation of gram-negative rods in specimens prior to culture may suggest *Haemophilus* or *Histophilus* infection. Isolation of such an organism is followed by demonstration of a growth factor requirement.

Organisms requiring X factor cannot convert delta-aminolevulinic acid to urobilinogen and porphyrin. The porphyrin test determines this ability and X factor requirement most reliably. Definitive assignment to a species usually requires additional tests.

Infectious coryza is diagnosed by culture or by serological means (agglutination, agar gel immunodiffusion, and hemagglutination-inhibition tests). The polymerase chain reaction with primers specific for *H. paragallinarum* (the HP-2 test) is quicker, and less expensive than classical cultural techniques (NAD-dependent and NAD-independent strains react in a similar manner in this test). *Ornithobacterium rhinotracheale* (see below) is a gram-negative rod-shaped bacterium that mimics haemophili (and other members of the family *Pasteurellaceae*), and is often isolated from the respiratory tracts of birds. It is not, however NAD-dependent (as are the classical strains of *H. paragallinarum*, see above, "Variability"). NAD-independent variants of *H. paragallinarum* are difficult to differentiate from *O. rhinotracheale*, except with the HP-2 test.

Treatment and Control

Most animal haemophili are susceptible to penicillin G, ceftiofur, and tetracyclines. *Histophilus somni* is susceptible to florphenicol, penicillin G, tilmicosin, and tetracycline. For the septicemic-meningoencephalitic form, timeliness and maintenance of treatment are critical.

For infectious coryza of fowl, erythromycin or sulfonamides can be administered in feed or water, but may also be controlled by elimination of carriers and immunization of individuals at risk. Poultry producers may depopulate infected flocks. When breeding stock must be preserved, flock additions are vaccinated at 16 weeks, four weeks before joining the infected flock.

Bacterins are of value in prevention of TEME but are less effective in other *Histophilus somni* infections.

ORNITHOBACTERIUM RHINOTRACHEALE

Ornithobacterium rhinotracheale is a gram-negative rod that resembles some members of the family *Pasteurellaceae*. It is a facultative anaerobe, whose growth is enhanced by carbon dioxide, is oxidase-positive, attacks carbohydrates fermentatively, and does not grow on MacConkey agar. It requires neither porphyrins/heme (factor X) nor nicotinamide adenine dinucleotide (NAD, NADP; factor V). It is important to note, however, that it is not a member of the family *Pasteurellaceae*, and in fact is not a member of any recognized group of microorganisms. Based upon the sequence of the DNA encoding the 16S ribosomal RNA, it is more closely related to *Riemerella* and *Capnocytophaga*. There are 12 serotypes (A–L), with A being the most common.

Ornithobacterium rhinotracheale causes (by unknown mechanisms) respiratory tract disease (sinusitis, airsacculitis, pneumonia) in birds (domestic and wild). In turkeys and chickens respiratory tract disease may be relatively mild, resulting in poor performance, or severe with increased mortality. Transmission is horizontal (aerosols, contaminated fomites) or vertical (it is unclear whether this is transovarian or cecal contamination of eggs).

With the appearance of NAD-independent strains of *Haemophilus paragallinarum* (see above) differentiation of *H. paragallinarum* from *O. rhinotracheale* is difficult by classical culture techniques. A polymerase chain reaction–based test (HP-2, see above) quickly and easily differentiates the two organisms.

Most isolates of *O. rhinotracheale* are susceptible to ampicillin, erythromycin, penicillin, spectinomycin, tetracycline, and tylosin. Vaccination with autogenous bacterins reduces morbidity.

15 Bordetella

Dwight C. Hirsh   Ernst L. Biberstein

Members of the genus *Bordetella* are gram-negative coccobacilli belonging to the family *Alcaligenaceae*. There are eight species described, some of which are important pathogens of humans and other animals (Table 15.1). All but one (*B. petrii*) are aerobic bacteria that are parasites of ciliated respiratory epithelium. *Bordetella petrii* is a facultative anaerobe that lives in the environment and has not been associated with disease. *Bordetella pertussis*, *B. parapertussis*, and *B. bronchiseptica* are very closely related, and probably belong to the same species. *Bordetella pertussis* (and, rarely, *B. parapertussis*) causes whooping cough in humans. Of veterinary importance, and the main topic of discussion in this chapter are *B. bronchiseptica*, which has been implicated in porcine Atrophic Rhinitis, canine kennel cough, and bronchopneumonia in many species, and *B. avium*, the cause of rhinotracheitis of birds (mainly turkeys).

Descriptive Features

Morphology and Staining

Bordetellae are pleomorphic gram-negative coccobacilli, about 0.5 μm X up to 2 μm in size.

Structure and Composition

The cell wall is typical of gram-negative bacteria being composed of lipopolysaccharide and protein. *Bordetella bronchiseptica* produces a capsule. Most if not all members of the genus produce fimbrial adhesins (pili). *Bordetella bronchiseptica* and *B. avium* are motile by peritrichous flagella.

Cellular Products of Medical Interest

With few exceptions, *B. pertussis*, *B. parapertussis*, *B. bronchiseptica*, and *B. avium* produce (or at least have the genes to produce) many of the same products important in the pathogenesis of disease (Table 15.2).

Adhesins. The role of adhesins, as in other microorganisms, is to allow the bacterium expressing them to adhere to cells lining a particular niche, as well as to the surface of so-called "target" cells prior to the initiation of disease (in some cases, niche and target cells may be the same). The expression of adhesins depends upon various environmental cues.

Bordetellae produce a number of structures that are responsible for adherence to host cells. These adhesins include fimbriae (or pili), filamentous haemagglutinin, pertactin, cell wall lipopolysaccharide, tracheal colonization factor, and pertussis toxin. All are positively regulated by the BvgAS regulon (see below, "Regulation of the Cellular Products of Medical Interest").

1. Fimbriae. Fimbriae are protein structures composed, in part, of subunits (pilins) responsible for adherence to receptors on host cells. *Bordetella* fimbriae adhere to ciliated epithelial cells of the respiratory tract. They are encoded by four structural genes *fim2*, *fim3*, *fim*X, and *fim*A that give rise to at least four serotypes (see below, "Variability").

2. Filamentous haemagglutinin. Fha (for *f*ilamentous *h*aem*a*gglutinin) is a protein adhesin that has at least three activities associated with various domains within the protein: adherence to ciliated epithelial cells of the respiratory tract and macrophages (by way of an "Arg-Gly-Asp" or RGD sequence targeting complement receptor 3 on host cells); adherence to ciliated epithelial cells of the respiratory tract and phagocytic cells (by way of a "carbohydrate recognition domain"); and a haemagglutinin.

3. Pertactin. Prn(for *p*e*r*tacti*n*) is an outer membrane protein that functions as an adhesin. Like Fha (see above), pertactin contains an "Arg-Gly-Asp" or RGD sequence. Though a particular host target cell has not been identified for Prn, it is likely that ciliated epithelial cells of the respiratory tract, as well as phagocytic cells are the targets for this adhesin.

4. Cell wall lipopolysaccharide. Cell wall lipopolysaccharide of *B. avium*, and by inference *B. pertussis*, *B. parapertussis*, and *B. bronchiseptica*, serves as an adhesin by binding to ciliated epithelium of the respiratory tract, and as a "shield" to cover the outer membrane protecting it from the action of membrane attack complexes generated by the complement system (see below).

5. Tracheal colonization factor. Tracheal colonization factor (Tcf) is a protein adhesin that binds to ciliated epithelial cells of the respiratory tract.

6. Pertussis toxin. Ptx (for *p*ertussis *tox*in) is both an ADP-ribosylating toxin (see below), and an adhesin. Following synthesis, a portion of Ptx is excreted from the bacterial cell, and a portion remains attached to its surface. It is the surface-associated portion that serves as the adhesin. The host cell types to

Table 15.1.   Members of the Genus *Bordetella* and Their Usual Source or Associated Condition

Species	Usual Source or Associated Condition
Bordetella pertussis	Whooping cough in human patients
B. parapertussis	Whooping cough–like condition in human patients; uncommon cause of pneumonia in sheep (sheep strains different from human strains)
B. bronchiseptica	Associated with Atrophic Rhinitis in swine; respiratory tract disease in a variety of animals
B. avium	Rhinotracheitis in poultry (especially turkeys)
B. hinzii	Normal flora of fowl
B. holmesii	Associated with upper respiratory tract disease, and septicemia in human patients
B. trematum	Associated with ear and wound infections in human patients
B. petrii	Environment

Table 15.2.   Distribution of Cellular Products of Medical Interest Within Selected Members of the Genus *Bordetella*

Product	B. pertussis	B. parapertussis	B. bronchiseptica	B. avium
Adenylyl cyclase	+	+	+	+
Brk	+	+	+	–
Capsule	–	–	+	–
DNT	+	+	+	+
Fha	+	+	+	–
Fimbria	+	+	+	+
Iron scavenging	+	+	+	+
LPS	+	+	+	+
Pertactin	+	+	+	?
Ptx	+	–a	–a	–
Tcf	+	–	–	?
Tracheal cytotoxin	+	+	+	+
Type III secretion system	+	+	+	+

aGenes encoding Ptx are present, but the toxin is not produced.

which Ptx adheres are ciliated epithelial cells of the respiratory tract, and phagocytic cells.

Capsule. The capsule plays many roles, the most important of which are interference with phagocytosis (antiphagocytic) and protection of the outer membrane from the deposition of membrane attack complexes generated by activation of the complement system.

Cell Wall. The cell wall of the members of this genus is one typical of gram-negative bacteria being composed of carbohydrates, lipids, and protein. Bordetellae possess lipopolysaccharide and outer membrane proteins that are important virulence determinants.

1. Lipopolysaccharide. The lipopolysaccharide (LPS) in the outer membrane is an important virulence determinant. Not only is the lipid A component toxic (endotoxin), but the length of the side chain in the O-repeat unit hinders the attachment of the membrane attack complex of the complement system to the outer membrane and imparts resistance to antimicrobial proteins (defensins) found in respi-

ratory tract secretions and within phagocytic cell granules. Lipopolysaccharide binds to lipopolysaccharide-binding protein, which transfers it to the blood-phase of CD14. The CD14-LPS complex binds to Toll-like receptor proteins (see Chapter 2) on the surface of macrophage cells triggering the release of proinflammatory cytokines. The composition of the LPS (presence or absence of the O-repeat portion, its length, and charge) influences the extent of protection against the complement system and antimicrobial peptides. LPS composition is regulated by the BvgAS regulon (see below, "Regulation of the Cellular Products of Medical Interest").

2. Outer membrane protein. Brk (for *Bordetella* resistance to killing) is an outer membrane protein. Brk imparts resistance to damage by the complement system (bestows the serum resistant phenotype). Brk is regulated by the BvgAS regulon (see below, "Regulation of the Cellular Products of Medical Interest").

Exotoxins. There are four exotoxins produced by the bordetellae that play important roles in diseases associated with members of this genus: tracheal cytotoxin, dermonecrotic toxin, adenylyl cyclase toxin, and pertussis toxin. All, except tracheal cytotoxin, which is a portion of the cell wall, are regulated by the BvgAS regulon (see below, "Regulation of the Cellular Products of Medical Interest").

1. Tracheal cytotoxin. Tracheal cytotoxin is a portion of the cell wall, and damages ciliated epithelial cells by interfering with DNA synthesis. It also binds to macrophages triggering the release of proinflammatory cytokines.
2. Dermonecrotic toxin. DNT (for *dermonecrotic toxin*) is a member of a family of toxins with similar structures and biological activity. The other "dermonecrotic" toxins include Pmt produced by *Pasteurella multocida* (see Chapter 12), and CNF1 and CNF2 produced by *Escherichia coli* (see Chapter 8). These toxins are so named because dermonecrosis follows their injection into the skin, an occurrence that does not occur naturally. DNT deaminates and transglutamates (preferred) the small GTP-binding protein Rho blocking its GTPase activity (i.e., GTPase activating proteins are unable to correctly bind to modified Rho). These modifications result in changes in the actin cytoskeleton of affected cells and inhibition of differentiation of osteoblasts in bone tissue.
3. Adenylyl cyclase toxin. Adenylyl cyclase toxin is a bifunctional protein with adenylyl cyclase as well as hemolytic activity. Adenylyl cyclase toxin enters the host cell, and following "activation" by calmodulin, increases the intracellular concentration of cAMP. Affected cells lose control of intracellular levels of cAMP resulting in an inability to regulate ion and fluid flow into and out of the "target" cell (respiratory tract epithelium). Loss of control of cAMP levels in phagocytic cells results in reduction of this cell's ability to phagocytose and kill. The hemolytic activity is associated with an RTX motif (*repeats in toxin*, so called because of the common feature of repeats in glycine-rich sequences within the protein, see also *Escherichia coli* haemolysin in Chapter 8, *Pasteurella/Mannheimia* leukotoxin in Chapter 12, *Actinobacillus* haemolysin in Chapter 13, *Moraxella* cytotoxin in Chapter 19). By virtue of the RTX-type toxin activity, adenylyl cyclase toxin is also a pore forming protein that targets neutrophils, macrophages, and lymphocytes.
4. Pertussis toxin. Pertussis toxin (Ptx) is an ADP-ribosylating toxin which ribosylates "activated" heterotrimeric G proteins (GTP-bound) rendering them incapable of returning to the inactive state (GDP-bound). "Activated" G proteins stimulate adenylyl cyclase leading to increased levels of intracellular cAMP. Abnormally high concentration of cAMP results in loss of fluid and ion flow into and out of the cell, and if the cell has phagocytic function, interference with uptake and intracellular killing. The role of Ptx as an adhesin is discussed above.

Iron Acquisition. Because iron is an absolute growth requirement, microorganisms must acquire this substance if they are to exist within the host. Bordetellae acquire iron by secreting a siderophore and utilizing siderophores made by other species of microorganism. In addition, they utilize the iron found in heme and hemoproteins.

Under conditions of iron starvation (as would occur in the host), bordetellae secrete a hydroxamate-type siderophore called *alcaligin*. Bordetellae also have the ability to utilize enterobactin, a siderophore produced by members of the family *Enterobacteriaceae*. These siderophores (alcaligin and enterobactin) remove iron from the iron-binding proteins of the host (transferrin and lactoferrin), making it available to the bacterium.

Heme and hemoproteins (albumin and hemopexin) are additional sources of iron. The outer membrane protein that binds these substances, BhuR (for *Bordetella heme uptake receptor*), is regulated by levels of available iron by means of the extracytoplasmic sigma factor Rhu (for *regulation of heme uptake*) and the Fur regulon (see *Escherichia coli*, Chapter 8).

Type III Secretion System. A Type III secretion system has been identified in the bordetellae (under the control of the BvgAS regulon, see below, "Regulation of the Cellular Products of Medical Interest"). The Type III secretion system consists of an assemblage of proteins (more than 20) that form a hollow tube-like structure through which effector proteins are "injected" into host "target" cells. As yet, *Bordetella* effector proteins have not been identified, but host "target" cells (tracheal epithelial cells, phagocytic cells) undergo apoptosis as a result of effector protein "injection" resulting in loss of epithelial integrity, and evasion of the immune system of the host (decreased phagocytosis, and decreased antigen processing which leads to reduced immune responses).

Regulation of the Cellular Products of Medical Interest. Bordetellae transcriptionally regulate the genes encoding products involved in the production of disease. These include the genes encoding all of the adhesins (fimbriae, filamentous haemagglutinin, pertactin, the character of the cell wall lipopolysaccharide, tracheal colonization factor, and pertussis toxin), pertactin, Brk, toxins (adenylyl cyclase, DNT, pertussis toxin), alcaligin, and the Type III secretion system. All are regulated by the products of the genes encoded in bvgA and bvgS (for *Bordetella virulence genes*) and are referred to as the BvgAS regulon. BvgS is a histidine kinase that acts as a "sensor" of environmental cues resulting in autophosphorylation of one of its histidine residues. This phosphate is then serially transferred to an aspartate residue, then to another histidine before being used to phosphorylate BvgA. Phosphorylated BvgA is a transcriptional activator of the genes encoding the products mentioned above. It is unclear exactly what the environmental cues are that are "sensed" by *Bordetella*. Growth at 37°C in low concentrations of $MgSO_4$ and nicotinic acid activates the regulon. Though growth at 37°C is compatible with a parasitic state, it is unclear what role $MgSO_4$ and nicotinic acid concentrations play in vivo.

Growth Characteristics

All but one of the species of *Bordetella* are strict aerobes deriving energy from oxidation of amino acids. *Bordetella petrii* (the exception) is a facultative anaerobe. *Bordetella bronchiseptica* and *B. avium* grow on ordinary laboratory media (35–37°C), including MacConkey agar, under atmospheric conditions; the former is inconsistently hemolytic on blood agar.

Biochemical Activities

Bordetella avium and *B. bronchiseptica* are catalase and oxidase positive, ferment no carbohydrates, and utilize citrate as an organic carbon source, but only *B. bronchiseptica* reduces nitrate and splits urea.

Resistance

Bordetella spp. are killed by heat or disinfectants. They are susceptible to broad-spectrum antibiotics and polymyxin, but not to penicillin. Their environmental survival is epidemiologically significant.

Variability

An assortment of typing schemes has been developed, mainly for epidemiological purposes.

At least four serotypes have been described for bordetellae based upon the Fim protein (see above, "Adhesins").

Bordetella bronchiseptica dissociates into four phases varying in colonial characteristics, hemolytic activity, suspension stability in saline, ease of colonization, and toxicity. Some strains appear to be host-specific.

Three serotypes, based on surface agglutinins, are recognized in *B. avium*.

Some 20 heat-labile (K) and heat-stable (O; 120°C/60min) antigens exist. Many are common to several species. Others are species- and type-specific.

Bordetella bronchiseptica from pigs appear different from the strains from dogs and horses (which are also different from each other).

Ecology

Reservoir

Bordetella spp. are mainly parasites of ciliated respiratory tract tissue. *Bordetella bronchiseptica* occurs in wild and domestic carnivores, wild and laboratory rodents, swine, rabbits, and occasionally horses, other herbivores, primates, and turkeys. Although probably not part of the resident flora, it is found in the nasopharynx of healthy animals.

Bordetella avium inhabits the respiratory tract of infected fowl, principally turkeys.

Transmission

Mammalian infections are primarily airborne, while in turkeys indirect spread via water and litter is common.

Pathogenesis

Mechanisms. Bordetellae "sense" various environmental cues leading to activation of the BvgAS regulon leading to up regulation of the various genes encoding the products discussed above (see above, "Cellular Products of Medical Interest"). Attachment of bordetellae to ciliated epithelial cells follows expression of adhesins (fimbriae, filamentous haemagglutinin, pertactin, cell wall LPS, tracheal colonization factor, pertussis toxin—see Table 15.2 for listing of which adhesins are produced by which bordetellae). Multiplication occurs (iron is scavenged from host iron-binding proteins—lactoferrin, transferrin—and from heme and hemoproteins; bordetellae outer membrane is protected from complement-generated membrane attack complexes by capsule, LPS, Brk) and inflammation is initiated (LPS; death of epithelial cells due to "injection" of effector proteins; tracheal cytotoxin). Inflammation and loss of the ability to control fluid and ion flow into and out of tracheal epithelial cells (increased production of cAMP from effects of increased activity of adenylyl cyclase) leads to increased mucus and fluid accumulation in the upper respiratory tract. Ciliated epithelial cells become ineffectual in clearing secretions (cilial paralysis due to increased levels of cAMP and cytoskeletal changes brought about by the action of DNT; death of ciliated cell due to tracheal cytotoxin, and the unidentified effector protein "injected" by way of the Type III secretion system). Unencapsulated bordetellae (all but *B. bronchiseptica*) adhere to inflammatory cells (by way of filamentous haemagglutinin, pertactin, and pertussis toxin), and release adenylyl cyclase (interferes with phagocytosis and killing), pertussis toxin (interferes with phagocytosis and killing), and "injection" of an effector protein (interferes with phagocytosis). If phagocytosis occurs, bordetellae survive within phagolysosomes (nature of their LPS) and also escape into endocytic compartments that do not lead to lysosomal fusion.

The consequences of *Bordetella*-induced changes in the ciliated portions of the respiratory tract are varied: depression of respiratory clearance mechanisms, facilitating secondary complications (e.g., pneumonia); in pigs, *B. bronchiseptica* provides nasal irritation, rendering the turbinates susceptible to the action of the dermonecrotic toxin (Pmt) of *Pasteurella multocida*, which has emerged as the primary agent of Atrophic Rhinitis ("progressive Atrophic Rhinitis," see Chapter 12). If *P. multocida* does not become involved, DNT as well as all of the products described above, produces a mild, reversible turbinate hypoplasia ("nonprogressive Atrophic Rhinitis"). Pneumonia, if this occurs, is due to inflammatory responses and the inability of host phagocytic cells and complement system to easily clear bordetellae.

Pathology. Destruction of ciliated respiratory epithelium is the hallmark of *Bordetella*-initiated disease. The process is a suppurative one affecting various portions of the tract (rhinitis, sinusitis, tracheitis). Compromise of the clearance mechanisms of the upper respiratory tract may lead to a suppurative pneumonia and airsacculitis with *Bordetella* itself or some other microorganism.

Disease Patterns

Swine. *Atrophic Rhinitis.* The progressive form of Atrophic Rhinitis is due to combined infection with *P. multocida* and *B. bronchiseptica*, and was discussed in Chapter 12. The nonprogressive form of this disease follows infection with *B. bronchiseptica* alone, and is transient and self-limiting.

Pneumonia. *Bordetella*-mediated compromise of the host defenses of the upper respiratory tract sometimes leads to secondary pneumonia associated with *B. bronchiseptica* or some other microorganism.

Dogs and Cats. *Canine Infectious Tracheobronchitis (Kennel Cough).* Kennel cough is associated with *B. bronchiseptica*. The natural disease is often accompanied by canine parainfluenza virus, canine adenoviruses 1 and 2, and canine herpes virus. While most dogs recover within a few weeks, the bacterium can persist for months. Transfer to susceptible cats has been demonstrated.

Pneumonia. *Bordetella bronchiseptica* is sometimes isolated from samples collected from pneumonic lungs, often from dogs with canine distemper.

Cats. *Bordetella bronchiseptica* produces a mild upper respiratory tract infection in cats, mainly those housed in colonies (upper respiratory tract infections in cats are also associated with herpes virus, calicivirus, *Mycoplasma*, *Chlamydophila*). Cats, like dogs, carry the organism asymptomatically (up to 19 weeks) following recovery. Transfer to susceptible dogs has been demonstrated.

Poultry. *Turkey Coryza.* Turkey poults infected with *B. avium* develop tracheobronchitis, sinusitis, and airsacculitis. Signs include nasal exudate, conjunctivitis, tracheal rales, and dyspnea. Morbidity is high, but mortality, except by secondary infection, is generally low (<5%). Recovery may begin after 2 weeks, although some illnesses may last 6 weeks.

Laboratory Animals. *Rabbit bordetellosis. Bordetella bronchiseptica* infections in rabbits are usually asymptomatic. However, in association with other infectious agents (e.g., *Pasteurella multocida*) may be involved with bronchopneumonia.

Epidemiology

Atrophic Rhinitis affects pigs under 6 weeks old, when osteogenesis and bone remodeling are most active. Affected pigs spread *B. bronchiseptica*. The ultimate sources are carrier sows, in which carrier rates decline with age.

Canine kennel cough usually affects young, nonimmune dogs that acquire it from clinically affected individuals, as well as recovered carriers.

Bordetella avium causes disease mainly in young poults. The contaminated environment is important in perpetuating the infection.

Immunologic Aspects

Pathogenic Factors

Depressed cell-mediated responses have been observed in experimental *B. avium* infections. Their relation to natural disease is undetermined. *Bordetella bronchiseptica* can para-sitize dendritic cells, which results in a decrease in immune responses due to inefficient antigen processing.

Protective Role

Local antibody is believed to prevent *B. bronchiseptica* colonization in dogs. No other immune responses have been shown to be protective.

Bordetella avium antiserum is ineffective in protecting turkeys, but maternal immunization reduces losses in challenged progeny. Antibody to adhesins prevents adherence to tracheal epithelia.

Immunization Procedures

Bacterins used on pregnant sows provide some colostral immunity to piglets, especially when including toxigenic *P. multocida* strains. Bacterin-toxoid preparations protect piglets.

Intratracheal administered live attenuated vaccine has been beneficial in kennel cough control.

Of *B. avium* vaccines, those using attenuated live organisms intratracheally have been most effective.

Laboratory Diagnosis

Nasal swabs (Atrophic Rhinitis), sediment of transtracheal washes (canine tracheobronchitis), and tracheal swabs (coryza of turkeys) are cultured on blood and MacConkey agars. Routine laboratory tests are used for identification. A polymerase chain reaction based assay utilizing primers designed to amplify various species-specific segments of DNA is available for determining the presence of bordetellae as well as for identification purposes.

Bordetella avium reacts like *Alcaligenes faecalis* in routine laboratory tests. Cellular fatty acid analysis differentiates the two. A microagglutination test is used for serodiagnosis.

Treatment and Control

The progressive form of Atrophic Rhinitis is not treatable. Preventive measures include maintenance of an aged sow herd with a low carrier rate; thorough disinfection and cleanup of farrowing houses and nurseries after each use; vaccination (see above); prophylactic use of sulfonamides in feed or water; and elimination of carrier sows based on nasal swab culture.

Canine tracheobronchitis responds inconsistently to antibiotics. Vaccination (see above), fumigation of kennels, adequate ventilation, and isolation of affected dogs are useful preventive practices. Tetracycline remains the drug of choice.

Bordetella avium is susceptible to tetracycline, erythromycin, and nitrofurantoin, but resistant to penicillin G, streptomycin, and sulfonamides. Mass medication and vaccination may prevent outbreaks without eliminating the infection.

16

Brucella

RICHARD L. WALKER

Brucellosis is an infectious bacterial disease caused by members of the genus *Brucella*. It is a disease of worldwide importance and affects a number of animal species. *Brucella* are obligate parasites, requiring an animal host for maintenance. Infections tend to localize to the reticuloendothelial system and genital tract with abortions in females and epididymitis and orchitis in males the most common clinical manifestations. Chronic infections are common.

DNA-DNA hybridization studies show that *Brucella* is a monospecific genus based on level of overall homology. The traditional species names for the different brucellas continue to be used in a biological species concept system based on host range, in addition to the presence of species-specific markers. The classical nomenclature is used in this chapter. Additional *Brucella* "species" have recently been described from marine mammals. The different *Brucella* species exhibit host preferences and vary in severity of the disease caused. Dye and phage susceptibility along with biochemical, cultural, and serologic characteristics are used to distinguish among species. The six traditional *Brucella* species are *B. abortus, B. canis, B. melitensis, B. neotomae, B. ovis,* and *B. suis.*

Many species of *Brucella* are capable of causing disease in humans. Infections are chronic and debilitating. The signs of brucellosis in humans are relatively nonspecific and individuals with brucellosis are sometimes labeled hypochondriacs because of the vague presenting clinical signs.

Descriptive Features

Morphology and Staining

Members of the genus *Brucella* are small, gram-negative coccobacilli measuring 0.6 to 1.5 μm by 0.5 to 0.7 μm in size. Cells are fairly uniform and can easily be mistaken for cocci. They are typically arranged singly but also occur in pairs or clusters. No capsules, flagella, or spores are produced; however, an external envelope has been demonstrated by electron microscopy around *B. abortus, B. melitensis,* and *B. suis. Brucella* stain red with Macchiavello and modified Ziehl-Neelsen stains.

Cellular Structure and Composition

Brucellae possess a typical gram-negative cell wall. Dominant surface antigens are located on the lipopolysac-charide. Specifically, the A and M antigens are found in varying concentrations among the different smooth *Brucella* species. The outer membrane contains other major surface antigens. The peptidoglycan layer (3 nm to 5 nm) is more prominent than that of *Escherichia coli.* The periplasmic space varies from 3 nm to 30 nm. The cytoplasmic membrane is a typical three-layered lipoprotein membrane. L-form variants are recognized and may play a role in persistent infections.

The mol% G + C of DNA is 58–59. Most *Brucella* species have two circular chromosomes. Plasmid DNA has not been demonstrated. The entire genomes of *Brucella suis* and *B. melitensis* have been sequenced and are likely to provide substantial insight into factors related to virulence and pathogenesis. The overall fatty acid composition is sufficiently unique to be useful for identification and taxonomic purposes.

Cellular Products of Medical Interest

Cell Wall. The cell wall of the members of this genus is one typical of gram negatives. The lipopolysaccharide (LPS) in the outer membrane is an important virulence determinant. Not only is the lipid A component toxic (endotoxin), but the length of the side chain in the O-repeat unit hinders the attachment of the membrane attack complex of the complement system to the outer membrane. LPS binds to lipopolysaccharide-binding protein (a serum protein), which in turn transfers it to the blood phase of CD14. The CD14-LPS complex binds to Toll-like receptor proteins (see Chapter 2) on the surface of macrophage cells triggering the release of proinflammatory cytokines. In addition, the cell wall LPS of brucellae aid in its survival within macrophages.

Erythritol. Erythritol (a four-carbon alcohol) is one of several "allantoic fluid factors" found in the gravid uterus, and appears responsible for the preferential localization to the reproductive tract of the pregnant animals. "Allantoic fluid factors" stimulate the growth of brucellae.

Outer Membrane Proteins. Porin proteins in the outer membrane are thought to stimulate delayed-type hypersensitivity and account for the varying susceptibility to dyes observed for the different species.

Miscellaneous Products. Production of adenine and guanine monophosphate by *Brucella* inhibits phagolysome fusion and activation of the myeloperoxidase-halide system. *Brucella* are able to inhibit apoptosis in infected macrophages, thereby preventing host cell elimination. Soluble protein products inhibit TNF-alpha production. The Vir (for *virulence*) operon encodes a Type IV secretion system, which appears to be involved with intramacrophage survival.

Growth Characteristics

On initial isolation, colonies are not apparent until 3 to 5 days' incubation. Most colonies are detected by 10 to 14 days, but in some cases incubation for up to 21 days is required. Growth is best in an aerobic environment at 37°C but occurs between 20°C and 40°C. Optimal pH is 6.6 to 7.4. *Brucella ovis* and some biovars of *B. abortus* require an increased concentration of CO_2. Enriched media with 5% serum are required by *B. abortus* biovar 2 and *B. ovis*.

Brucella colonies have a characteristic bluish color when examined with obliquely transmitted light. Colonies have smooth or nonsmooth morphologies that are determined by the presence or absence, respectively, of the polysaccharide side chain in the lipopolysaccharide. These morphologic variations are the result of spontaneous mutation and are influenced by specific growth factors. Smooth colonies are white, convex with an entire edge, and have a creamy consistency. Nonsmooth colonies have intermediate, rough, or mucoid forms. Rough colonies are dull yellow, opaque, and friable. They are difficult to suspend in solution and agglutinate spontaneously. The mucoid colonies are similar to the rough colonies except for having a glutinous texture.

Resistance

Brucellae survive freezing and thawing. Under proper environmental conditions, they survive for up to 4 months in milk, urine, water, and damp soil. Most disinfectants active against other gram-negative bacteria kill *Brucella*. Pasteurization effectively kills *Brucella* in milk.

Diversity

The *Brucella* genome appears to be very stable. Strains associated with a specific animal host have a unique genomic organization.

The colony morphology of *Brucella* varies from rough to smooth forms (see "Growth Characteristics," above). *Brucella abortus, B. melitensis, B. suis,* and *B. neotomae* are typically isolated in the smooth form but can develop rough forms on subsequent laboratory passage. *Brucella ovis* is always in a rough form. Isolates of *B. canis* have a mucoid appearance. In general, smooth strains of *Brucella* are more virulent than rough strains.

Variations in CO_2 requirement, H_2S production, urease production, susceptibility to differing concentrations of certain dyes (thionin and basic fuchsin), and susceptibility to naturally or mutagen-derived bacteriophages account for diversity among species and biovars within species. The different species of *Brucella* vary in host preference and degree of virulence within and among animal species.

Ecology

Zoologic and Geographic Reservoirs

As obligate parasites, *Brucella* require an animal reservoir. Host preference is exhibited by the different *Brucella* species; however, a broad host range has been demonstrated for some species. Survival time outside the host is variable and depends on temperature and moisture. Colder weather extends survival time.

Cattle are the preferential host for *B. abortus*. Other animals, including bison, camels, and yaks, are commonly infected. The different biovars of *B. abortus* have different geographic distributions. Biovars 1 and 2 have a worldwide distribution, while biovar 3 is predominantly found in India, Egypt, and Africa.

Swine are the preferential host for *B. suis* biovar 1. This biovar is widely distributed. Biovar 2 is found in swine and wild hares (*Lepus timidus*), predominately in western and central Europe. *Brucella suis* biovar 3 is predominately recovered from midwestern North America in the United States. Biovar 4 affects reindeer and caribou in Alaska, Canada, and Siberia.

Brucella melitensis infects goats and sheep worldwide except for North America, Australia, and New Zealand. Camels, alpacas, and llamas are also infected.

Brucella ovis infections are limited to sheep and *B. canis* infections are limited to dogs. Both have a worldwide distribution. *Brucella neotomae* has only been found in the wood rat (*Neotoma lepida*) with geographic distribution limited to the Salt Lake Desert of Utah. Recently, *B. melitensis* and *B. suis* have become established in cattle in some Middle Eastern and South American countries, respectively.

The newly recognized *Brucella* species found in marine mammals also show host preferences similar to other *Brucella* species. Marine *Brucella* species (proposed species—*B. cetaceae* and *B. pinnipediae*) have been found in a number of species of sea mammals and are considered host-adapted and enzootic in large populations of these animals. Pathology is typically minimal and the marine *Brucella* species are currently considered opportunists or secondary pathogens.

Transmission

Brucella are disseminated by direct or indirect contact with infected animals. Ingestion is the most common route of entry, although exposure through the conjunctival and genital mucosa, skin, and respiratory routes occurs. The major source for exposure to *B. abortus* in cattle and *B. melitensis* in sheep and goats is through aborted fetuses, the placenta, and postabortion uterine fluids. Aborted tissue and fluids are also a common means for transmission of *B. suis* and *B. canis*. Genital infections in cattle routinely clear within 30 days after calving and cows are not considered infectious for other cattle after that time. Genital infections in swine, in some cases, persist longer than those in cattle.

Ingestion of milk from infected cattle and goats is another source for infection of calves and kids. Direct transfer in utero has also been documented.

Infections of the accessory sex glands of males allows for dissemination of organisms through the semen. Infections can occur in the accessory sex organs without testicular or epididymal lesions being present. Venereal transmission of *B. suis* in swine, *B. ovis* in sheep, and *B. canis* in dogs is common. Urine is another vehicle for disseminating *B. canis* to other dogs.

Insects may play a minor role in transmission and maintenance of infection in a herd. Face flies have been shown to take up and excrete *Brucella* in their feces.

Pathogenesis

Mechanisms. Following exposure, *Brucella* penetrate intact mucosal surfaces. In the alimentary tract, the epithelium covering the ileal Peyer's patches are a preferred site for entry. After penetrating mucosal barriers, organisms may be engulfed by phagocytic cells. *Brucella* are internalized in macrophages by generalized membrane ruffling and macropinocytosis. Various mechanisms are employed by *Brucella* to allow for survival inside phagocytic cells. Some of the genes for intracellular survival are actually shared with plant pathogens and endosymbionts. *Brucella* are capable of surviving and multiplying inside macrophages by modifying the phagosome maturation process and creating an intracellular environment suitable for multiplication. Acidification of the phagosome induces the *virB* promoter for the VirB complex, an important virulence factor. The VirB operon appears to encode a Type IV secretion system and is likely involved in intracellular trafficking and macropinocytosis. Phagosome maturation is arrested at steps between acidification and phagolysosome fusion.

Intracellular survival in macrophages and, to a lesser extent, neutrophils is enhanced by suppressing the myeloperoxidase-H_2O_2-halide system. Superoxide dismutase and catalase production may play a role in defense against oxidative killing. Stress proteins have been demonstrated in *Brucella*, however their role in virulence is considered marginal. These proteins are thought to play a role in protecting organisms from hydrolytic enzymes, oxygen radicals, and myeloperoxidase killing systems in the phagolysosome. The lipopolysaccharide of *Brucella* is directly associated with virulence and is thought to play a role in enhancing intracellular survival. Production of adenine and guanine monophosphate by *Brucella* inhibits phagolysome fusion and activation of the myeloperoxidase-halide system. *Brucella* are able to inhibit apoptosis in infected macrophages, thereby preventing host cell elimination. Soluble protein products inhibit TNF-alpha production. It is believed that the variations in virulence observed among the *Brucella* species may, in part, be related to the greater ability of some species to avoid host defenses.

Following entry into the host, *Brucella* organisms, either free in the extracellular environment or in phagocytic cells, localize to regional lymph nodes. There they proliferate and infect other cells or are killed and the infection is terminated. Some cattle appear to be innately resistant to infection. This resistance is related to the macrophages' ability to contain the organisms. From the regional lymph nodes, *Brucella* disseminate hematogenously and localize in the reticuloendothelial system and reproductive tract.

There is preferential localization to the reproductive tract of pregnant animals. Unknown factors in the gravid uterus, collectively referred to as *allantoic fluid factors*, stimulate the growth of *Brucella*. Erythritol is considered to be one of these factors.

Experimental infection studies have demonstrated that, at the cellular level, *Brucella* localizes into the cisternae of the rough endoplasmic reticulum of trophoblasts of the placentome. Infection subsequently spreads to the fetus. The exact mechanism of abortion is unclear; however, likely possibilities are that abortion results from 1) interference with fetal circulation due to the existing placentitis, 2) the direct effect of endotoxin, and/or 3) fetal stress resulting from the inflammatory response in fetal tissue.

Although less is known about the factors involved in localization of *Brucella* in the reproductive tract of males, the presence of growth stimulating compounds may be a factor. The prolonged bacteremia observed with some of the *Brucella* species accounts for the greater likelihood for extragenital manifestations to occur in animals infected with those species.

Pathology. There are grossly visible lesions in the placenta associated with *Brucella* abortions. Intercotyledonary thickening with a yellow gelatinous fluid is present. The cotyledons are frequently necrotic, yellow-gray in color, and covered with a thick brown exudate. The degree of necrosis varies among the *Brucella* species with *B. melitensis* infections in goats being most severe. The aborted fetus is frequently edematous. Abomasal contents may be turbid and have a lemon-yellow color. The most common histologic findings in the fetus are bronchitis and bronchopneumonia with a predominately mononuclear cell infiltrate. In general, *Brucella* induce a granulomatous-type inflammatory reaction.

In males palpable enlargement of the epididymis, especially involving the tail portion, is common. Epididymal lesions are characterized by hyperplasia and hydropic degeneration of tubular epithelium. Resulting extravasation of sperm leads to the formation of a spermatic granuloma (Fig 16.1). In bulls with orchitis the scrotum is swollen, largely due to an inflammation of the tunica and fibrinopurulent exudate in the tunica vaginalis. The testicular parenchyma becomes necrotic and is sometimes replaced by pus. Pathology of the accessory sex organs includes prostatitis in dogs and fibrinopurulent seminal vesiculitis in bulls.

Extragenital tract pathology includes lymphocytic endophthalmitis in dogs (*B. canis*), purulent or fibrinopurulent synovitis in swine (*B. suis*), osteomyelitis in dogs and swine (*B. canis* and *B. suis*), necrotizing and purulent bursitis in horses (*B. abortus*), and hygroma development in cattle (*B. abortus*).

Disease Patterns. The primary clinical manifestations of brucellosis are related to the reproductive tract. In general, animals do not exhibit overt systemic illness. In females, abortion is the most common presentation. No premonitory signs are usually apparent. Abortion in cattle commonly occurs in the fifth month of gestation or later. Retained placenta is a possible sequela. Females usually abort only once, presumably due to acquired immunity. *Brucella melitensis* infections in goats and sheep are similar

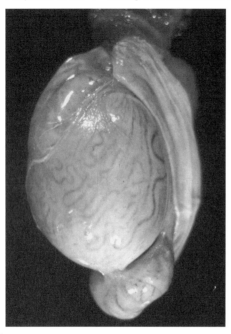 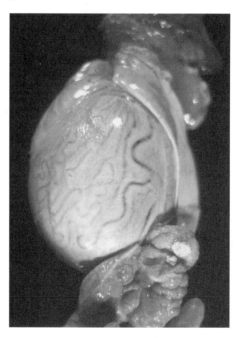

to *B. abortus* in cattle except that acute mastitis develops in goats infected with *B. melitensis*. The mastitis in goats presents with palpable nodules in the udder and milk that is clotted and watery. Abortions in swine can occur at any time in gestation and are related to time of exposure. Abortions in dogs due to *B. canis* occur around 50 days of gestation. *Brucella ovis* infections in sheep only rarely result in abortions in ewes.

In males, epididymitis and orchitis are the most common presenting signs. Lesions are usually unilateral but may be bilateral. Semen examination reveals increased numbers of neutrophils in acute cases. Neutrophils are few in number in more chronic infections. *Brucella ovis* infections in rams predominately affect the epididymis with testicular lesions being uncommon. Palpable lesions in the epididymis of mature rams are frequently the result of infection with *B. ovis*, whereas epididymitis in yearlings and ram lambs are usually caused by a variety of other organisms. In bulls, infection with *B. abortus* frequently involves the testicle. Dogs infected with *B. canis* develop scrotal swelling as a result of fluid accumulation in the tunica. Scrotal dermatitis may develop because of constant licking of the scrotum. Infections of the male genital tract result in decreased fertility and, in some cases, sterility.

Extragenital manifestations develop in many animal species. Swine infected with *B. suis* may develop arthritis, especially in the large joints of the limbs, or lumbar spondylitis. Lesions in the lumbar vertebrae result in tissue necrosis that puts pressure on the spinal cord and can lead to posterior paralysis. Dogs infected with *B. canis* can develop meningoencephalitis, osteomyelitis, discospondylitis, and anterior uveitis. Ocular manifestations in dogs may be the initial presenting sign for canine brucellosis.

Chronic infections with *B. abortus* in cattle can result in hygromas. Horses infected with *B. abortus* develop "poll evil" or "fistulous withers" and present with fistulous tracts originating from the atlantal or supraspinous bursas, respectively. Infections in horses usually result from contact with infected cattle.

Brucellosis in humans is primarily a disease of the reticuloendothelial system. A mild lymphadenopathy, splenomegaly, and hepatomegaly may be detected. Onset of signs occurs within 2 to 3 weeks of exposure. Clinical signs are nonspecific and include alternating fever and chills with night sweats, fatigue, muscle and joint pains, and backaches. Depression and insomnia are common. Specific clinical manifestations of infections include arthritis, osteomyelitis and endocarditis.

Epidemiology

Humans acquire infections by handling tissues containing *Brucella* organisms. *Brucella melitensis* is considered the most virulent species for humans followed by *B. suis*, *B. abortus*, and *B. canis*. *Brucella ovis* and *B. neotomae* do not infect humans. Common sources for infection are aborted fetuses, placentas, and postabortion uterine fluids, all of which contain large numbers of organisms. Veterinarians, ranchers, and slaughterhouse workers are particularly at risk for acquiring infections.

The prolonged bacteremic phase of *B. suis* infections in swine poses a special risk for slaughterhouse workers handling infected tissues. Individuals who participate in the hunting of feral swine are also at risk for contracting *B. suis* infections. Relatively few cases of infections in humans due to *B. canis* have been reported. Individuals at risk are kennel workers and breeders coming in contact with contaminated fluids from infected dogs.

Infected animals also shed organisms in the milk. Raw milk or raw milk products of bovine or caprine origin are ready sources for infections in humans. Marine mammal *Brucella* species have caused intracerebral granulomas in humans.

Accidental self-inoculation with live *Brucella* vaccine strains can result in disease. Human-to-human transmission is rare.

Characteristics of Infection in Animal Populations. Susceptibility to infection depends on age, sex, breed, and pregnancy status. Younger animals tend to be more resistant, and frequently clear infections, although latent infections do occur. Less than 3% of animals infected at birth remain infected as adults. Sexually mature animals are much more susceptible to infection, regardless of gender. Most animals infected as adults remain infected for life.

Herd size and animal density are directly related to prevalence of disease and difficulty in controlling infection in a population. Calving practices also play a major role in the spread of brucellosis. Separate calving pens allow for minimizing exposure of uninfected animals. Whether a herd raises its own replacement animals or purchases replacement animals affects the potential for introduction into the herd.

In contrast to cattle, where bulls play a relatively minor role, boars are more likely to be a source for introducing *Brucella* into a swine herd. Both venereal transmission and exposure to aborted fetuses and fetal membranes are important for maintaining infections in a herd. Confinement of breeding swine in common pens or lots provides the ideal setting for spreading infection. Management practices directed at eliminating infected boars and minimizing exposure to aborted tissue greatly reduce the incidence of disease in commercial swine operations. Feral swine serve as a reservoir for *B. suis* and are more commonly infected than commercial swine in some countries. In some European countries where *B. suis* biovar 2 is found, the European hare acts as a source for infection in swine.

Dissemination of *B. ovis* in sheep occurs during the breeding season. Older rams are more likely to be infected than yearlings. Introduction of an infected ram during the breeding season can lead to rapid spread of infection within the flock. Transmission occurs when an uninfected ram breeds a ewe recently bred by an infected ram. The ewe acts mainly as a mechanical vector for transmitting infection. Homosexual activity of rams is another means of spreading infection among rams.

Dogs in suburban areas are least likely to be infected with *B. canis*. Prevalence of infection is greatest in economically depressed areas. Close confinement settings such as kennels increase the likelihood for transmitting infections.

Immunologic Aspects

Immune Mechanisms in Pathogenesis

Evidence indicates that antibodies against *Brucella* play both a protective and detrimental role. IgM antibodies, which appear initially after infection, and low levels of IgG will cause complement-mediated lysis of *Brucella*. Elevated levels of IgG antibodies, however, appear to act as blocking antibodies that modulate the ability of the complement membrane attack complex to lyse cells. This may account for resistance to complement-mediated lysis in the face of high specific antibody levels and the lack of correlation between protection and high antibody titers. The blocking antibodies are opsonizing and promote uptake by phagocytes where *Brucella* have developed mechanisms for survival and proliferation.

Phagocytic cells unable to eliminate *Brucella* play a role in dissemination of organisms to other parts of the body and in persistence of infection.

IgA autoantibody has been demonstrated in dogs infected with *B. canis* and may explain some of the observed effect on fertility.

Mechanisms of Resistance and Recovery

Effective immunity is primarily cellular in nature. Specifically sensitized T lymphocytes release cytokines that activate macrophages, which in turn control *Brucella* by reactive oxygen intermediates. *Brucella* can activate NK cells by inducing antigen-presenting cells to secrete IL-12. NK cells can then kill infected target cells. A more effective immunity develops when animals are infected prior to sexual maturity.

Artificial Immunization

Cattle are immunized with either nonviable (*B. abortus* 45/20) or attenuated live (*B. abortus* strains 19 and RB51) vaccines. These products provide protection from abortion, the major mode of dissemination, but not from infection. A single dose at 3 to 7 and 4 to 12 months of age is required with *B. abortus* strain 19 and strain RB51, respectively. Two doses 6 weeks apart in animals over 6 months of age are required with *B. abortus* 45/20. Adult cow vaccination is sometimes performed as a regulatory effort to control infection in a herd. Strain 19 is occasionally shed in the milk and can cause abortions in cattle. Adult vaccination with *B. abortus* strain RB51 only rarely causes abortion. Bulls should not be vaccinated because orchitis can develop. The type of vaccine used is generally established by the particular country's regulatory agency in charge of brucellosis control. Recently, in a number of regulatory programs *B. abortus* strain RB51 has replaced strain 19 as the approved calfhood vaccine because it does not interfere with serologic evaluation.

Brucella melitensis Rev 1, a partially attenuated vaccine, is used to control brucellosis in goats and sheep caused by *B. melitensis*. A killed product, *Brucella melitensis* H38, is also available.

Bacterins for control of *B. ovis* are available, but their efficacy is limited. *Brucella melitensis* Rev 1 has been used to protect against *B. ovis* infections in sheep; however, it cannot be used in countries free of *B. melitensis* because the antibody titers interfere with serologic evaluations for *B. melitensis* infection.

Vaccination is not practiced for control of disease caused by *B. suis* or *B. canis*.

Laboratory Diagnosis

Specimens

Great care should be employed when working with infected tissues and cultures in the laboratory. All *Brucella* cultures should be handled following biosafety level 3 practices because of the potential for laboratory infection. All laboratory procedures should be performed in a manner that prevents aerosolization, and all work should be conducted in a biological safety cabinet.

Appropriate samples for diagnosis of brucellosis depend on the animal species affected, species of *Brucella* involved, and clinical presentation. Abscess material, semen, and vaginal fluids associated with recent abortions are useful for recovering organisms antemortem. Milk samples from cattle and goats are used in antemortem isolation attempts and for immunodiagnostic evaluation. In dogs, blood cultures are useful for isolation of *B. canis* because of the prolonged bacteremia that occurs. Serum is used for serologic evaluation.

Samples collected at necropsy should include spleen, liver, udder, and multiple lymph nodes, including the supramammary, retropharyngeal, internal iliac, lumbar, and mesenteric lymph nodes. The supramammary lymph node is superior to other lymph nodes for isolating *Brucella* from dairy cattle. Abomasal fluid and lungs of the aborted fetus and the placenta are the preferred specimens in the case of abortion. In males the epididymis, testicle, and accessory sex organs are examined.

Direct Examination

Gram stains of fetal stomach contents from an aborted fetus and the placenta reveal large numbers of gram-negative coccobacilli. Using carbol fuchsin rather than safranin as a counter-stain in the gram-staining procedure makes organisms more easily detectable. Modified Ziehl-Neelsen and Macchiavello stains are also used to demonstrate *Brucella*. Organisms can be detected in semen but are usually in low numbers. *Brucella* is difficult to detect by direct examination in other samples, especially from chronically infected animals.

Isolation

Tissues are cultured directly on solid media. Milk cultures are performed by centrifuging milk at 5900 to 7700 x g for 15 minutes or by allowing for gravity cream separation to occur overnight. Both the cream layer and sediment, if the centrifugation technique is used, should be plated on solid media. Commonly used media include serum dextrose, tryptose, and brucella (Albimi) agars.

If contamination is likely to be a problem, isolation attempts should be made using media containing actidione (30 mg/L), bacitracin (7500 U/L), and polymyxin B (1800 U/L). Selective media are used both with and without the incorporation of ethyl violet (1:800,000) (Fig 16.2). Cultures should be incubated at 37°C in 10% CO_2 for a minimum of 10 days and up to 21 days in highly suspicious cases.

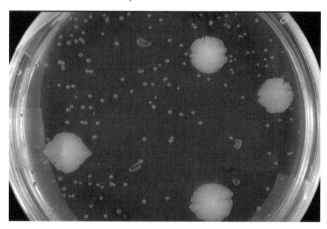

FIGURE 16.2.   *Culture plate from the supramammary lymph node from a cow that reacted positive for serum antibodies to* Brucella abortus. *Numerous* Brucella *colonies are growing on the selective* Brucella *media with ethyl violet. Four large colonies of another bacteria are also present.*

Animal inoculation is the most sensitive method for detection of *Brucella* and is sometimes necessary when very low numbers of organisms are present. Guinea pigs are the most sensitive laboratory animals for this purpose. Two guinea pigs are inoculated and at 3 and 6 weeks postinoculation an animal is sacrificed. Serum is examined for antibodies and tissues are cultured for organisms.

Identification

Presumptive identification of *Brucella* species requires demonstrating colonies of gram-negative coccobacilli that are nonhemolytic, catalase positive, and oxidase positive (except for *B. ovis* and some strains of *B. abortus*). Most species, except *B. ovis*, are strongly urease positive. Glucose and lactose are not fermented by any of the species. Agglutination in unadsorbed antismooth *Brucella* serum helps in presumptive identification of smooth strains.

Definitive identification is usually performed by a *Brucella* reference laboratory. A fluorescent antibody test is used for rapid identification. Urease production, CO_2 requirement, H_2S production, oxidation of metabolic substrates, agglutination in monospecific antisera, growth in the presence of varying concentration of thionin, and basic fuchsin and phage typing are used to determine species and biovars within species (Fig 16.3). *Brucella abortus* strain 19 can be differentiated from field strains of *B. abortus* by its lack of requirement for CO_2 for growth and inhibition by 5 mg/ml penicillin or 1 mg/ml of erythritol. Strain RB51 can be differentiated from field strains and strain 19 by demonstrating its resistance to rifampin (200 µg/ml), staining with crystal violet, and agglutination with acriflavin.

Polymerase chain reaction (PCR) methods have been described for differentiation of *Brucella* species. PCR-restriction fragment length polymorphism, particularly of the *omp*2 gene, has proven particularly useful. A deletion in the *ery* locus can be used to differentiate Strain 19 from

FIGURE 16.3. *Lysis of a confluent lawn of* Brucella abortus *with increasing tenfold dilutions of Tbilisi phage (B. abortus specific phage). The "routine test dilution" used is the highest dilution showing confluent lysis where phage is applied. At the 10⁻⁵ dilution, individual plaques are becoming apparent.*

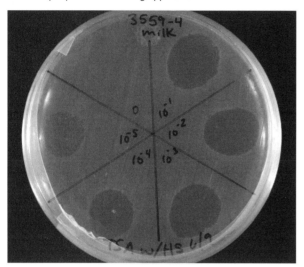

FIGURE 16.4. Brucella *milk ring test for detection of antibodies in milk. In a negative sample, the added, stained Brucella antigen remains dispersed in the milk portion and the cream layer is white (left). In a positive sample, the antibodies react with stained antigen and the complex rises to the top in the cream layer. The cream layer appears purple (right).*

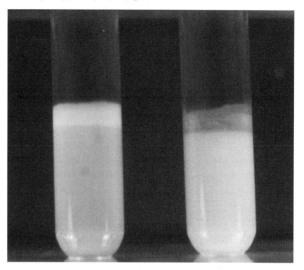

field strains of *B. abortus* and the presence of an insertion sequence in the *wboA* gene, which encodes a glycotransferase, can be used to differentiate Strain RB51 from field strains.

Immunodiagnosis

Antibody detection is commonly used for diagnosing brucellosis and in control programs. Samples tested include blood, milk, and occasionally semen. A number of immunodiagnostic tests have been developed for cattle. These tests detect different classes and types of antibodies and vary in their sensitivity and specificity. Individual blood samples can be tested by tube agglutination, plate agglutination, rose bengal plate, or card tests. Other tests include the buffered plate agglutination assay, rivanol agglutination, complement fixation, and enzyme-linked immunosorbent assay (ELISA).

Frequently, highly sensitive but less specific tests are used for screening purposes and are followed by more specific tests for confirmation purposes. A similar approach to that used in cattle is employed when testing goats and sheep for *B. melitensis*. Sera are screened with a test such as the rose bengal test and results confirmed with a more specific test.

Milk is screened with the *Brucella* milk ring test, which identifies specific antibodies in milk. The test is performed on bulk tank milk samples as a means of screening dairy herds. Stained *Brucella* antigen is added to milk. If antibodies are present, agglutinated antigen is buoyed to the top by the rising cream and a purple ring develops at the top of the tube (Fig 16.4).

Serologic tests are commonly used to identify infected swine herds and monitor herd status. These tests are less accurate when testing individual pigs because some in-

fected swine do not have detectable antibody titers. Herds can be screened by the brucellosis card test. Tests such as rivanol agglutination and 2-mercaptoethanol agglutination are used for confirmation.

Rams are tested for antibodies to *B. ovis* using either a complement fixation test or ELISA.

For canine brucellosis, screening is performed with a rapid slide agglutination test (RSAT). The RSAT is sensitive but not very specific, therefore positive results should be confirmed with additional tests that are more specific. An agar gel immunodiffusion test using cytoplasmic antigen is more specific but not as sensitive as the RSAT and is used as a confirmatory test.

Nonculture Detection Methods

A number of nonculture methods, including PCR, immunoperoxidase staining, DNA probes, and coagglutination, have been described for detection of *Brucella* in tissues and fluids.

Treatment

As a general rule, treatment of infected livestock is not attempted because of the high treatment failure rate, cost, and potential problems related to maintaining infected animals in the face of ongoing eradication programs. Tetracycline and dihydrostreptomycin have been used to treat *B. ovis* infections in rams with variable results. Once a palpable epididymal lesion is present, antibiotic treatment will not be beneficial. The presence of abscesses and fibrosis in tissues of the accessory sex organs makes penetration with antibiotics to these areas difficult.

Treatment of dogs with brucellosis requires a prolonged

course of antibiotic therapy. The combination of dihydrostreptomycin and tetracycline or minocycline for a 2-to-4-week period is commonly used. Fluoroquinolones may also be useful; however, only limited information about their effectiveness is available. Treatment failures are common. Treatment should also consist of neutering affected animals. Treatment is not recommended in canine breeding colonies. In this case, infected dogs should be culled.

Control and Prevention

Approaches at control and prevention of brucellosis depend on the animal species involved, *Brucella* species, management practices, and availability and efficacy of vaccines. Approaches used to control brucellosis include 1) immunization alone, 2) testing and removal of infected animals in conjunction with an immunization program, and 3) testing and removal of infected animals without immunization.

Control by Immunization Alone

Immunization by itself reduces the number of abortions and, thereby, reduces potential for exposure. By itself, immunization will not result in eradication of the infection in a herd. Immunization alone should be considered as a means of controlling the level of disease only.

Immunization Followed by Test and Slaughter

Control of bovine brucellosis routinely employs a combination of vaccination of females and a test and slaughter program. Cattle are vaccinated at a young age and evaluated with immunodiagnostic tests when they reach sexual maturity and vaccination titers have diminished. Vaccination with strain 19 is approximately 70% effective on an individual basis but more effective when evaluated on a herd basis. In experimental challenge, vaccination with strain RB51 provided protection similar to vaccination with strain 19. Any animals identified as infected are culled from the herd and slaughtered. Routine testing is done by the milk ring test in dairy cattle or blood tests from beef cattle at slaughter. A similar program is followed with *B. melitensis* infections in sheep and goats.

Test and Slaughter Without Immunization

Immunization control programs are not used for swine brucellosis. The most successful method of control is depopulation of the entire herd and restocking with uninfected replacement animals. Methods other than depopulation, such as removing only adult animals and retaining weanlings, are less successful. Removal of only the serological reactors will not control infection in the herd. Confinement operations and closed herds make establishing and maintaining a swine herd free of brucellosis readily achievable. In some instances, depopulation is practiced with *B. melitensis* infections in sheep and goats.

Control Methods for *Brucella ovis*

Removing infected rams and preventing new infections in rams are the main means of controlling *B. ovis* infection in a flock. Practices that allow for introduction of infected rams into a flock, such as loaning of rams, should be avoided. Yearling rams should be maintained separately from mature rams. All rams should be palpated for epididymal lesions at least twice a year before breeding season and rams with palpable lesions culled. Serologic tests (ELISA, CF) are used to identify infected rams without lesions. Serologic testing should be performed a minimum of two times before rams are turned in to breed ewes. Vaccination can be employed but its efficacy is limited and it interferes with serologic interpretation. No effort is made to control infections in ewes. Ewes, although playing a role in transmission of infection at breeding, are only transiently infected and naturally eliminate the infection by the next breeding season.

Control Methods for *Brucella canis*

Prevention of canine brucellosis involves serologic testing of dogs prior to breeding. Males are also evaluated by palpating for epididymal and testicular lesions. In breeding colonies with brucellosis, infected animals identified by serologic tests are removed. Repeat serologic testing is performed to identify previously undetected infected animals. Until at least three negative test results are obtained, a kennel should not be considered free of brucellosis. Kennel areas should be thoroughly disinfected with quaternary ammonium compounds or iodophors.

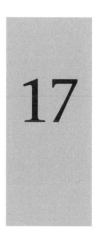

17

Burkholderia mallei and *Burkholderia pseudomallei*

Dwight C. Hirsh   Ernst L. Biberstein

Members of the genus *Burkholderia* are gram-negative, aerobic rods. As of this writing, there are 24 species belonging to this genus, most of which live in soil and/or produce disease in plants. Members of the *B. cepacia* complex produce disease in compromised human patients (e.g., those with cystic fibrosis; chronic granulomatous disease). Two members of this genus, *B. mallei* (the cause of "glanders" primarily in equids) and *B. pseudomallei* (the cause of "melioidosis" in a variety of species) are important in veterinary medicine, and are the topics of discussion in this chapter. Both produce pyogranulomatous disease.

BURKHOLDERIA MALLEI

Burkholderia mallei is a gram-negative, aerobic rod that causes "glanders," once a widespread disease of *Equidae,* and remains important only in Asia (Mongolia and China) with pockets of activity in India, Iraq, Turkey, and the Philippines. Glanders is a systemic pyogranulomatous disease varying in acuteness and severity. It also affects members of the cat family and occasionally dogs, goats, camels, sheep, and humans.

Descriptive Features

Morphology and Staining

Burkholderia mallei are gram-negative rods 0.5 μm wide and variable in length.

Structure and Composition

Burkholderia mallei produces a carbohydrate capsule. The cell wall is typical of gram-negative bacteria composed of lipopolysaccharide and protein. Being nonmotile, flagella are not produced (differentiating it from *B. pseudomallei* which is motile).

Cellular Products of Medical Interest

Capsule. The only demonstrable function the capsule plays in disease produced by *B. mallei* is to protect the outer membrane from membrane attack complexes generated following activation of the complement system (which is manifest as a serum-resistant phenotype). Mutants generated by insertional inactivation of the genes encoding the capsule are avirulent.

Cell Wall. The cell wall of *B. mallei* is typical of gram-negative bacteria. The lipopolysaccharide (LPS) in the outer membrane is an important virulence determinant. Not only is the lipid A component toxic (endotoxin), but the length of the side chain in the O-repeat unit hinders the attachment of the membrane attack complex of the complement system to the outer membrane. Lipopolysaccharide binds to lipopolysaccharide-binding protein (a serum protein), which transfers it to the blood-phase of CD14. The CD14-LPS complex binds to Toll-like receptor proteins (see Chapter 2) on the surface of macrophage cells triggering the release of proinflammatory cytokines.

Miscellaneous Products. Burkholderia mallei possess a cluster of genes encoding a Type III secretion system (an assemblage of more than 20 proteins that form a hollow tube-like structure through which effector proteins are "injected" into host "target" cells). Effector proteins have not been characterized, however, nor has a "target" cell been identified.

Proteases, lipases, and a phospholipase C have been demonstrated in the culture fluids of *B. mallei*. None of these products have been shown to play a significant role in disease.

Growth Characteristics

The organism grows best on media containing glycerol or blood. Nonhemolytic colonies develop in 48 hours or more at 20°C to 41°C. They range from mucoid to rough in five possible forms. Confluent growth is common. *Burkholderia mallei* does not grow on MacConkey agar or at 42°C.

Biochemical Characteristics

Burkholderia mallei is aerobic and oxidase and catalase-positive; it reduces nitrates and hydrolyzes urea. Glucose is attacked oxidatively.

Resistance

Resistance is unremarkable, although in dark, damp, and cool environments the agent can survive for months. Aminoglycosides, chloramphenicol, fluoroquinolones, macrolides, sulfonamides, and tetracyclines inhibit B. mallei in vitro.

Ecology

Reservoir

Infected *Equidae* are the reservoir.

Transmission

Exposure occurs via contaminated feed, water, and fomites, and sometimes through inhalation and wounds. Infectious material originates mostly in the respiratory tract or skin lesions.

Pathogenesis

Pathology. The basic nodular lesion is made up initially of neutrophils, fibrin, and red cells. The neutrophils degenerate and the central necrotic area becomes surrounded by epithelioid and giant cells and by lymphocytes embedded in granulation tissue. Near epithelial surfaces, ulceration is common. Strain variations determine the suppurative vs. granulomatous predominance in lesions.

Mechanisms. Although toxins are suspected in pathogenesis, the mechanisms are uncertain. Primary lesions form at the point of entry—the pharynx, for example. Infection spreads along lymphatics, producing nodular lesions on the way to lymph nodes and the bloodstream, which disseminates the agent. Metastatic lesions form in the lungs or other organs, such as spleen, liver, and skin, producing cutaneous glanders ("farcy"). Lesions in the nasal septum may be primary, hematogenous, or secondary to a pulmonary focus.

Disease Patterns

Glanders. Acute infections are characterized by fever, nasal discharge, and lymphadenitis of head and neck, with swelling along the upper respiratory tract. They tend to end fatally in about two weeks and predominate in donkeys and felids, less so in mules.

In horses, protracted chronic and subclinical infections are typical; signs, if present, include occasional fever, persistent respiratory problems, skin abscesses ("farcy buds"), and nodular induration of cranial lymph nodes.

Human exposures are traced to acutely ill horses and may lead to acute or chronic infections. All acute infections and 50% of chronic ones were fatal prior to the advent of effective antimicrobials.

Epidemiology

The persistence of glanders depends on an infected horse population. Susceptible nonequids acquire glanders from infected horses or horsemeat, and appear to be dead-end hosts.

Immunologic Aspects

Humoral and cell-mediated responses occur.

Apparent recovery from glanders, including loss of dermal hypersensitivity, has been observed under natural conditions, but without increased resistance to reinfection.

No method of immunization is known.

Laboratory Diagnosis

Nodular contents are cultured on blood or glycerol agar. They may be examined for gram-negative rods and by immunofluorescence.

Guinea pigs and hamsters are highly susceptible to fatal infection with virulent strains.

Any suspect isolates should be submitted to a qualified reference laboratory. Differentiation from B. pseudomallei is important.

Serologically, glanders is diagnosed by complement fixation tests employing aqueous bacterial extracts as antigen. The intradermo-palpebral mallein test detects cell-mediated hypersensitivity, which indicates infection and has served as a basis for glanders eradication. Mallein is a heat extract of old B. mallei broth cultures.

A polymerase chain reaction–based assay that utilizes primers specific for B. mallei is available for detection and identification.

Treatment and Control

Although glanders is treatable by many antimicrobics (see above), treatment is inappropriate in countries committed to glanders eradication. Equine imports from endemic areas are mallein-tested, and reactors are destroyed.

BURKHOLDERIA PSEUDOMALLEI

Burkholderia pseudomallei are aerobic gram-negative, facultative intracellular rods that cause a pyogranulomatous disease called "melioidosis," a disease superficially resembling glanders. Important distinctions are that 1) melioidosis affects a wide host range and 2) the agent is a saprophyte (an endosymbiont of amoebae living in the environment), whose prevalence is unaffected by elimination of infected animals.

Descriptive Features

Morphology and Staining

Burkholderia pseudomallei are gram-negative rods 0.5 μm wide and variable in length.

Structure and Composition

Burkholderia pseudomallei produces a carbohydrate capsule. The cell wall is typical of gram-negative bacteria composed of lipopolysaccharide and protein. Being motile, flagella are produced (differentiating it from *B. mallei* which is nonmotile).

Cellular Products of Medical Interest

Adhesin. *Burkholderia pseudomallei* adheres to amoebic trophozoites prior to uptake (and by inference adherence to phagocytic cells). Adherence is by means of the flagellar protein Fli (for *flagellin*).

Capsule. The only demonstrable function the capsule has been shown to play in *B. pseudomallei* is to protect the outer membrane from membrane attack complexes generated following activation of the complement system (which is manifest as a serum-resistant phenotype). Mutants generated by insertional inactivation of the genes encoding the capsule are avirulent.

Cell Wall. The cell wall of *B. pseudomallei* is typical of gram-negative bacteria. The lipopolysaccharide (LPS) in the outer membrane is an important virulence determinant. Not only is the lipid A component toxic (endotoxin), but the length of the side chain in the O-repeat unit hinders the attachment of the membrane attack complex of the complement system to the outer membrane. Lipopolysaccharide binds to lipopolysaccharide-binding protein (a serum protein), which transfers it to the blood-phase of CD14. The CD14-LPS complex binds to Toll-like receptor proteins on the surface of macrophage cells triggering the release of proinflammatory cytokines.

Miscellaneous Products. The chromosome of *B. pseudomallei* possess at least one Pathogenicity Island (a cluster of genes encoding virulence determinant(s), an integrase protein, a specific insertion site, and mobility) encoding a Type III secretion system (an assemblage of more than 20 proteins that form a hollow tube-like structure through which effector proteins are "injected" into host "target" cells). However, effector proteins have not been characterized, nor has their "effect" been delineated. A "target" cell has not been identified.

Proteases, lipases, and a phospholipase C have been demonstrated in the culture fluids of *M. pseudomallei* grown in vitro. None of these products have been shown to play a significant role in disease production.

Growth Characteristics

Unlike *B. mallei*, *B. pseudomallei* grows on MacConkey agar, in the presence of 2% sodium chloride, and at 42°C.

Resistance

Burkholderia pseudomallei is killed by disinfectants and does not survive chilling and freezing in biologic specimens. It is generally susceptible in vitro to fluoroquinolones, tetracyclines, chloramphenicol, trimethoprim-sulfamethoxazole, and novobiocin.

Ecology

Reservoir

Burkholderia pseudomallei is considered a soil and water dweller (most likely an endosymbiont of amoebae). Although most prevalent between 20° northern and southern latitude, extratropical foci do exist, for example, in France, Iran, China, and North America.

Transmission

Ingestion, wound infection, and possibly arthropod bites introduce infection. In humans, consumption of infected animal products and airborne infection may be significant.

Pathogenesis

Mechanisms. Being an endosymbiont of amoebae, *B. pseudomallei* is adapted to survive within phagocytic cells of the host. Microorganisms are taken up by a process of "coiling" phagocytosis and survive within the cell by being resistant to lysosomal contents (e.g., defensins), and by escaping phagosomes and phagolysosomes. Actin-based motility has been observed within phagocytic cells (see Chapters 11 and 33), and actin-associated "budding" occurs from affected to nonaffected cells. Host cells infected with *B. pseudomallei* release proinflammatory cytokines, and undergo apoptosis.

Pathology. The lesions are primarily pyogranulomatous. Small abscesses tend to coalesce, developing into larger suppurative foci or granulomas.

Disease Patterns

Melioidosis. This disease is typically systemic. Manifestations depend on the extent and distribution of lesions. The equine disease may mimic glanders. In cattle, acute and chronic infections can localize in lung, joints, and uterus. Arthritis and lymphadenitis occur in sheep. Goats suffer loss of condition, respiratory and central nervous system disturbances, arthritis, and mastitis. Similar signs are seen in swine, along with abortions and diarrhea. Dogs develop a febrile disease with localizing suppurative foci.

Epidemiology

Clinical disease is usually sporadic. The host range in mammals is virtually unlimited, and avian cases are reported. Human infections range from the rapidly fatal to the subclinical. A wet environment, such as a swampy terrain or rice paddies, is related to exposure.

Immunologic Aspects

Complement-fixing and indirect hemagglutinating antibodies are produced during infections. Cell-mediated hypersensitivity has been demonstrated in infected goats. Successful vaccination of horses and zoo animals is reported.

Laboratory Diagnosis

The methods for isolating and identifying *B. mallei* apply to *B. pseudomallei*. Chilling and freezing of specimens should be avoided. Motility, growth on citrate, growth at 42°C, and reduction of nitrates to gaseous nitrogen distinguish *B. pseudomallei* from *B. mallei*. A polymerase chain reaction-based assay utilizing primers specific for *B. pseudomallei* is available for detection and identification.

Treatment and Control

Antimicrobial susceptibilities should be verified by laboratory tests. Fluoroquinolones and the tetracyclines are considered drugs of choice. Vaccines are not commercially available.

18 *Francisella tularensis*

DWIGHT C. HIRSH   ERNST L. BIBERSTEIN

Members of the genus *Francisella* are gram-negative, aerobic, rods. There are two species: *F. tularensis*, and *F. philomiragia*. There are four subspecies of *F. tularensis*: *tularensis* (previously known as biotype A, or as subspecies *nearctica*); *holartica* (previously known as biotype B, or as subspecies *palaearctica*); *novicida*; and *mediasiatica*. *Francisella tularensis* subspecies *tularensis* and subspecies *holartica* are facultatively intracellular pathogens of humans and, under limited epidemiologic conditions, occasionally infect domestic animals (sheep, horses, swine, carnivores) producing the disease tularemia. *Francisella philomiragia* and *F. tularensis* subspecies *novicida* and subspecies *mediasiatica* are of uncertain animal pathogenicity.

Descriptive Features

Morphology and Staining

Francisella tularensis is a gram-negative coccobacillus, measuring less than 1 µm in any dimension. They can pass filter membranes of 600 nm porosity. In older cultures, more pleomorphism develops. Giemsa stain is preferred.

Cellular Anatomy and Composition

Francisella tularensis produces a capsule composed of lipids (50–70%), amino acids, and carbohydrates. It possesses a gram-negative cell wall, whose lipopolysaccharide portion (endotoxin) has substantially less toxic activity than the lipopolysaccharide found in the cell walls of other gram-negative microorganisms.

Cellular Products of Medical Interest

Capsule. Capsules protect the outer membrane from the membrane attack complex of the complement cascade. Since capsules of other microorganisms inhibit attachment to, and ingestion by, phagocytic host cells, it is unclear what the role (aside from protecting the outer membrane from complement components) of a capsule is for *F. tularensis*, an intracellular parasite (see below).

Cell Wall. The cell wall of the members of this genus is one fairly typical of gram-negative bacteria. The lipopolysaccharide (LPS) in the outer membrane is an important virulence determinant. Not only is the lipid A component toxic (endotoxin), but the length of the side chain in the O-repeat unit hinders the attachment of the membrane attack complex of the complement system to the outer membrane. Lipopolysaccharide binds to lipopolysaccharide-binding protein, which transfers it to the blood-phase of CD14. The CD14-LPS complex binds to Toll-like receptor proteins on the surface of macrophage cells triggering the release of proinflammatory cytokines. As mentioned above ("Cellular Anatomy and Composition"), the potency of lipopolysaccharide of *F. tularensis*, as compared to other gram-negative microorganisms, is much less. Neither the reason nor the role for this is known.

Acid Phosphatase (Acp). The Acp (for *acid phosphatase*) of *F. tularensis* suppresses the respiratory burst of phagocytic cells, especially neutrophils.

Products of the Intracellular Growth Locus (Igl). The 23 kDa protein, termed Igl (for *intracellular growth locus*), is associated with the prevention of fusion of phagosomes (containing *F. tularensis*) with lysosomes. However, acidification of the phagosome still occurs, facilitating iron acquisition from intracellular iron stores. How these events occur is not known. Igl also prevents secretion of proinflammatory cytokines by infected macrophages.

Macrophage Growth Locus (Mgl). The Mgl (for *macrophage growth locus*) proteins are associated with prevention of the fusion of phagosomes (containing *F. tularensis*) with lysosomes. However, acidification of the phagosome occurs, facilitating iron acquisition from intracellular iron stores. How these events occur is not known.

Growth Characteristics

Francisella tularensis is a fastidious aerobe. The preferred medium is glucose-cysteine-blood-agar. Two to four days of incubation (35–37°C) produce grayish, viscous, oxidase-negative colonies 1 to 4 mm in diameter. Tests for acidification of certain carbohydrates and citrulline ureidase activity permit subdivision of the *F. tularensis* into biotypes A (now designated subspecies *tularensis*) and B (subspecies *holartica*), which differ in geographic distribution, host specificity, and virulence for humans (see "Epidemiology," below).

Francisella tularensis survives cold temperatures for months in water, soil, and animal tissues.

Ecology

Reservoir

The reservoirs of *F. tularensis* are infected lagomorphs (hares, rabbits; subspecies *tularensis*) and rodents (sub-

117

species *holartica*). Some have suggested that *F. tularensis* is an endosymbiont of free-living amoeba.

Transmission

The more virulent subspecies *tularensis* (predominant in North America) is transmitted largely by ticks and hemophagous insects. Surface waters contaminated by rodents are sources of infection with the less virulent subspecies *holartica* (predominant in Eurasia). Ingestion of infected prey spreads *F. tularensis* to the predator. Sheep on the western ranges of North America are infected by way of ticks. Transmission by animal bite has been documented. Humans are commonly infected by contact (percutaneous, conjunctival, inhalation, ingestion).

Pathogenesis

Following the infectious event (bite, inhalation, ingestion), *F. tularensis* comes in contact with tissue fluids (complement proteins) followed by initiation of an inflammatory response (chemistry of cell wall). Complement proteins (especially the membrane attack complex) are ineffectual due to the presence of the capsule. Early arriving neutrophils do not easily eliminate the organism (suppression of the respiratory burst by Acp; it is unclear whether the capsule plays a role at this stage). Intracellular growth occurs following phagocytosis by macrophages (made possible by a suppressed respiratory burst by Acp, lack of fusion of phagosomes and lysosomes by Igl and Mgl proteins, and iron acquisition from iron-binding proteins within the phagosome under acid conditions). Intracellular growth of *F. tularensis* results in apoptotic death of the macrophage. Liberation of the microorganism is followed by another "round" of phagocytosis. Endotoxemia (see Fig 8.1) follows if the infectious process reaches the disseminated phase.

Epidemiology

Tularemia is a northern disease, its southern limits being Mexico and Mediterranean Africa. Seasonal peaks reflect vector activity and contact with the reservoir. Waterborne infections predominate in fall and winter. *Francisella tularensis* subspecies *tularensis* is predominant in North America, and *F. tularensis* subspecies *holartica* is predominant in Europe and Asia.

Immunologic Aspects

Solid, largely cell-mediated immunity follows recovery in humans. Animals in endemic areas carry antibody. Its relation to immunity is unrelated. A live attenuated vaccine (e.g., LSV for *live* strain *vaccine*) is used in humans at risk.

Laboratory Diagnosis

Demonstration of the organism in exudates is by Romanovsky-type stains (Wright's or Giemsa), immunofluorescence, and culture. Isolation is facilitated by injection of suspect material into mice or guinea pigs.

Rising serum tube agglutination titers (1:>80) are evidence of infection.

DNA primers are available for the diagnosis and identification of *Francisella* by the polymerase chain reaction.

See "Growth Characteristics" earlier in this chapter for isolation medium.

Treatment and Control

Aminoglycosides (especially streptomycin) are effective drugs for treating human tularemia, but due to toxicity other antimicrobials are preferred. The fluoroquinolones have been used successfully, and are a safe alternative to the aminoglycosides. Tetracycline has been effective in animals. Other antimicrobials (macrolides, beta lactams, chloramphenicol) are less effective. Control measures are aimed at limiting tick exposure and access to contaminated feed and water.

19 *Moraxella*

Dwight C. Hirsh   Ernst L. Biberstein

Members of the genus *Moraxella* are gram-negative rods and cocci belonging to the family *Moraxellaceae*. The genus *Moraxella* is subdivided into two subgenera, *Moraxella* (containing the rod-shaped members of the genus) and subgenus *Branhamella* (the coccoid members). There are 14 members of this genus (see Table 19.1), most of which are associated with diseases of human patients. From a veterinary perspective, *Moraxella* subgenus *Moraxella bovis* (hereafter referred to as *Moraxella bovis*) is the most important member of the group. *Moraxella bovis* is the cause of infectious bovine keratoconjunctivitis (IBK), the most common occular disease of cattle.

Descriptive Features

Morphology and Staining

Moraxellae are short, plump gram-negative rods, 11.5 μm X 1.5 to 2.5 mm, and are often arranged in pairs ("diplobacilli") or short chains (Fig 19.1).

Structure and Composition

The cell wall is typical of gram-negative bacteria being composed of lipopolysaccharide and protein. The lipopolysaccharide of moraxellae does not contain O-repeat units, in contrast to many other gram-negative microorganisms (e.g., members of the family *Enterobacteriaceae*).

The fimbrial adhesins (pili) of *M. bovis* are virulence determinants and can be lost in subculture (see below, "Variability"). Capsules may be present on fresh isolates.

Cellular Products of Medical Interest

Adhesins. The role of adhesins, as in other microorganisms, is to allow the bacterium expressing them to adhere to cells lining a particular niche, as well as to the surface of so-called "target" cells prior to the initiation of disease (in some cases, niche and target cells may be the same). *Moraxella bovis* produces a type 4 pilus (fimbria) that adheres to conjunctival and corneal epithelial cells. This pilus is similar to those of *Pseudomonas aeruginosa*, *Neisseria gonorrhoeae*, *Dicholobacter nodosus*, *Pasteurella multocida*, and *Vibrio cholerae*. Mutants unable to produce this adhesin are avirulent.

Capsule. The capsule plays many roles, the most important of which are interference with phagocytosis (antiphagocytic), and protection of the outer membrane from the deposition of membrane attack complexes generated by activation of the complement system.

Cell Wall. The cell wall of the members of this genus is one typical of gram-negative bacteria (except for the absence of the O-repeat unit). The lipopolysaccharide (LPS) in the outer membrane is an important virulence determinant. LPS binds to lipopolysaccharide-binding protein (a serum protein), which transfers it to the blood-phase of CD14. The CD14-LPS complex binds to Toll-like receptor proteins (see Chapter 2) on the surface of macrophage cells triggering the release of proinflammatory cytokines.

Exotoxins. The most noteworthy toxin produced by *M. bovis*, is an RTX (repeats in *t*oxin, so called because of the common feature of repeats in glycine-rich sequences within the protein) type of cytotoxin (see also *Escherichia coli* haemolysin, Chapter 8, *Pasteurella/Mannheimia* leukotoxin, Chapter 12, *Actinobacillus haemolysin,* Chapter 13, adenylyl cyclase toxin of *Bordetella*, Chapter 15). This cytoxin, sometimes referred to as "hemolysin" due to its behavior on blood agar plates, has been termed Mbx (for *Moraxella b*ovis *t*oxin). Mbx is a pore-forming toxin with specificity for conjunctival and corneal epithelial cells, and neutrophils. Mutants unable to produce Mbx are avirulent.

Iron Acquisition. Because iron is an absolute growth requirement, microorganisms must acquire this substance if they are to exist within the host. Moraxellae acquire iron from the iron-binding proteins of the host (transferrin and lactoferrin) by expressing Tbp and Lbp (for *t*ransferrin- and *l*actoferrin-*b*inding *p*roteins, respectively) on their surface. Tbp and Lbp bind their respective proteins giving moraxellae access to iron.

Miscellaneous Products. A number of proteins with toxic activities are produced in vitro by *M. bovis*. These include complement-degrading proteases, lipases, phosphoamidases, peptidases, and proteases. There is little evidence showing that any of these play a role in vivo.

Growth Characteristics

Moraxella bovis grows best at 35°C in the presence of serum and blood. No growth occurs on MacConkey agar or anaerobically. In 48 hours, fresh isolates produce flat, hemolytic, friable colonies, about 1 mm in size that corrode the agar and autoagglutinate when suspended in saline.

Biochemical Activities

Moraxella bovis is oxidase-positive, nonfermenting, and catalase-variable. Nitrates and urea are not attacked, but proteins are digested.

Table 19.1.   Members of the Genus *Moraxella* and Their Usual Source or Associated Condition

Species	Usual Source or Associated Condition
Moraxella atlantae (CDC Group M-3)	Septicemia in human patients
M. boevrei	Respiratory tract of normal goats
M. bovis	Infectious keratoconjunctivitis in cattle (IBK)
M. cuniculi (Neisseria cuniculi)	Respiratory tract of rabbits
M. canis	Respiratory tracts of normal dogs and cats
M. caprae	Respiratory tracts of normal goats and sheep
M. catarrhalis (N. catarrhalis)	Middle ear infections in children; upper respiratory tract infections in human patients
M. caviae (N. caviae)	Respiratory tract of guinea pigs
M. lacunata	Conjunctivitis and keratitis in human patients
M. lincolnii	Respiratory tract of human patients
M. nonliquefaciens	Respiratory tract of normal human patients; blood, cerebral spinal fluid, and lungs of compromised human patients
M. ovis (N. ovis)	Keratoconjunctivitis in sheep
M. osloesis	Nematodes; various conditions in human patients
M. phenylpyruvica	Respiratory tract of normal human patients; blood stream of compromised human patients

FIGURE 19.1.   Moraxella bovis *in the cornea of an experimentally infected calf. There is evidence of digestion of corneal substance around the bacterial cells. Scanning electron micrograph, 22,000X. (Photograph courtesy of Dr. G. Kagonyera.)*

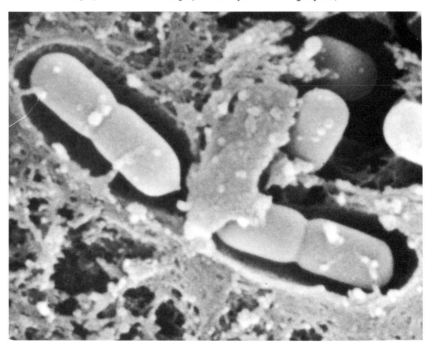

Resistance

Resistance to physical and chemical agents is not remarkable. It is usually susceptible to commonly used antibiotics.

Variability

In culture, *M. bovis* undergoes colonial dissociation (phase variation) producing smooth butyrous colonies composed of cells, which lack pili (due to inversion of the pilin encoding gene) and infectivity, and are less autoagglutinable. Pili are immunogenically diverse, and this trait is responsible for a classification scheme based on serological similarities. Nonhemolytic variants are nonpathogenic.

Ecology

Reservoir

Moraxella bovis occurs worldwide on the bovine conjunctiva and upper respiratory mucosa, often without clinical manifestations.

Transmission

Dissemination is by direct and indirect contact, including flying insects and possibly other airborne transmission.

Pathogenesis

Mechanisms. Disease produced by *M. bovis* is closely linked to cytoxin (Mbx) and pili. Attachment (pili) to conjunctival epithelium is followed by destruction (Mbx) of conjunctival and corneal cells. Growth of *M. bovis* in the conjunctival and corneal lesions leads to inflammation (gram-negative cell wall). Mbx-mediated lysis of neutrophils amplifies inflammation and tissue destruction.

Environmental factors implicated include ultraviolet irradiation, flies, dust, and woody pasture plants, all of which contribute to irritation of the target tissues. Concurrent infections with viruses, such as bovine herpesvirus 1 (infectious bovine rhinotracheitis virus) and adenovirus, mycoplasma (*Mycoplasma bovoculi*), bacteria (*Listeria monocytogenes*), and nematodes (*Thelasia*), may complicate the disease.

Disease Pattern and Pathology

Infectious Bovine Keratoconjunctivitis (IBK). IBK begins with invasion of conjunctiva and cornea by *M. bovis*, resulting in edema and a predominantly neutrophilic inflammatory response. It may progress from mild epiphora and corneal clouding to production of severe edema, corneal opacities, vascularization, ulceration, and rupture leading to uveal prolapse and panophthalmitis (see Fig 72.2). Healing of the ulcers proceeds from the periphery and requires several weeks. Central scarring may persist for months. Though a self-limiting disease, losses occur because vision-impaired animals do not forage and lose condition.

Epidemiology

IBK is a highly infectious disease, mostly of beef cattle. Young animals are preferentially affected, probably due to lack of acquired immunity. Lack of eyelid pigmentation and prominent placement of eyes are apparent predisposing factors, as is vitamin A deficiency.

Prevalence is greatest during summer and early fall, when environmental stresses are maximal.

Immunologic Aspects

Antibodies of all isotypes are produced during infection, with secretory IgA predominating locally. Temporary resistance to reinfection follows recovery. The relative roles in immunity and recovery of general vs. local responses and humoral vs. cell-mediated responses are unsettled.

Experimental bacterins and fimbrial antigens stimulate resistance, optimally to homologous challenge. Apparently, fimbrial proteins, Mbx, and proteolytic enzymes have protection-inducing activity. Fimbrial vaccines are commercially available.

Laboratory Diagnosis

The agent may be demonstrated in smears of exudate, most convincingly by immunofluorescence (by using antibody specific for *M. bovis* antigens). Exudate is cultured on blood agar and *Moraxella* are identified by colonial characteristics, oxidase activity, hemolysis, proteolysis, and failure to ferment carbohydrates. Specific fluorescent antibody conjugates can be applied directly to suspect colonies on plates for identification even of dissociant colonies (epifluorescence). Polymerase chain reaction–based assays utilizing *M. bovis*–specific primers are available for detection and identification.

Treatment and Control

Affected animals should be placed in a dark stall, free from dust and flies. Topical corticosteroids may relieve the inflammation, while antimicrobial drugs, given topically or systemically, may be beneficial. Long-acting tetracycline or florfenicol are considered the drugs of choice.

Fimbrial vaccines are the most promising specific prophylactics.

20 Pseudomonas

Dwight C. Hirsh

Members of the genus *Pseudomonas* are gram-negative, aerobic rods. Of the many recognized species of *Pseudomonas*, only *P. aeruginosa* is of veterinary importance. Previously named pseudomonads of veterinary importance, *P. mallei* and *P. pseudomallei*, have been moved to the genus *Burkholderia* (see Chapter 17).

Pseudomonas aeruginosa is very rarely involved with primary disease, although it is extremely important in clinical medicine. Most strains are resistant to the commonly used antimicrobial agents and are therefore sometimes difficult to eliminate when they contaminate a compromised site.

Descriptive Features

Morphology and Staining

The organisms are gram-negative rods, 0.5 to 1.0 µm by 1.5 to 5.0 µm.

Cellular Anatomy and Composition

Pseudomonads produce a typical gram-negative cell wall, surrounded by a carbohydrate-containing capsule. All members of the genus are motile by means of polar flagella. Pili (fimbrial adhesins) are produced.

Cellular Products of Medical Interest

Adhesins. *Pseudomonas aeruginosa* produces several products that serve as adhesins. These include a fimbrial adhesin that has affinity for certain glycoproteins on epithelial cells. In addition, there are non-fimbria adhesins, an outer membrane protein with affinity for mucin, and another, the lipopolysaccharide of the cell wall that has affinity for chloride channel proteins.

Capsule. The capsule protects the outer membrane from the membrane attack complex of the complement cascade. The capsule also inhibits attachment to, and ingestion by, phagocytic host cells.

Cell Wall. The cell wall of the members of this genus is one typical of gram-negative bacteria. The lipopolysaccharide (LPS) in the outer membrane is an important virulence determinant. Not only is the lipid A component toxic (endotoxin), but the length of the side chain in the O-repeat unit hinders the attachment of the membrane attack complex of the complement system to the outer membrane. Lipopolysaccharide binds to lipopolysaccha-ride-binding protein, which transfers it to the blood-phase of CD14. The CD14-LPS complex binds to Toll-like receptor proteins (see Chapter 2) on the surface of macrophage cells triggering the release of proinflammatory cytokines.

Iron-Acquiring Systems. Iron is an absolute growth requirement for all living things. *Pseudomonas aeruginosa* produces the iron-acquiring siderophores pyochelin and pyoverdin, as well as using the siderophores produced by other bacteria living in its environment (e.g., enterobactin and aerobactin). These products are used to remove iron from host iron-binding proteins.

Exotoxins. *Pseudomonas aeruginosa* produces a number of protein exotoxins: exotoxin A, exotoxin S, exotoxin T, exotoxin U, exotoxin Y, elastase, and a number of other proteins with biological activity (proteases, phospholipases). Exotoxins S, T, U, and Y are "injected" into host cells by way of a Type III secretion apparatus (an assemblage of proteins—more than 20—that form a hollow tube-like structure through which effector proteins are "injected" into host "target" cells):

1. Exotoxin A. Exotoxin A inhibits protein synthesis by ribosylation of elongation factor-2 (EF-2) following receptor-mediated endocytosis.
2. Exotoxins S and T. Exotoxins S and T ribosylate host cell GTP-binding proteins, interrupting cell functions relying on the actin cytoskeleton, e.g., phagocytosis.
3. Exotoxin U. Exotoxin U is cytotoxic, but the mechanism is undefined.
4. Exotoxin Y. Exotoxin Y is an adenylyl cyclase that raises the amount of intracellular cAMP to damaging levels.

Miscellaneous Products. *Pseudomonas aeruginosa* produces bacteriocins (pyocins) and pigments (pyocyanins). Pyocins are useful epidemiologically for tracing epidemics within the hospital environment. Pyocyanin has toxic activity and is used as an aid in the laboratory identification of *P. aeruginosa*. Pyocyanin reacts with oxygen to form reactive oxygen radicals that are toxic to eukaryotic and prokaryotic organisms. *Pseudomonas aeruginosa* protects itself from the toxic effects of pyocyanin by increasing synthesis of catalase and superoxide dismutase.

Product Regulation. Regulation of the expression and excretion of cellular products involved in the pathogenesis of disease produced by *P. aeruginosa* is complex. Secretion of products that are secreted by way of the Type III secretion apparatus (exotoxins S, T, U, and Y) is initiated following bacteria-host cell interaction. The remaining bacterial cell products are under the control of the "quorum sensing" system of *P. aeruginosa*. The genes that encode these products are expressed when concentrations of bacterially produced homoserine lactones reach a threshold level (a "quorum"). All *P. aeruginosa* cells excrete homoserine lactones, but the concentration is too low to trigger virulence gene expression until a critical number of bacterial cells is reached. Finally, exotoxin A and an endoprotease are also regulated by levels of pyoverdin. When free iron concentrations are low (as would be the case in vivo), these two proteins are expressed and excreted.

Growth Characteristics

Pseudomonas aeruginosa is an obligate aerobe, deriving energy from the oxidation of organic materials and using oxygen as a terminal electron acceptor. It grows on all common media over a wide range of temperatures: 4°C to 41°C.

Ecology

Reservoir

Most members of the genus *Pseudomonas* live in soil and water. *Pseudomonas aeruginosa* may also be found in the feces of normal animals, but not as a member of the normal flora (i.e., they are transients).

Transmission

Environmental or endogenous exposure is constant, and most infections are secondary to compromised host defenses.

Pathogenesis

Mechanisms. Pseudomonas aeruginosa contaminates areas of the body that possess reduced numbers of normal flora. Disruption of the normal flora is almost always due to antimicrobial agents. Since *P. aeruginosa* is resistant to most commonly used antimicrobial agents, it will replace the normal flora. If the site colonized is compromised or contiguous to a compromised site, there is risk of infection of the site. Tissue destruction follows initiation of inflammation (cell wall), and liberation of exotoxin(s) and pyocyanin.

Pseudomonas aeruginosa is also isolated from certain sites of animals that have no history of antimicrobial therapy.

Disease Patterns

Dog (Cat). Conditions in which *P. aeruginosa* is associated include otitis externa, lower urinary tract infection, and pyoderma.

Horse. Conditions in which *P. aeruginosa* is associated include metritis (vaginitis) secondary to prolonged treatment with antimicrobial agents, keratitis, and conjunctivitis following treatment of corneal ulcers with topical steroid-antibiotic mixtures.

Bovine. Conditions in which *P. aeruginosa* is associated include mastitis (uncommon).

Miscellaneous. Pseudomonas aeruginosa is an uncommon cause of septicemia in immunocompromised animals, but a frequent cause of bacteremia in human beings with burns, leukemia, or cystic fibrosis.

Epidemiology

The organism is ubiquitous in the environment. Disease determinants therefore lie largely with the hosts and their immediate environment. In a veterinary hospital, however, a number of situations favor selection of this organism. *Pseudomonas aeruginosa* thrives in wet, poorly aerated environments within the hospital, especially in surgery areas within support bags that have not been properly dried, in hoses on anesthetic machines that have not been cleaned and dried properly, or in disinfectant solutions that have not been changed frequently. These situations result in an increase in the number of pseudomonads in the environment of the compromised animal (site), thereby increasing the risk of infection (contamination).

Immunologic Aspects

Specific immune responses do not seem to play much of a role in pathogenesis or resistance, though artificial protection has been shown to occur in animals vaccinated with extracts of the organism or exotoxin A. The most important consideration is to decrease the risk of infection by reducing the concentration of the organism in the environment of the patient, in addition to reducing the extent of compromise, for example, by cleaning and drying an infected ear.

Laboratory Diagnosis

Pseudomonas aeruginosa grows well on blood agar medium. The colonies are somewhat large, >1 mm in diameter, gray (gunmetal), rough, usually with a zone of hemolysis. A plate containing *P. aeruginosa* has a characteristic odor, reminiscent of corn tortillas. Besides being oxidase-positive, a trait that sets it apart from members of the family *Enterobacteriaceae*, it turns triple sugar iron agar slightly alkaline (without gas), utilizes glucose oxidatively, grows at 42°C, and forms a blue-green, chloroform-soluble pigment, pyocyanin. Resistance to some antimicrobials is due to permeability barrier of the *Pseudomonas* cell wall, and to others because of inactivation due to products encoded by plasmid-based genes (R plasmids).

Treatment and Control

Treatment involves correction of compromise and, if necessary, the use of an antimicrobial agent. *Pseudomonas aeruginosa* is usually susceptible to gentamicin, tobramycin, amikacin, carbenicillin, ciprofloxacin, and ticarcillin-clavulanic acid, and these agents are used for the treatment of soft tissue infections. In the canine urinary tract, tetracycline achieves concentrations sufficient to kill most isolates. Most pseudomonads are susceptible to levels achieved by antimicrobial agents in otic preparations: enrofloxacin, neomycin, polymyxin, chloramphenicol, and

gentamicin. It should be noted that there are no in vitro tests that predict susceptibility/resistance of an isolate from infectious processes that will be treated topically (e.g., the ear).

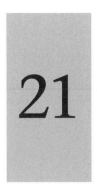

21

Taylorella equigenitalis

ERNST L. BIBERSTEIN   DWIGHT C. HIRSH

Members of the genus *Taylorella* are gram-negative, facultatively anaerobic rods. The genus contains two species, *T. equigenitalis*, the cause of contagious equine metritis (CEM), and *T. asinigenitalis*, an inhabitant of the genital tract of clinically normal male donkeys. Because of its clinical and economic importance, *T. equigenitalis* will be discussed in detail. Because of its phenotypic similarity to *T. equigenitalis*, *T. asinigenitalis* will be briefly described.

TAYLORELLA EQUIGENITALIS

Taylorella equigenitalis causes an acute, suppurative, self-limiting disease of the uterus of mares called contagious equine metritis (CEM). The disease results in temporary sterility, is highly communicable, and is followed by long-term asymptomatic carriage of the agent. Stallions develop no signs of illness but may remain carriers of the agent indefinitely. The disease is geographically limited at present.

Descriptive Features

Morphology and Staining

Taylorella equigenitalis is a gram-negative coccobacillus, about 0.8 μm by 5 to 6 μm in size.

Structure and Composition

Taylorella equigenitalis produces a carbohydrate capsule and a cell wall that is typical of gram-negative bacteria being composed of lipopolysaccharide and protein. It is inconsistently piliated. It shares some antigens with *Haemophilus*, *Pasteurella*, and *Brucella*.

Cellular Products of Medical Interest

Capsule. The capsule protects the outer membrane from the membrane attack complex of the complement cascade. The capsule also inhibits attachment to and ingestion by phagocytic host cells.

Cell Wall. The cell wall of *T. equigenitalis* is typical of gram-negative bacteria. The lipopolysaccharide (LPS) in the outer membrane is an important virulence determi-

nant. Not only is the lipid A component toxic (endotoxin), but the length of the side chain in the O-repeat unit hinders the attachment of the membrane attack complex of the complement system to the outer membrane. Lipopolysaccharide binds to lipopolysaccharide-binding protein (a serum protein), which transfers it to the blood-phase of CD14. The CD14-LPS complex binds to Toll-like receptor proteins (see Chapter 2) on the surface of macrophage cells triggering the release of proinflammatory cytokines.

Growth Characteristics

Taylorella equigenitalis is a facultative anaerobe that grows optimally at 37°C under 5% to 10% carbon dioxide on chocolate agar (see Chapter 14) in a rich base (Columbia, Eugon). After 48 hours of incubation, colonies have a diameter of 1 mm and may enlarge further upon longer incubation. They are shiny, smooth, grayish-white, waxy, and sometimes pleomorphic.

The organism is oxidase, catalase, and phosphatase-positive and produces no acid from carbohydrates.

The agent is unrelated to other gram-negative bacteria.

Resistance

The resistance of *T. equigenitalis* is not remarkable. Samples on swabs can be shipped in transport medium under refrigeration and successfully cultured within 48 hours of collection.

Most antibiotics except streptomycin inhibit *T. equigenitalis*, although they are strain-susceptible to this antibiotic. Trimethoprim-sulfamethoxazole, lincomycin, and clindamycin are sufficiently well tolerated to have been included in selective isolation media.

Variability

Apart from harboring streptomycin-susceptible variants, the species appears to be antigenically homogeneous, though some strains (as defined by DNA analysis, see below) appear more virulent than others as measured by entry into cells in vitro.

Molecular methods such as Random Amplification of Polymorphic DNA (RAPD) and pulsed field gel electrophoresis of restriction endonuclease-digested DNA have identified different strains of *T. equigenitalis*.

Ecology

Reservoir

Taylorella equigenitalis is a parasite exclusively of the equine genital tract. Antibodies to the agent but no infections have been found in cattle and humans.

The reservoir is in Europe, but the agent has been recovered from animals with CEM in Japan, Australia, and North America.

Transmission

Taylorella equigenitalis is sexually transmitted, although its occurrence in newborn and virgin animals suggests alternative means of transmission.

Pathogenesis

Within a few days of exposure, a purulent endometritis develops with variable amounts of exudate. The main damage is to uterine epithelium (exclusive of glands), which becomes covered by neutrophilic exudate. The cellular infiltrate in the endometrial stroma is predominantly mononuclear. Epithelium is eroded or undergoes severe degenerative changes. The uterine infection usually subsides spontaneously within several weeks. Endometrial repair is complete and there is no lasting impairment of breeding performance. Infection has been demonstrated in placentas and newborn foals, but abortions have been few.

There is no fever or other sign of illness. The only effect may be failure of conception. Alternatively, there may be a mucoid to mucopurulent vulvar discharge of variable abundance some days after service; internal examination reveals a cervicovaginal exudate of uterine origin. External signs of disease disappear within 2 weeks, although the uterine infection may persist longer.

Epidemiology

Inapparent persistence of *T. equigenitalis* is frequent in recovered mares and in stallions in endemic areas. The foci of carriage in mares are the clitoridal fossa and sinuses; in stallions, the foci are the prepuce, urethra, and the urethral fossa and sinus.

Dissemination of infection is tied to breeding operations and the movement and use of infected animals.

Immunologic Aspects

Recovered animals show increased resistance for several months, manifested by milder signs and lower numbers of bacteria when reinfected. The mechanism of resistance is uncertain.

Complement-fixing serum antibody appears late in the first week and rises for 3 weeks after experimental exposure. Duration of titers in mares varies, but tests are consistently positive during the third to the seventh week postinfection. Titers are apparently unrelated to the carrier status. Antibody is present in vaginal mucus, but its relation to infection is unknown.

Bacterins do not prevent infection, but do reduce its severity.

Laboratory Diagnosis

Diagnosis of CEM and carrier identification require demonstration of *T. equigenitalis* in the genital tract. In clinical cases, the agent can be demonstrated in the uterine exudate by Gram stain.

Definitive identification of an infected animal requires replicate cultures of appropriate specimens (see under "Treatment and Control," below) on chocolate Eugon agar (prepared with horse blood) with and without added streptomycin. A third medium incorporating clindamycin and trimethoprim permits growth of all strains. Plates are examined daily from the second to the seventh days of incubation (see "Growth Characteristics," above). Gram-negative, oxidase-positive, and catalase-positive organisms from suspect colonies must be confirmed serologically. Any identification of *T. equigenitalis* should be considered tentative until confirmed by a competent reference laboratory.

A polymerase chain reaction (PCR)–based assay has been developed and found to be more sensitive than traditional culture techniques used to identify affected animals and to identify isolates.

Serological testing (CF) may be done on suspect mares between the fifteenth and fortieth day postbreeding.

Treatment and Control

Uterine infusions of disinfectants or antimicrobics and systemic antibiotic treatment are used in attempts to reduce the severity and duration of illness and perhaps abort the carrier state. Their benefit has been questioned.

Topical treatment of affected mares consists of a cleansing of the clitoridal fossa with 2% chlorhexidine followed by liberal application of nitrofurazone ointment (0.2%). The prepuce, urethral sinus, and fossa glandis of stallions imported into the United States of America from countries in which CEM is known to exist are cultured. The stallions are then bred to two uninfected mares, which subsequently are sampled three times for culture of clitoridal fossa and clitoridal sinuses. In mares to be imported, each of these sites is cultured repeatedly throughout one estrus.

Some countries require surgical obliteration of the clitoridal sinuses in imported mares.

In CEM-endemic countries, attempts at control have included mandatory veterinary examinations, negative cultures of all animals intended for breeding, and supervision of the movement of horses.

TAYLORELLA ASINIGENITALIS

Taylorella asinigenitalis is a gram-negative, facultatively anaerobic rod that is phenotypically similar to *T. equigeni-*

talis. At the present time the only way the two microorganisms can be differentiated is by a polymerase chain reaction that utilizes especially designed primers.

Taylorella asinigenitalis appears to reside in the genital track of donkey jacks. It can be transmitted to mares by natural service, but not by artificial means. Depending upon the strain of *T. asinigenitalis* that is used, some affected mares develop clinical disease that is similar to CEM. However, mares do test positive when the complement fixation test is used to identify animals infected with *T. equigenitalis*. This, coupled with the fact that isolates of *T. asinigenitalis* and *T. equigenitalis* are similar phenotypically, makes identification of horses with *T. equigenitalis* (an economically devastating disease) difficult. At this time, the significance (other than making control of CEM more difficult) of *T. asinigenitalis* is not known.

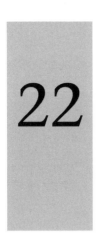

22 Spiral-Curved Organisms I: *Borrelia*

Rance B. LeFebvre

Borreliae are spirochetes transmitted and maintained primarily by ticks. The infections they cause have blood-borne phases accompanied or followed by general and localized manifestations.

Animal pathogens include *B. anserina*, the fowl spirochetosis agent; *B. theileri*, a mild pathogen mainly of cattle; and *B. burgdorferi* sensu lato, comprised of three genospecies, the cause of Lyme disease in dogs, horses, cattle, and humans. Tick-borne relapsing fever borreliae of humans (*B. hermsii, B. parkeri, B. turicata*) occur asymptomatically in feral mammals, birds, and reptiles.

Descriptive Features

Morphology and Staining

Borreliae are gram-negative but stain poorly. For demonstration by light microscopy, silver, or Romanovsky-type strains (Giemsa, Wright's) are best (Fig 22.1). Dark field examination reveals spirals and motility.

Cellular Anatomy and Composition

Borreliae have a structure like other spirochetes, with an outer sheath encasing the axial fibrils consisting of 15 to 20 endoflagella (depending on species).

Members of the genus *Borrelia* are unique among prokaryotes in that they have a linear double-stranded chromosome of approximately 900 kbp and a multiplicity of linear and circular plasmids that may in fact constitute components of the genome.

Cellular Products of Medical Interest

Cell Wall. Members of the genus *Borellia* have a gram-negative cell wall. The lipopolysaccharide (LPS) in the outer membrane is an important virulence determinant. Not only is the lipid A component toxic (endotoxin), but the length of the side chain in the O-repeat unit hinders the attachment of the membrane attack complex of the complement system to the outer membrane. LPS binds to lipopolysaccharide-binding protein (a serum protein), which in turn transfers it to the blood phase of CD14. The CD14-LPS complex binds to Toll-like receptor proteins (see Chapter 2) on the surface of macrophage cells triggering the release of proinflammatory cytokines.

Hemolysin. Hemolysin activity has been associated with *B. burgdorferi*.

Growth Characteristics

Of the borreliae pathogenic for animals, *B. anserina* is propagated in embryonated hen's eggs, and *B. burgdorferi* sensu lato is cultivated at 33°C on modified Kelly's medium (BSK), an enriched serum broth made selective by inclusion of kanamycin and 5-fluorouracil.

The organisms are slow-growing microaerophiles (doubling times of 12 to 18 hours). They ferment glucose and possibly other carbohydrates.

Survival of borreliae is about a week at room temperature in blood clots, several months at 4°C, and indefinite at less than 20°C.

Variability

A number of genes encoding outer surface proteins have been identified in several *Borrelia* species. The antigenic variability available to the spirochetes is utilized for immune evasion in the relapsing fever borreliae. Lyme disease spirochetes are also equipped to express a wide range of outer surface proteins. Though not utilized as with the relapsing fever borreliae, an immune evasion function of these antigens may still be involved in their maintenance and expression.

Ecology

Reservoir and Transmission

Pathogenic borreliae of animals are vectored by ticks. Ticks become infected at some stage in their life cycle by feeding on infected animals. Some vertical (transovarian, maternal) transmission occurs. Other arthropods may serve as short-term vectors. Infection occurs by wound contamination, usually during feeding by infected ticks. Passage via placenta, milk, and urine has been documented. With birds, infection may occur by coprophagia and cannibalism.

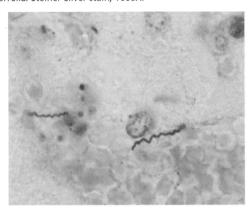

FIGURE 22.1. *Section of liver from a horse showing presence of Borrelia. Steiner Silver stain, 1000X.*

Pathogenesis

Endotoxin is incriminated in the pathogenesis of relapsing fever and probably other borrelioses. Hemolysin activity has been described in Lyme disease spirochetes.

ANIMAL BORRELIOSES

BORRELIA ANSERINA

Borrelia anserina causes fowl spirochetosis in chickens, turkeys, geese, ducks, pheasants, pigeons, canaries, and some species of wild birds. Onset of disease is marked by fever, depression, and anorexia. Affected birds are cyanotic and develop a greenish diarrhea. Later signs may include paralysis and anemia. Mortality ranges from 10% to almost 100%. Necropsy reveals splenomegaly and widespread hemorrhages. The enlarged liver may contain necrotic foci. Peripheral blood is often sterile.

Avian spirochetosis occurs on all continents and in all ages of birds. The young suffer high mortality rates and die at earlier, septicemic stages of infection. Following an outbreak, the agent generally disappears from the flock within 30 days.

The leading vector, *Argas persicus*, can remain infected for over a year and can pass the agent transovarially.

Temporary immunity, apparently antibody mediated, follows recovery. Antisera confer protection for several weeks. Inactivated vaccines made from infected blood or egg-propagated *B. anserina* are beneficial.

Spirochetes are demonstrable in blood by darkfield microscopy, stained smear, or immunofluorescence. Suspect material (i.e., blood, spleen, or liver suspension) may be inoculated into the yolk sac of 5-to-6–day embryonated eggs. Spirochetes will appear within 2 or 3 days. Antigen or antibody may be demonstrated in agar gel diffusion tests.

Borrelia anserina is susceptible to penicillin G, tetracycline, chloramphenicol, streptomycin, kanamycin, and tylosin. Immune serum has protective potential and bacterins produce long-lasting immunity.

Control of ectoparasites is essential.

BORRELIA THEILERI

Borrelia theileri causes a mild febrile anemia, most often in African and Australian cattle, and occasionally in sheep and horses. The disease is associated with several species of ixodid ticks. The pathogenic mechanism(s) is not understood. Most information comes from field cases, which may be complicated by other tick-borne infections. Although not routinely treated, animals respond to tetracycline. Tick control is advisable.

LYME BORRELIOSIS

Lyme disease is caused by *B. burgdorferi* sensu lato, a pathogenic spirochete. Genetic analysis now defines three genospecies, *B. burgdorferi* sensu stricto, *B. garinii*, and *B. afzelii*. *Borrelia burgdorferi* sensu stricto is the predominant pathogen of North America.

Distribution and Transmission

Endemic areas include the North American Atlantic states, as well as Minnesota and Wisconsin; parts of the North American South and far West; most of continental Europe and Britain; Russia; Asia; Japan; and parts of New South Wales in Australia. May through October is the time of peak prevalence. Increasing spread of the disease is attributed to increased deer populations, increasing human movement into rural areas, and the dissemination of infected ticks by migratory birds. The agent is harbored by several ixodid ticks (primarily *Ixodes scapularis* and *I. pacificus* in North America). The tick has a 2-year life cycle comprised of a larval, nymph, and adult stage, requiring a blood meal at each molt. Deer mice, white-footed mice, and other small rodents serve as reservoirs for the spirochete. *Borrelia burgdorferi* has been isolated from the urine of dogs and cows as well as milk from infected cows, potentially serving as alternate routes for exposure and infection.

Human Lyme borreliosis, caused by *B. burgdorferi*, typically begins with a skin lesion (erythema migrans) often followed weeks or months later by neural, cardiac, and arthritic complications. Endotoxin, hemolysin, immune complexes, and immunosuppression may be involved in pathogenesis.

In other animals, dogs are most often affected, with manifestations of polyarthritis, fever, and anorexia the most common signs. Malaise, lymphadenopathy, carditis, and renal disease have also been noted in dogs. Similar signs have also been reported in domestic cats, though feline borreliosis is rare.

Borreliosis also occurs in horses and cattle. In horses, polyarthritis, ocular and neural involvement, and foal mortality have been reported.

Diagnosis

Diagnosis involves demonstration of the agent in tissues and fluids (darkfield, immunofluorescence microscopy), antibody in serum or other fluids (indirect immunofluorescent test, enzyme-linked immunosorbent assay, ELISA), or DNA amplification of tissue or fluid samples using genus specific DNA primers and the polymerase chain reaction.

Culture is laborious and often unrewarding. However, culturing ear punch biopsies from infected dogs and mice has proven to be reliable. Culture of synovial fluid from affected joints is also possible. BSK is a good isolation medium. The spirochetes grow best at 33°C.

Treatment and Control

Tetracycline, doxycycline, enrofloxacin, erythromycin, and penicillin G are generally effective, although not invariably so. Tick control is vital.

Immunologic Factors

A humoral immune response appears essential for protection against *B. burgdorferi* infection. Most animals appear to self-immunize with no apparent clinical manifestations subsequent to exposure to the spirochete.

Artificial Immunization

Antibodies produced in response to vaccination with *B. burgdorferi* have proven effective in preventing infection of laboratory animals. These observations have led to the development of a commercially available whole cell bacterin for use in canines. Subunit vaccines comprised of outer surface protein A (OspA) are also commercially available. Protective immunity for these vaccines is not 100%. Protective immunity also appears to be of short duration and limited in range, probably due to considerable heterogeneity in the OspA antigen. It has been demonstrated that the OspA antigen is synthesized by *B. burgdorferi* only while in the mid-gut of the tick vector. Its synthesis is turned off during the first 24 hours of a blood meal as the spirochetes migrate toward the tick's mouth and subsequent inoculation into the mammalian capillary. Thus, OspA subunit vaccines function in a two-step process. Vaccinated mammals serve as antibody factories to OspA which in turn must be delivered to the midgut of a feeding tick to neutralize the spirochetes at this site.

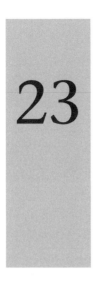

23

Spiral-Curved Organisms II: *Brachyspira (Serpulina)*

Dwight C. Hirsh

Members of the genus *Brachyspira* are gram-negative, spiral-shaped obligately anaerobic bacteria belonging to the family *Spirochaetaceae*. *Brachyspira hyodysenteriae* is the causative agent of swine dysentery, a disease of actively growing pigs. *Brachyspira pilosicoli* (*Anguillina coli*) is associated with intestinal spirochetosis of pigs in the post-weaning period, dogs, birds, and humans (usually those that are immunocompromised). *Brachyspira aalborgi* is a rare cause of human spirochetosis. Other brachyspiras with uncertain pathogenic potential include *B. intermedia* and *B. murdochii*. *Brachyspira innocens*, found in feces of symptomatic as well as asymptomatic pigs, has little if any pathogenic potential. "*Brachyspira canis*" is often found in the intestinal content of symptomatic as well as asymptomatic dogs.

Descriptive Features

Morphology and Staining

Brachyspira hyodysenteriae and *B. pilosicoli* are loosely coiled spirochetes, 6 to 11 μm long by 0.25 to 0.35 μm in width (Fig 23.1). Another very similar brachyspira, *B. innocens* (the so-called small spirochete), is often found in the feces of pigs with signs of dysentery as well as in normal feces. *Brachyspira innocens* measures 5 to 7 μm by 0.2 μm tightly coiled.

The brachyspiras are gram-negative, but this characteristic is not used to identify or detect them. Romanovsky-type stains (e.g., Wright's, Giemsa) are more useful in demonstrating these organisms in smears.

Cellular Anatomy and Composition

Cells are typical of spirochetes. The axial filament of *B. hyodysenteriae* is made up of 8 to 12 flagella inserted at either end; *B. innocens* has 10 to 13 flagella, and *B. pilosicoli* 4 to 6.

Cellular Products of Medical Interest

Cell Wall. The brachyspiras possess a gram-negative cell wall. The lipopolysaccharide (LPS) in the outer membrane is an important virulence determinant. Not only is the lipid A component toxic (endotoxin), but the length of the side chain in the O-repeat unit hinders the attachment of the membrane attack complex of the complement system to the outer membrane. Lipopolysaccharide binds to the plasma protein lipopolysaccharide-binding protein, which then binds to CD14. The CD14-LPS complex binds to a Toll-like receptor (see Chapter 2) on the surface of macrophage cells, triggering the release of proinflammatory cytokines.

Cytoxin/Hemolysin. The protein, Tly (for cytoxin/hemolysin) is responsible for the strong beta-hemolysis displayed by *B. hyodysenteriae* in vitro (the degree of hemolysis in vitro is often used to differentiate *S. hyodysenteriae*, which is strongly beta-hemolytic, from *B. innocens* and *B. pilosicoli*). This protein is a virulence determinant in vivo. Mutants that are unable to produce Tly are less virulent. Tly is a pore-forming cytotoxin affecting host target cells (goblet cells and colonic epithelial cells).

Hemolysin. Another hemolysin, Hly (for hemolysin) has been described, but its relation to virulence is unclear.

Flagella. Flagella, though present on virulent as well as avirulent brachyspiras, appear necessary for virulence. This trait is related to movement through the intestinal mucus to gain access to target cells in the large intestine. It has also been shown that virulent strains have an affinity for intestinal mucus.

Growth Characteristics

All members of the genus *Brachyspira* are obligate anaerobes.

Brachyspira hyodysenteriae is strongly beta-hemolytic, a trait that has been used by some to differentiate it from *B. innocens* and *B. pilosicoli*, which are weakly beta-hemolytic (Fig 23.2).

Brachyspira hyodysenteriae and *B. pilosicoli* are resistant to high concentrations of spectinomycin, a characteristic useful in isolating these organisms from feces. *Brachyspira hyodysenteriae* and presumably *B. pilosicoli* remain infective for long periods if enclosed within organic material in temperatures of 5°C to 25°C. They do not withstand drying or direct sunlight.

FIGURE 23.1.   Brachyspira hyodysenteriae *in a colonic scrapping of a pig with swine dysentery. Victoria Blue 4R stain, 1000X.*

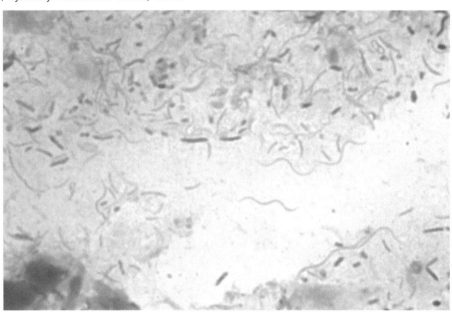

FIGURE 23.2.   Brachyspira hyodysenteriae *growing on a blood agar plate.*

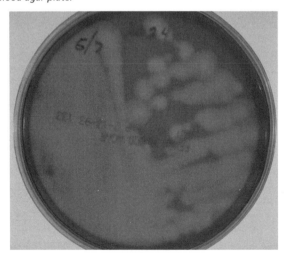

Variability

There are at least twelve serotypes of *B. hyodysenteriae*. Fingerprinting isolates by means of restriction-length polymorphisms of whole-cell DNA, DNA encoding ribosomal RNA, DNA encoding specific genes (e.g., flagellin), and multilocus enzyme electrophoresis has demonstrated the heterogeneity of members of this species as well as the others (*B. innocens* and *B. pilosicoli*).

Ecology

Reservoir and Transmission

The reservoir for *B. hyodysenteriae* is the gastrointestinal tract of pigs, especially asymptomatic carriers of the organism (animals recovered from the disease). The agent has been isolated from the feces of dogs, rats, and mice living on farms where the disease exists. Transmission is through the fecal-oral route.

Brachyspira pilosicoli has been isolated from dogs, birds, and humans. There is evidence that humans may acquire *B. pilosicoli* from affected dogs.

Pathogenesis

Brachyspira hyodysenteriae multiplies and produces disease in the colon (swine dysentery). It appears that *B. hyodysenteriae* alone will not produce disease. Other bacteria normally found in the colon of pigs, such as *Bacteroides vulgatus, B. fragilis, Fusobacterium necrophorum, Campylobacter coli*, a *Clostridium* sp., and *Listeria denitrificans*, have been shown to be involved in this supporting role. Superficial coagulation necrosis with epithelial cell erosion is observed. Edema, hyperemia, hemorrhage, and influx of polymorphonuclear neutrophil leukocytes (PMNs) into the mucosa and submucosa are seen. There is failure of colonic absorption. Inflammation, brought about by cytotoxin-mediated destruction of colonic target cells (goblet cells initially, then enterocytes), may induce a secretory diarrhea. DNA sequences encoding known enterotoxins have not been found in *B. hyodysenteriae*.

The signs of disease are rather typical. Affected pigs will void gray to strawberry-colored feces, become dehydrated,

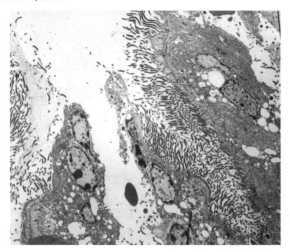

FIGURE 23.3.   Brachyspira pilosicoli *in the intestinal tract of a pig with intestinal spirochetosis. Transmission electron micrograph, about 40,000X.*

and, in the extreme, be acidotic and hyperkalemic. Temperature generally remains normal. Morbidity rates in susceptible pigs will be close to 90%, with mortality in untreated herds of approximately 20% to 40%. Duration of illness ranges from few days to several weeks. Survivors may be permanently stunted and remain asymptomatic shedders. There is no easy way to detect such animals.

Intestinal spirochetosis of pigs (post-weaning period), dogs, birds, and humans is associated with *B. pilosicoli*. This disease is characterized by a mild, persistent diarrhea and low mortality. Biopsies of affected colon show large clumps of spirochetes adhering "end on" to the intestinal epithelium (Fig 23.3).

Immunologic Aspects

Little is known about the immunologic factors of these diseases. Pigs recovered from swine dysentery are resistant to reinfection. Bacterins have met with some success in reducing the severity of the disease in affected swine.

Laboratory Diagnosis

Sample Collection

Fecal samples from affected animals showing signs of the disease are used to detect *B. hyodysenteriae* and *B. pilosicoli*.

Direct Examination

Smears of fecal material are stained with a Romanovsky-type stain (e.g., Wright's, Giemsa) or carbol fuchsin. Ob-

servation of large, loosely coiled spirochetes in diarrheal feces is presumptive evidence of infection with *B. hyodysenteriae* (swine dysentery) or *B. pilosicoli* (intestinal spirochetosis) (see Fig 23.1). *Brachyspira innocens* may be present in samples from pigs with swine dysentery, but these will be smaller and have tighter coils, a distinction that is sometimes difficult to make.

Isolation/Detection

Isolation of *B. hyodysenteriae* and *B. pilosicoli* from fecal samples is accomplished by inoculation onto blood agar plates containing spectinomycin (400 µg/ml). The plates are incubated 24 to 48 hours in an anaerobic environment containing 10% carbon dioxide. Colonies of *B. hyodysenteriae* will be small and strongly beta-hemolytic; those of *B. pilosicoli* will not be as strongly hemolytic (see Fig 23.2).

A multiplex polymerase chain reaction (PCR) assay using primers designed to detect the DNA of common diarrhea-associated microorganisms (*B. hyodysenteriae, Lawsonia intracellularis,* and *Salmonella*) has been described.

Identification

Brachyspira hyodysenteriae must be differentiated from *B. innocens*. This is best done by gas chromatographic analysis of volatile fatty acids or by DNA probing/analysis. Unfortunately these techniques do not lend themselves to performance in a busy diagnostic laboratory. Therefore, observing the strength of the beta-hemolysis, fructose fermentation (*B. innocens* will be positive), and indole production (*B. hyodysenteriae* will be positive) are traits used to make the distinction. Though the hemolysis trait seems to be relatively stable, the other tests are somewhat variable and misidentifications are possible. *Brachyspira pilosicoli* hydrolyzes hippurate; *B. innocens* does not. *Brachyspira pilosicoli* is differentiated from "*B. canis*" by molecular means (sequence of the gene encoding the 16S rRNA combined with multilocus enzyme electrophoresis).

Treatment, Control, and Prevention

Drugs shown to be effective in treating swine dysentery and intestinal spirochetosis in swine include organic arsenicals, tylosin, gentamicin, nitrofurazone, virginiamycin, and lincomycin. These have been used at low prophylactic levels, but it should be kept in mind that drugs used routinely to prevent the disease will ultimately lose their effectiveness. Metronidazole is the recommended treatment for dogs with intestinal spirochetosis.

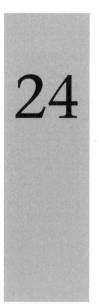

24

Spiral-Curved Organisms III: *Campylobacter, Arcobacter, Lawsonia*

Dwight C. Hirsh

Members of the genera *Campylobacter, Arcobacter,* and *Lawsonia* are gram-negative, curved rods. They are associated with diseases of the reproductive and intestinal tracts. Taxonomically, *Campylobacter* and *Arcobacter* (previously classified within the genus *Campylobacter*) are members of the family *Campylobacteriaceae. Lawsonia* does not appear to be related phylogenetically to any other species of pathogenic bacteria.

Descriptive Features

Morphology and Staining

Members of the genera *Campylobacter, Arcobacter,* and *Lawsonia* are gram-negative, slender, curved rods that measure 0.2 to 0.5 μm by 0.5 to 5 μm. When two or more bacterial cells are placed together, they form S or gullwinged shapes that may appear as "spirals" (Fig 24.1).

Cellular Anatomy and Composition

Members of the genera *Campylobacter, Arcobacter,* and *Lawsonia* have typical gram-negative cell walls, capsules, and flagella.

CAMPYLOBACTER

Members of the genus *Campylobacter* are implicated in enteric and reproductive diseases of animals. Though the genus contains 15 species, only a few have been implicated in disease. These include *C. fetus, C. jejuni, C. coli, C. concisus, C. helveticus, C. hyointestinalis, C. mucosalis, C. lari,* and *C. upsaliensis.*

Two species of *Campylobacter* are important in regard to the genital tract and reproductive performance: *C. fetus* and *C. jejuni. Campylobacter fetus* has two subspecies: *venerealis* and *fetus.* The disease produced by these organisms is sometimes referred to as *vibriosis* because the agents were

once classified as members of the genus *Vibrio.* They are not.

Campylobacter jejuni and *C. coli* are major causes of gastroenteritis in people and nonhuman primates, and have been found in fecal samples from dogs and cats with diarrhea. *Campylobacter jejuni* is the more commonly isolated of the two. Though *C. coli* occurs in high numbers in swine dysentery and was once thought to be the causative agent, the disease is caused by *Brachyspira (Serpulina) hyodysenteriae* (see Chapter 23). Both *C. coli* and *C. jejuni* may occur in feces of normal animals.

Campylobacter concisus has been associated with gastrointestinal disease of humans.

Campylobacter helveticus has been recovered from the feces of dogs and cats with diarrhea.

Campylobacter hyointestinalis and *C. mucosalis* were once implicated as contributors to the swine proliferative enteritis complex. This disease is caused by *Lawsonia intracellularis* (see below), a microorganism that produces this disease in conventional pigs in pure culture, something neither *C. hyointestinalis* nor *C. mucosalis* will do.

Campylobacter lari, isolated from the feces of asymptomatic gulls (from which it gets its name), has also been isolated from the feces of various hosts, including dogs, birds, and horses. Its role in disease is uncertain.

Campylobacter sputorum is sometimes isolated from the prepuce of bulls or vagina of cattle, but are not considered significant.

Campylobacter upsaliensis has been isolated from feces of dogs and cats with diarrhea. Enteric disease and abortion have been associated with this microorganism in humans.

Descriptive Features

Cellular Products of Medical Interest

Adhesin. Campylobacter jejuni involved with enteric disease produce a mannose-resistant adhesin that binds to a fucose-containing receptor on the target cell (epithelial cells of the small intestine).

FIGURE 24.1.   Campylobacter fetus *subspecies* fetus *in the stomach fluid of an aborted lamb. Gram stain, 1000X.*

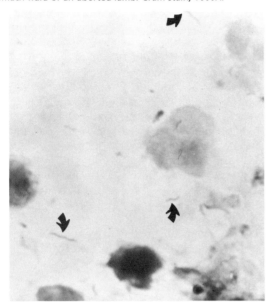

FIGURE 24.1.   Campylobacter fetus *subspecies* fetus *in the stomach fluid of an aborted lamb. Gram stain, 1000X.*

Capsule. The glycoprotein capsule protects the outer membrane from the membrane attack complex of the complement cascade. The capsule also inhibits attachment to, and ingestion by, phagocytic host cells.

Cell Wall. The cell wall of the members of this genus is one typical of gram-negative bacteria. The lipopolysaccharide (LPS) in the outer membrane is an important virulence determinant. Not only is the lipid A component toxic (endotoxin), but the length of the side chain in the O-repeat unit hinders the attachment of the membrane attack complex of the complement system to the outer membrane. Lipopolysaccharide binds to the serum protein, lipopolysaccharide-binding protein, which transfers it to the blood-phase of CD14. The CD14-LPS complex binds to Toll-like receptor proteins (see Chapter 2) on the surface of macrophage cells triggering the release of proinflammatory cytokines.

Enterotoxin. Campylobacter jejuni involved with enteric disease secrete a toxin with similar activity to cholera toxin and the heat-labile toxin (LT) of *Escherichia coli* (see Chapter 8) by increasing intracellular levels of cAMP and cytoskeletal rearrangements. Both toxins are immunologically related and bind to the same ganglioside (GM1) on the surface of the target cell. *Campylobacter coli* and *C. lari* produce uncharacterized substances with cytotonic and cytotoxic activity.

Cytotoxins. Campylobacter jejuni involved with enteric disease produce a number of proteins with cytotoxic activity. These cytotoxins include a heat and trypsin labile protein of 70 kDa in size which is neutralized by antibody to shiga-like toxin (see Chapter 11); a 73 kDa protein, termed Cia (for *Campylobacter* invasion antigen) that is inserted into the target epithelial cell allowing subsequent invasion of the cell (a Type III secretion system may be involved, see below); a protein active on Vero tissue culture cells; a pro-

tein that increases intracellular cAMP followed by cell death (a cytolethal distending toxin, see Chapter 8); a protein that has hemolytic activity (hemolysin); and a protein that was shown to induce hepatitis in mice (hepatotoxin). All of these toxic compounds have a tenuous association with the disease process in humans and other animals.

Miscellaneous Products. Campylobacter jejuni possess a Type III secretion system (an assemblage of proteins—more than 20—that form a hollow tube-like structure through which effector proteins are "injected" into host "target" cells). The proteins involved with this system, Cia (for *Campylobacter* invasion antigens) are responsible for triggering the uptake of *C. jejuni* after adherence to intestinal epithelial cells.

Growth Characteristics

Campylobacter spp. are microaerophilic (with the exception of *C. hominis* which appears to be obligately anaerobic), requiring an atmosphere containing 3% to 15% oxygen and 3% to 5% carbon dioxide for growth. Some, such as *C. jejuni*, grow at 42°C, a characteristic that is useful for its selectivity in isolation from intestinal sources. Unlike members of the family *Enterobacteriaceae*, they are oxidase-positive. They do not ferment or oxidize carbohydrates, generating energy from oxidation of amino acids or tricarboxylic acid intermediates through the respiratory pathway. Though they possess catalase and superoxide dismutase, these enzymes are overwhelmed by the excess of hydrogen peroxide and superoxide anions formed when they are grown in the presence of atmospheric concentrations of oxygen.

Variability

Campylobacter fetus subspecies *fetus* contains two serovars, A-2 and B, based on heat-stable surface antigens. Strains with both antigens occur. *Campylobacter fetus* subspecies *venerealis* has two serovars, A-1 and A-sub 1. The serovars differ not only with respect to heat-stable surface antigen (A) but also culturally and biochemically. *Campylobacter jejuni* possesses one serovar C, based on a heat-stable surface antigen. *Campylobacter jejuni* has twenty-two serovars as determined by analysis of extractable heat-labile antigens (Lior scheme) or twenty-three serovars by utilizing extractable heat-stable antigens (Penner scheme).

Ecology

Reservoir

Campylobacter fetus subspecies *venerealis*. The reservoir of *C. fetus* ssp. *venerealis* is the preputial crypts of the bull (main) and the vagina of carrier animals (rare after one to two breeding seasons without re-exposure).

Campylobacter fetus subspecies *fetus*. The reservoir for *C. fetus* ssp. *fetus* is the intestinal tract of infected (recovered) sheep (perhaps through contamination from a colonized gallbladder).

Campylobacter jejuni. The reservoir for *C. jejuni* is the intestinal tract of normal animals (especially young ruminants, various birds, asymptomatic dogs and cats) or animals that have had the disease.

Other Campylobacters. The sources of *C. lari, C. helveticus,* and *C. upsaliensis* are not known but are presumed to be the intestinal tract of infected individuals. Feces from healthy puppies and kittens have been shown to contain *C. upsaliensis.*

Transmission

Reproductive Disease. Acquisition of campylobacters affecting the reproductive tract occurs either venereally (*C. fetus* ssp. *venerealis,* cattle) or by ingestion (*C. fetus* ssp. *fetus* and *C. jejuni,* sheep and goats, rarely cattle).

Enteric Disease. Acquisition of campylobacters associated with enteric disease (*C. jejuni, C. coli*) occurs by the fecal-oral route, direct or indirect, and is probably the main mode of spread.

Pathogenesis

Reproductive Disease (Cattle). The agent *C. fetus* ssp. *venerealis* is introduced into a susceptible female by an infected bull at coitus. The organisms remain at the cervicovaginal junction until the end of estrus. This is probably a consequence of the increased blood supply and active polymorphonuclear neutrophil leukocytes (PMNs) seen in the reproductive tract during this time. The organisms multiply at this site and, when conditions are suitable, move into the uterus. Further multiplication and perhaps active invasion result in inflammation of the uterus with resultant endometritis and cessation of pregnancy. The animal will return to estrus. This process continues until the female makes an immune response sufficient to eliminate the agent from the uterus. Subsequently, the endometritis subsides, and the animal conceives and pregnancy goes to term. Sporadic abortions sometimes occur.

Clinically, there are signs of repeat breeding and extended cycles (10-to-60–day cycles; 21 days is normal), which are usually manifested in an infected herd as prolonged calving intervals and extended calving periods. In addition, the herd bull will show loss of condition. The herd, if it remains closed, develops immunity, and calving intervals gradually return toward normal. This process takes years, however, and the economic consequences of the disease are disastrous.

Reproductive Disease (Sheep and Goats). These species are infected following ingestion of *C. fetus* ssp. *fetus* or *C. jejuni.* Following ingestion, the organism somehow gains entry into the bloodstream and localizes in the pregnant uterus, especially in the latter stages of pregnancy. Incubation may be as long as 2 months. A placentitis develops along with infection of the fetus (amniotic fluid) and abortion results. The placenta, fluids, and fetus contain large numbers of the organism and act as a source of infection for susceptible animals. Abortions, when they occur, are usually in "storms" occurring in great numbers relatively suddenly following a few scattered abortions. Cattle are rarely infected with *C. fetus* ssp. *fetus* and, when they are, sporadic abortions are observed.

Enteric Disease. *Campylobacter jejuni* adheres to cells of the small intestine, especially the distal segments. The organism multiplies and invades the target epithelial cell (Cia), with resultant inflammation. It is uncertain whether the toxins elaborated by *C. jejuni* are responsible for the disease. However, the LT-like toxin is thought to deregulate the adenylyl cyclase system as described for enterotoxigenic *E. coli* (see Chapter 8). At the same time, the cytotoxin destroys the mucosal epithelium. The inflammatory response elicited by *Campylobacter* interaction with the target epithelial cells, and the chemistry of the cell wall leads to the development of diarrhea. Diarrhea follows prostaglandin synthesis by the recruited PMNs (and perhaps by the affected host cells), as well as activation of various inositol-signaling pathways within affected host cells. The net result is the secretion of chloride ions and water. The bactericidal effects of serum destroy *C. jejuni* that escape into the lymphatics and into the systemic circulation. Diarrheal feces containing cell debris and mucus are produced, and products of the inflammatory response are seen in direct smears. Mucus and blood are sometimes seen grossly.

Epidemiology

Reproductive Disease (Cattle). The disease is seen mainly in beef cattle, since the agent is effectively killed by techniques used to prepare and store semen for insemination in the dairy industry.

Reproductive Disease (Sheep and Goats). The gallbladder of sheep, and presumably goats, may become colonized with *Campylobacter.* If this occurs, these animals become a source of infectious organisms for susceptible stock.

Enteric Disease. In addition to producing disease of the reproductive tract of animals, members of the genus *Campylobacter* are a significant cause of human disease. *Campylobacter jejuni* is one of the leading causes of gastroenteritis in human beings. Human beings in developed societies acquire *C. jejuni* from symptomatic or asymptomatic companion animals (dogs and cats) and from food such as raw milk, water, and poultry products. Most sporadic cases probably arise from consumption of improperly handled poultry or contact with infected pets, whereas large outbreaks most often occur from contact with raw milk or contaminated water. The feces of approximately 10% of asymptomatic dogs and approximately 5% of asymptomatic cats are found to contain *C. jejuni.* This percentage may be higher in animals acquired from animal shelters. The ceca of approximately 50% of chickens sampled contain *C. jejuni.* At slaughter, these organisms contaminate the environment and, as a consequence, almost as many chicken carcasses found in stores will be contaminated. From 2% to 100% of cattle may be healthy shedders of *C. jejuni,* a circumstance that may explain outbreaks of campylobacter-induced diarrheal disease following ingestion of unpasteurized milk.

Immunologic Aspects

Reproductive Disease (Cattle). Development of an active immune response results in the uterus being cleared of the organism. Specific serum IgG and IgM function by initiating the complement cascade (IgG and IgM) and by acting as opsonizing agents (IgG). In the latter case, these antibodies bind to the antigenic determinants composing the capsular antigens, resulting in the phagocytosis and subsequent destruction of the agent. Secretory IgA, IgG, and IgM specific for surface structures bind and prevent the adherence of the organism to the surface of the epithelium. All isotypes, if specific for the flagellar antigens, prevent movement of more organisms from the vagina. Animals clear the entire tract of the agent if they are not reinfected. Clearance rarely takes more than one year. The mechanism responsible for clearing is unknown but is probably due to the fact that the campylobacters have to deal with an immune response as well as the normal flora of the vagina.

The disease can be controlled by vaccinating heifers or cows with bacterins or by eliminating carrier animals, including the bull. Bulls do not carry the organism efficiently until they are older than about five years. The most commonly held explanation is that the preputial crypts of older bulls are deeper and more hospitable than the shallower crypts found in younger bulls.

Reproductive Disease (Sheep and Goats). Sheep and goats are immune following abortion. The basis for this immunity is mainly antibody of the IgM and IgG types. These antibodies bind to the surface of the agent while it is in the bloodstream, resulting in removal by phagocytic cells in the liver and spleen. Antibody bound to the surface also initiates the complement cascade leading to lysis of the agent. The immune response is also effective in killing organisms that had reached the placenta but had not yet produced enough damage to terminate pregnancy.

Enteric Disease. Circulating antibody develops as a result of infection. The disease is self-limiting due to the combined effects of secretory antibody and the normal flora.

Laboratory Diagnosis

Sample Collection

Reproductive Disease (Cattle). Samples for culture or observation are best taken from the prepuce of the bull. Smegma is collected by aspiration into the tip of an insemination pipette. If the female is to be cultured, samples are collected from the anterior vagina. With either sex, 10% of the herd or 20 animals (whichever is greater) are sampled for diagnostic testing.

Reproductive Disease (Sheep and Goats). Samples from the liver and the abomasum of the aborted fetus are most rewarding. The placenta and fluids of the abortus are usually too contaminated.

Enteric Disease. Fecal samples are taken for the diagnosis of *C. jejuni* infections.

Direct Examination

Reproductive Disease (Cattle). The low numbers of campylobacters together with the high numbers of organisms of the normal flora make it difficult to observe the campylobacters (small curved rods) in stained smears (Gram or Romanovsky). Fluorescent antibody-stained preparations have proven useful in detection. Campylobacters exhibit a characteristic "tumbling" motility when observed in wet mounts of affected material.

Reproductive Disease (Sheep and Goats). Gram (carbol fuchsin as counterstain) or Romanovsky-stained preparations of stomach contents from aborted fetuses often demonstrate the agent (see Fig 24.1). Such findings, in conjunction with doughnut-shaped necrotic foci sometimes found on the liver, help support the diagnosis (see Fig 74.5). Examination of wet mounts of affected material is sometimes useful.

Enteric Disease. Stained (Gram stain with carbol fuchsin as counterstain; Romanovsky-type stain) smears of fecal material will reveal numerous slender, curved rods in most cases of diarrhea produced by *C. jejuni*.

Isolation

Reproductive Disease (Cattle). Smegma, vaginal fluid, or stomach contents are plated onto media that contain antimicrobial agents (vancomycin, polymyxin B or C, and trimethoprim are commonly added to decrease the growth of noncampylobacters; amphotericin B is included in some formulations to inhibit growth of fungi). The plate is incubated at 37°C in an atmosphere containing 6% oxygen and 5% to 10% carbon dioxide. Plates are examined in 48 hours.

Reproductive Disease (Sheep and Goats). Abomasal contents and liver (aborted fetus) are plated onto blood agar plates (with or without antimicrobials, depending upon the degree of contamination). The plates are incubated at 37°C in an atmosphere containing 6% oxygen and 5% to 10% carbon dioxide. Plates are examined in 48 hours.

Enteric Disease. Campylobacter jejuni and *C. coli* are best isolated from affected intestinal samples on selective media containing antimicrobial agents (e.g., Campy-CVA containing cefoperazone, vancomycin, and amphotericin B). The plates are incubated at 37°C, or at 42°C when isolation of *C. jejuni* or *C. coli* from feces is attempted, in an atmosphere of 6% oxygen and 5% to 10% carbon dioxide.

Identification

Isolation of a gram-negative, curved rod that is oxidase-positive is presumptive evidence that a member of the genus *Campylobacter* (or "*Arcobacter*," see below) has been isolated. Though there are a number of fermentation reactions that have been described for the identification of *Campylobacter*, these are tedious and time consuming. Methods based on detection of specific DNA sequences may be used for identification (e.g., generation of fragments of a certain size following amplification of specific DNA sequences by polymerase chain reaction, or determining the sequence of the gene encoding ribosomal RNA). Likewise, analyses of cell wall fatty acids have been useful.

Serodiagnosis

Serodiagnosis is sometimes used in the diagnosis of reproductive disease involving *Campylobacter*-associated disease in cattle. In particular, the disease can be diagnosed by tests of cervicovaginal mucus for antibody to campylobacter antigens. For collection, a tampon is placed in the vagina near the cervix. Following removal, the mucus is collected and diluted serially. Agglutinins appear in the cervicovaginal mucus in 3 to 80 days of infection and persist for approximately 7 months. Samples are collected 4 to 5 days after estrus or 1 to 2 days before. Samples taken at estrus are too dilute due to the excess mucus. The presence of blood invalidates the test. Antibody to *C. fetus* can also be detected by using an enzyme-linked immunosorbent assay (ELISA). Reportedly, this test can be run on samples collected during estrus and will be positive within 18 to 40 days after infection.

Treatment

Reproductive Disease (Cattle). Bulls can be treated parenterally with streptomycin. For topical treatment, an aqueous solution of penicillin and streptomycin is instilled into the prepuce. Vaccination of bulls has been reported to clear the carrier state.

The disease is best controlled by prevention. Sound husbandry practices reduce the chances of introducing the organism into the herd. The use of young bulls that have tested negative when bred to a virgin heifer, and barring of replacement heifers or cows originating from herds with unknown history, are means to keep out campylobacters. Once the agent is in the herd, a number of alternatives are available. The least acceptable to the producer is to rest the herd for one breeding season and cull the bulls. This eliminates the organism from the females and removes a source of the organism when breeding resumes. Artificial insemination is a very effective way to control and eliminate the disease from a herd. Antibiotic treatment of females is unrewarding, but bacterins are used to prevent the disease in herds in which it is endemic. Vaccination is performed yearly.

Reproductive Disease (Sheep and Goats). Administering antibiotics can stop abortion storms. The most effective is penicillin G. Aborting ewes should be isolated from those that are apparently unaffected.

Administering a bacterin prior to breeding can prevent the disease.

Enteric Disease. The enteritis produced by *C. jejuni* is most often self-limiting. Macrolide antibiotics (clarithromycin, erythromycin, tylosin) remain the drugs of choice for treatment of *C. jejuni* diarrhea. Tetracyclines are effective when macrolides cannot be used, although tetracycline-resistant strains exist (R plasmid–based). Most campylobacters from animals are susceptible to fluoroquinolone antibiotics. However, due to the high rate of mutational resistance campylobacters have to this group of antibiotics, a resistance that sometimes occurs while animals are being treated, fluoroquinolones are not the drugs of choice. In addition, diarrhea due to *C. jejuni* most often occurs in younger animals, most too young to be safely treated with this group of drugs.

Control in the veterinary hospital and kennel requires meticulous adherence to hygienic measures, such as handwashing, cleaning, and disinfection protocols.

There are no immunizing preparations that will prevent enteritis produced by *C. jejuni.*

ARCOBACTER

Members of the genus *Arcobacter* are associated with diarrheal conditions (calves), mastitis in cattle, and reproductive disease of livestock, especially swine. The genus *Arcobacter* (at one time designated as *Campylobacter*-like organisms) contains three species with pathogenic potential for humans and other animals: *A. cryaerophilus, A. butzleri,* and *A. skirrowii.*

Descriptive Features

Cellular Products of Medical Interest

Virtually nothing is known about the cellular products of *Arcobacter,* aside from a typical cell wall (see above, "*Campylobacter*").

Growth Characteristics

Members of the genus *Arcobacter* are aerotolerant, a trait that separates them from *Campylobacter.* They grow over a wide temperature range, and some strains of *A. butzleri* grow at 42°C.

Ecology

Reservoir

The reservoirs of *Arcobacter* are presumably the intestinal tracts and the immediate environment of affected animals (calves with diarrhea, cattle with mastitis, aborted pig fetuses). Asymptomatic swine, cattle, and poultry may serve as an important reservoir for humans.

Transmission

It is unknown how animals acquire arcobacters, though ingestion or entry through other mucosal surfaces are likely possibilities.

Pathogenesis

Little is known regarding the interactions of *Arcobacter* with the host.

Epidemiology

Very little is known about the epidemiology of the diseases associated with *Arcobacter* infection. The organism is probably an inhabitant of the intestinal tract of asymptomatic swine, cattle, and poultry.

Immunologic Aspects

The immune response of affected animals to *Arcobacter* has not been clarified.

Laboratory Diagnosis

Sample Collection

Arcobacters have been isolated from stomach contents, kidney, and placenta of aborted swine fetuses. Fecal samples are taken for the diagnosis of *Arcobacter*-associated diarrhea.

Direct Examination

Gram (carbol fuchsin as counterstain) or Romanovsky-type (e.g., Wright's, Giemsa) stained preparation of stomach contents, kidney impressions, or placental fluids often demonstrate the agent in affected swine fetuses. Little is known regarding the usefulness of direct smears in the diagnosis of *Arcobacter*-associated diarrhea. An important distinction is differentiating *Arcobacter* from *Campylobacter*—difficult without specific antibody (e.g., fluorescently labeled antibody).

Isolation

The same media used to isolate *Campylobacter* is successful for *Arcobacter*. *Arcobacter* does not require the same atmospheric environment as do campylobacters. They will, however grow in a microaerophiliic atmosphere.

Identification

Isolation of a gram-negative, curved rod that is oxidase-positive is presumptive evidence that a member of the genus *Campylobacter* (see above) or *Arcobacter* has been isolated. Though there are a number of fermentation reactions that have been described for the identification of *Arcobacter*, these are tedious and time consuming. Methods based on detection of specific DNA sequences have proven useful for identification (e.g., generation of fragments of a certain size following amplification of specific DNA sequences by polymerase chain reaction, or determining the sequence of the gene encoding ribosomal RNA). Likewise, analyses of cell wall fatty acids have been useful.

Treatment

The arcobacters, *A. butzleri* and *A. cryaerophilus*, are resistant to the macrolide antibiotics but susceptible to the tetracyclines and fluoroquinolones. Whether these microorganisms have the same resistance problems as with the campylobacters is unknown.

Treatment of arcobacter-associated conditions in swine is poorly documented. Use of autologous bacterins has shown promise.

LAWSONIA

The genus *Lawsonia* contains only one species, *L. intracellularis*, previously known as *ileal symbiont intracellularis*. It is an obligate intracellular microorganism causing proliferative enteritis of swine. The microorganism is also associated with a similar condition in birds (emus, ostriches), blue fox, deer, dogs, horses, rabbits, and rodents ("wet tail" of hamsters).

Descriptive Features

Cellular Products of Medical Interest

Adhesins. Lawsonia intracellularis expresses a surface protein, LsaA (for *Lawsonia* surface antigen) that is responsible for the attachment to and entry into target cells (the apical surface of immature intestinal epithelial cells).

Cell Wall. The cell wall of the members of this genus is one typical of gram-negative bacteria. The lipopolysaccharide (LPS) in the outer membrane is an important virulence determinant. Not only is the lipid A component toxic (endotoxin), but the length of the side chain in the O-repeat unit hinders the attachment of the membrane attack complex of the complement system to the outer membrane. Lipopolysaccharide binds to the serum protein, lipopolysaccharide-binding protein, which transfers it to the blood-phase of CD14. The CD14-LPS complex binds to Toll-like receptor proteins (see Chapter 2) on the surface of macrophage cells triggering the release of proinflammatory cytokines.

Growth Characteristics

Lawsonia intracellularis has not been grown in lifeless media.

Ecology

Reservoir

The reservoirs of *L. intracellularis* are the intestinal tracts and the immediate environment of affected animals.

Transmission

Infection occurs following the ingestion of an animal product contaminated with infected feces.

Pathogenesis

Following ingestion, *L. intracellularis* associates with and is internalized (endocytosis involving actin polymerization) by immature (crypt) cells of the distal small intestine (due in part to Lsa). After internalization, the microorganisms escape from the vacuole into the cell cytoplasm where multiplication and spread to adjacent cells occurs. There is as yet no evidence to suggest that *L. intracellularis* utilizes actin polymerization (see Chapters 11 and 33) as a means of propulsion and spread through the cell cytoplasm. Affected cells proliferate resulting in the characteristic lesions associated with this disease. An inflammatory response in most cases is minimal. Swine proliferative enteritis is a disease complex involving a number of intestinal abnormalities: intestinal adenomatosis, necrotic enteritis, regional ileitis, and proliferative hemorrhagic enteropathy. Thickening of the ileal wall, but including, on occasion, segments on either side, characterize the disease.

Epidemiology

Lawsonia intracellularis is widely distributed among swine herds worldwide (some estimates run as high as 50% of herds are infected). The disease is most often apparent as poor performance. Affected pigs ("weaners" and growing pigs), infected while nursing or shortly thereafter, do not make target weights. Overt manifestations of disease (diarrhea, often bloody) are not a common presentation, and are often brought about by stressful situations. However, infection of mature pigs commonly results in clinical disease.

Immunologic Aspects

Both humoral and cellular immune responses are generated following infection of susceptible species. There is some suggestion that an immunosuppressive phenomenon may account for the progression of the disease. A diminished inflammatory response that is commonly observed supports this notion.

Laboratory Diagnosis

Sample Collection

Scrapings of affected intestine are used to diagnose proliferative enteritis. Likewise, formalin-fixed tissues acquired from affected sites are also used.

Direct Examination

Impression smears of the intestine of swine with proliferative enteritis contain small curved rods within the cells lining the area. The silver stains, such as Warthin-Starry, or a modified acid-fast stain (use 0.5% acetic acid for 30 seconds for decolorization) are sometimes used to demonstrate organisms in this site. Immunohistochemical methods are used to detect the presence of the microorganism in fixed tissue.

Isolation

Lawsonia intracellularis has not been grown in lifeless media. However, DNA methods (DNA probes, or the use of DNA primers to amplify *Lawsonia*-specific sequences by using the polymerase chain reaction) have been developed that enable the detection of this microorganism in tissue or feces.

Identification

The nature of the lesion, together with the results of direct smear examination, is presumptive evidence that *L. intracellularis* is involved. Methods utilizing DNA analysis are quick, easy, and specific.

A multiplex polymerase chain reaction (PCR) assay using primers designed to detect the common diarrhea-associated microorganisms affecting swine (*B. hyodysenteriae*, *Lawsonia intracellularis*, and *Salmonella*) has been described.

Treatment

Clinical trials have shown that the tetracyclines are most effective in treating disease produced by *L. intracellularis*. Alternate drugs include tiamulin and tylosin.

Excluding the organism from swine herds is at present the most desirable method of control. There is a relationship between herd size and occurrence of the diseases (smaller the herd, less disease). Thus, a small "all in, all out" herd type management system seems the most efficient way to prevent this disease.

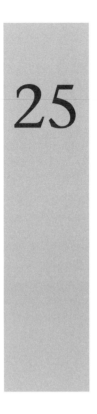

25

Spiral-Curved Organisms IV: *Helicobacter*—The Spiral Shaped Microorganisms of the Gastrointestinal Tract and Liver

JAMES G. FOX

Gastric spiral shaped microorganisms have been noted in humans and other animals for more than a century. After the discovery of *Helicobacter pylori* in diseased gastric tissue of humans in 1982, helicobacters have been cultured from the stomachs of ferrets, non-human primates, dogs, cats, hamsters, cheetahs, dolphins, whales, and harp seals. These gram-negative, microaerophilic curved to spiral-shaped bacteria isolated from gastric mucosa of humans and other animals during the last 20 years have created a great deal of interest because of their causal role in gastric disease. The type species, *H. pylori* colonizes the stomach of 20 to 95% of adult human populations worldwide. This microorganism causes persistent, active, chronic gastritis and peptic ulcer disease in humans and also has been linked to the development of gastric adenocarcinoma and gastric mucosal–associated lymphoma. In addition to gastric helicobacters, an increasing number of species of *Helicobacter* have been isolated from the lower gastrointestinal tract of mammals and birds. At least 27 members of the genus *Helicobacter* have been identified and named (Table 25.1). Members of the genus *Helicobacter* are taxonomically distinct from the genus *Campylobacter*, which also have spiral morphology and grow under microaerophilic conditions, as well reside in the gastrointestinal tract. The complete genomes of both *H. pylori* and *H. hepaticus* have been sequenced.

Descriptive Features

Morphology and Staining

Members of the genus *Helicobacter* have a vast array of morphologies, ranging from spirals (e.g., *H. pylori*, 0.5–1.0 by 2.5–5 µm), to slightly bent rods (e.g., *H. mustelae*, 0.5 by 2

µm). All express flagella differing in number and distribution (Table 25.2), and except for *H. pullorum* and *H. rodentium*, the flagella are sheathed.

Cellular Products of Medical Interest

The cellular products of medical interest listed below are for *H. pylori* (the most studied of the helicobacters), unless otherwise stated. It is assumed that other helicobacters will have similar traits and characteristics.

Adhesins. Adhesins are proteins that mediate adherence to target cells in the gastrointestinal tract and to cells comprising the niche for the strain. *Helicobacter pylori* expresses at least two adhesins with specificity for gastric epithelia:

1. Sialic acid-binding adhesin (SabA). SabA (for *s*ialic *a*cid-*b*inding *a*dhesin) binds to sialylated glycoproteins on the surface of gastric epithelial cells.
2. Blood group antigen-binding adhesin (BabA). BabA (for *b*lood group *a*ntigen-*b*inding *a*dhesin) binds to fucosylated blood group antigens found on gastric epithelial cells (Lewis blood group).

Cell Wall. The lipopolysaccharide (LPS) in the outer membrane is an important virulence determinant. Not only is the lipid A component toxic (endotoxin), but the length of the side chain in the O-repeat unit hinders the attachment of the membrane attack complex of the complement system to the outer membrane. LPS binds to lipopolysaccharide-binding protein (a serum protein), which in turn transfers it to the blood phase of CD14. The CD14-LPS complex binds to Toll-like receptor proteins (see Chapter 2) on the surface of macrophage cells triggering the release of proinflammatory cytokines

cag *Pathogenicty Island.* cag (for *c*ytotoxin-*a*ssociated *g*ene product) Pathogenicity Island (a cluster of genes en-

Table 25.1.   Habitats of *Helicobacter* species

Helicobacter taxon	Source(s)	Primary Site	Secondary Site
HUMAN			
H. bizzozeronii[a]	Human, cat, dog, cheetah, primates, wild rats	Stomach	
H. canis	Human, cat, dog	Intestine	Liver (dog)
H. canadensis	Human, wild geese	Intestine	
H. cinaedi	Human, hamster, macaque, dog	Intestine	Blood, brain, joint (human)
H. fennelliae	Human	Intestine	
H. pullorum	Human, chicken	Intestine	Liver (chicken)
H. pylori	Human, macaque, cat	Stomach	
Flexispira (Helicobacter) taxon 8[b]	Human, dog, sheep, mouse	Intestine	Placenta/fetus (sheep) Blood (humans)
H. winghamensis	Human	Intestine	
NONHUMAN			
H. aurati	Hamster	Stomach, intestine	
H. acinonychis	Cheetah	Stomach	
H. bilis	Mouse, dog, rat, cat	Intestine	Liver (mouse)
H. cetorum	Dolphins, whales	Stomach	
H. cholecystus	Hamster	Gallbladder	
H. felis	Cat, dog	Stomach	
H. ganmani	Mouse	Intestine	
H. hepaticus	Mouse	Intestine	
H. marmotae	Cat, woodchuck	Intestine	Liver/woodchuck
H. mesocricetorum	Hamster	Intestine	
H. muridarum	Mouse, rat	Intestine	
H. mustelae	Ferret, mink	Stomach	
H. pametensis	Birds, swine	Intestine	
H. rodentium	Mouse	Intestine	
H. salomonis	Dog	Stomach	
H. suis	Pigs	Stomach	
H. typhlonius	Mouse	Intestine	
H. trogontum	Rat	Intestine	

[a] Likely the same as "*H. heilmannii*." "*Helicobacter heilmannii*" (formerly *Gastrospirillum hominis*) has the same phenotype as listed here for *H. bizzozeronii*. Only a single "*H. heilmannii*" strain has been isolated by culture, and thus it has not been included in Table 1.
[b] Formerly regarded as "*Flexispira rappini*"—now has been subgrouped into ten taxa.

coding virulence determinant[s], an integrase protein, a specific insertion site, and mobility) encodes the Cag protein (see below), and a Type IV secretion system, which mediates translocation of Cag into host cells.

Cytolethal Distending Toxin. A cytolethal distending toxin is produced by *H. hepaticus*, *H. bilis*, *H. marmotae*, *H. pullorum*, and *H. cinaedi*. This protein produces significant in vitro cytopathic effects in cell lines and causes cell cycle arrest. It is not known what effect this cytotoxin has in vivo.

Cytotoxin Associated Gene Product (Cag). Cag (for *cytotoxin-associated gene* product) is a protein encoded in the *cag* Pathogenicity Island (see above). Cag is secreted, and subsequently phosphorylated by gastric epithelial cells. The phosphorylated product leads to polymerization of cellular actin resulting in disruption of cellular function.

Flagella. Motility is vital for *H. pylori* to find its way through mucus in order to adhere to gastric epithelial cells.

Urease. Urease hydrolyzes urea (secreted by gastric epithelial cells) forming ammonium ions. Ammonium ions neutralize stomach acid, thereby allowing the microorganism to live in the gastric environment. Urease also stimulates the production of inflammation.

Vacuolating Cytotoxin (Vac). Vac (for *v*acuolating *c*ytotoxin) is responsible for disruption of the epithelial cell barrier stimulating an inflammatory response.

Miscellaneous Products. Gastric helicobacters colonize the mucosa and induce an inflammatory response. Levels of reactive oxygen species are thereby increased. *Helicobacter pylori* minimizes oxidative damage by producing superoxide dismutase and catalase. The *rec*A gene products play a role in repair of damaged DNA.

Table 25.2. Characteristics That Differentiate *Helicobacter* Species[a]

Helicobacter taxon	Catalase Production	Nitrate Reduction	Alkaline Phosphatase	Urease	Indoxyl Acetate Hydrolysis	γ-Glutamyl Transferase	Growth At 42C	Growth With 1% Glycine	Resistance to[b]: Nalidixic Acid	Cephalothin	Flagella
HUMAN											
H. bizzozeronii[c]	+	+	+	+	+	+	+	–	R	S	Bipolar
H. canis	–	–	+	–	+	+	+	–	S	I	Bipolar
H. canadensis	+	+/–	–	–	+	–	+	+	R	R	Mono/Bipolar
H. cinaedi	+	+	–	–	–	–	–	+	S	I	Bipolar
H. fennelliae	+	–	+	–	+	–	–	+	S	S	Bipolar
H. pullorum	+	+	–	–	–	ND[d]	+	–	R	S	Monopolar
H. pylori	+	–	+	+	–	+	–	–	R	S	Monopolar
Flexispira (Helicobacter) taxon 8[e]	+/–	–	–	+	–	+	+	–	R	R	Bipolar
H. winghamensis	–	–	–	–	+	ND	–	+	R	R	Bipolar
NONHUMAN											
H. acinonychis	+		+	+		+			R	S	Bipolar
H. aurati											
H. bilis	+	+	–	+	–	+	+	+	R	R	Bipolar
H. cholecystus	+	+	+	–	–	–	+	+	I	R	Monopolar
H. felis	+	+	+	+	–	+	+	–	R	S	Bipolar
H. aurati	+	–	–	+	+	+	+	–	S	R	Bipolar
H. hepaticus	+	+	–	+	+	–	–	+	R	R	Bipolar
H. marmotae	+	–	+	+	–	–	–	+	R	R	Bipolar
H. mesocricetorum	+	+	+	–	ND	–	+	–	S	R	Bipolar
H. muridarum	+	–	+	+	+	+	–	–	R	R	Bipolar
H. mustelae	+	+	+	+	+	+	+	–	S	R	Peritrichous
H. pametensis	+	+	+	–	–	–	+	+	S	S	Bipolar
H. rodentium	+	+	–	–	–	–	+	+	R	R	Bipolar
H. salomonis	+	+	+	+	+	+	–	ND	R	S	Bipolar
H. trogontum	+	+	–	+	–	+	+	ND	R	R	Bipolar

[a] All *Helicobacter* species are oxidase–positive and lack the ability to oxidize or ferment carbohydrates in routine reactions.

[b] Resistance is determined by disk diffusion. Isolates are incubated for several days at 37°C on blood-containing medium containing 30 µg antibiotic disks. Microaerophilic conditions are typically used, and exact incubation times vary between organisms. Resistance (R) is defined as the complete absence of an inhibition zone, whereas intermediate (I; zones usually <15 mm) and susceptible (S; zones usually >20 mm in diameter) isolates have visible inhibition zones of various sizes.

[c] Likely the same as "*H. heilmannii*." "*Helicobacter heilmannii*" (formerly *Gastrospirillum hominis*) has the same phenotype as listed here for *H. bizzozeronii*. Only a single "*H. heilmannii*" strain has been isolated by culture, and thus it has not been included in this table.

[d] ND, not determined.

[e] Formerly regarded as "*Flexispira rappini*"—now has been subgrouped into ten taxa.

Growth Characteristics

Because helicobacters are fastidious, selective media are used for isolation. A commercially available medium consists of brucella agar with 10% horse blood as well as vancomycin (10 mg/l), polymyxin B (2500 units/l) and trimethoprim (5 mg/l). Fresh media are recommended for optimal growth. Specific *Helicobacter* sp. also may have different antibiotic susceptibilities; therefore, selection of antibiotics in culture media may determine the success of isolation. The organisms do not grow under aerobic or anaerobic conditions and achieve optimum growth in a high humidity with microaerophilic conditions (10% CO_2, 80% N_2, 10% H_2).

Variability

Helicobacter pylori exhibits a high degree of genomic heterogenicity, due in part to nucleotide substitutions among strains. However, *H. pylori* lacks a SOS mutagenesis pathway, and the large number of nucleotide substitutions are probably due to mechanisms such as replication fidelity deficiencies or mismatch repair defects.

Ecology

Reservoirs

Gastric helicobacters reside in the gastric mucus layer of a variety of mammals. Enterohepatic helicobacters' ecological niches are the crypts of the colon and cecum, and in some cases, the organism also colonizes the bile canaliculi of the liver. Animals maintained in closed colonies—reared in pounds or kennels, for example—often have prevalence rates of gastric helicobacters approaching 100%. Some helicobacters colonize specific hosts while others are capable of infecting a number of different animal species. Mammals, and birds in some cases, may be reservoirs for zoonotic transmission to humans (see "Zoonotic Potential," below).

Since the original observation of helicobacters in mice in the 1990s, it is now known that *Helicobacter* spp. are prevalent in many rodent colonies both commercial and academic, throughout the world. They are also increasingly isolated from the intestines of humans, other mammals, and birds. Though the epizootiology of these enteric infections is unknown, the bacteria apparently persist in the intestine for the life of mice, other rodents, and perhaps other animals as well.

Transmission

Both oral-oral and fecal-oral routes are probably operable in transmission of gastric helicobacters. Transmission of intestinal helicobacters is via the fecal oral route. There is continued controversy whether viable, but non-culturable, coccoid forms of helicobacter exist in the environment, and if present, whether they are important in transmission to susceptible hosts.

Pathogenesis

Although it is now known that both urease and flagella are necessary to sustain colonization of *Helicobacter* spp. in the gastric mucus, mechanisms are being actively explored to explain the chronic inflammation induced by some helicobacters. These include several putative bacterial virulence factors, (adhesins, Cag, LPS, Vac, and urease, together with certain proteins expressed by genes located on the *cag* Pathogenicity Island), which in the persistently infected host, initiate sustained production of proinflammatory cytokines.

Pathology

Helicobacter felis and *"H. bizzozeronii"* (*"H. heilmannii"*) have been associated with gastric histopathology in laboratory-reared beagle dogs. When these bacteria were observed in low numbers e.g., in the fundus of the stomach, the organism was considered innocuous; however, in large numbers, as seen in the cardia and fundic pyloric junction, the organism may induce lymphoreticular hyperplasia and may cause premature senescence of parietal cells. The presence of gastric *Helicobacter*-like organisms (GHLOs) is often accompanied by reduction in mucus content of sur-

face epithelia, occasional intraepithelial leukocytes, and some degenerating glands. Of the glandular epithelia cells, only the parietal cells are markedly altered. Abnormal findings include vacuolation, enlarged size, and nuclear degeneration consisting of both karyolysis and karyorrhexis. The presence of large numbers of *H. pylori* in the gastric mucosa of commercially reared cats is associated with a lymphofollicular gastritis, characterized by lymphoid aggregates and diffuse inflammation in the deep mucosa and lamina propria.

Helicobacter pylori colonizes the gastrointestinal tract of gnotobiotic dogs orally challenged with this microorganism. Such dogs are colonized with *H. pylori* in all parts of the stomach examined: cardia, fundus, antrum, and pyloric antrum; the fundus is the most heavily colonized. Focal to diffuse lymphoplasmacytic infiltrates with follicle formation and focal infiltration of neutrophils and eosinophils in the gastric lamina propria are observed. Also, gnotobiotic dogs orally inoculated with *H. felis* have the organism recovered from all areas of the stomach, with colonization being heaviest in the body and antrum. Occasionally, *H. felis* is observed within the canaliculi of gastric parietal cells.

Experimentally, *"H. bizzozeronii"* (*"H. heilmannii"*) causes mucosa-associated lymphoma in mice and is linked with the same diseases in humans.

The histopathological changes occurring in the stomach closely coincided in topography with the presence of *H. mustelae*. A superficial gastritis present in the body of the stomach shows that *H. mustelae* is located on the surface of the mucosa but not in the crypts. In the distal antrum, inflammation occupies the full thickness of the mucosa, the so-called diffuse antral gastritis described in humans. In this location *H. mustelae* is seen at the surface, in the pits, and on the superficial portion of the glands. In the proximal antrum and the transitional mucosa, a precancerous lesion, focal glandular atrophy, and regeneration is present, in addition to those lesions seen in the distal antrum.

The liver lesion present in naturally *H. hepaticus*-infected mice progressively increases in severity. It is an inflammatory and necrotizing lesion, which involves the hepatic parenchyma, the portal triads, and importantly, the small intralobular hepatic venules. The widespread, multifocal hepatitis and single cell to coalescing hepatocellular necrosis appears to be random in distribution. Within both the parenchymal perivascular lesion and the affected portal triads, variable degrees of oval, Ito, and Kupffer cell hyperplasia are present. There is an age-associated increase in cell proliferation in infected animals, which is not seen in uninfected control mice. Liver cell proliferation is more pronounced in male mice than in age-matched female mice. The increased levels of hepatocyte proliferation indices in *H. hepaticus*-infected male mice are consistent with the observation of increased hepatomas and hepatocellular carcinomas observed in *H. hepaticus*-infected aged A/JCr male mice. More recently, it has been demonstrated that the B6C3F1 and B6AF1 hybrids are susceptible to *H. hepaticus*-induced liver tumors, indicating liver tumor formation susceptibility is a dominant trait. *Helicobacter canis* has also been observed in a dog liver with multifocal hepatitis, in a liver of a rhesus monkey with hepatitis, and in woodchucks with hepatitis. *Helicobacter hepaticus* and *H. bilis* infection are associated with inflammatory bowel disease in immunodeficient mice and only infrequently in *H. hepaticus* infected immunocompetent mice. The immune response to *H. hepaticus* infection appears to be T helper-1–mediated since splenocytes produced large amounts of interferon (when stimulated with *H. hepaticus* antigens. Normally, humans and other animals remain hyporesponsive or tolerant to their own enteric flora. In patients with inflammatory bowel disease, tolerance is disrupted as individuals become "hyper-responsive" to endogenous enteric antigens. IL-10 is a T helper-2 cytokine with anti-inflammatory and T helper-1 suppressive effects, and the lack of IL-10 manifests predictably as an unopposed T helper-1 immune response. The IL-10$^{-/-}$ mice reared conventionally present with enterocolitis, but subsequent rearing in specific pathogen-free (SPF) facilities restricted the inflammation to the colon, whereas in germ-free IL-10$^{-/-}$ there is no lower bowel inflammation. Thus, enteric bacterial antigens including *H. hepaticus* contribute to the induction of colitis and more recently induction of colon cancer in rag mice and TGFß1 deficient mice.

Disease Features

Ferrets. Helicobacter mustelae is routinely present in ferrets (*Mustela putorius furo*) with gastritis and peptic ulcers. Ferrets infected with *H. mustelae*, are recognized clinically by vomiting, melena, chronic weight loss, and lowered hematocrit. Acute episodes of gastric bleeding can also be noted on occasion. *Helicobacter mustelae* has also been demonstrated within the pyloric mucosa of ferrets with pyloric adenocarcinoma and mucosa-associated lymphoma of the stomach.

Swine. Swine with gastric disease have a higher prevalence of *H. suis* (closely related to "*H. heilmannii*" type 1) associated with gastric ulcers located in the parsoesophagea.

Nonhuman Primates. *Helicobacter pylori* has been isolated from nonhuman primates, particularly macaques. The presence of *H. pylori* in gastric mucosa of infected monkeys is often accompanied by a lymphocytic plasmacytic gastritis that apparently persists. Clinical signs have not been described. Primates are also commonly colonized with large gastric spiral "*H. heilmannii*"-like organisms. Most recently enteric helicobacter have been isolated from macaques and cotton top tamarins with idiopathic colitis.

Dogs and Cats. Clinical signs in pet animals, attributable to *Helicobacter*-associated gastritis may or may not be present. *Helicobacter pylori* has been identified in 100% of the stomachs examined from a group of specific pathogen free, asymptomatic cats, obtained from a commercial vendor.

Helicobacter canis has been isolated from feces of normal and diarrheic dogs and normal cats. This microorganism has also been isolated from the liver of a puppy diagnosed as having an active, multifocal hepatitis. *Helicobacter canis* has also been cultured from the feces of children and adult humans suffering from gastroenteritis.

Helicobacter marmotae, originally isolated from the diseased liver of woodchucks, has also been isolated and characterized from the feces of cats, as has been *H. bilis.*

Helicobacter cinaedi and *H. fennelliae*, have been linked to proctitis and colitis in immunocompromised humans, and septicemia in neonates. Of interest is the recent isolation, based on cellular fatty acid analysis, of *H. cinaedi* from the feces of dogs, a cat, and rhesus monkeys. *Helicobacter fennelliae* has also been identified in the feces of a dog and a macaque.

Sheep. "*Flexispira rappini*" was first isolated from a human patient with diarrhea. In the same household, the bacterium was isolated from the feces of a young asymptomatic dog. A similar bacterium has been cultured from aborted ovine fetuses and was given the provisional name "*Flexispira rappini.*" Apparently "*F. rappini*" crosses the placenta in pregnant sheep, induces abortions, and causes acute hepatic necrosis in the fetus. Experimentally, "*F. rappini*" causes abortions and necrotic hepatitis in guinea pigs. Analysis of the DNA encoding the 16S rRNA shows that this microorganism belongs in the genus *Helicobacter.*

Helicobacters of Rodents. To date, 12 species of *Helicobacter* have been isolated from the intestinal tract and/or livers of rodents; two of these, *H. hepaticus* and *H. bilis* have been isolated from the ceca, colons, and livers of mice.

Helicobacter muridarum colonizes the lower intestinal tract of rats and mice, and under certain circumstances colonizes the gastric tissue of mice and induces a gastritis.

"*Flexispira rappini*" colonizes the colons and ceca of mice.

Helicobacter cinaedi and *H. mesocricetorum* colonizes the intestinal tract of asymptomatic hamsters.

Helicobacter aurati is isolated from hamsters with severe gastritis.

Helicobacter trogontum and *H. bilis* have been isolated from the colons of rats, *H. rodentium, H. typhlonius,* and *H. ganmani* from the colons and ceca of mice and *H. cholecystus* has been cultured from diseased gallbladders of hamsters. Clinical signs in infected rodents have not been noted, except in immunocompromised mice infected with *H. hepaticus* or *H. bilis* where diarrhea and/or rectal prolapse may be present.

Helicobacters in Birds. *Helicobacter pametensis* is a urease-negative enteric helicobacter isolated from wild bird and porcine feces.

Helicobacter pullorum has been isolated from ceca of asymptomatic chickens, the livers and intestinal contents of chickens with hepatitis, and feces of humans with gastroenteritis. There is speculation that *H. pullorum* may be the microbial agent responsible for the syndrome termed *avian vibrionic hepatitis* described in both chickens and turkeys. Though *Campylobacter jejuni* has been suggested as an etiological agent in this disease, studies conducted to ascertain whether *C. jejuni* (derived from humans or chickens) produces hepatopathy have failed. Most recently, wild geese have been identified as reservoirs for *H. canadensis*, a helicobacter first identified in diarrheic humans and misclassified as *H. pullorum.*

Zoonotic Potential

Helicobacter pylori-infected cats have been screened by culture and polymerase chain reaction (PCR) for the presence of *H. pylori* in salivary secretions, gastric juice, gastric tissue, and feces. *Helicobacter pylori* was cultured from salivary secretions in 6 of 12 (50%) cats and from gastric fluid samples in 11 of 12 (91%) cats. Isolation of *H. pylori* from feline mucosal secretions suggest a zoonotic risk from exposure to personnel handling *H. pylori*-infected cats in vivaria. However, to date, there is no indication based on several epidemiological studies that pets pose increased risk of *H. pylori* zoonotic transmission to humans.

Because *"H. heilmannii"* (*"H. bizzozeronii"*) and to a lesser extent *H. felis* colonize a small percentage of humans with gastritis, and no environmental source for these bacteria has been recognized, pets in several published reports have been implicated in zoonotic transmission of these microorganisms. In Germany, a recent survey of 125 individuals infected with GHLOs provided information in a questionnaire regarding animal contact. Of these patients, 70% had contact with one or more animals (as compared with 37% in the "normal" population). More than a threefold preponderance of males over female patients with GHLOs was recorded.

Since *H. cinaedi* has been isolated from humans and the normal intestine flora of hamsters, it has been suggested that pet hamsters serve as a reservoir for transmission to humans. Also given that *H. canis*, *Flexispira* (*Helicobacter*) *rappini*, *H. pullorum*, and *H. canadensis*, have been isolated from animals and diarrheic humans, the probability that these helicobacters are also zoonotic agents exists.

Immunologic Aspects

A variety of serologic tests have been used to measure the increased anti-*H. pylori*–specific IgG and IgA antibody found in humans with different types of gastritis and duodenal or gastric ulcers. The most popular tests have been an enzyme-linked immunosorbant assay (ELISA) using glycine-extracted antigen or whole-cell sonicates of the bacteria. The severity of gastritis in terms of inflammatory response does not correlate with levels of antibody. Specific serum IgG antibodies to gastric helicobacters in animals have also been used to diagnose those both naturally and experimentally infected with *Helicobacter* spp. Analyses of serum and mucosal secretions by ELISA in *H. pylori* naturally infected cats reveals an *H. pylori*-specific IgG response, and elevated IgA anti-*H. pylori* antibody levels in salivary and local gastric secretions. Like humans, though helpful in diagnosis, neither secretory nor serum antibody responses are protective.

Helicobacter hepaticus has apparently developed strategies to evade host immune responses similar to those of gastric helicobacters. *Helicobacter hepaticus* infected A/JCr mice with hepatitis have a persistent IgG antibody response to this microorganism, which does not confer protection. Younger mice, whose intestinal crypts are colonized with *H. hepaticus*, but without appreciable hepatitis, do not have elevated IgG antibody to *H. hepaticus*.

Laboratory Diagnosis

Direct Examination

In addition to using a Gram stain on homogenized gastric tissue for a rapid, presumptive diagnosis, the urease activity of these gastric bacteria is utilized. A diagnostic test for urease is commercially available that detects urease activity in gastric tissue within 15 minutes to 3 hours. Thus, a gastric biopsy can be minced and placed directly into urea broth and a positive reaction obtained in 1 hour.

Gastric brushing cytology can be performed during routine endoscopy. Cells and mucus that adhere to the brush are applied to a glass slide, air-dried and stained with a Giemsa stain. For visualization of gastric helicobacters, oil immersion magnification (100X) is used. Phase microscopy is also helpful in establishing a tentative diagnosis.

Isolation and Identification

Helicobacters can now be isolated routinely from the gastric tissue of infected humans, ferrets, nonhuman primates, and increasingly from other laboratory, domestic, and wild animals. It is more difficult to isolate *H. felis* from dogs and cats, and until very recently *H. bizzozeronii* (*"H. heilmannii"*), the large gastric spiral, was uncultivable. However, this organism has now been isolated from both dogs and humans. *Helicobacter salomonis* has been isolated from dog stomachs as well. When attempting to grow *H. felis*, *H. bizzozeronii*, and *H. salomonis*, it is very important to use moist plates, which are incubated lid uppermost. These species do not form distinct colonies, but rather bacterial growth consists of a very fine spreading film, which could easily be dismissed as water stains. Another limiting factor in isolation of gastric *Helicobacter* spp. from animals and humans is the necessity of obtaining gastric biopsies. The organisms are not routinely cultured from gastric juice or feces. Enterohepatic helicobacters can be isolated on the same selective antibiotic media used to isolate gastric helicobacters. Also, the use of 0.45 µ or 0.65 µ filters to selectively filter feces helps minimize contamination from other enteric organisms during primary culture on selective agar. Higher hydrogen levels in the gas mixture—i.e., 10%—enhances recovery of the enterohepatic helicobacters. It is now recognized that helicobacters and campylobacters can be a mixed infection and isolated from the same feces of both animals and humans. Polymerase chain reaction (PCR)–based assays may therefore be required in many cases to verify whether mixed infections exist in the same host.

Figure 25.1 and Table 25.2 outline the various phenotypic characteristics of various helicobacters that are used to isolate and identify helicobacters from gastric biopsies.

Molecular Methods

DNA primers specific for genes encoding various proteins specific for helicobacters, as well as primers specific for segments of DNA encoding the 16S rRNA, have been described and used for demonstration in samples and identification by the use of the polymerase chain reaction.

Figure 25.1. *Isolation of* Helicobacter *from gastric biopsies.*

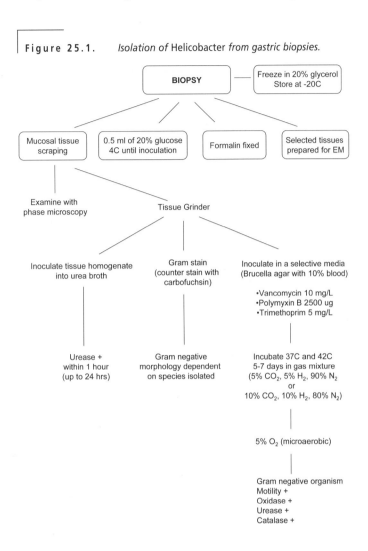

Treatment and Control

Helicobacter pylori. A triple-therapy regimen consisting of amoxicillin and metronidazole, or tetracycline and metronidazole, in combination with bismuth subsalicylate given for 2 to 3 weeks has proven to be efficient in eradication of *H. pylori.* Indeed, this antimicrobial regimen, plus ranitidine, has proven successful in treating patients with ulcer disease. In studies comparing this treatment to those patients receiving ranitidine alone, ulcers not only healed faster, but the recurrence of ulcers was significantly less than the antibiotic-treated group where *H. pylori* had been eradicated. Recently, therapy regimens using proton pump inhibitors (e.g., omeprazole) in combination with other antibiotics also have shown considerable efficacy in eradicating *H. pylori.* Several reports describing antimicrobial therapy in domestic dogs and cats with gastritis have failed to eradicate the large gastric spiral organisms from the stomach of infected animals.

Other Helicobacters. Antimicrobial susceptibility testing of *H. cinaedi* indicates that tetracycline, chloramphenicol, and various aminoglycosides should be effective in treating infections with this microorganism. Apparent relapses of *H. cinaedi* bacteremia have occurred in people treated with ciprofloxacin despite its previous use to treat *H.*

cinaedi infection successfully. The occurrence of in vitro resistance of isolates of *H. cinaedi* to ciprofloxacin suggests that fluoroquinolones should be used with caution.

"*Flexispria (Helicobacter) rappini*"–like organisms have been isolated from immunocompetent and immunoincompetent (X-linked agammaglobulinemia) children. These isolates have had variable susceptibility to a number of antimicrobials. However, most isolates have shown susceptibility to imipenem, metronidazole, minocycline, and rifampin, and intermediate sensitivity to doxycycline.

Studies in ferrets indicate that the triple therapy consisting of amoxicillin (30 mg/kg), metronidazole (20 mg/kg), and bismuth subsalicylate (17.5 mg/kg) (Pepto-Bismol original formula, Proctor & Gamble) three times a day for 3 to 4 weeks has successfully eradicated *H. mustelae.* Dosages of clarithromycin and ranitidine bismuth citrate that successfully eradicated *H. mustelae* were 12.5 and 24 mg/kg of body weight per os every 8 hrs, respectively for a 14-day period.

Helicobacter hepaticus–infected mice receiving triple therapy consisting of amoxicillin, metronidazole, and bismuth 3x daily for 2 weeks by gastric intubation eradicated the microorganism. Use of antibiotic impregnated dietary wafers has not been successful in eradicating this microorganism.

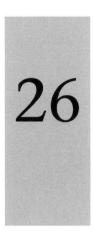

26

Spiral-Curved Organisms V: *Leptospira*

Rance B. LeFebvre

Leptospirae are spirochetes that are morphologically and physiologically uniform but serologically and epidemiologically diverse. Domestic animals most commonly affected are dogs, cattle, swine, and horses. Canine leptospirosis manifestations are septicemic, hepatic, and renal disease. In cattle and swine, septicemic illness is largely confined to the young, while abortion is the principal manifestation in adults. Abortion and recurrent uveitis (moon blindness, or periodic ophthalmia) are the most common manifestations in horses. California sea lions are susceptible to acute, septicemic leptospiral infections. Other host species, though susceptible to infection, develop clinical signs less frequently. Leptospirosis in humans is typically an acute febrile disease.

Taxonomy studies, based on DNA analyses, have led to the description of eight pathogenic species: *Leptospira borgpetersenii, L. inadae, L. interrogans sensu stricto, L. kirschneri, L. meyeri, L. noguchii, L. santarosae,* and *L. weilee.* Notwithstanding, leptospires are classified and referred to by their antigenic composition. They are currently sorted into 23 serogroups. Leptospire isolates placed within these serogroups are further characterized and identified antigenically as unique serovarieties (serovars), of which there are more than 200. Reference to these organisms is typically by genus and serovar in clinical settings, (i.e., *Leptospira* serovar *canicola* is the accepted designation of the most common canine pathogen found in North America. Other serovars important in North America and their principal hosts and clinical hosts (in parentheses) are:

icterohaemorrhagiae: rodents (dogs, horses, cattle, swine)
grippotyphosa: rodents (dogs, cattle, swine)
canicola: dogs (swine, cattle)
pomona: cattle, swine (horses, sheep, sea lions)
hardjo: cattle
bratislava: swine (horses, sea lions)

Descriptive Features

Morphology and Staining

Leptospirae (from the Greek *leptos,* meaning "thin") are tightly coiled spiral organisms. Because they stain poorly, they require darkfield or phase contrast microscopy for visualization. The spirals are best demonstrated by electron microscopy. Typical cells have a hook at each end making them S- or C-shaped. Wet mounts reveal them to be motile.

Leptospirae are gram-negative but stain poorly and thus, unrecognizable in routinely fixed, stained smears. They can be demonstrated by fluorescent antibody or silver impregnation (Fig 26.1).

Cellular Anatomy and Composition

Leptospiral cells consist of an outer sheath, axial fibrils ("endoflagella"), and a cytoplasmic cylinder. The outer sheath combines features of a capsule and outer membrane. A cell membrane and the peptidoglycan layer of the cell wall cover the cytoplasmic cylinder.

Cellular Products of Medical Interest

Cell Wall. Members of the genus *Leptospira* have a gram-negative cell wall. The lipopolysaccharide (LPS) in the outer membrane is an important virulence determinant. Not only is the lipid A component toxic (endotoxin), but the length of the side chain in the O-repeat unit hinders the attachment of the membrane attack complex of the complement system to the outer membrane. LPS binds to lipopolysaccharide-binding protein (a serum protein), which in turn transfers it to the blood phase of CD14. The CD14-LPS complex binds to Toll-like receptor proteins (see Chapter 2) on the surface of macrophage cells triggering the release of proinflammatory cytokines

Hemolysin. The hemolysin (a cytotoxin) produced by some serovars *Leptospira* is a sphingomyelinase C.

Growth Characteristics

Leptospirae are obligate aerobes, which grow optimally at 29°C to 30°C. Generation time averages about 12 hours. No growth occurs on blood agar or other routine media. Traditional media are essentially rabbit serum (10%), in solutions of peptones, vitamins, electrolytes, and buffers. Some newer media have substituted polysorbates and bovine albumin substituted for rabbit serum. Protein is not required. Unlike most prokaryotes, leptospirae are not able to synthesize pyrimidines and thus 5-fluorouracil is added to growth media as an inhibitory agent to contaminating bacteria and fungi.

FIGURE 26.1. Leptospira interrogans, *serovar pomona in the renal tubules of a pig. Levaditi silver stain, 1000X.*

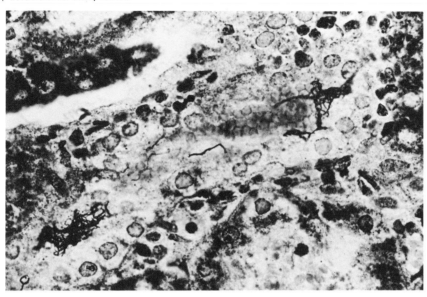

Most media are fluid or semisolid (0.1% agar). In fluid media, little turbidity develops. In semisolid media, growth is concentrated in a disc—called a "dinger zone"—about 0.5 cm below the surface.

Biochemical Reactions

Leptospirae are oxidase and catalase-positive; many have lipase activity. Some produce urease. Identification beyond genus is based on serology. Species-specific DNA primers in conjunction with the polymerase chain reaction (PCR) have also been developed for a more accurate characterization of pathogenic leptospirae.

Resistance

Leptospirae are killed by drying, freezing, heat (50°C for 10 minutes), soap, bile salts, detergents, acidic environments, and putrefaction. They persist in a moist, temperate environment at neutral to slightly alkaline pH (see "Epidemiology," below).

Variability

More than 200 serovars of parasitic leptospirae exist. They vary in host and geographic distribution, and in pathogenicity.

Ecology

Reservoir

Members of the genus *Leptospira* inhabit the tubules of mammalian kidneys. They have been isolated from birds, reptiles, amphibians, and invertebrates, but the epidemiologic significance of such associations is not established.

Rodents are the most frequent leptospiral carriers, with wild carnivores ranking second. No mammal can be excluded as a possible host. Typically reservoir hosts show minimal, if any, signs of disease.

Transmission

Exposure is through contact of mucous membranes or skin with urine-contaminated water, fomites, or feed. Other sources are milk from infected cows and genital secretions from cattle and swine of either sex.

Pathogenesis

Clinical and pathological manifestations suggest toxic mechanisms. Filtrates of tissue fluids from experimentally infected animals contain cytotoxic factors that produce vascular lesions similar to those seen with leptospirosis.

The spirochetes enter the bloodstream subsequent to mucous membrane or reproductive inoculation, colonizing particularly liver and kidney, where they produce degenerative changes. Other affected organs may be muscles, eyes, and meninges, where a nonsuppurative meningitis may develop. Hemorrhages result from damaged vascular endothelium. All serovars produce these changes to varying degrees. *Leptospira* serovar *pomona* in cattle causes intravascular hemolysis due to a hemolytic exotoxin. Autoimmune phenomena may also contribute to this condition. Secondary changes include icterus due to liver damage and blood destruction, and acute, subacute, or chronic nephritis due to renal tubular injury. The cellular exudates contain predominantly lymphocytes and plasma cells. In surviving animals, leptospirae are removed from circulation with the appearance of antibody but persist in the kidneys for many weeks (see Fig 26.1).

Disease Patterns

Most leptospiral infections run an inapparent course probably due to infection of the animal by a host-adapted serovar. Clinical infections manifesting overt signs are primarily due to non-host-adapted serovar infections. These occur mainly in dogs, cattle, and swine; increasingly in sea lions; occasionally in horses, goats, and sheep; and exceptionally in cats.

Canine. Leading serovars involved are *icterohaemorrhagiae* and *canicola*, with the latter the more common. Increasing numbers of dogs with acute renal failure due to serovars *grippotyphosa*, *pomona*, and *bratislava* infections are being reported.

The most acute form affects young pups preferentially, producing fever without localizing signs, and is commonly fatal within days. Hemorrhages are often apparent antemortem on mucous membranes and skin, or manifested by epistaxis or by bloodstained feces and vomitus. Icterus is absent.

The icteric type runs a slower course, and hemorrhages are less conspicuous. Icterus is prominent. Renal localization causes nitrogen retention, while renal casts and leukocytes appear in the urine.

The uremic type, centered in the kidneys, results subsequent to either of the types of infections described above or may develop in their absence. It may be acute and rapidly fatal with signs of gastrointestinal upsets, uremic breath, and ulcerations in the anterior alimentary tract; or it may run a slow course with delayed onset. The relationship of leptospirosis to chronic interstitial nephritis leading to uremic death is controversial.

Cattle. The predominant manifestation of bovine leptospirosis is abortion, usually late term, but may occur at any time following infection. Abortion is due to primary fetal death rather than placental infection. Fetal retention with progressive autolysis is common. Abortions due to serovar *hardjo*, the host-adapted serovar for cattle, are primarily a problem of heifers in dairies due to management practices that differ between beef cattle and dairy operations. *Leptospira* serovar *hardjo* infections affect calves in utero, leading either to abortion or "weak-calf syndrome." These infections are often subclinical or may be marked by "milk-drop syndrome," reproductive failure, and infertility. Chronic infection of the kidneys and the shedding of leptospirae in urine are common.

Acute leptospirosis due to serovar *pomona* affects mostly calves and sometimes adult cattle. It is marked by fever, hemoglobinuria, icterus, anemia, and a fatality rate of 5% to 15%.

Swine. The serovars implicated in porcine leptospirosis include serovars *pomona*, *icterohaemorrhagiae*, *canicola*, *tarassovi*, *bratislava*, and *muenchen*. As in bovine leptospirosis, septicemia with icterus and hemorrhages occurs, especially in piglets, while abortion and infertility are the manifestations in sows.

Horses. Equine leptospirosis is due most often to serovars *pomona*, *grippotyphosa*, and *icterohaemorrhagiae*. Signs in natural infections have been fever, mild icterus, and abortion. Leptospirosis is involved in equine recurrent uveitis (periodic ophthalmia, moon blindness; see "Immunologic Factors," below). *Leptospira* serovar *pomona* and an as yet unidentified leptospira have been cultured from the aqueous humor of horses with clinical signs of this disease.

Miscellaneous Species. In small ruminants, leptospirosis, usually due to serovar *pomona*, resembles that seen in cattle. Infections with serovars *hardjo* and *grippotyphosa* also occur. Epidemics due to serovar *pomona* have caused high mortality among California sea lions periodically since the 1940s.

Humans. Humans are susceptible to all serovars with no host-adapted strains identified. Infections cause fever, icterus, muscular pains, rashes, and nonsuppurative meningitis, manifestations varying somewhat with the serovars involved. A malignant form, most often associated with serovar *icterohaemorrhagiae*, can cause fatal liver or renal disease.

Epidemiology

The many tolerant hosts and the protracted shedder state perpetuate leptospirosis. Indirect exposure depends on mild and wet conditions, which favor environmental survival of leptospirae. More direct transfer occurs by urine aerosols in milking barns and cattle sheds or by canine courting habits, which may explain the male bias of canine leptospirosis.

Contaminated bodies of water are important sources of infection to livestock, aquatic mammals, and humans. Animal handlers, sewer workers, field hands, miners, and veterinarians are at increased risk of exposure.

Immunologic Factors

Immune Mechanisms of Disease

Immunologic mechanisms may relate to some features of leptospiral disease:

1. The hemolytic anemia characteristic of septicemic leptospirosis due to servar *pomona* in ruminants is associated with the presence of cold hemagglutinins, suggesting an autoimmune process. The relative roles of this and the bacterial hemolysin are uncertain.

2. Canine chronic interstitial nephritis is considered by many a postleptospiral lesion. A leptospiral etiology is suggested by a frequent history of leptospirosis and the presence of leptospiral antibody, particularly in urine. An immune-based etiology is attractive, as antirenal antibody has been demonstrated in infected dogs.

3. Evidence of a leptospiral basis for equine recurrent uveitis (periodic ophthalmia, moon blindness) rests in part on leptospiral antibody and its relative titers in serum and aqueous humor. The condition has been reproduced in horses and dogs experimentally by using leptospiral antigens.

Mechanisms of Resistance and Recovery

Recovery from acute leptospirosis coincides with the cessation of septicemia and the appearance of circulating antibodies, usually during the second week of infection. Protective antibodies are of IgM and IgG isotypes and are directed mainly at the outer sheath antigens.

Agglutinating antibodies, which persist after recovery, is not an indication of immunity nor of the shedder state, which may exist in the presence or absence of antibody.

Immunity following recovery is generally solid and serovar-specific. Repeated abortions due to serovar *hardjo* have been reported in cows, probably due to weak immune response to this bovine-adapted serovar.

Artificial Immunization

Vaccination with bacterins is used in dogs (bivalent containing serovars *icterohaemorrhagiae* and *canicola*). A bivalent bacterin containing serovars *grippotyphosa* and *pomona* is also commercially available. These bacterins are comprised of killed, whole-cell leptospires. Toxic components of these products, such as endotoxin, may be responsible for the adverse reactions reported in dogs.

In North America, cattle and swine are vaccinated with a pentavalent bacterin containing the most common North American serovars (*hardjo, grippotyphosa, pomona, icterohaemorrhagiae,* and *canicola*), with the addition of serovar *bratislava* and a second serovar *hardjo* component in some vaccines. Humans who are at risk may opt for vaccination as well. Protection is serovar-specific and temporary, requiring at least annual boosters. Vaccination prevents overt disease but not necessarily infection.

Laboratory Diagnosis

Diagnosis of leptospirosis must be established by laboratory confirmation.

Sample Collection

From living subjects, blood, urine, cerebrospinal fluid, uterine fluids, and placental cotyledons are examined. Blood is usually negative after the first febrile phase. Milk is destructive to leptospirae and not a promising source for cultures. Urine should always be tested.

From cadavers, including aborted fetuses, kidneys are the most likely organs to harbor leptospirae. In septic fatalities (including abortions) many organs, especially the liver, spleen, lung, brain, and eye, may contain the agent.

Culturing is done promptly after sample collection.

Direct Examination

Methods of direct visual demonstration are wet mounts, examined by darkfield (or phase) microscopy, immunofluorescent stains, and silver impregnation of fixed tissue.

Routine darkfield microscopy should be limited to urine. Other body fluids contain artifacts morphologically similar to leptospirae. Brief, low-speed centrifugation clears the specimen of interfering particles but will not sediment leptospirae. Methods using formalinized urine have been described, but they destroy motility, which aids in the identification of leptospirae. Negative results of direct examinations do not rule out leptospirosis.

Fluorescent antibody has been used on fluids, tissue sections, homogenates, organ impressions, and, most effectively, on aborted bovine fetuses, where examination of kidney is most rewarding. Silver-impregnated sections must be interpreted with caution, because argyrophilic tissue fibrils mimic leptospirae.

DNA amplification using the polymerase chain reaction together with specific DNA primers has become an excellent diagnostic tool for detecting the presence of leptospirae in animal tissues and fluids.

Isolation and Identification

The medium of Ellinghausen, McCullough, Johnson, and Harris (EMJH medium) is a good isolation medium, especially for serovar *hardjo*, the slowest growing of the common serovars. Replicate inoculations are made into EMJH medium with and without selective inhibitors (5-fluorouracil, neomycin, cycloheximide). Cultures are examined microscopically at intervals during incubation for up to several months.

Animal inoculation (hamsters or guinea pigs) eliminates minor contaminants from the primary inoculum, which is injected intraperitoneally. Blood is drawn periodically for culture starting a few days after inoculation. After 3 to 4 weeks, the animals are killed and their kidneys examined and cultured for leptospirae. If infected with leptospirae, they will have developed antibody. Any isolate recovered by these methods can be identified morphologically as a member of the genus *Leptospira*. Definitive identification is carried out by reference laboratories.

Serology

Direct examination is often unreliable and culture laborious, expensive, and slow. Serology is the most common diagnostic method. The microscopic agglutination test employing live antigen is most widely used. Others include macroscopic plate and tube agglutination tests, complement fixation tests, and enzyme-linked antibody assays. Paired samples are preferred: one collected at first presentation and one 2 weeks later. If leptospirosis was the problem, a fourfold or greater rise in titer should have occurred in the interval. In bovine abortion, these relations may not hold. This is due to the fact that serovar *hardjo* infections of cattle elicit a very weak immune response that is probably due to their adaptation to this animal species.

Treatment and Control

Leptospirae are susceptible to penicillin G, fluoroquino-lones, tetracycline, chloramphenicol, streptomycin, and erythromycin. Treatment, to be of benefit, must be instituted early, possibly even prophylactically in cases of known exposure. Doxycycline is used to treat humans pro-phylactically. However, evidence of leptospiral infection in the kidneys and reproductive tracts of cattle subsequent to antibiotic treatment is not uncommon.

Vaccination generally prevents disease. It does not prevent infection nor shedding, although it does reduce its extent.

27 *Staphylococcus*

Dwight C. Hirsh   Ernst L. Biberstein

Staphylococci are spherical gram-positive bacteria that divide in several planes to form irregular clusters. They are present in the upper respiratory tract and on other epithelial surfaces of all warm-blooded animals. Four of some 20 species are of veterinary importance: *S. aureus, S. intermedius, S. hyicus,* and *S. schleiferi* subspecies *coagulans*. *Staphylococcus aureus* is a common pyogenic agent in humans and several animal species. *Staphylococcus intermedius* is the leading pus-forming bacterium in dogs. *Staphylococcus hyicus,* which is found in several species, causes exudative epidermidis of swine and sometimes, bovine mastitis. *Staphylococcus schleiferi* subspecies *coagulans* (along with *S. intermedius*) is sometimes associated with otitis externa of dogs. *Staphylococcus sciuri and S. xylosus* (and rarely *S. epidermidis*) are universally present on skin and some mucous membranes, but are rarely pathogenic. Pathogenic staphylococci usually produce the enzyme coagulase (see below).

Descriptive Features

Morphology and Staining

Staphylococci are 0.5 to 1.5 μm in diameter and generally stain strongly gram-positive. In exudates they form clusters, pairs, or short chains (Fig 27.1). Spores and flagella are absent. Encapsulation is variable.

Structure and Composition

The cell wall consists of proteins and polysaccharides. One protein ("clumping factor," "bound coagulase") is usually present in *S. aureus* and *S. intermedius*. Clumping factor interacts in vitro with fibrinogen to produce an agglutination-like reaction. Another, Protein A, produces aggregation by combining with the Fc fragment of immunoglobulins. The predominant polysaccharide is teichoic acid linked to peptidoglycan. Its alcohol moiety is ribitol in *S. aureus,* and glycerol in *S. epidermidis* and *S. intermedius*. Carotenoid pigments in the cell membrane can impart a "golden" (Latin: "aureus") color to colonies of *S. aureus*. A capsule is sometimes produced by *S. aureus,* and often a "pseudocapsule," a loosely associated carbohydrate structure, is produced by strains causing bovine mastitis.

Cellular Products of Medical Interest

Most of what follows has been determined for *S. aureus,* the most intensively studied species of staphylococcus.

Presumably, the other species have similar traits and characteristics that make them potentially pathogenic.

Adhesins. Staphylococci produce a number of surface proteins that bind to a variety of extracellular matrix proteins of the host (fibronectin, fibrinogen, collagen, vitronectin, laminin). These "adhesins" have been termed *MSCRAMMs* (*m*icrobial *s*urface *c*omponents *r*ecognizing *a*dhesive *m*atrix *m*olecules). Staphylococci produce a number of different adhesins, giving some strains affinity for a certain tissue types (bone, kidney, bladder).

Capsule. *Staphylococcus aureus* produces 11 serologically distinct polysaccharide capsules. The genes encoding capsule production are located on a *Staphylococcal Cassette Chromosome Genetic Element (SCCcap).* SCCs satisfy the characteristics outlined for defining a Pathogenicity Island: a cluster of genes encoding virulence determinant(s), an integrase protein, a specific insertion site, and mobility. The capsule is thought to act in preventing phagocytosis.

Cell Wall. The cell wall of the members of this genus is one typical of gram-positive bacteria. The lipoteichoic acids and peptidoglycan of the gram-positive cell wall interact with macrophage cells resulting in the release of proinflammatory cytokines.

Enterotoxins/Pyrogenic Toxin Superantigens. Coagulase-positive staphylococci produce a group of exotoxins of similar size and three-dimensional shape. These include 11 enterotoxins (SE, for *s*taphylococcal *e*nterotoxin) A–M (there is no F nor J), and the toxic shock syndrome toxin (TSST-1). The genes encoding these toxins are located on Pathogenicity Islands (SEB, SEC, SEK-M, TSST-1), prophages (SEA, SEE), or plasmids (SED). All are small proteins (20,000 to 30,000 in molecular weight) and dissimilar in primary amino acid sequence, but remarkably similar in shape. They are resistant to heat and digestive enzymes. The SEs, which are usually ingested as a preformed toxin, act by binding to an undefined receptor in the wall of the intestinal tract triggering reflex stimulation of the vomiting center. Both SEs and TSST-1 are superantigens, and part of the systemic symptomatology may be related to the cytokine "storm" that results from the interaction of T lymphocyte receptors, macrophages, and these toxins which are released in vivo (TSST-1 crosses mucus membranes, the SEs do not).

Exfoliative Toxins. *Staphylococcus aureus* produces two exfoliative toxins (sETA, ETB), and *S. hyicus* produces three antigenically different exfoliative toxins (shETA-C). The genes encoding the ETs of *S. aureus* are located either on a

FIGURE 27.1. Staphylococcus aureus *in urinary sediment from a cat. Gram stain, 1000X.*

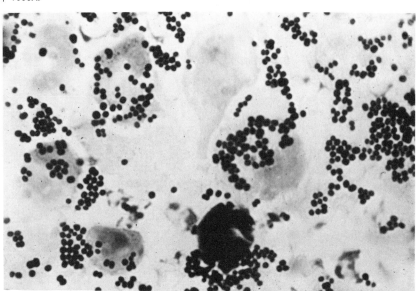

prophage (sETA) or plasmid (ETB). The exfoliative toxins are atypical glutamate-specific serine proteases. They target the intercellular adhesion protein, desmoglein (a cadherin), found only in the epidermis. Whether the exfoliative toxins are superantigens, is unsettled.

Hemolytic Toxins. There are four hemolytic toxins (alpha, beta, gamma, and delta), so-called because of their action on erythrocytes in vitro. Hemolysis is not a property observed during the disease process. The hemolytic toxins are expressed singly, in combination, or not at all. They differ antigenically, biochemically, and in their effect on the erythrocytes of various species. The genes encoding the hemolytic toxins are located on the chromosome:

1. Alpha toxin. Alpha toxin acts on membrane lipids, is hemolytic in vitro, is mitogenic, is lethal to rabbits following intravenous injection, and is necrotizing upon intradermal injection. The major effect in vivo is related to its insertion into membranes. The toxin is excreted as monomers, which come together in the host cell membrane to form a cylinder through which ions flow. Loss of membrane integrity in a variety of cell types results in untoward effects on the host. At high concentrations alpha toxin initiates target-cell death by necrosis (ion and ATP depletion). In lower concentrations, apoptosis is triggered. In certain instances, coagulase-positive staphylococci are internalized by nonprofessional phagocytes (endothelial cells, some epithelial cells), but escape the endosome to multiply within the cytoplasm. Endosomal escape is thought to be associated with alpha hemolysin-mediated lysis of the endosomal membrane.

2. Beta toxin. Beta toxin, a phospholipase C is prevalent in animal strains. Beta toxin produces broad zones of "hot-cold lysis" on sheep or cattle blood agar at 37°C, a partial hemolysis ("water-stain" appearance) that occurs and goes to completion on further incubation at lower temperatures (Fig 27.2). Its role in vivo is unclear, but damage to host cell membranes is a reasonable assumption.

3. Gamma toxin. Gamma toxin is a bicomponent toxin composed of two proteins that combine to form an active moiety. This toxin stimulates degranulation of phagocytic cells, thereby intensifying in-

FIGURE 27.2. Staphylococcus *beta toxin activity on bovine blood agar. For explanation, see text.*

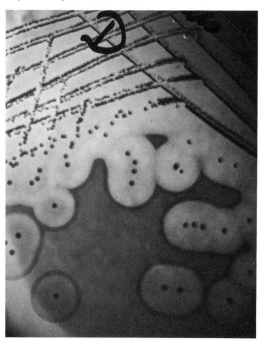

flammatory responses and tissue damage. Gamma toxin is not observed surrounding colonies growing on blood agar plates since it is inhibited by agar, but virtually all strains of coagulase-positive staphylococci produce the toxin.

4. Delta toxin. Delta toxin lyses cells of various species by a detergent-like action but is inhibited by serum. Like gamma toxin, almost all strains of coagulase-positive strains produce this toxin. Its role in disease, however, is undefined.

Iron Acquisition. Staphylococci with pathogenic potential (i.e., coagulase-positive strains) grow better in iron-restricted conditions (as would occur in vivo), as compared to those staphylococci with less potential (coagulase-negative strains). Under iron-limiting conditions, the coagulase-positive strains produce siderophores, aurochelin and staphyloferrin, which are responsible for iron acquisition from extracellular sources (transferrin, lactoferrin). Staphylococci also utilize the siderophores produced by other bacteria, specifically enterobactin and aerobactin from gram-negative organisms.

Leukocidin. Like gamma hemolysin, leukocidin, also known as the Panton-Valentine toxin, is a bicomponent toxin. In fact, some of the proteins encoded at the locus containing the genes for gamma hemolysin, form a part of leukocidin. Leukocidin stimulates the degranulation of phagocytic cells, thereby intensifying inflammatory responses and tissue damage.

MprF (Multiple Peptide Resistance Factor). MprF bestows resistance to the action of defensins through the lysinylation of phospholipids in the cell membranes of coagulase-positive staphylococci. Not only does this permit survival within defensin-containing phagolysosomes (this does not protect against oxygen-dependent killing, however), it allows existence within niches that are bathed in defensins (upper respiratory tract, intestinal tract, genital tract).

Miscellaneous Products. Staphylococci produce a plethora of other products that may or may not have a role in disease production. These products include lipases, serine proteases, thiol proteases, metaloproteases (aureolysin), esterases, deoxyribonucleases, staphylokinase (a plasminogen activator), hyaluronidase, and phospholipases. Urease, an enzyme produced by coagulase-positive staphylococci is associated with the production of uroliths in the canine bladder. Coagulase, an enzyme that causes plasma coagulation in vitro and aids in the identification of the pathogenic species: *S. aureus, S. intermedius, S. schleiferi* ssp. *coagulans,* and some *S. hyicus,* probably has little, if any role in vivo.

Regulation of the Cellular Products of Medical Interest. The production of many of the products involved with pathogenesis of staphylococcal disease is regulated by way of a quorum-sensing, global-regulatory system. Aside from the iron-regulated products, most if not all of the products of interest are regulated by the *agr-sar* (for *accessory gene regulator, staphylococcal accessory gene regulator,* respectively) system. This system is comprised of a series of genes (*agr*A-D, and *sar*A) whose products "sense" and respond to a thiolactone-containing pheromone (*Auto*inducing

Peptide Pheromone or AIP, which is the modified product encoded by the *agr*D gene) produced by other staphylococci in the immediate environment. Each staphylococcal cell produces a basal level of AIP, and will produce more, when a certain environmental concentration of AIP is attained (quorum sensing). AIP induces the formation of RNAIII (not its translated product) that regulates the transcription of many of the genes involved with staphylococcal disease (global regulation). Thus, when the numbers of staphylococci increase to a certain mass, the increased amount of AIP directs the up regulation (by way of RNAIII) of certain genes (those encoding hemolysins, enterotoxins, exfoliative toxins, leukotoxins, lipases, serine esterase, deoxyribonuclease, staphylokinase, hyaluronidase, phospholipase, and capsule production), while down regulating those gene products that are made when AIP is made in lesser amounts (adhesins).

Growth Characteristics

Staphylococci grow overnight on common laboratory media, over a wide temperature range, and atmospheric conditions producing on agar smooth opaque colonies over 1 mm in diameter.

Biochemical Characterization

Staphylococci are catalase-positive, facultative anaerobes that attack carbohydrates oxidatively and fermentatively.

Resistance

Staphylococci withstand drying (especially in exudates) for weeks, heating up to 60°C for 30 minutes, pH fluctuations from 4.0 to 9.5, and salt concentrations of 7.5%, which are used in selective media for isolation of staphylococci.

Staphylococci are inhibited by bacteriostatic dyes (e.g., crystal violet), bile salts, disinfectants like chlorhexidine, and many antimicrobial drugs.

Variability

Colonies vary from smooth (S) to rough (R). G ("gonidial") and L (wall-less) variants reflect progressive cell wall loss produced by unfavorable environmental conditions, such as antibiotic treatment.

Isolates can be "typed" by their susceptibilities to bacteriophage lysis. Phage-typing sets have been developed for human, bovine, and avian *S. aureus.*

Resistance to beta-lactam antimicrobics is due to possession of a plasmid-encoded penicillinase (beta-lactamase), or the presence of a Staphylococcal Cassette Chromosome Genetic Element containing the gene that encodes a penicillin-resistant penicillin-binding protein (SCC*mec*). *Tolerance,* a rarer form of penicillin resistance, is attributed to failure of autolytic cell wall enzymes. Intrinsic penicillin resistance may be due to changes in penicillin-binding proteins (enzymes responsible for cell synthesis, see Chapter 4).

Resistance to other antimicrobics is common.

Ecology

Reservoir

Coagulase-positive species *S. aureus* and *S. intermedius* inhabit the distal nasal passages, external nares, and skin, especially near mucocutaneous borders such as the perineum, external genitalia, and bovine udder. They also occur as transients in the gastrointestinal tract.

Coagulase-negative staphylococci, especially *S. sciuri and S. xylosus* (and rarely *S. epidermidis*) are predominant among the resident skin flora but also colonize the upper respiratory tract. In swine, this generalization applies to *S. hyicus*, a species potentially pathogenic, especially for piglets.

Staphylococci are found worldwide in warm-blooded animals. Interspecies spread (e.g., humans to cows, dogs to humans) appears to be limited.

Transmission

Staphylococci spread by direct and indirect contact. Many animal infections are probably endogenous, that is, caused by a resident strain.

Pathogenesis

Mechanisms. The deposition of staphylococcal cells into a normally sterile site is the first step in the infectious process. Presumably, the numbers of staphylococci at this stage would be few, and the amount of AIP (see above, "Regulation of the Cellular Products of Medical Interest"), low. Thus, expression of adhesins (MSCRAMMs) results in adherence to extracellular matrix proteins. Inflammation is initiated by cell wall constituents (peptidoglycans and lipoteichoic acids), and by deposition of complement proteins on the bacterial cell surface leading to the generation of split products that are chemotactic and anaphylotoxic. At this stage, the infecting strain may be eliminated, or not, depending upon bacterial factors (inoculum size, virulence of the strain) and host factors (strength of the innate immune system, underlying disease or defects such as the extent of tissue damage). If the infecting strain is not controlled and eliminated, their numbers increase so that the concentration of AIP rises leading to the down regulation of adhesins, and the up regulation of capsule and toxins. Siderophore production aids in the acquisition of iron. The capsule prevents further phagocytosis; the toxins aggravate tissue damage by destroying recruited inflammatory cells (membrane active toxins, and triggering degranulation). The predominant pattern of staphylococcal pathogenesis is suppuration and abscess formation. Systemic effects may be the result of superantigen activity.

Cell-mediated immune phenomena intensify inflammatory responses in some staphylococcal infections while spatially confining them. In some forms of canine pyoderma (juvenile pyoderma, folliculitis), cell- and antibody-mediated hypersensitivity may be induced.

The enterotoxin-induced diseases (food poisoning) are not prominent in animals (though so-called "garbage can enteritis" may be staphylococcal enterotoxin-induced in

dogs). Toxic shock syndrome does not commonly occur (if at all) in the veterinary species.

The exfoliative toxins may play a role in exudative dermatitis of pigs. A condition resembling staphylococcal scalded-skin syndrome has been described in dogs.

Pathology. The typical lesion is the *abscess*, an inflammatory focus in which participating cells have been destroyed by the combined effects of bacterial and inflammatory cell activity. This confrontation between leukocytes and microorganisms produces pus, a mixture of host cell debris and bacteria, living and dead. In an abscess, pus is surrounded by intact leukocytes and fibrin strands. Unless the pus is drained, a fibrous capsule will gradually be formed. In chronic, ulcerative staphylococcal wound infections ("botryomycosis"), fibrous elements predominate, interspersed with pockets of suppuration.

Disease Patterns

Although all warm-blooded animals can be clinically affected by coagulase-positive staphylococci, the prevalence and form of such interactions vary among host species. The more common presentations are listed, and it should be kept in mind that staphylococci can affect any organ or tissue.

Dog and Cat.   The term *canine pyoderma* covers many clinical pictures, all of which include some degree of pyogenic skin inflammation associated with bacterial infection. *Staphylococcus intermedius* is the chief bacterium implicated. Its contribution and the degree of suppuration are variable. In chronic and recurrent forms, cell-mediated hypersensitivity and immune complexes are thought to be involved. Host aspects, including genetic, endocrine, and immunological factors, may play an important part.

Osteomyelitis (especially discospondylitis) and arthritis are frequently associated with *S. intermedius*.

Mastitis is frequently associated with *S. intermedius*.

Otitis externa is usually a mixture of yeast (*Malassezia*, see Chapter 45) and bacteria. The bacteria frequently associated with this condition are *S. intermedius* and *S. schleiferi* ssp. *coagulans*.

Triple Phosphate (struvite, apatite) urolithiasis is almost always infectious, with *S. intermedius* as the etiologic agent. Other bacteria frequently found include *Pseudomonas* (see Chapter 20), *Proteus* (see Chapter 7), and *Enterococcus* (see Chapter 28).

Ruminant.   As a leading cause of bovine mastitis, *S. aureus* rivals *Streptococcus agalactiae* (see Chapter 28). Infection occurs via the teat canal, and the course of the infectious process varies from subclinical to acute suppurative, gangrenous, or chronic, depending on the infecting strain, infecting dose, and host resistance. Bovine mastitis is sometimes caused by coagulase-negative staphylococci, notably *S. epidermidis*, *S. hyicus*, *S. xylosus*, and *S. sciuri*.

Tick pyemia of lambs, resulting from inoculation of indigenous skin *S. aureus* by tick bites, may be acute with toxemic death, or chronic with disseminated abscess formation. It is often linked with tick-borne fever (caused by the rickettsial agent *Anaplasma phagocytophila*, Chapter 43).

Abscess disease of sheep, resembling caseous lymphadenitis (which is caused by *Corynebacterium pseudotuberculosis*, Chapter 31) is caused by an anaerobic subspecies of *S. aureus*.

Equine. Mastitis in mares is frequently associated with *S. aureus*.

Pectoral abscesses are sometimes associated with *S. aureus* (*Corynebacterium pseudotuberculosis* is far more common, however).

Spermatic cord abscesses after castration are sometimes associated with *S. aureus*.

Porcine. Exudative epidermitis (greasy pig disease) due to *S. hyicus* affecting young pigs (7 weeks). It is often systemic and rapidly fatal, affecting the lungs, lymph nodes, kidneys, and brain. Skin lesions are characterized by a thick, grayish-brown exudate (Fig 27.3), especially around the face and ears.

Avian. "Bumblefoot" of gallinaceous birds is a chronic pyogranulomatous process in the subcutaneous tissues of the foot resulting in thick-walled swellings on one or more joints. This condition is associated with trauma together with *S. aureus*.

Staphylococcosis in turkeys, a bacteremia localizing in joints and tendon sheaths, is often produced by *S. aureus*.

Epidemiology

Staphylococcal diseases (e.g., pyoderma, otitis externa, urinary tract and wound infections) often arise endogenously. Studies on humans suggest widespread staphylococcal colonization within hours of birth. Clinical infections appear to be decisively determined by host factors.

In bovine mastitis, staphylococci may enter the gland during milking. Management practices and milking hygiene influence prevalence significantly.

Transmission of *S. aureus* between animals and humans occurs infrequently.

Prolonged environmental survival of staphylococci permits their indirect transmission.

Immunologic Aspects

Possible immune mechanisms in pathogenesis have already been cited.

Recovery and Resistance

Clearance of staphylococci depends chiefly on phagocytosis. Humoral factors are apparently important because agammaglobulinemic individuals suffer frequent infections. Cell-mediated factors contribute to localization and resolution of lesions.

Recovery from staphylococcal infection confers no lasting resistance.

Artificial Immunization

The benefits of vaccination are doubtful. Commercial or autogenous whole-culture preparations, toxoids plus bacterins, are used prophylactically on dairy cattle and sometimes in small animal dermatology to treat persistent infections. Although successes have been reported, controlled evaluations are lacking.

Use of staphylococcal phage lysates and nonspecific stimulants of cell-mediated immunity in cases of nonre-

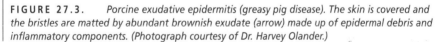

FIGURE 27.3. *Porcine exudative epidermitis (greasy pig disease). The skin is covered and the bristles are matted by abundant brownish exudate (arrow) made up of epidermal debris and inflammatory components. (Photograph courtesy of Dr. Harvey Olander.)*

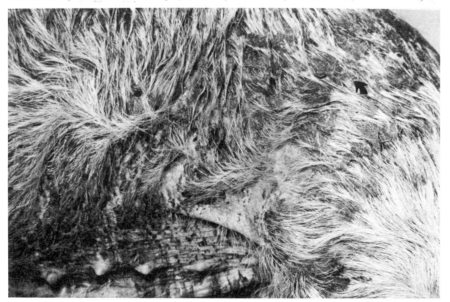

sponsive pyoderma awaits support by adequate clinical or experimental evidence.

Laboratory Diagnosis

Sample Collection

Aspirates from unopened lesions, in sterile syringes or sterile containers, are preferred. Swabs in transport media are acceptable. Milk is collected into containers under sterile precautions. Blood and urine culture routines are appropriate for staphylococcal isolation.

Direct Examination

On gram-stained films, staphylococci appear as gram-positive cocci in pairs, clusters, or short chains (see Fig 27.1). In specimens from skin pustules, they may be sparse.

Isolation and Identification

Bovine blood agar is best for the detection of beta toxin ("water stain" appearance), which is diagnostic for coagulase-positive staphylococci (*S. aureus*, *S. intermedius*, and *S. schleiferi* ssp. *coagulans*; see Fig 27.2). Colonial appearance is as described. Biochemical tests are used to identify staphylococcal isolates. Commercial kits are available.

Treatment and Control

Abscesses are drained of pus. For the most superficial forms of pyoderma, topical application of mild antiseptics (3% hexachlorophene) may be adequate.

Extensive, inaccessible, and disseminated processes require systemic treatment. Staphylococci are commonly resistant to penicillin G, streptomycin, and tetracycline. Usually effective antimicrobics include penicillinase-resistant penicillins, fluoroquinolones, chloramphenicol, cephalosporins (first generation), vancomycin, lincosamides (lincomycin and clindamycin), the macrolides (erythromycin, azithromycin, clarithromycin), and trimethoprim-sulfas. Clavulanic acid inactivates the beta-lactamase produced by *S. aureus* and *S. intermedius*, therefore cell wall antibiotics containing this substance are protected (e.g., clavulanic acid/amoxicillin). The penicillinase-resistant penicillin cloxacillin is effective in treating staphylococcal mastitis, especially in dry cows.

For staphylococcal cystitis, penicillins remain effective because of their high urinary concentrations. Cloxacillin is used topically and systemically on exudative epidermitis due to *S. hyicus*.

A controversial approach to prevention of staphylococcal infections in infants utilizes "bacterial interference": the implantation of a nonvirulent strain to preclude colonization by virulent staphylococci. The method shows promise for control of staphylococcosis in turkeys.

28 *Streptococcus* and *Enterococcus*

DWIGHT C. HIRSH   ERNST L. BIBERSTEIN

STREPTOCOCCUS

Streptococci are gram-positive cocci occurring in pairs and chains; they show considerable ecologic, physiologic, serologic, and genetic diversity. There are 55 recognized species within the genus, but only a handful is regularly associated with diseases of veterinary importance. These, along with the historically important streptococci mainly affecting primates are shown in Table 28.1.

The streptococci are superficially "grouped" by how they grow on blood agar plates. Effects on sheep or bovine blood agar are used to divide streptococci into three types:

Alpha-hemolytic streptococci (α) do not lyse erythrocytes but produce a zone of green discoloration around the colonies (change the hemoglobin to methemoglobin). Most commensal streptococci of animals are alpha-hemolytic. Streptococci that do this are sometimes referred to as "viridans streptococci." They are not hemolytic in the true sense of the word.

Beta-hemolytic streptococci (ß) lyse erythrocytes and produce a "clear" zone around the colonies. Most pathogenic types are beta-hemolytic.

Gamma streptococci (γ) are nonhemolytic. Most are non-pathogenic.

Descriptive Features

Morphology and Staining

Streptococci vary from spherical to short bacillary cells, about 1μm in diameter. Division occurs in one plane, producing pairs and chains. Chain formation is variable, though some species (e.g., *S. equi* subspecies *equi*) are consistent chain formers (Figs 28.1, 28.2).

Young cultures are gram-positive. In exudates and older cultures (>18 hours) organisms often stain gram-negative.

Structure and Composition

Streptococci have a typical gram-positive cell wall composed of proteins and polysaccharides. Capsules are made by some species. Cell wall polysaccharides (C-substance) are sometimes used in streptococcal identification (see below, "Variability").

Cellular Products and Activities of Medical Interest

Adhesins. Streptococci produce a number of surface proteins that bind to a variety of extracellular matrix proteins of the host (fibronectin, fibrinogen, collagen, vitronectin, laminin). These "adhesins" have been termed MSCRAMMs (*m*icrobial *s*urface *c*omponents *r*ecognizing *a*dhesive *m*atrix *m*olecules). Some MSCRAMMs, specifically those that bind fibrinogen (M protein, others, see below, "Cell Wall"), impart an antiphagocytic property to the streptococcal particle. "Coating" of streptococcal cells with this host protein, is thought to result in the "covering" of sites for complement activation (and thus decrease opsonization) as well as those recognized by serum proteins (collectins/ficollins) that opsonize foreign particles. The hyaluronic acid capsule of *S. pyogenes* is an adhesin (as well as imparting antiphagocytic effects, see below), with affinity for human epithelial cells via CD44, a hyaluronic acid–binding glycoprotein. Whether the hyaluronic acid capsules of streptococci of veterinary importance also act as adhesins is unclear. Other adhesins are responsible for binding of streptococci to host cells. Psa (for *p*neumococcal *s*urface *a*dhesin) is a lipoprotein found on *S. pneumoniae*, *S. equi* ssp. *equi*, and *S. equi* ssp. *zooepidemicus* and is responsible for adherence to cells lining the upper and lower airways).

Capsule. Some species of streptococci produce a capsule. Streptococcal capsules are composed of hyaluronic acid. Hyaluronic acid, also a constituent of mammalian connective tissue, is poorly antigenic and does not readily bind complement components (and is thus, antiphagocytic). Hyaluronic acid capsules may also serve as an adhesin (see above).

Cell Wall. The gram-positive cell wall contains proteins and polysaccharides that are of medical interest. The lipoteichoic acids and peptidoglycan of the gram-positive cell wall interact with macrophage cells resulting in the release of proinflammatory cytokines. A fibrillar surface protein, termed the M protein (a MSCRAMM) imparts antiphagocytic properties by binding fibrinogen (see above).

Pyrogenic Toxin Superantigens. Most of what is known about the *streptococcal pyrogenic exotoxins* (SPEs) involves those produced by *Streptococcus pyogenes* (a Group A, beta-hemolytic streptococcus affecting people, see Table 28.1 and below, "Variability"). *Streptococcus pyogenes* produces several SPEs: SPEA, C, G–I, J, and Z (SPEF has been

Table 28.1.   Streptococci of Veterinary Interest

Species	Lancefield Group	Host Species Affected[a]	Principal Diseases	Remarks
Streptococcus. pyogenes	A	Humans, rodents (dairy cattle)	Pharyngotonsillitis, pyoderma, erysipelas, puerperal fever, rheumatic fever, glomerulonephritis (mastitis)	Poststreptococcal immune sequelae. More than 50 serotypes (β)[b]
S. agalactiae	B	Dairy cattle[c] (sheep, goats) humans[c] (cats, dogs)	Mastitis Neonatal infections	5 serotypes (α, β, γ)
S. dysgalactiae ssp equisimilis	C	Swine, horses (humans, dogs)	Miscellaneous suppurative conditions	8 serotypes (β)
S. dysgalactiae ssp. dysgalactiae	C	Dairy cattle	Mastitis	3 serotypes (α, γ)
S. equi ssp. equi	C	Horses	"Strangles"	1 serotype (β)
S. equi ssp.zooepidemicus	C	Horses (fowl, dogs, ruminants, lab animals, humans)	Secondary pneumonias, miscellaneous suppurative conditions, genital and neonatal conditions	15 serotypes (β)
Enterococcus spp.[d]	D	All species	Many opportunistic infections, canine urinary tract infections, chicken septicemia	Normal gut flora (α, γ)
S. porcinus	E	Swine	Jowl abscesses	6 serotypes (β)
S. canis	G	Carnivores	Feline lymphadenitis, miscellaneous pyogenic conditions of dogs and cats, humans[e]	(β)
S. suis	R (=type 2) S (=type 1) RS T ungroupable	Swine (humans—R)	Neonatal infections, septicemias, pneumonia (humans—septicemia, arthritis, meningitis)	React with group D antiserum (α, γ)
S. uberis	—	Cattle	Mastitis	(α, γ)
S. pneumoniae	—	Primates (lab animals, cattle)	Pneumonia, septicemia (mastitis, calf septicemia, meningitis)	More than 80 serotypes (α)

[a] Parentheses indicate that species is affected, but only rarely.
[b] Type of hemolysis on sheep blood agar.
[c] Cattle and human strains are different.
[d] This genus has been proposed based on nucleic acid studies. Not all group D streptococci belong to it (e.g., *S. bovis, S. equinus*).
[e] Canine and human strains appear different.

shown to be a DNase). Some streptococci of veterinary importance, *S. equi* ssp. *equi* for example, have been shown to produce SPEs as well (see below). The genes encoding the SPEs are chromosomally located. The SPEs are superantigens, and part of the systemic symptomatology may be related to the cytokine "storm" that results from the interaction of T lymphocyte cell receptors, macrophages, and these toxins.

Miscellaneous Products. The streptococci produce a number of proteins in vitro with "toxic" activity. These so-called toxins may or may not play a role in disease production and include a peptidase that degrades C5a (Scp for *s*treptococcal *c*ysteine *p*rotease), the hemolysins responsible for beta-hemolysis on sheep blood agar plates (streptolysins O and S), hyaluronidase, DNases (e.g., SPEF, which is a DNase), NADases, proteases (e.g., SPEB which is a cysteine protease), and streptokinases (a fibrinolysin). Streptolysins O and S are membrane active substances and may serve in vivo to damage cell membranes (they are made in vivo since antibodies are produced to these substances by patients that have streptococcal disease). Streptolysin O and suilysin O (produced by *S. suis*) are cholesterol-binding cytolysins (see for example, listerial listeriolysin O, Chapter 33; clostridial perfringolysin O, Chapter 36; and arcanobacterial pyolysin, Chapter 29). These toxins bind to cholesterol-containing rafts in the eukaryotic cell membrane, forming a pore, resulting in death of the cell.

Regulation of the Cellular Products of Medical Interest. Expression of virulence-related genes in *S. pyogenes* is regulated by at least three global systems (whether these systems occur in other streptococci is unknown). The first is a "growth-phase related signal" that is undefined, but certain genes (including those encoding streptolysin S and DNases) are up regulated during stationary phase, while others (including those encoding capsule, streptokinase, streptolysin O, and a protein called *m*ultigene regulator in *g*roup *A* streptococci or Mga) are up regulated during late exponential phase of growth. The second system involves regulation by Mga. Mga itself is regulated by growth phase as well as other undefined environmental cues. Mga up regulates the genes encoding the M protein, and Scp. Finally, a third system involves the protein Cov (*c*ontrol *o*f *v*irulence). Cov down regulates all of the genes that were up regulated by growth phase, except Mga. The gene encoding Cov, like Mga, responds to undefined environmental cues.

Growth Characteristics

Streptococci have fairly exacting growth needs best satisfied by media containing blood or serum.

FIGURE 28.1. Streptococcus equi *subsp.* equi *in pus from cervical lymph node of a horse. Gram stain, 1000X.*

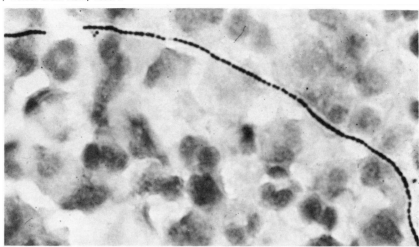

FIGURE 28.2. Streptococcus equi *subsp.* zooepidemicus *in cervical exudate from a mare. Gram stain, 1000X.*

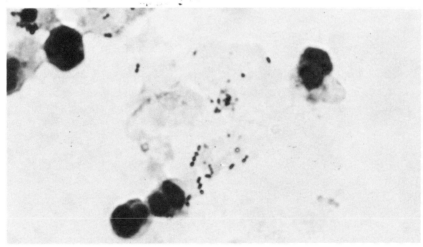

After overnight incubation at 37°C, streptococci produce clear colonies, usually less than 1 mm in diameter. Encapsulated forms, such as *S. equi* ssp. *equi*, produce larger, mucoid colonies.

Pathogenic species grow best at 37°C.

Biochemical Activities

Streptococci are catalase-negative facultative anaerobes, deriving energy from fermentation.

Resistance

Beta-hemolytic streptococci can survive in dried pus for weeks. They are killed at 55°C to 60°C in 30 minutes, and inhibited by 6.5% sodium chloride and 40% bile (except *S. agalactiae*), 0.1% methylene blue, and low (10°C) and high (45°C) temperatures. Members of the genus *Enterococcus*

tolerate these conditions (see below). Viridans streptococci vary with respect to heat and bile resistance. Only *S. pneumoniae* is bile-soluble. Streptococci tolerate 0.02% sodium azide, which is used in streptococcal isolation media.

Pathogenic streptococci are usually susceptible to penicillins, cephalosporins, macrolides, chloramphenicol, and trimethoprim-sulfonamides; they are often resistant to aminoglycosides, fluoroquinolones, and tetracycline.

Variability

Rebecca Lansfield developed the serological method used to group streptococci based upon serologic similarities of cell wall polysaccharide. This method is called Lansfield serologic grouping. Groups are designated by capital letters (A to V). Serologic subdivisions exist in most streptococcal species except *S. equi* ssp. *equi* (see Table 28.1). *Streptococcus pyogenes* has some 70 immunotypes, based on M and other proteins, while *S. pneumoniae* has over 80 capsular types. In *S. pyogenes*, change from rough (matte) to smooth accompanies loss of M protein and virulence. Cell wall deficient forms (L forms) also occur.

Ecology

Reservoir

Most streptococci of veterinary interest live commensally in the upper respiratory, alimentary, and lower genital tract.

Transmission

Those streptococci that are contagious (*S. equi* ssp. *equi*, *S. porcinus*, and *S. agalactiae*) are transmitted by inhalation or ingestion, sexually, congenitally, or indirectly via hands and fomites.

Pathogenesis

Mechanisms. The relation of streptococcal products to pathogenesis is largely speculative, with the following exceptions. The capsule of *S. pneumoniae* is a proven virulence factor. M protein is an important virulence determinant, and antibody to it is protective. Other antiphagocytic cell constituents and cytotoxins of streptococci are probable virulence factors.

Streptococci trigger inflammatory processes that lead to suppuration and abscess formation.

Pathology. The basic pathologic process resembles that of staphylococcal infection, i.e., the typical lesion is an *abscess*, an inflammatory focus in which participating cells have been destroyed by the combined effects of bacterial and inflammatory cell activity. This confrontation between leukocytes and microorganisms produces pus, a mixture of host cell debris and bacteria, living and dead. In an abscess, pus is surrounded by intact leukocytes and fibrin strands. Unless the pus is drained, a fibrous capsule will gradually be formed.

Disease Patterns

Equine. Strangles is a highly contagious rhinopharyngitis caused by *S. equi* subspecies *equi* (hereafter referred to as *S. equi*). After deposition on the mucous membranes of the upper respiratory tract, *S. equi* adheres to epithelial cells by way of MSCRAMMs (M protein, fibronectin-binding protein, fibrinogen-binding protein, Psa) and hyaluronic acid capsule. Adherence triggers internalization and subsequent localization in the subepithelial spaces. Cell wall constituents as well as pyrogenic exotoxins (SPEH and SPEI) initiate an acute inflammatory response. Capsule, M protein, and Scp protect *S. equi* from opsonization and phagocytosis. Streptolysins may act to destroy host cells by damaging their membranes. Systemic symptomatology may be due to the superantigen effects of pyrogenic exotoxins (SPEH and SPEI). Other "toxins" may contribute to the process by digesting DNA (DNases), fibrin (streptokinase), and hyaluronic acid (hyaluronidase). The disease is

marked by a serous or purulent nasal discharge, diphasic temperature rise, local pain, cough, and anorexia. In regional lymph nodes, abscesses develop, which typically rupture and drain within two weeks. Recovery follows. The overall mortality rate is under 2%. Complications include pyemic dissemination to meninges, lungs, pericardium, and abdominal viscera, or extension to the guttural pouches. Purpura hemorrhagica, a Type III hypersensitivity manifested by subcutaneous swellings, mucosal hemorrhages, and fever, may follow the acute disease by about three weeks.

Bacterial pneumonia/pyothorax in horses is almost always associated with a beta-hemolytic streptococcus with *S. equi* ssp. *zooepidemicus* (hereafter referred to as *S. zooepidemicus*) being the most commonly isolated. In addition, a gram-negative microorganism (*Actinobacillus* is the most common, see Chapter 13) is frequently found along with *S. zooepidemicus*. The infectious process is endogenous. The microorganisms involved are part of the normal flora of the upper respiratory tract, which then contaminate a compromised lung (e.g., following an episode of viral pneumonia). *Streptococcus zooepidemicus* (plus the others) are deposited in the lung and initiate or amplify a preexisting inflammatory process (cell wall constituents, pyrogenic exotoxins). The intensity of the inflammatory response is not as extreme as with the response initiated by *S. equi*, nor are the constitutional signs as severe. However, it is presumed that the mechanisms involved in the pathogenesis are similar. Pyothorax is probably an extension of the pneumonic process just described. Like pneumonia, *S. zooepidemicus* is the most common isolate, combined with a gram-negative species. Unlike pneumonia, an obligate anaerobe (*Bacteroides* or *Fusobacterium* are the most common, see Chapter 35) is frequently found as well.

Genital tract diseases in horses are associated with *S. zooepidemicus*, which is frequently associated with cervicitis and metritis. Infections in newborn foals, which are often umbilical infections (navel ill, pyosepticemia, joint ill, polyarthritis) disseminate via the bloodstream to joints and the renal cortex. The microorganisms originate from the genital tract of the dam (they are a part of her normal flora).

Beta-hemolytic streptococci (*S. zooepidemicus* is the most common) are associated with a variety of miscellaneous conditions in horses including osteomyelitis, arthritis, abscesses, and wounds. All are endogenous, with the infecting strain arising from the normal flora.

Swine. Cervical lymphadenitis of swine (jowl abscess) is a contagious disease affecting swine. This condition is associated with *S. porcinus* (previously known as "Group E *Streptococcus*"). The disease is analogous to strangles but clinically less dramatic and frequently not diagnosed until slaughter. Its most damaging aspect is carcass condemnation.

Secondary pneumonias in swine are sometimes associated with *S. dysgalactiae* ssp. *equisimilis*.

Streptococcus suis, *S. dysgalactiae* ssp. *equisimilis* and streptococci belonging to Groups L and U cause neonatal septicemia, pneumonia, arthritis, and meningitis. The exotoxin, suilysin, a cholesterol-binding cytolysin (see above, "Cellular Products and Activities of Medical Interest"), is produced by *S. suis*. It has been proposed that this cytotoxin is active in vivo and may account for some of the tissue damage associated with this disease.

Ruminants. The leading agent of streptococcal mastitis is *S. agalactiae*. Less frequent causes are *S. dysgalactiae* ssp. *dysgalactiae* (hereafter referred to as *S. dysgalactiae*) and *S. uberis*.

Dogs and Cats . Secondary pneumonias affecting dogs and cats are sometimes associated with *S. canis*.

Laboratory cats occasionally experience cervical lymphadenitis from which *S. canis* is isolated (see Fig 67.5). The condition probably arises endogenously being precipitated by an unknown event.

Streptococcus canis is associated with septicemia in newborn puppies.

Streptococcus canis has been associated with a toxic shock–like syndrome and necrotizing fasciitis in dogs. No virulence-associated traits have been defined as they have for similar conditions seen in humans affected with *S. pyogenes*.

Primates. *Streptococcus pneumoniae* is a leading cause of pneumonia, septicemia, and meningitis in primates. Pneumococcal pneumonia in monkeys runs an acute course with high mortality rates. The lesions are those of a fibrinous pleuropneumonia. Recent shipment and viral infection are common antecedents.

Miscellaneous Species. Cervical lymphadenitis in guinea pigs is caused by *S. zooepidemicus* ssp. *zooepidemicus*.

Septicemic disease in fish from freshwater aquaculture farms and from salt-water environments has been associated with *S. iniae*, a beta-hemolytic streptococcus without a Lansfield designation. People handling (cleaning/necropsy) affected fish are at risk of developing cellulitis, endocarditis, or arthritis presumably following self-inoculation.

Septicemic disease in seals is associated with *S. phocae*, a beta-hemolytic streptococcus that reacts to Lansfield group antisera C and F.

Septicemic disease and dermatitis in opossums is associated with *S. didelphis*, a beta-hemolytic streptococcus without affiliation with known Lansfield groups.

Epidemiology

Healthy individuals may carry all the streptococci discussed, and many infections are probably endogenous and stress-related. Neonatal infections are commonly maternal in origin.

Strangles and porcine lymphadenitis are contagious diseases preferably affecting young animals (past infancy). *Streptococcus equi* and *S. porcinus* are spread by contaminated food, drinking water, or utensils and by recovered animals, which may remain clinically healthy shedders for months. Milking equipment, unskilled attempts at intramammary medication, and unsanitary milking practices often spread *Streptococcus agalactiae* among dairy cows.

Animal streptococci have limited public health significance. The Group B streptococci that cause disease in human infants are apparently distinct from bovine strains, but infections with *S. zooepidemicus* have been traced to infected milk, and *S. suis* (Type 2) has caused serious infections in swine handlers. The Group G streptococci affecting dogs (*S. canis*) are apparently different from the Group G streptococci affecting human patients.

Immunologic Aspects

Immune Mechanisms of Disease

Human poststreptococcal diseases (rheumatic fever, acute glomerulonephritis) are attributed to immunopathogenic mechanisms. Similarly, equine purpura hemorrhagica following strangles is probably immune complex–mediated.

Recovery and Resistance

The main defenses against streptococcal infections are phagocytic, and the antiphagocytic M protein elicits protective antibodies. Animals recovered from strangles and cervical lymphadenitis are at least temporarily immune to reinfection.

Polysaccharide capsules of *S. agalactiae* and *S. pneumoniae* evoke the formation of opsonizing antibody. In streptococcal pneumonia, their appearance determines recovery from infection. In bovine mastitis, no useful immunity develops: Cows, unless treated, remain infected. Experimental evidence suggests that anticapsular IgG_2-type antibody is protective.

All immunity is serotype-specific.

Artificial Immunization

A whole-cell bacterin and an M protein vaccine are available for vaccination against strangles. Neither is uniformly effective, and often elicits local reactions at the injection site. An intranasal avirulent live vaccine that stimulates essential local antibody responses appears promising. Feeding live avirulent cultures has produced immunity to porcine jowl abscesses.

Laboratory Diagnosis

Sample Collection

Aspirates from unopened lesions, in sterile syringes or sterile containers, are preferred. Swabs in transport media are acceptable. Milk is collected into containers under sterile precautions.

Direct Examination

Smears of exudates or sediments of suspect fluids are fixed and gram stained. Streptococci appear as gram-positive cocci in pairs, short chains, and in some instances very long chains (typically seen in pus aspirated from cervical lymph nodes of horses infected with *S. equi*—see Fig

28.1). Streptococci have a tendency to lose their gram-positivity and sometimes stain weakly gram-positive or gram-negative.

Culture

Exudates, milk, tissue, urine, transtracheal aspirates, and cerebrospinal fluid are cultured directly on cow or sheep blood agar. Incubation at 37°C in 3% to 5% CO_2 is preferable. Streptococcal colonies, smooth or mucoid, will appear in 18 to 48 hours. It is sometimes difficult to distinguish alpha from beta hemolysis. Intact erythrocytes remain adjacent to alpha- but not to beta-hemolytic colonies. Beta-hemolytic strains consistently lyse red cells in blood broth; alpha-hemolytic strains of animal origin generally do not.

Identification relies on a combination of classical techniques (determination of Lansfield grouping and biochemical tests), and molecular techniques (e.g., determination of the sequence of DNA encoding the 16S ribosomal DNA, or using species specific primers in the polymerase chain reaction). Commercial kits are available for both purposes. Other useful diagnostic tests include the following:

1. The CAMP phenomenon (named after *C*hristie, *A*tkins, and *M*unch-*P*etersen) reflects hemolytic synergism between staphylococcal beta toxin and a *S. agalactiae* toxin (CAMP protein sometimes referred to as cocytolysin). A beta toxin-producing staphylococcus is inoculated across the equator of a sheep or bovine blood agar plate. At right angles to this line, and approximately 0.5 cm from it, a suspect *S. agalactiae* is inoculated. After incubation, hemolysis by CAMP-positive bacteria will be enhanced in the beta-toxin zone (Fig 28.3). The combined action of these two toxins on sheep or bovine blood agar produces larger and clearer zones of hemolysis than either agent alone (see Fig 28.3). This reaction has diagnostic value.

2. Bacitracin sensitivity. Bacitracin disks (0.04 units) inhibit growth of *S. pyogenes* on blood agar. This reaction is not entirely consistent or specific.

3. Bile esculin agar tests the ability of 40% bile-salt-tolerant bacteria to hydrolyze esculin, a characteristic of those belonging to Lansfield Group D.

4. Optochin sensitivity. Growth of *S. pneumoniae*, but not other alpha-hemolytic streptococci, is inhibited around disks impregnated with optochin (ethyl hydrocuprein hydrochloride).

Treatment and Control

Localized suppurative conditions are drained of pus.

For systemic treatment, penicillin G and ampicillin are effective on most beta-hemolytic and viridans streptococci. Cephalosporins, chloramphenicol, and trimethoprim-sulfas are alternatives. Streptococcal endocarditis is treated with combined penicillin and gentamicin. Susceptibility to fluoroquinolones is unpredictable. Streptococcal toxic shock and necrotizing fasciitis are treated with peni-

FIGURE 28.3.   *CAMP phenomenon on bovine blood agar. The dark line across the field is growth of* Staphylococcus aureus *surrounded by a zone of beta-toxin activity. Growing in lines at right angles to it are, left to right: a viridans streptococcus,* Streptococcus agalactiae, *another viridans streptococcus,* Streptococcus equi *subsp.* zooepidemicus, *and* Streptococcus agalactiae. *See text for discussion of CAMP phenomenon. (Photograph courtesy of Dr. Richard Walker.)*

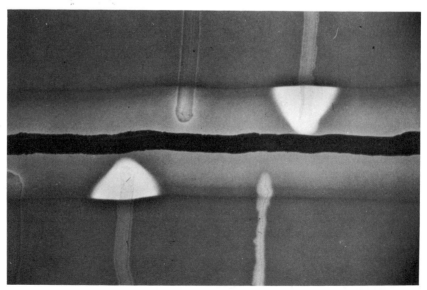

cillin G and clindamycin (clindamycin decreases toxin production, and penicillin G is bactericidal).

Penicillins (intramammary) are effective for treating mastitis due to *S. agalactiae* and most other streptococci. For the many available alternatives, a specialty text should be consulted. Important aspects of mastitis control lie in the area of sanitation and herd management.

For strangles, it is most beneficial to treat exposed and affected animals prior to abscess formation and to continue treatment past the febrile stage. Inappropriate or inadequate therapy of strangles is blamed for prolonging the illness and causing "bastard strangles" (widespread abscess formation with systemic manifestations). Populations at risk may be vaccinated. Affected or suspected horses should be rigorously isolated.

ENTEROCOCCUS

Enterococci were once classified as Group D streptococci. Unlike most true members of the genus *Streptococcus*, these microorganisms possess phenotypic traits (resistance to salt, bile, methylene blue, and growth at increased temperatures) that set them apart. Molecular genetic analysis showed that they are unique, and prompted the establishment of a new genus, *Enterococcus*. There are 28 species in the genus, most of which live in the intestinal tracts of mammals and birds. They are mainly opportunists that infect compromised sites to produce disease. There are some (*E. durans*, *E. hirae*, and *E. villorum*) that have been associated with intestinal disease in neonatal animals (piglets, foals, calves, puppies, kittens) as well as adult dogs and cats (though only the isolates from piglets have been subjected to the genetic analyses needed to definitively determine the identity of the isolates). Enterococci are either alpha- or gamma-hemolytic on sheep or cattle red blood cell–containing blood agar plates (see above, "Streptococcus").

Descriptive Features

Morphology and Staining

Enterococci vary from spherical to short bacillary cells, about 1 μm in diameter. Division occurs in one plane, producing pairs and chains.

Structure and Composition

Enterococci have a typical gram-positive cell wall composed of proteins and polysaccharides. Polysaccharide capsules are made by some species. Most enterococci possess Lancefield Group D carbohydrate.

Cellular Products and Activities of Medical Interest

Much of what is known regarding cellular products and activities of medical interest comes from study of *E. faecalis* and *E. faecium*, the most common enterococci producing disease in human patients. Presumably, some (if not all) of what is known about these two species also applies to the other members of the genus.

Aggregation Substance. Aggregation substance is a surface protein that promotes adherence of enterococci to each other (to form aggregates) and to epithelial surfaces (an adhesin).

Capsule. Some enterococci produce a polysaccharide capsule. The capsule discourages association with phagocytic cells by interfering with complement deposition and imparting a relative hydrophilicity to the microbe's surface. It is unlikely that the capsule is made while enterococci associate with enterocytes in the intestinal tract.

Cell Wall. Enterococci posses a typical gram-positive cell wall. Cell wall peptidoglycan and lipoteichoic acids initiate an inflammatory response following their interaction with macrophages.

Cytolysin. Cytolysin is a cytotoxin whose mechanism of cell destruction is not understood. It is also a hemolytic toxin, lysing human and horse red blood cells (but not sheep or bovine red blood cells, red blood cells most often used in blood agar plates). Cytolysin production is under the control of a quorum-sensing system.

Extracellular Superoxide. Some enterococci secrete a superoxide that appears to afford some protection against killing by phagocytic cells.

Gelatinase. Some enterococci produce a gelatinase that is marginally related to virulence.

Iron Acquisition. Enterococci produce a hydroxamate type of siderophore in response to low levels of iron.

Growth Characteristics

Enterococci produce clear to gray colonies 1–2 mm in diameter (either alpha- or gamma-hemolytic) after overnight incubation at 37°C, though they will grow between 10 to 45°C. Enterococci will grow in 6.5% sodium chloride, 40% bile, and in 0.1% methylene blue.

Biochemical Activities

Enterococci are catalase-negative facultative anaerobes, deriving energy from fermentation.

Resistance

Enterococci are hardy microorganisms able to survive in the environment for extended periods of time. They are able to grow in 6.5% sodium chloride and 40% bile, 0.1% methylene blue, and low (10°C) and high (45°C) temperatures. They are intrinsically resistant to the beta-lactam antibiotics (including cephalosporins and penicillinase-resistant penicillins), aminoglycosides, clindamycin, fluoroquinolones, and the trimethoprim-sulfonamides (they are effective scavengers of thymidine found in exudates, thereby bypassing the effect of the trimethoprim-sulfonamides). They are able to acquire resistance to high levels of beta-lactams, high levels of aminoglycosides, the glycopeptides (vancomycin), tetracycline, erythromycin, fluoroquinolones, rifampin, and chloramphenicol. Selection of vancomycin-resistant strains by the growth promoter avoparcin is discussed below (see below, "Epidemiology," and Chapter 4).

Ecology

Reservoir

Enterococci live in the intestinal tract of mammals and birds as part of the normal flora of these species. Whether the enterococci associated with "primary" disease, *E. durans, E. hirae, E. villorum,* as opposed to opportunistic-type disease, are members of the normal flora, is unknown.

Transmission

Enterococci that are associated with opportunistic disease are part of the normal flora of the host. It is unknown whether this is true for *E. durans, E. hirae,* and *E. villorum.*

Pathogenesis

Except for *E. durans, E. hirae,* and *E. villorum*–associated disease, endogenous enterococci infect a compromised site (e.g., urinary bladder, moist external ear canal, catheter). The cell wall peptidoglycan and lipoteichoic acids initiate an inflammatory response. Capsule, cytolysin, and superoxide potentate the inflammatory processes.

Enterococcus durans, E. hirae, and *E. villorum* associate with the villi (from tip to crypt) of the small intestine of affected animals (see below). Associated diarrhea does not appear to be due to an enterotoxin or epithelial cell damage.

Disease Patterns

Dogs and Cats. Otitis externa is usually the result of infection (bacteria and a yeast, *Malassezia,* see Chapter 45) of a compromised external ear canal. The bacteria involved are usually an environmental species (e.g., *Pseudomonas* and *Proteus,* see Chapters 20 and 7, respectively) or a member of the patient's normal flora (e.g., *Enterococcus, Staphylococcus intermedius,* see Chapter 27).

Enterococcus is a common isolate from dogs with lower urinary tract infections (see Fig 74.2B).

Enterococcus spp. (*E. durans, E. hirae, E. villorum*) are associated with diarrhea in puppies, kittens, and adult dogs and cats.

Almost any compromised site may be contaminated with an enterococcus.

Horse. *Enterococcus* spp. (*E. durans, E. hirae, E. villorum*) are associated with diarrhea in foals.

Enterococcus spp. should be expected in any condition that results from contamination of a compromised site with fecal material (e.g., street nail/sole abscess, wound).

Cattle. *Enterococcus* spp. (*E. durans, E. hirae, E. villorum*) are associated with diarrhea in calves.

Enterococcus spp. should be expected in any condition that results from contamination of a compromised site with fecal material (e.g., wound).

Swine. *Enterococcus* spp. (*E. durans, E. hirae, E. villorum*) are associated with diarrhea in piglets.

Enterococcus spp. should be expected in any condition that results from contamination of a compromised site with fecal material (e.g., wound).

Miscellaneous Species. *Enterococcus* spp. (*E. durans, E. hirae, E. villorum*) are associated with diarrhea in infant rats.

Epidemiology

Most of the infectious processes from which enterococci are isolated are due to contamination with members of the normal flora. In hospital settings, nosocomial spread (e.g., fomites, hands of care givers, soles of shoes) to compromised sites is an important issue. The epidemiology of the diarrhea-associated enterococci (*E. durans, E. hirae, E. villorum*) is unknown.

Vancomycin-resistant strains of enterococci are a serious problem in human medicine, because members of this genus (especially *E. faecalis,* and *E. faecium*) are major contributors to nosocomially acquired disease. Enterococci as a group are very resistant to antimicrobial agents (see above, "Resistance"). Vancomycin (a glycopeptide antibiotic) is one of the few effective drugs for treatment of such infectious processes. Vancomycin-resistant strains of enterococci arose in Europe after the initiation of feeding of another glycopeptide avoparcin (a growth promoter) to food-producing animals. Though at first the vancomycin-resistant strains were limited to the intestinal tract of animals fed this antibiotic, they soon spread, as did the genes encoding vancomycin resistance (*van*A), to the human intestinal tract. In the United States (where avoparcin was not allowed), injudicious use of vancomycin in human hospitals resulted in the same effect, i.e., an increase in selective pressure resulting in an increase in colonization by vancomycin-resistant enterococci (especially in hospitals).

Laboratory Diagnosis

Sample Collection

Aspirates from unopened lesions, in sterile syringes or sterile containers, are preferred. Swabs in transport media are acceptable. Urine samples are obtained by antepubic cystocentesis (bladder tap), catherization, or midstream catch.

Direct Examination

Stained (Gram's or Romanovsky-type such as Wright's or Giemsa) smears of exudates are examined. Urine can be examined unstained or stained (Gram's or Romanovsky-type). Histopathologic sections of small intestine obtained from animals with associated enterococcal enteritis are needed to demonstrate characteristic adherence of coccal forms to villi.

Culture

Samples are streaked onto the surface of blood agar plates and incubated at 37°C overnight in air (because enterococci are facultative anaerobes, any atmosphere will suffice). Enterococci produce clear to gray colonies 1–2 mm in diameter (either alpha- or gamma-hemolytic). Preliminary identification entails testing for the production of catalase (negative), and ability to grow in 6.5% sodium chloride and 40% bile. Most isolates can be speciated by using commercially available kits, sequencing the gene encoding the 16S ribosomal RNA, or a combination of both.

Treatment and Control

Correction of the underlying condition is the most important aspect of treatment of most situations from which enterococci are isolated. In some instances, removal of the compromise is enough to initiate host-elimination of enterococci (because they do not have potent virulence determinants). This is an important concept because enterococci tend to be quite resistant to antimicrobials (see above, "Resistance"). Too, in those infectious processes that have a polymicrobic etiology (along with the compromise), success can be achieved by correction of the compromise and antimicrobic therapy aimed at the other (usually more susceptible) microorganisms.

Enterococci isolated from the lower urinary tract of dogs are usually susceptible to urine concentrations of amoxicillin-clavulanate, chloramphenicol, and tetracycline. Even though most urinary strains of enterococci test susceptible to trimethoprim-sulfonamides, care should be taken in interpreting in vitro test results because of the thymidine-savaging ability of this group of microorganisms.

Enterococci associated with otitis externa in dogs are dealt with by correcting the underlying compromise and use of any of the otic preparations that contain an antimicrobial (topical concentrations of most incorporated antimicrobics usually far exceed the minimal inhibitory concentration needed to inhibit growth of enterococci).

Treatment options of diarrheal disease associated with *E. durans*, *E. hirae*, or *E. villorum* are undefined.

ABIOTROPHIA AND *GRANULICATELLA* (NUTRITIONALLY VARIANT STREPTOCOCCI)

Members of the genera *Abiotrophia* and *Granulicatella* were discovered as small colonies growing as satellites around other bacterial colonies when samples obtained from normal human mucosal surfaces (eyes, genital tract, mouth, respiratory tract) were inoculated onto blood agar plates. The bacteria comprising these colonies were gram-positive, catalase-negative cocci requiring vitamin B_6 for growth (satisfied by the addition of 0.002% pyridoxal hydrochloride to media). These microorganisms were provisionally termed "nutritionally variant streptococci," but later placed into the genera *Abiotrophia* and *Granulicatella* based upon the sequence of the gene encoding the 16S ribosomal RNA.

Clinically, members of these genera have been isolated from the bloodstream, abscesses, dental plaque, joints, corneal ulcers, and cardiac valve vegetations of human patients. They have been isolated from the genital tracts, respiratory tracts, abscesses, and eyes of horses and ruminants.

29

Arcanobacterium

DWIGHT C. HIRSH   ERNST L. BIBERSTEIN

Members of the genus *Arcanobacterium* are pleomorphic, non–spore-forming, nonmotile gram-positive bacilli. In shape, members of this genus are "diphtheroids" (see Chapter 31), and many were at one time included within the genus *Corynebacterium* (e.g., *C. pyogenes*) as well as the genus *Actinomyces* (e.g., *Actinomyces pyogenes*). Sequence analysis of the gene encoding the 16S ribosomal RNA revealed that the genus *Arcanobacterium* is the appropriate place for these microorganisms.

Of the five members of the genus, *Arcanobacterium pyogenes* is the main species of veterinary importance, being involved in suppurative processes of ruminants and swine. Other arcanobacteria of note include *A. phocae*, *A. pluranimalium*, and *A. hippocoleae* isolated from the respiratory tract of seals, the spleen of a harbor porpoise and the lung of a deer, and from an equine vaginal exudate, respectively.

ARCANOBACTERIUM PYOGENES

Descriptive Features

Morphology and Staining

Arcanobacterium pyogenes is a small, gram-positive, pleomorphic rod (0.5 μm by up to 2 μm; Fig 29.1) that lacks capsules and metachromatic granules. The instability of the gram-positive reaction is comparable to that of streptococci.

Structure and Composition

Its cell wall peptidoglycan contains lysine, rhamnose, and glucose. Unlike members of the genera *Corynebacterium* and *Rhodococcus,* it does not contain mycolic acids.

Cellular Products of Medical Interest

Cell Wall. The lipoteichoic acids and peptidoglycan of the gram-positive cell wall interact with macrophage cells, resulting in the release of proinflammatory cytokines.

Exotoxins. Arcanobacterium pyogenes produces a number of proteins with toxic properties:

1. Pyolysin O. PLO (for *pyolysin O*) is produced by all strains of *A. pyogenes* (see also, streptococcal streptolysin O, Chapter 28; listerial listeriolysin O, Chapter 33; and clostridial perfringolysin O,

Chapter 36). It is a pore-forming, cholesterol-dependent cytolysin that is a major virulence determinant for this species (mutants deficient in this protein have reduced virulence; antibodies to it are protective). PLO binds to cholesterol-containing rafts in the eukaryotic cell membrane, forming a pore, resulting in death of the cell. PLO is also responsible for the hemolysis observed when *A. pyogenes* is grown on blood containing media. How PLO acts in vivo is not known, but it is assumed that it damages host cell membranes.

2. Neuraminidases. *Arcanobacterium pyogenes* produces at least two neuraminidases, Nans (for *N*-acetylneuraminyl hydrolases). How the Nans work in vivo is not clear, but they appear to be involved in adhesion of the microorganisms to host cells.

3. Miscellaneous products. Several proteins with proteolytic activity in vitro have been demonstrated, as well as a DNase. What roles, if any, these other "toxins" play in the pathogenesis of disease are not known.

Growth Characteristics

Arcanobacterium pyogenes is a facultative anaerobe requiring enriched media and up to 40 hours to produce discernible colonies on blood agar. Growth occurs optimally at 37°C and produces translucent, hemolytic colonies up to 1 mm in size.

Biochemical Activities

Arcanobacterium pyogenes is catalase-negative, ferments lactose, and digests protein (gelatin, casein, coagulated serum).

Resistance

Arcanobacterium pyogenes is susceptible to drying, heat (60°C), disinfectants, and beta-lactam antibiotics. It is resistant to sulfonamides, and increasingly so to tetracycline.

Ecology

Reservoir

Arcanobacterium pyogenes is found on mucous membranes (including the rumen and stomach) and skin of susceptible species.

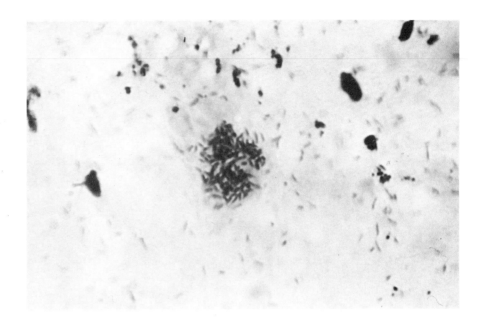

FIGURE 29.1. *Arcanobacterium pyogenes in pus from sheep lung. Gram stain, 1000X.*

Transmission

Most infections are probably endogenous. In "summer mastitis," cow-to-cow spread, aided by flies, is thought to occur.

Pathogenesis

Mechanisms. Arcanobacterium pyogenes causes suppurative processes, usually complicated by other potentially pathogenic commensals, especially non-spore-forming anaerobes (*Bacteroides, Fusobacterium, Porphyromonas, Prevotella, Peptostreptococcus*, see Chapter 35). Pyolysin O (PLO) is a major virulence determinant (supported by the finding that antibodies to PLO are protective, and mutants deficient in PLO are avirulent). Deposition of *A. pyogenes* (from a contiguous surface or from the immediate environment) into a normally sterile site initiates an inflammatory response (adherence, by way of Nans, cell wall constituents, action of PLO). The exudate (pus) consists of bacteria, neutrophils (live or dead), and host cell debris.

Pathology. The lesions are abscesses, empyemas, or pyogranulomas. Abscesses are often heavily encapsulated. Any offensive odors are contributions of anaerobic participants.

Disease Patterns

Cattle. *Arcanobacterium pyogenes* is involved in most purulent infections of traumatic or opportunistic origins, which may be local, regional, or metastatic. Common localizations are the lung, pericardium, endocardium, pleura, peritoneum, liver, joints, uterus, renal cortex, brain, bones, and subcutaneous tissues. In other susceptible species (sheep, goats, wild ruminants, swine) similar lesions may be found.

Arcanobacterium pyogenes causes abortion and mastitis in cattle. "Summer mastitis" is a communicable disease among pastured dairy cattle during their dry period. It often takes a destructive course, causing abscess formation and sloughing. Bacteria implicated in its etiology include *A. pyogenes, Streptococcus dysgalactiae* ssp. *dysgalactiae* (see Chapter 28), and non–spore-forming anaerobes (see Chapter 35).

Epidemiology

Because *A. pyogenes* is a permanent resident of susceptible species, disease prevalence is sporadic and governed by precipitating stress or trauma.

"Summer mastitis" is most prevalent in northern Europe. It is spread by flies attracted to traumatized teats.

Immunologic Aspects

Immune responses to *A. pyogenes* are not well understood. Infection or vaccination confers no useful resistance. The usefulness of pyolysin as a vaccine remains to be demonstrated, but toxoids produced from PLO are protective in laboratory animals.

Laboratory Diagnosis

Gram-stained smears from tissues or exudates reveal gram-positive pleomorphic rods (see Fig 29.1) often mixed with other bacteria. Material suspected of containing *A. pyogenes* is cultured on blood agar. Routine methods are used to identify this microorganism. Primers designed to amplify *A. pyogenes*-specific DNA by the polymerase chain reaction have been described.

Treatment and Control

Incision and drainage of abscesses are essential. Although many antibiotics, including all penicillins, are active in vitro, medical treatment alone is usually disappointing due to inadequate drug delivery to the lesions.

30 Bacillus

DWIGHT C. HIRSH   ERNST L. BIBERSTEIN

Members of the genus *Bacillus* are gram-positive, spore-forming, facultatively anaerobic rods that typically inhabit soil and water. Some species cause diseases of insects. The only consistent pathogen of vertebrates, including humans, is *B. anthracis*, the causative agent of anthrax. *Bacillus anthracis* is a close relative of *B. cereus* that causes canine and human food poisoning.

BACILLUS ANTHRACIS

Descriptive Features

Morphology and Staining

Cells of *B. anthracis* are gram-positive, nonmotile, roughly rectangular rods with square ends (about 1 µm by 3 to 5 µm). Chains of rods are common. Spores within the cell cause no swelling. A capsule is formed in vivo, or under appropriate condition in vitro.

Cellular Composition

The capsule consists of a D-glutamyl polypeptide. The cell wall is largely polysaccharide. Covering the cell wall is a proteinaceous paracrystalline structure (S-layer). When *B. anthracis* produces a capsule, the S-layer lies between it and the rest of the cell wall. No virulence properties have been ascribed to the S-layer or its proteins.

Cellular Products of Medical Interest

Capsule. The vegetative form of *B. anthracis* produces a capsule composed of a D-glutamyl polypeptide. The genes encoding this structure are on a plasmid called pXO2. The expression of the genes encoding the capsule are under control of two regulatory gene products, AtxA and AcpA (for *a*nthrax *tox*in *a*ctivator and *a*nthrax *cap*sule *a*ctivator, respectively) which respond to environmental cues (see below, "Regulation of Cellular Products of Medical Interest"). The capsule enables the vegetative form to avoid phagocytosis. The genes encoding AtxA and AcpA are on the plasmids, pXO1 (see below, "Lethal Toxin") and pXO2, respectively.

Toxins. A number of toxins are made by *B. anthracis*. The most important of these in the production of disease are the lethal toxin and the edema toxin:

1. Lethal toxin. The genes encoding the lethal toxin (LeTx for *le*thal *tox*in) are found on a plasmid termed pXO1. LeTx is a binary toxin composed of "protective antigen" (PA) and "lethal factor" (LF). PA is responsible for binding of LeTx to "target cells," while LF is responsible for its toxic activity. PA and LF associate only after PA has been oligomerized on the "target" cell surface (see below). LF is a zinc metalloprotease that inactivates mitogen-activated protein kinase kinases (MAPK kinases), resulting in the disruption of signaling pathways within the affected cell (macrophages appear to be the principal cell that LT affects, even though it enters several others). PA binds to cell surface receptors on a variety of cell types. It is activated by furins on the cell surface resulting in oligomerization, which is followed by internalization of LT (as well as edema factor, see below). At low concentrations, the LeTx-macrophage interaction results in a cytokine "storm" leading to multiorgan dysfunction, similar to what occurs during endotoxemia (see Fig 8.1). That is, under the influence of LeTx, macrophages become hyperresponsive and produce large amounts of tumor necrosis factor (TNF), interleukin (IL)-1, and IL-6 resulting in increased vascular permeability (TNF on endothelium), increased intravascular clotting (TNF on endothelium), attraction of inflammatory cells (TNF/IL-1 signaling endothelium to produce IL-8 and macrophage chemotactic factor), release of acute phase proteins (IL-6 on liver), endogenous pyrogen (TNF, IL-1, IL-6 on brain), and somnogenic (TNF, IL-1 on brain). At higher concentrations, LeTx produces apoptotic death of affected macrophages. Production of LeTx is under control of the regulatory gene product, AtxA (for *a*nthrax *tox*in *a*ctivator), which responds to as yet unknown environmental cues (see below, "Regulation of Cellular Products of Medical Interest"). AtxA is also encoded on pOX1.

2. Edema toxin. The genes encoding the edema toxin (EdTx for *ed*ema *tox*in) are found on a plasmid termed pXO1. EdTx is a binary toxin composed of "protective antigen" (PA) and "edema factor" (EF). PA is responsible for binding of EdTx to "target cells," while EF is responsible for its toxic activity. PA and EF associate only after PA has been oligomerized on the "target" cell surface (see below). EF is a calmodulin-dependent adenylyl cyclase that in-

creases levels of cAMP within the affected cell causing electrolyte and fluid loss. PA binds to cell surface receptors on a variety of cell types. It is activated by furins on the cell surface resulting in oligomerization, which is followed by internalization of EF (as well as lethal factor, see above). Production of EdTx is under control of the regulatory gene product, AtxA (for *anthrax toxin activator*), which responds to as yet unknown environmental cues (see below, "Regulation of Cellular Products of Medical Interest"). AtxA is also encoded on pOX1.

3. Miscellaneous "toxins." Several homologues of proteins shown to be important in virulence of other microorganisms have been discovered in the DNA sequence of the genome of *B. anthracis*. These include genes encoding proteins important in survival within phagolysosomes and on mucosal surfaces (Inh and MprF), escape from phagolysosomes, and phagocytic cells (anthrolysins), and iron acquiring products (Dlp).

   a. Inh and MprF. The genome of *B. anthracis* contains the genes encoding the homologues of Inh (for *immune inhibitor protein*) in *Bacillus cereus*, and MprF (for *multiple peptide resistance factor*) in *Staphylococcus* (see Chapter 27), which have been shown to bestow resistance to defensins (found within the phagolysosome, and in secretions bathing mucosal surfaces) by lysinylation of phospholipids in the bacterial cell membranes.

   b. Anthrolysins. The genome of *B. anthracis* contains the genes encoding anthrolysins (also referred to as *anthralysins*), which are homologues of several phospholipase C and cholesterol-binding cytolysins (anthrolysin O) in other pathogenic bacteria (see also clostridial perfringolysin O, Chapter 36; streptococcal streptolysin O, Chapter 28; listerial listeriolysin O, Chapter 33; and arcanobacterial pyolysin, Chapter 29). The phospholipases are pore-forming cytolysins, and anthrolysin O, also a pore-forming toxin, binds to cholesterol containing rafts in the eukaryotic cell membranes. Though a definitive role has yet to be determined, there is strong evidence that the anthrolysins are responsible for lysis of phagolysosome containing *B. anthraces* followed by the liberation of the microorganism into the cytoplasm of the affected cell, as well as lysis of the cell membrane leading to liberation into the extracellular environment. Note too, that the anthrolysins have hemolytic activity. This activity is demonstrable under conditions not used in the clinical laboratory for isolation and identification of *B. anthracis* (it is typically "nonhemolytic" under clinical laboratory conditions).

   c. Dls. The genome of *B. anthracis* contains the genes encoding Dlp (for *Dps like protein*) which is an iron-binding protein homologue of that found in *Escherichia coli* called Dps (for *DNA protecting protein under starved conditions*).

4. Regulation of the Cellular Products of Medical Interest. There are two proteins, AtxA and AcpA (for *anthrax toxin activator* and *anthrax capsule activator*, respectively) that are produced in response to environmental cues. What these cues are in vivo is unknown. Under the appropriate conditions, however, AtxA increases the production of LeTx, EdTx, and proteins involved in the "escape" from phagolysosomes and macrophages (presumably the anthrolysins). AcpA production is amplified under increased amounts of CO_2 (5% or greater). AtxA acts synergistically with AcpA in this regard.

Growth Characteristics

Bacillus anthracis is a facultative anaerobe and grows on common media between 15°C and 40°C. Colonies reach a diameter of 2 mm or greater in 24 hours at 37°C. Colonies grown in air have a dull surface and wavy margin formed by strands of bacterial chains ("medusa-head"). Cells are nonencapsulated. Colonies grown in greater than 5% carbon dioxide on serum agar containing 0.7% bicarbonate are mucoid and consist of encapsulated bacteria (Fig 30.1).

Sporulation occurs under abundant oxygen, but not while inside the animal. Organisms in infected tissue or fluids exposed to air sporulate after several hours.

Biochemical Activities

Reactions differentiating *B. anthracis* from *B. cereus*, its nearest relative and a frequent contaminant, are summarized in Table 30.1.

Resistance

Vegetative cells in unopened carcasses may survive for up to 1 to 2 weeks, but spores can persist for decades in a stable, dry environment. Spores are killed by autoclaving (121°C/15 min) and dry heat (150°C/60 min), but not by boiling (100°C) for less than 10 minutes. They are not highly susceptible to phenolic, alcoholic, and quaternary ammonium disinfectants. Aldehydes, oxidizing and chlorinating disinfectants, beta-propiolactone, and ethylene oxide are more useful. Heat fixation of smears does not kill spores.

Variability

Colonial and pathogenic variability may be caused by environmental manipulation or spontaneous mutations. Under natural conditions the bacterium is antigenically uniform.

Ecology

Reservoir

The soil is the source of anthrax infection for herbivores. Other species, including humans, are exposed via infected animals and animal products.

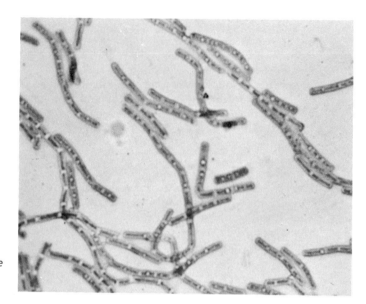

FIGURE 30.1.   Bacillus anthracis *grown on calcium carbonate agar under 20% carbon dioxide for capsule production. McFadyean capsule stain, 1000X.*

Table 30.1.   Differentiation of *Bacillus anthracis* from *Bacillus cereus*[a]

	B. anthracis	B. cereus
Motility	−	d+[b]
Hemolysis (sheep blood agar)	±	+++
Reduction of methylene blue	±	+++
Fermentation of salicin	−	+
Growth at 45°C	−	+
Mucoid colonies on bicarbonate agar under 20% CO_2	+	−
Susceptible to gamma phage	+	−

[a] Modified after Burdon KL. Rapid isolation and identification of *Bacillus anthracis*. Presented at the Symposium on Anthrax in Man, Philadelphia, October 1954.
[b] Different strains exist, with most being motile.

Transmission

The endospore is the "infectious unit." Infection takes place by ingestion of contaminated feed or water or via wound infection and arthropod bites.

Human infections occur via skin wounds (malignant carbuncle), inhalation (e.g., "wool-sorter's disease") and, exceptionally, ingestion, which is also the likely exposure for predators.

Pathogenesis

Mechanisms. Spores are acquired from the environment (e.g., soil, animal products, see above, "Transmission"). They are phagocytosed by macrophages (polymorphonuclear neutrophil leucocytes do not appear to play a role in the disease process). The spores germinate within the phagolysosome compartment. Vegetative bacteria, responding to cues, produce the regulatory proteins AtxA and AcpA, which in turn up regulate the production of

LeTx, EdTx, capsule, and other putative toxins (anthrolysins, iron-acquiring products, defensin-resistance factors). Inh and MprF aid in the survival of *B. anthracis* while it is in the phagolysosome. Anthrolysins permit escape from first the phagolysosome, and then the macrophage itself. Production of LeTx triggers the hyperproduction of cytokines leading to multiple organ dysfunction, shock, and depletion of clotting factors (see Fig 8.1), as well as apoptotic death of affected macrophages. EdTx produces severe fluid and electrolyte imbalances, resulting in localized edema and systemic shock. The capsule discourages further association of the vegetative form with phagocytic cells.

Pathology. In tissue, spores germinate and the vegetative form proliferates, producing gelatinous edema. Inflammatory reactions are minimal. Infection disseminates to reticuloendothelial sites. When these are saturated, a terminal bacteremia occurs, with enormous numbers of organisms in circulation. Postmortem findings are widespread hemorrhages; a black, engorged, friable spleen; tarry, nonclotting blood; and absence of rigor mortis. Bleeding at body orifices is common.

Disease Pattern

Ruminants.   The process described above is typical for the most susceptible species—cattle and sheep. The course, following an incubation period of 1 to 5 days, ranges from a few hours to 2 days. Some animals die without overt clinical signs. Others develop high fever, agalactia, and they may abort. There is congestion of mucous membranes, hematuria, hemorrhagic diarrhea, and often-regional edema. These forms are regularly fatal. Occasional animals show just localized edema or an ulcerative skin lesion and recover.

Horses.   Horses develop colic and diarrhea; edema also occurs, particularly of dependent parts and at the point of infection (e.g., the intestine or the throat) where it may cause death by asphyxiation. Alternatively, the course may be septicemic, as in ruminants.

Swine. In swine, localization in pharyngeal tissues is typical. An ulcerative lesion at the portal of entry is associated with regional lymphadenitis. Obstructive edema may cause death. Ulcerative hemorrhagic enteritis and mesenteric lymphadenitis sometimes occur.

Carnivores. Carnivores (including mink) are rarely affected; when they are, the disease pattern is similar to that in swine, although massive exposure through tainted meat may trigger septicemia.

Humans. In humans, percutaneous introduction of spores causes "malignant carbuncle" (pustule), a local ulcerative inflammatory lesion covered by a black scab (eschar). Possible complications are subcutaneous edema and septicemia. The case fatality rate is 10% to 20%. A shock-like state precedes death. Inhalation anthrax (e.g., "woolsorter's disease") produces pulmonary edema, hemorrhagic pneumonia, and sometimes meningitis. Mortality rates approach 100%.

Epidemiology

A soil rich in calcium and nitrate, with a pH range of 5.0 to 8.0, favors sporulation and bacterial proliferation at temperatures above 15.5°C (60°F), especially after flooding. The geography and seasonality of outbreaks reflect such circumstances. In cattle, sheep, and possibly horses, outbreaks begin with a few cases contracted from the soil. After excretions and postmortem discharges seed the area, secondary cases occur. Floods and industrial effluents from rendering works, tanneries, carpet mills, brush factories, or wherever else carcasses are salvaged may contaminate areas. Bone meal, an animal feed supplement, is a common vehicle in nonendemic areas. Carnivores (mink) are usually exposed via infected meat.

Human exposures are contracted in occupations dealing with animals and animal-derived material such as imported hides, wool, and bone. Anthrax occurring under industrial conditions is often the lethal airborne version.

Immunologic Aspects

Hyperimmune sera can prevent and alleviate disease. Antibacterial and antitoxic factors are thought to be involved. In most species, immunity is directed against the protective antigen. Capsular polypeptide fails to stimulate protective antibody.

Artificial immunization of livestock has utilized mostly modified live spore vaccines. Currently these are derived from avirulent (noncapsulated) mutants. The most widely used is the Sterne vaccine (a strain of *B. anthracis* that lacks the pXO2 plasmid). A cell-free vaccine consisting of concentrated culture filtrate has been used on humans exposed to industrial anthrax. It produces temporary protection against cutaneous infection. Protective antigen, produced by microorganisms into which the encoding gene has been placed, shows promise, as do plants into which the PA encoding gene has been cloned.

Laboratory Diagnosis

Sample Collection

During sample collection, precautions against contamination of the environment are important. Blood may be aspirated from a superficial vessel. Aqueous humor has the added advantage of remoteness from sources of early postmortem contamination. For direct examination, bloody discharges from orifices are sampled.

If the carcass has been opened, spleen material may be collected.

Direct Examination

Blood and organ smears are stained by Gram stain and a capsule stain such as McFadyean's methylene blue. Chains of encapsulated, gram-positive, non–spore-forming rods (see Figs 30.1 and 67.1) suggest *B. anthracis*. Contaminant *Bacillus* spp. are usually not encapsulated and lack the clipped, squared-off appearance of anthrax bacilli. Fluorescent antibody helps in the differentiation.

Isolation and Identification

Bacillus anthracis grows on all common media. Presumptive identification can be made by the characteristics outlined in Table 30.1 and the "string of pearls" test (the characteristic blebbing that occurs when *B. anthracis* contacts penicillin). Definitive identification is by specific bacteriophage (gamma phage). Fluorescent antibody and lectins of appropriate specificities are helpful. *Bacillus cereus* is a commonly encountered contaminate that is similar to *B. anthracis* in appearance. These two microorganisms can be differentiated using various tests (see Table 30.1).

Experimental animals (mice, guinea pigs) are injected subcutaneously with suspect material. Death from anthrax occurs after 24 hours. Lesions include hemorrhages, gelatinous exudate near the inoculation site, and an engorged spleen. The encapsulated agent is demonstrable in blood and tissue.

Immunodiagnosis

Bacillus anthracis antigens can be demonstrated in extracts of contaminated products by a precipitation test using high-titered antiserum (Ascoli test).

Molecular Techniques

Various gene sequences have been targeted in the design of primers that are used to amplify segments of DNA by using the polymerase chain reaction. Examples include portions of the gene encoding the 16S ribosomal RNA, and parts of pOX1 and pOX2.

Treatment, Prevention, and Control

Bacillus anthracis is susceptible to penicillins, chloramphenicol, streptomycin, tetracycline, fluoroquinolones, and erythromycin. Treatment should continue for at least 5 days. In some areas, antiserum is given simultaneously. Antiserum is not available in the United States. In acute anthrax, antimicrobial treatment is often unsuccessful.

Populations at risk are vaccinated annually.

When an outbreak or a case of anthrax has occurred, animal health authorities are notified to supervise control measures. Carcass disposal involves incineration (preferred) or deep burial (>6.5 ft) under a layer of quicklime (anhydrous calcium oxide). Surviving sick animals are isolated and treated. Susceptible stock are vaccinated. The premises are quarantined for 3 weeks subsequent to the last established case. Milk from infected animals is discarded under appropriate precautions. Barns and fences are disinfected with lye (10% sodium hydroxide). Boiling for 30 minutes will kill spores on utensils. Surface soil is cleared of spores by treatment with 3% peracetic acid solution at the rate of 8 liters (2 gal) per square meter. Some other material can be gas-sterilized with ethylene oxide.

Prevention of anthrax exposure through animal products imported from endemic areas requires disinfection of such material as hair and wool by formaldehyde. Bone meal is sterilized by dry heat (150°C/3 h) or steam (115°C/15 min).

BACILLUS CEREUS

Bacillus cereus can cause opportunistic infections, most notably abortions and bovine mastitis. This is often acutely gangrenous and rapidly fatal or destructive to entire quarters. Frequent initiators are udder surgery and intramammary medications.

Bacillus cereus is also responsible for several forms of human food poisoning manifested by diarrhea or vomiting, the former being associated with various foods, the latter mostly with rice. Toxins are involved: an emetic toxin (cereulide) and three secretory enterotoxins (HBL, NHE, T).

31

Corynebacterium

Dwight C. Hirsh   Ernst L. Biberstein

Members of the genus *Corynebacterium* are pleomorphic, non–spore-forming, nonmotile gram-positive bacilli. Corynebacteria occur in packets of parallel ("palisades") or crisscrossing cells ("Chinese letters") that include coccoid, rod, club, and filamentous shapes. This pattern is called *diphtheroid* after the type species *C. diphtheriae*, which is the cause of human diphtheria (Fig 31.1).

Of the more than 30 species included in the genus, two are regularly associated with diseases of veterinary importance: the facultatively intracellular bacterium *C. pseudotuberculosis* (the cause of abscesses in ruminants and horses), and *C. renale* (the cause of disease of the ruminant urogenital tract). Briefly mentioned in this chapter are *Actinobaculum suis* (at one time called *Eubacterium suis* and *Corynebacterium suis*), the cause of urinary tract infection of sows, and *C. auricanis*, associated with otitis externa and dermatitis in dogs.

CORYNEBACTERIUM PSEUDOTUBERCULOSIS

Descriptive Features

Morphology and Staining

Corynebacterium pseudotuberculosis (Fig 31.1) is a typical diphtheroid. The cells range from coccoid to filamentous, 0.5μm by >3.0 μm, are non–acid-fast and nonencapsulated, and often contain granules.

Structure and Composition

The cell wall is typical of gram-positive bacteria, with the addition of meso-diamino-pimelic acid (DAP), arabinogalactan, and mycolic acids (branched chained fatty acids with a chain length for members of the genus *Corynebacterium* of C_{22}–C_{38}). The cell wall contains a high concentration of lipids.

Cellular Products of Medical Interest

Cell Wall. The gram-positive cell wall contains polysaccharides and lipids that are of medical interest. The lipoteichoic acids and peptidoglycan of the gram-positive cell wall interact with macrophage cells resulting in the release of proinflammatory cytokines. The high concentration of lipids contributes to intraphagocytic survival and leukotoxicity.

Exotoxins. *Corynebacterium pseudotuberculosis* produces at least two exotoxins: a phospholipase D and a serine protease.

1. Phospholipase D (PLD). PLD (a sphingomyelinase related to the toxin of the brown recluse spider) is a membrane-active toxin with activity on endothelial cells, lyses erythrocytes by activating complement, produces dermal necrosis, and is lethal to a variety of experimental animals. In vitro, PLD lyses sheep and bovine erythrocytes, inhibits beta toxin of *Staphylococcus aureus* (Fig 31.2) and *Clostridium perfringens* alpha toxin (see Chapter 36), and potentiates hemolytic activity of "*R. equi* factors" (see Chapter 34) (Fig 31.3).
2. Serine Protease. The role played by the serine protease is unknown, but antibodies to it are protective.

Iron Acquisition. *Corynebacterium pseudotuberculosis* possess a cluster of four genes, *fag*A–D (for *Fe* acquisition *g*ene) encoding proteins that are involved with iron uptake. The uptake system is similar to the one used by enterobactin (a catechol-type of siderophore found in members of the family *Enterobacteriaceae*). Deletion of this gene results in a decrease in virulence.

Growth Characteristics

Corynebacterium pseudotuberculosis is a facultative anaerobe. It grows best on media containing blood or serum. At 48 hours on blood agar (35–37°C), colonies are off-white, dull, faintly hemolytic, and about 1 mm in diameter. They can be pushed across the agar without disintegrating (some describe this as pushing a "hockey puck"), and disperse poorly in liquids.

Biochemical Activities

The agent is catalase-positive. Some carbohydrates are fermented.

Resistance

Disinfectants and heat (60°C) kill *C. pseudotuberculosis*, but organisms survive well where moisture and organic matter abound. Penicillins (including ceftiofur), erythromycin, chloramphenicol, lincomycin, tetracycline, enrofloxicin, and trimethoprim-sulfonamide are inhibitory in vitro. The agent is resistant to aminoglycosides.

FIGURE 31.1.   Corynebacterium pseudotuberculosis *in pus from an equine chest abscess. Note club shapes, palisading, "Chinese letter" patterns, pleomorphism. Gram stain, 1000X.*

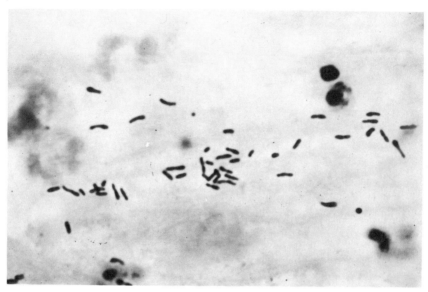

FIGURE 31.2.   *Inhibition of staphylococcal beta toxin (phospholipase C) activity on bovine blood agar by* Corynebacterium pseudotuberculosis *exotoxin (phospholipase D).*

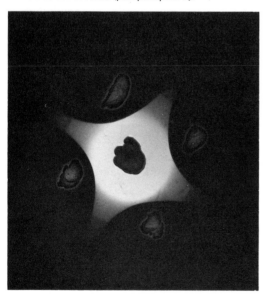

FIGURE 31.3.   *Synergistic hemolysis by* Corynebacterium pseudotuberculosis *(center) and* Rhodococcus equi *(periphery). Hemolysis is maximal where the diffusion zones of the two organisms overlap.*

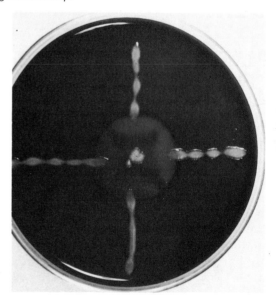

Variability

There are two biotypes that differ biochemically, serologically, and epidemiologically: the "equine biotype," which isolates from equine, and most bovine sources reduce nitrates to nitrites (nitrate-positive); and the "ovine biotype," which isolates from ovine, caprine, and some bovine sources do not (nitrate-negative).

Ecology

Reservoir

The ovine biotype (see above, "Variability") *C. pseudotuberculosis* is found in lesions, the gastrointestinal tract of normal sheep, and the soil of sheep pens. The reservoir of the equine type is not known.

Transmission

Sheep become infected through breaks in the skin (e.g., wounds acquired during shearing), goats probably following trauma related to butting, and horses following breaks in the skin (e.g., biting flies).

Pathogenesis

Mechanisms. Corynebacterium pseudotuberculosis is a facultatively intracellular parasite whose resistance to phagolysosomal disposal is related to its surface lipids.

Virulence is attributed to PLD (and perhaps the serine protease) and cell wall lipids. Both the cell wall and the exotoxins initiate and amplify an inflammatory response. PLD damages neutrophils, macrophages, and endothelial cells.

Following infection, abscesses form but remain localized when exotoxin and/or protease are absent or neutralized.

Pathology. Neutrophilic infiltration and endothelial damage characterize early changes. The lesions are abscesses. Distribution, progress, and appearance differ with species and routes of inoculation, but lymphatic involvement is consistent. The nature of the pus varies largely with age of the lesion, which grossly appears creamy to dry and crumbly ("cheesy"). Old abscesses consist of dead macrophages with peripheral neutrophils, giant cells, and fibrous tissue. Lesions almost always contain just *C. pseudotuberculosis*.

Disease Patterns

Equine. Ulcerative lymphangitis of horses (rarely cattle) ascends the lymphatics, usually of the hind limbs, starting at the fetlock. Its progress toward the inguinal region is marked by swelling and abscesses, which rupture to leave ulcers along its course. Hematogenous dissemination is rare. Areas other than extremities are occasionally affected. Contagious acne (Canadian horse pox) is an uncommon equine folliculitis due to *C. pseudotuberculosis* infection.

Pectoral abscess is also called "pigeon fever" and "breastbone fever." *Corynebacterium pseudotuberculosis* causes abscesses, usually in the muscles of the chest and caudal abdominal region of horses. The infective mechanism is not understood, but the seasonal peak (autumn) and geographic restriction (mainly California) suggest an arthropod vector. The lesions of cutaneous ventral habronemiasis and a midventral dermatitis due to horn fly (*Haematobius irritans*) activity are possible portals of entry. Signs such as swelling, pain, and lameness depend on the location and size of the abscesses. Septicemia occurs rarely, but may result in abortions, renal abscesses, debilitation, and death. The superficial lesions resolve slowly after drainage.

Sheep and Goats. Caseous lymphadenitis of sheep and goats is usually traced to a break in the skin. After introduction, the agent elicits a diffuse inflammation, followed by the formation of an abscess that coalesces and undergoes encapsulation. Inflammatory cells traverse the capsule peripherally, adding a layer of suppuration and a new capsule. Several such cycles give the lesions, especially in sheep, an "onion ring" appearance (Fig 31.4). Old lesions acquire thick, fibrous capsules. The general health is unaffected unless dissemination occurs to other lymph nodes, viscera, or the central nervous system, causing progressive debilitation (thin ewe syndrome). Most forms of infection are chronic.

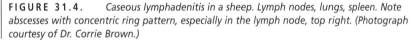

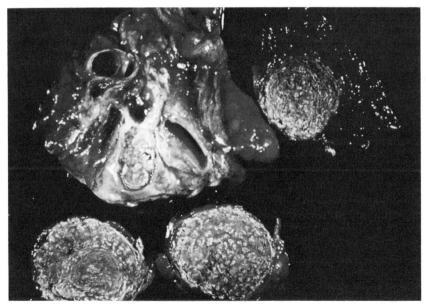

FIGURE 31.4. *Caseous lymphadenitis in a sheep. Lymph nodes, lungs, spleen. Note abscesses with concentric ring pattern, especially in the lymph node, top right. (Photograph courtesy of Dr. Corrie Brown.)*

Cattle. Cattle occasionally develop skin infections with lymph node involvement. Such episodes are often acute and can be epidemic. The most common site is the lateral body wall, suggesting that trauma initiates the disease by producing breaks in the skin.

Human Beings. A relatively benign lymphadenitis may result following infection in human patients. These infections generally follow animal contact (e.g., sheep shearers).

Epidemiology

The current view is that *C. pseudotuberculosis* is an animal parasite and only an accidental soil inhabitant. In sheep, shearing, docking, and dipping are significant factors in the spread of infection. In goats, direct contact, ingestion, and arthropod vectors must be considered. The prevalence of infection increases with age. Caseous lymphadenitis is one of the important bacterial infections of small ruminants.

The hypotheses concerning equine exposure have been considered. No age predilection has been noted. Ulcerative lymphangitis is thought to reflect poor management and is uncommon nowadays. "Pigeon fever" is limited to the far western United States. Annual prevalence varies, seeming highest after a wet winter.

Immunologic Aspects

The roles of antibody and cell-mediated responses that occur during the infectious process are undefined. Antitoxin limits dissemination of abscesses. Caseous lymphadenitis can be progressive, and equine abscesses recur.

Bacterin-toxoid combinations prevent dissemination (not infection) in sheep for at least a year and evoke protective responses in goats and horses. Purified serine protease in adjuvant elicits a protective response in sheep. Mutants constructed by knocking out specific genes that encode products related to virulence (e.g., PLD; aromatic amino acid production) result in a modified live product that elicits antibody and cell-mediated immune responses. These modified live vaccines are effective immunizing products.

Laboratory Diagnosis

Intracellular or extracellular diphtheroid-shaped organisms may be demonstrable in stained direct smears of material from lesions (see Fig 31.1).

Blood agar plates inoculated with abscess material and incubated for 24 to 48 hours (35–37°C) produce small, off-white, faintly hemolytic colonies that can be pushed intact ("hockey puck effect") over the agar surface.

Inhibition of staphylococcal beta toxin (see Fig 31.2) and synergistic hemolysis with *R. equi* (see Fig 31.3) confirm identification of *C. pseudotuberculosis*. Suppression of these reactions by antibody (supplied by serum from an infected animal) forms the basis of serodiagnostic tests (synergistic hemolysis inhibition test).

Other tests utilize agglutination, complement fixation, indirect hemagglutination, hemolysis inhibition, gel diffusion, and toxin neutralization. Members belonging to this genus can be identified following analysis of cell fatty acid analysis (this method has not been as useful in speciation within the genus). Genus- and species-specific primers have been developed to amplify DNA by using the polymerase chain reaction.

Treatment and Control

In sheep and goats, antibiotic treatment is ineffective. Control is aimed at limiting exposure by segregation or culling of affected animals and at scrupulous sanitary care during activities like shearing, dipping, and surgical procedures. Bacterin-toxoid combinations may be helpful in limiting infections. Modified-live products show promise.

Equine abscesses are handled surgically. Prolonged penicillin therapy is used to prevent or treat disseminated disease.

CORYNEBACTERIUM RENALE GROUP

Diphtheroid bacteria, traditionally called *Corynebacterium renale* but actually constituting three species (see below), colonize the lower genital tract of cattle and sometimes sheep. Associated diseases are bovine pyelonephritis and ovine posthitis ("pizzle rot"). At one time, *C. renale* was considered to be comprised of three serotypes (Type I, II, and III). Subsequent DNA analysis revealed that each serotype constituted a separate species: *C. renale* (Type I), *C. cystidis* (Type II), and *C. pilosum* (Type III); together they are referred to as the *C. renale* Group.

Descriptive Features

Morphology and Staining

Members of the *C. renale* Group are typical diphtheroids. The cells range from coccoid to filamentous, are non–acid-fast, nonencapsulated, and often contain granules.

Structure and Composition

The cell wall is typical of gram-positive bacteria, with the addition of meso-diamino-pimelic acid (DAP), arabinogalactan, and mycolic acids (branched chained fatty acids with a chain length for members of the genus *Corynebacterium* of C_{22}–C_{38}).

Cellular Products of Medical Interest

Adhesin. Members of the *C. renale* Group express a fibrillar protein adhesin (pili, fimbriae) on their surfaces.

Cell Wall. The gram-positive cell wall contains polysaccharides, and lipids that are of medical interest. The lipoteichoic acids and peptidoglycan of the gram-positive cell wall interact with macrophage cells resulting in the release of proinflammatory cytokines.

Urease. Members of the *C. renale* Group produce urease, which is associated with the virulence of this group.

Growth Characteristics

Members of the *C. renale* Group are facultative anaerobes capable of growing on most common laboratory media as nonhemolytic, opaque, off-white colonies that develop within 48 hours at 37°C on blood agar.

Biochemical Activities

Members of the *C. renale* Group have impressive urease activity, which is demonstrable in most strains within minutes of contact with its substrate. Glucose is slowly acidified, other carbohydrates variably so. All strains are catalase-positive. Members of the *C. renale* Group produce a protein, renalin, which results in a positive CAMP test (see *Streptococcus agalactiae*, Chapter 28).

Resistance

The agents are not particularly resistant to heat, disinfectants, or antimicrobial agents.

Ecology

Reservoir

Members of the *C. renale* Group inhabit the lower genital tract of cattle and sometimes other ruminants. Occasionally they are implicated in urinary tract disease of sheep, horses, dogs, and nonhuman primates. No human infections are known. Distribution is global.

Transmission

Organisms pass between animals by direct and indirect contact. Many clinical cases are probably endogenous.

Pathogenesis

Adhesin-mediated attachments to urothelium and urea hydrolysis are considered critical in pathogenesis. Urea breakdown with production of ammonia initiates an inflammatory process, high alkalinity in urine (pH 9.0), and suppression of antibacterial defenses, possibly through complement inactivation by ammonia.

Pathology. A chronic inflammatory process successively involves the bladder, ureter(s), renal pelvis, and renal parenchyma in pyelonephritis in cattle. A similar inflammatory response occurs in small ruminants, but is usually localized to the distal urethra.

Disease Patterns

Cattle.   Bovine pyelonephritis is an ascending urinary tract infection, beginning with cystitis, proceeding to ureteritis

and pyelonephritis. Rectal palpation reveals thickened bladder and ureteral walls, distended ureters, and enlarged kidneys with obscured lobulations. Early cases show pollakiuria, hematuria, and increasing degrees of abdominal pain. Chronic infections progress to debilitation and death due to uremia.

Small Ruminants.   Ovine posthitis ("pizzle rot"), the more common form of infection in sheep, is a necrotizing inflammation of the prepuce and adjacent tissues in wethers or rams. Disease develops in the presence of the urealytic agent in an area constantly irrigated with urine. Ammonia is thought to initiate the inflammatory process. A similar condition occurs in goats. Only *C. renale* and *C. pilosum* have been found in ovine posthitis.

Epidemiology

Bovine pyelonephritis is found mostly in cows near parturition, appearing as an opportunistic infection by a commensal organism. Bulls are rarely affected, but are commensal hosts of all three types and the sole commensal source of *C. cystitidis* (Type III).

"Pizzle rot" occurs typically in animals on rich legume pasture that is high in proteins, which increase urea excretion, and estrogens, which cause preputial swelling and urine retention in the sheath.

Immunologic Aspects

No useful immunity develops in the course of the infection. Serum antibody is present and antibody coating (mostly IgG) of bacteria in urine occurs in bovine pyelonephritis (not cystitis).

No immunizing agents exist.

Laboratory Diagnosis

Gross examination of urine may reveal the presence of red blood cells and high alkalinity (pH 9.0). Microscopically, packets of pleomorphic gram-positive diphtheroid rods are seen (Fig 31.5). The agent is readily cultured from sediment. A generous inoculum of colonial growth planted in one spot on a Christensen's urea agar slant will produce an alkaline shift, indicating urea hydrolysis, within minutes of inoculation. A diphtheroid isolate from urine capable of producing this reaction and fermenting glucose probably belongs to the *C. renale* Group.

Treatment and Control

Members of the *C. renale* group are susceptible to penicillin, but antimicrobic therapy is successful only in the early stage of the infection.

Ovine posthitis is treated by surgical care of lesions, local antiseptic applications, dietary restriction, and testosterone administration.

FIGURE 31.5. Corynebacterium renale *in urinary sediment of a cow with pyelonephritis. Note "diphtheroid" configurations, including palisades and "Chinese letters." Gram stain, 3000X.*

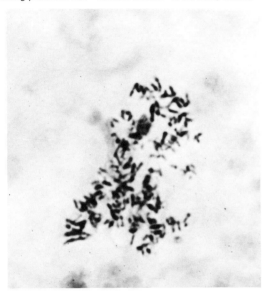

ACTINOBACULUM (EUBACTERIUM, CORYNEBACTERIUM) SUIS

Actinobaculum suis, is an anaerobic diphtheroid, which was first described as *Corynebacterium suis*. It is associated with urinary tract infection of sows (see Fig 74.3). Like bovine pyelonephritis, the disease is an apparently ascending infection by an urealytic diphtheroid agent, limited to females and often related to breeding operations, pregnancy, and parturition. Boars are frequent carriers. The disease is recognized primarily in Britain and continental Europe but also in North America, Australia, and Hong Kong. Treatment is rarely successful.

CORYNEBACTERIUM AURICANIS

Corynebacterium auricanis is a typical diphtheroid isolated from various disease processes in dogs, mainly otitis externa and pyoderma. It has been isolated from the vagina of normal canines.

32 *Erysipelothrix*

RICHARD L. WALKER

Erysipelothrix rhusiopathiae is the type species of the genus and is the species of primary importance. A second species, *E. tonsillarum*, has been described for some strains previously designated as serotypes of *E. rhusiopathiae*. *Erysipelothrix tonsillarum* is biochemically and morphologically similar to *E. rhusiopathiae* but is genetically distinct by DNA-DNA homology. *Erysipelothrix tonsillarum* is only occasionally involved in clinical disease and is nonpathogenic for swine. An additional species, *E. inopinata,* has recently been described.

Erysipelothrix rhusiopathiae can be isolated from a wide variety of environmental settings as well as from the alimentary tract and lymphoid tissue of healthy animals. The disease, erysipelas, occurs in various animal species, with swine the most frequently and severely affected. Other susceptible animals include turkeys and sheep. Clinical presentations include septicemia, a generalized skin form, arthritis, and vegetative endocarditis. In humans, the most commonly recognized form of infection is *erysipeloid*, a self-limiting infection of the skin, usually involving the hand.

Descriptive Features

Morphology and Staining

Erysipelothrix rhusiopathiae is a gram-positive, nonmotile, non–acid-fast, non–spore-forming bacillus, which measures 0.2 to 0.4 μm by 0.8 to 2.5 μm in size. On subculture, rough colonies may develop and produce filamentous forms 60 μm or more in length.

Structure and Composition

Erysipelothrix rhusiopathiae exhibits a cell wall typical of gram-positive organisms. It contains murein of the B 1 delta type. The diamino acid of cell wall peptidoglycan is lysine. The DNA base composition is 36–40 mol% G + C. A polysaccharide capsule has been described and related to virulence. Little is known about the surface proteins of *Erysipelothrix*. A protective protein, SpaA, shares similarities in the C-terminal region with choline-binding proteins of *Streptococcus pneumoniae.*

Cellular Products of Medical Interest

Adhesin. See "Neuraminidase," below.
Capsule. Erysipelothrix rhusiopathiae produces a polysaccharide capsule, which protects the microorganism from phagocytosis.

Cell Wall. The cell wall of the members of this genus is one typical of gram-positive bacteria. The lipoteichoic acids and peptidoglycan of the gram-positive cell wall interact with macrophage cells resulting in the release of proinflammatory cytokines.

Neuraminidase. Neuraminidase production varies directly with virulence of *E. rhusiopathiae.* Cleavage of sialic acid residues on endothelial cells leads to thrombus formation. Neuraminidase is also responsible for adherence to cell surfaces.

Miscellaneous Products. Most strains of *E. rhusiopathiae* produce hyaluronidase and coagulase, but there does not appear to be a relationship between virulence and these enzymes.

Growth Characteristics

Growth is best on media supplemented with glucose. *Erysipelothrix rhusiopathiae* is a facultative anaerobe preferring an environment containing 5% to 10% CO_2. Optimal growth occurs at 30°C to 37°C and at a pH of 7.2 to 7.6; however, it is capable of growing over a temperature range of 5°C to 42°C and a pH range of 6.7 to 9.2.

Resistance

Erysipelothrix rhusiopathiae is resistant to drying and withstands salting, pickling, and smoking. It survives for up to 6 months in swine feces and fish slime at cool temperatures. It is killed by moist heat (55°C) in 15 minutes, but grows in the presence of potassium tellurite (0.05%), crystal violet (0.001%), phenol (0.2%), and sodium azide (0.1%). *Erysipelothrix rhusiopathiae* is susceptible to penicillin, cephalosporin, clindamycin, and fluoroquinolones but is resistant to novobiocin, sulfonamides, and aminoglycosides. Resistance to erythromycin, oleandomycin, oxytetracycline, and dihydrostreptomycin has been observed. Resistance is apparently not plasmid-mediated.

Variability

Common heat-labile antigens account for cross-reactions between strains. Heat-stable, somatic antigens account for the existence of at least 23 serotypes. No relationship between host species and serotype has been recognized. Serotypes 3, 7, 10, 14, 20, 22, and 23 exhibit a higher degree of DNA-DNA homology with the type strain of *E. tonsillarum* than with the type strain of *E. rhusiopathiae*. Cultures dissociate on passage from convex, circular, smooth colonies with entire edges to rough colonies with undulate edges. L-forms have been reported.

Ecology

Reservoir

Erysipelothrix rhusiopathiae is often recovered from sewage effluent, abattoirs, surface slime of fresh and saltwater fish, and soil. It has been recovered from over 50 species of mammals and 30 species of wild birds, and it can be isolated from the tonsils of apparently healthy swine, the most prominent reservoir.

Transmission

Transmission among animals is mostly by ingestion of contaminated material (surface water, fish meal). Wound infections and arthropod bites are other possible routes.

Pathogenesis

Mechanisms. Strains of *E. rhusiopathiae* vary in virulence. Virulent strains produce high levels of neuraminidase, which is considered an important virulence factor in acute septicemic infections. Neuraminidase cleaves sialic acid present on cell surfaces, leading to vascular damage and hyaline thrombus formation. Neuraminidase plays a role in bacterial attachment and invasion into cells. Antibodies to neuraminidase are protective against experimental infections in mice. The presence of capsules has been described and appears to play a role in resistance to phagocytosis by polymorphonuclear leukocytes. Survival inside professional phagocytes is important for pathogenicity. In the presence of normal serum, acapsular mutants do not survive inside phagocytes, whereas encapsulated organisms survive and multiply. In the presence of immune sera, organisms are readily killed.

Partial immunity of the host and low virulence of strains are felt to account for the localized skin form in swine.

Localization of *E. rhusiopathiae* in joints of swine leads to fibrinous exudation and pannus formation. Subsequent damage to the articular cartilage and an immunologic response to persistent bacterial antigens in synovial tissue and chondrocytes are responsible for the chronic articular changes.

Valvular endocarditis, presumably initiated by bacterial emboli and vascular inflammation, results in chronic changes and damage to the heart valves.

Pathology. Pigs dying from acute erysipelas infections exhibit hemorrhages of the gastric serosa, skeletal and cardiac muscles, and renal cortex. Congestion of lungs, liver, spleen, skin, and urinary bladder is frequent. Vascular damage with microthrombi is observed microscopically. A mononuclear infiltrate predominates in most cases. Raised, pink to purple cutaneous lesions result from vasculitis, thrombosis, and ischemia.

In joints, acute synovitis often proceeds to more chronic articular changes. Synovial membranes become hyperplastic and villous and are infiltrated with mononuclear cells. Spreading of granulation tissue over articular surfaces and erosion of articular cartilage may occur. Ankylosis of the joint may be the ultimate outcome. Localization to intervertebral disks leads to a destructive diskospondylitis.

In valvular endocarditis, the mitral valve is most commonly involved with development of large, valvular vegetations due to fibrin deposition and connective tissue proliferation. Emboli may produce infarcts in the spleen and kidney.

In turkeys, the pathology associated with erysipelas infections is generally marked by congestion and intramuscular and subpleural hemorrhages (Fig 32.1). The liver and spleen are often swollen and the abdominal fat is petechiated. A swollen, cyanotic snood and diffuse reddening of the skin are frequent.

Disease Patterns

Swine.   Swine with the septicemic form present with fever, anorexia, depression, vomition, stiff gait, and reluctance to walk. Urticarial lesions in the skin may be palpable before becoming visible. They may be pink or, in severe cases, purplish, especially on the abdomen, thighs, ears, and tail. In severe cases, the skin becomes necrotic and is sloughed. If untreated, this form has a high mortality rate.

In a less severe form of erysipelas in swine, lesions are limited to the skin but may be accompanied by a mild fever. Skin lesions are red to purple rhomboidals— "diamond skin disease." Lesions may progress to necrosis or resolve, leaving a mild scruffiness to the skin. Mortality is seldom associated with this form.

Localization to certain tissues leads to chronic forms, which may occur as sequelae to the acute stages or without previous illness. A vegetative endocarditis is manifested by signs of cardiac insufficiency or sudden death. Arthritis is the other chronic form seen in swine. Signs include limping, stiff gait, and enlargement of the affected joints. Infrequently, sows abort due to *Erysipelothrix* infection.

Birds.   Erysipelas in birds, especially turkeys, is usually a septicemia. Turkeys develop a cyanotic skin, become

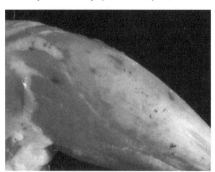

FIGURE 32.1.   *Multiple petechial hemorrhages on the muscle surface of a turkey with an* Erysipelothrix *septicemia.*

droopy, and may subsequently die. A swollen cyanotic snood, if present, is considered almost pathognomonic. Mortality rates range from 2% to 25%. Chronic manifestations include vegetative endocarditis and arthritis. Turkeys with endocarditis appear weak and emaciated or die suddenly without prior signs. Other affected avian species include chickens, chukars, ducks, emus, parrots, peacocks, and pheasants.

Sheep. Polyarthritis is the most common presentation of *E. rhusiopathiae* infection in sheep. Entry is thought to be through the umbilicus or wounds associated with castration, docking, or shearing. Affected animals have a stiff gait and, often, swollen joints. They may have trouble getting up and down. A cutaneous infection following dipping also occurs in sheep. Pneumonia has been described in ewes.

Miscellaneous Species. *Erysipelothrix rhusiopathiae* causes arthritis and endocarditis in dogs. *Erysipelothrix tonsillarum* can also be a canine pathogen and has been isolated from dogs with endocarditis. Septicemia and urticaria due to *E. rhusiopathiae* have been reported in dolphins. Human infections of skin and subcutis are called *erysipeloid* and are seen mostly in animal and fish-handlers. Septicemia, endocarditis, and polyarthritis are rare. Human "erysipelas" is a streptococcal infection.

Epidemiology

Pigs less than 3 months and over 3 years of age are least susceptible. Variable passive and active immunity probably accounts for age-related susceptibility. Predisposing factors include environmental stress, dietary change, fatigue, and subclinical aflatoxicosis.

In turkeys, the male is most frequently infected, possibly through fight wounds. Insemination of hens with contaminated semen is an important source of infection.

Immunologic Aspects

Immune Mechanisms in Pathogenesis

Persistence of antigen in the joint tissue acts as a chronic stimulus for immune reaction and development of arthritis. In addition, an autoimmune process secondary to the erysipelas infection may be responsible for some of the chronic joint changes.

Mechanisms of Resistance and Recovery

Cell-mediated and humoral responses occur, directed at neuraminidase, protective surface protein, and other cell wall components. Serum opsonins apparently play a decisive role. Phagocytosis is carried out primarily by mononuclear phagocytes.

Artificial Immunization

Attenuated vaccines and bacterins have been used for vaccination in swine. While effective against the acute forms, neither type appears to be highly protective against chronic erysipelas. Attenuated vaccines are given orally, parenterally, or, in some countries, by aerosol. Whole-cell bacterins and soluble antigen are given subcutaneously or intramuscularly. Most commercial vaccines are prepared from serotype 2. Certain strains have been refractory to vaccine-induced immunity. Formalin-inactivated, aluminum-hydroxide–absorbed bacterins appear to be effective in turkeys.

Laboratory Diagnosis

Specimens

Specimens are collected from appropriate sites according to signs. Blood cultures from several affected animals are useful in diagnosing septicemia. Necropsy specimens include liver, spleen, kidney, heart, and synovial tissue. Recovery of the organisms from skin lesions is also possible. In the more chronic forms, cultures from joints or heart valves are less successful.

Direct Examination

Specimens are examined by Gram stain for the presence of gram-positive rods. A negative result does not preclude infection.

Culture

Samples are plated on blood agar and incubated at 37°C in 10% CO_2. Colonies are often nonhemolytic and pinpoint after 24 hours' incubation. At 48 hours, a greenish hemolysis may be apparent. *E. rhusiopathiae* is catalase- and oxidase-negative and nonmotile. Inoculation of triple sugar iron agar slants will show an acid reaction and H_2S production along the stab line (Fig 32.2). A "pipe cleaner" type of growth occurs in gelatin stab cultures of rough colonies held at room temperature for 3 to 5 days. *Erysipelothrix rhusiopathiae* does not hydrolyze esculin or urea, reduce nitrates, or produce indole. Fermentative activity is weak. Fermentable carbohydrates include glucose, lactose, levulose, and dextrin. *Erysipelothrix tonsillarum* usually ferments saccharose while *E. rhusiopathiae* does not.

Selective media containing various aminoglycosides and vancomycin may be used to isolate *E. rhusiopathiae* from contaminated tissue. Other selective media contain sodium azide (0.1%) and crystal violet (0.001%).

Serology is of little value in diagnosing erysipelas infections. Polymerase chain reaction assays have been described for diagnostic use.

Treatment, Control, and Prevention

Treatment with penicillin for at least 5 days is effective against the acute forms of erysipelas in swine. Tetracycline and tylosin are alternatives, although resistance to oxytetracycline and some macrolides has been reported. Antiserum (equine origin) is sometimes used in conjunc-

FIGURE 32.2.   *Hydrogen sulfide production by* Erysipelothrix rhusiopathiae *along stab line in triple sugar iron agar slant.*

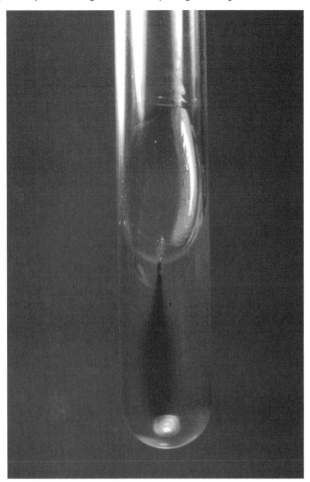

tion with antibiotic therapy. Treatment of chronic forms is less successful.

Good sanitation and nutrition are beneficial in preventing outbreaks. Infected carcasses should be disposed of in a proper manner and replacement animals isolated for at least 30 days before introduction into the herd. Vaccination is recommended in areas with previous history of erysipelas.

In turkeys, penicillin is the drug of choice. Subcutaneous injection of penicillin and vaccination with erysipelas bacterin are recommended, if practicable. Penicillin in the drinking water for 4 to 5 days has been effective in controlling some outbreaks. Injectable erythromycin is a recommended alternative treatment.

Good management practices including preventing fighting among toms, ensuring proper insemination practices of turkey hens, rotating turkey ranges away from contaminated areas, and using vaccination in areas with a history of erysipelas are useful preventive and control measures.

33

Listeria

RICHARD L. WALKER

Listeriosis is an infectious disease affecting humans and many species of animals and birds. Of six recognized species of *Listeria*—*L. innocua, L. ivanovii, L. grayi, L. mono-cytogenes, L. seeligeri,* and *L. welshimeri*—*L. monocytogenes* and *L. ivanovii* are important pathogens. Two subspecies of *Listeria ivanovii* are recognized—subspecies *ivanovii* and subspecies *londoniensis.*

Ruminants are the most frequently affected domestic animals. Principal forms of listeriosis include septicemia, encephalitis, and abortion. In sheep and cattle, abortion is the usual manifestation of *L. ivanovii* infections. Listeriosis occurs worldwide, especially in temperate climates.

Descriptive Features

Morphology and Staining

Listeria are gram-positive, non–acid-fast, non–spore-forming, acapsular rod-shaped bacteria, which measure 0.5 to 2 µm by 0.4 to 0.5 µm.

Structure and Composition

Listeria has a typical gram-positive cell wall. Meso-diaminopimelic acid is the major diamino acid. Cell wall polysaccharides determine O-antigen. Peritrichous flagella and motility are present at 22°C. Motility is poor at 37°C.

Cellular Products of Medical Interest

ActA. ActA protein is important in intracellular movement by actin polymerization and is also thought to play a role in cell trophism (adhesion) and invasion.

Adhesins. See "Internalins," below, and "ActA," above.

Cell Wall. The cell wall of the members of this genus is one typical of gram-positive bacteria. The lipoteichoic acids and peptidoglycan of the gram-positive cell wall interact with macrophage cells resulting in the release of proinflammatory cytokines.

Hemolysin. See "Listeriolysin O," below.

Internalins. Internalins are surface proteins responsible for adhesion and entry into target cells.

Listeriolysin O. LLO (for *l*isteriolysin O) is a pore-forming, cholesterol-dependent cytolysin that is a major virulence determinant for this species (mutants deficient in this protein have reduced virulence; antibodies to it are protective). The major role for LLO is in the release of *L. monocytogenes* from the phagosome into the cytosol following phago-

some acidification, under which conditions LLO is most active. Other roles include lysis of ferritin vacuoles and perhaps its affect on secondary vesicles formed during *L. monocytogenes* movement from cell to cell. LLO is also thought to induce apoptosis in hepatocytes. Ivanolysin, another cholesterol-dependent cytolysin, is the counterpart in *L. ivanovii*. See also, streptococcal streptolysin O, in Chapter 28; clostridial perfringolysin O, in Chapter 36; and arcanobacterial pyolysin, in Chapter 29.

Phospholipases C. Phosphatidylinositol-specific phospholipase C and a lecithinase are important in mediating membrane lysis.

Miscellaneous Products. A bile salt hydrolase may promote survival and persistence of *Listeria* in the intestinal lumen. A protein, termed p60, may play a role in adherence to target cells.

Growth Characteristics

Listeria are facultative anaerobes that grow best under reduced oxygen and increased carbon dioxide concentration. Growth occurs at 4°C to 45°C, with an optimum at 30°C to 37°C. Simple laboratory media support growth, preferably at an alkaline or neutral pH. On sheep blood agar, most strains of *L. monocytogenes* produce a narrow zone of hemolysis. Colonies are usually 1 to 2 mm in diameter and appear blue-green in obliquely transmitted light on solid media such as tryptose agar. Colonies of *L. ivanovii* typically produce a larger and more intense zone of hemolysis.

Listeria tolerates 0.04% potassium tellurite, 0.025% thallium acetate, 3.75% potassium thiocyanate, 10% NaCl, and 40% bile in media. Most strains grow over a pH range of 5.5 to 9.6. It has greater heat tolerance than other non–spore-forming bacteria; however, short-time high-temperature pasteurization is effective at killing *Listeria*.

Variability

There are 16 recognized serovars in the genus *Listeria* based on somatic (O) and flagellar (H) antigens. There is no correlation between serovars and species, except that strains of serovar 5 are *L. ivanovii*. No relationship between serovars and host specificity has been recognized. Various nucleic acid-based methods have been used to further discriminate between *Listeria* strains for epidemiologic analysis and strain tracking purposes. Whole genome sequencing of species within the genus has recently identified numerous genes found in virulent species but absent in avirulent species.

Smooth and rough colonial variants occur. In rough colonies, filaments 20 μm or more in length may be observed. L-forms develop on media containing penicillin and have been isolated from clinical cases in humans.

Ecology

Reservoir

Listeria have a worldwide distribution and have been isolated from soil, silage, sewage effluent, stream water, and over 50 species of animals, including ruminants, swine, horses, dogs, cats, and various species of birds. In some areas, up to 70% of humans are reported to be asymptomatic fecal carriers. Many isolates from environmental samples, previously called *L. monocytogenes*, would now be identified as one of the nonpathogenic species based on current taxonomic criteria.

Transmission

Soil contamination and ingestion of contaminated feed are the primary modes of transmission of *Listeria*. Poor quality silage, with a pH greater than 5.5, is commonly implicated and accounts for listeriosis often being referred to as "silage disease." An asymptomatic carrier can be a source for further contamination of the environment and, therefore, an indirect source of infection.

Pathogenesis

Mechanisms. Exposure to *Listeria* occurs via the oral route. Most *Listeria* are destroyed by gastric acids. Use of antacids and H2 blockers increases survival rate and are considered risk factors for developing listeriosis. Intestinal translocation appears to be a passive process that can involve both intestinal epithelial cells and M-cells overlying Peyer's patches. Internalin, a surface protein, and its interaction with host cell receptors mediate entry. After passage through the intestinal barrier, *Listeria* can be observed in phagocytic cells within the lamina propria. Further dissemination occurs via the bloodstream. Various bacterial ligands have been identified for adherence and include proteins of the multi-gene internalin family, ActA and p60. Nonphagocytic cells can internalize listeriae through a zipper-type mechanism. After internalization, listeriae escape from the phagosome, become associated with actin filaments in the cytoplasm, and propels itself to the cell's plasma membrane via polar assembly of actin filaments (ActA). In this way, it is able to pass to neighboring cells in plasma membrane protrusions and thus avoid host defense mechanisms.

An alternative route of entry has been proposed for CNS infections through damaged oral, nasal, or ocular mucosal surfaces via the neural sheath of peripheral nerve endings, particularly the trigeminal nerve. It is postulated that centripetal migration along cranial nerves leads to infection of the central nervous system. Organisms have been demonstrated in the myelinated axons of the trigeminal nerve and cytoplasm of medullary neurons. The lack of visceral involvement supports a route other than hematogenous although a primary hematogenous route cannot be discounted.

Pathology. With central nervous system involvement, the cerebrospinal fluid may be cloudy and the meningeal vessels congested. Occasionally, areas of softening in the medulla are seen. Histologically, perivascular cuffing predominated by lymphocytes and histiocytes is commonly observed (Fig 33.1). Focal necrosis and microglial and neutrophilic infiltrates are seen in parenchymal tissue. Resulting microabscesses are characterized by liquefaction of the neuropil. The rhomboencephalon area of the brain is most commonly involved.

In the septicemic form, multifocal to diffuse necrosis in the liver (Fig 33.2) and, less frequently, the spleen may be noted.

In the aborted fetus of ruminants, gross lesions are minimal. Autolysis is usually present as a result of the dead fetus being retained for a period before being expelled.

Disease Patterns

Clinical outcome depends on the number of organisms ingested, pathogenic properties of the strain of *Listeria,* and the immune status of the host. Septicemia, encephalitis, and abortion are the major disease forms.

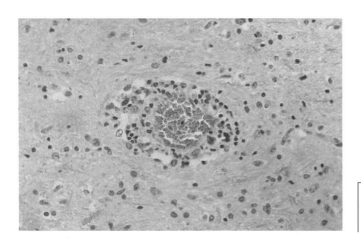

FIGURE 33.1.   *Section from the brain of a cow with the encephalitic form of listeriosis. Perivascular cuffing is present (H&E).* Listeria monocytogenes *was isolated.*

FIGURE 33.2.   *Section of liver from a 5-week-old foal that died of* Listeria monocytogenes *septicemia. A severe, diffuse necrotizing hepatitis was present.*

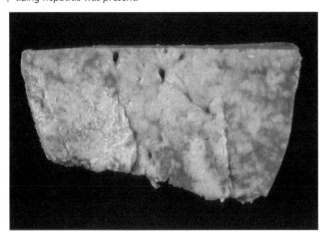

Monogastrics and Neonates.   The septicemic form marked by depression, inappetence, fever, and death is the most common in monogastric animals and in neonates.

Chinchillas.   Chinchillas are particularly susceptible to listerial septicemia.

Horses.   Septicemia in neonates is the most common presentation in horses.

Ruminants.   *Encephalitis.* The encephalitic form, sometimes called *circling disease* is the most common form in ruminants. In cattle, it is subacute to chronic. Signs include depression, anorexia, and tendency to circle in one direction, head pressing or turning of the head to one side, unilateral facial paralysis, and bilateral keratoconjunctivitis. Similar signs are seen in sheep and goats, but the course is more acute and frequently fatal.

Abortion. Abortion is common in ruminants, but also occurs in other species. Abortion is usually late term—after 7 months in cattle and 12 weeks in sheep. The fetus may be macerated or delivered weak and moribund. Retained placenta and metritis may result. Systemic signs are rare in the cow unless the fetus is retained and triggers a fatal septicemia. Although abortion is usually sporadic, abortion rates of up to 10% have been noted. It is uncommon to find the encephalitic form and abortions occurring in a single outbreak.

Conjunctivitis. Conjunctivitis in ruminants without associated abortions has been related to feeding on contaminated silage in elevated feed bunkers.

Humans.   In humans, meningitis is the most common of the three major forms of listeriosis. Still other disease manifestations include infective endocarditis, oculoglandular disease, and dermatitis.

Epidemiology

The widespread distribution of environmental and animal-associated occurrence of *Listeria* makes localizing the source of a particular outbreak difficult. Contaminated silage is a classic source of infection. Other sources include particularly organic refuse (e.g., poultry litter). Stress factors predisposing to clinical disease include nutritional deficiencies, environmental conditions (including elevated iron concentrations), underlying disease, and pregnancy. Cases are usually sporadic and may involve up to 5% of cattle herds or 10% of sheep flocks over a two-month period of time. Listeriosis in animals usually occurs in the winter and spring.

Most human cases occur in urban environments in the summer. There are occasional reports of listerial dermatitis in veterinarians and others after handling tissues from listerial abortions. Otherwise, animals are unlikely direct sources of human infections. Human epidemics have been traced to food sources of animal origin, including milk, Latin-style cheeses, hot dogs, and liver paté. Coleslaw made from cabbage originating on a farm with recent history of ovine listeriosis was the source in one outbreak. In many instances, postprocessing contamination is found to be the source for *Listeria* contamination. Frequently there is also opportunity for selective growth of *L. monocytogenes* to occur during long periods of refrigeration.

Immunologic Aspects

The majority of human cases of listeriosis are associated with immunosuppressed individuals, the elderly, the very young, and pregnant women. Likewise in animals, neonates and pregnant animals are predisposed; however, in some cases a predisposing immunosuppressive factor is not apparent.

As a facultatively intracellular parasite, *Listeria* is primarily contained by cell-mediated responses. Humoral factors may play some limited role in host defense.

No immunizing preparations have met with significant success. Killed preparations have been ineffective, while live attenuated vaccines afforded some protection in sheep.

Laboratory Diagnosis

Specimens

Laboratory diagnosis is based upon isolation of the organism. Spinal fluid, blood, brain tissue, spleen, liver, abomasal fluid, and/or meconium are cultured, depending on signs, lesions, and tissues available.

Direct Examination

A direct smear of infected tissue may reveal numerous gram-positive rods in septicemias and abortions; however, fewer numbers of organisms are typically observed in the encephalitic form (Fig 33.3). Negative findings are inconclusive. Immunohistochemical staining with specific antisera is also useful in diagnosing encephalitic listeriosis.

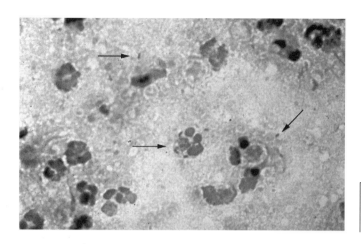

FIGURE 33.3.   *Gram-stained impression smear from the brain stem of a goat with listeriosis. Rare to small numbers of gram-positive, regular rods are present (arrows).*

Isolation

Samples are plated on sheep blood agar and incubated at 35°C in 10% CO_2. Isolation of *L. monocytogenes* from brain tissue may be enhanced by pour plate methods. After the initial isolation attempts, remaining tissue is stored at 4°C for "cold enrichment." Such tissue is subcultured weekly for up to 12 weeks. Cold enrichment is not necessary for isolation from listerial abortions or septicemias.

For samples where contamination is likely, enrichment and the use of selective media (lithium chloride-phenylethanol-moxalactam medium, Oxford medium, or PALCAM *Listeria* selective medium) are advisable. Various DNA-based and antigen capture methods for detection of *Listeria* have been described, especially for detection in food products.

Identification

Typical colonies consisting of gram-positive, regular rods are suggestive. *Listeria* is catalase-positive, motile at 25°C, and hydrolyzes esculin. *Listeria monocytogenes* is CAMP-positive when cross-streaked with a beta-toxin producing *Staphylococcus aureus* on 5% washed sheep blood agar. A similar phenomenon is observed when *L. ivanovii* is cross-streaked with *Rhodococcus equi*. A weak CAMP-like reaction is sometimes observed between *L. monocytogenes* and *R. equi*. (Fig 33.4). In semisolid motility media incubated at room temperature, a characteristic umbrella pattern of motility develops 3 mm to 4 mm below the surface, due to the microaerophilic nature of *Listeria* (Fig 33.5). An end-over-end tumbling type of motility with intermittent periods of quiescence is seen in hanging drop preparations. Acid is produced from glucose and l-rhamnose but not d-mannitol or d-xylose by *L. monocytogenes*. *Listeria ivanovii* differs by fermenting d-xylose but not l-rhamnose. Fluorescent antibody staining or agglutination with specific antiserum is helpful.

Mouse inoculation causes death within 5 days, with necrotic foci present in the liver. This procedure differentiates *L. monocytogenes* from nonpathogenic species of *Listeria*; however, it is rarely necessary for definitive identification.

Immunodiagnosis

Serology has not been useful for diagnosis due to the prevalence of positive titers in apparently normal animals and cross-reactions with *Staphylococcus aureus, Enterococcus faecalis,* and *Arcanobacterium pyogenes*.

FIGURE 33.4.   *Positive CAMP reactions of* Listeria monocytogenes *(LM) with* Staphylococcus aureus *(SA) and* L. ivanovii *(LIV) with* Rhodococcus equi *(RE). A weak reaction is seen between* L. monocytogenes *and* R. equi. *No reaction is detected with* L. innocua *(LIN). The variation in the degree of intensity of hemolysis of* L. monocytogenes *compared to* L. ivanovii *is apparent.* Listeria innocua *is not hemolytic.*

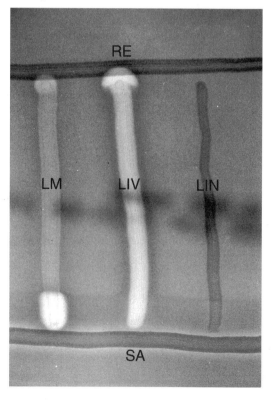

FIGURE 33.5.   *Umbrella-type motility of* Listeria monocytogenes *in semi-solid motility media incubated at room temperature.*

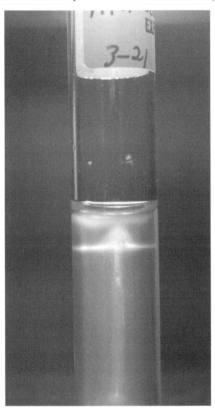

FIGURE 33.5.   *Umbrella-type motility of* Listeria monocytogenes *in semi-solid motility media incubated at room temperature.*

Treatment, Control, and Prevention

Listeria monocytogenes is susceptible in vitro to penicillin, ampicillin, erythromycin, tetracycline, and rifampin. Chlortetracycline and penicillin may be effective in timely treatment of cattle with meningoencephalitis. Treatment of sheep has been less successful. In human patients, the combination of ampicillin and an aminoglycoside (gentamicin) is the primary treatment approach.

Control measures include reduction or elimination of feeding of silage, particularly poor-quality silage. All forms of stress should be minimized. Affected animals should be isolated and infected material disposed of properly.

Vaccination has not proven to be highly successful and may not be warranted due to the sporadic nature of the disease.

34 Rhodococcus

Dwight C. Hirsh   Ernst L. Biberstein

Members of the genus *Rhodococcus* are pleomorphic, non–spore-forming, nonmotile, facultatively anaerobic gram-positive bacilli. There are 15 members of the genus *Rhodococcus*, but only *R. equi* is regularly associated with disease of animals, particularly equine foals, where it causes pneumonia. *Rhodococcus equi* is a facultative intracellular parasite of macrophages.

RHODOCOCCUS EQUI

Descriptive Features

Morphology and Staining

Rhodococcus equi cells measure about 1 μm by up to 5 μm. In smears, strongly gram-positive rods and cocci (some being misshapen appearing as "watermelon seeds") are observed. They are encapsulated and are sometimes weakly acid-fast.

Structure and Composition

The cell walls contain meso-diamino-pimelic acid (DAP), arabinogalactan, and mycolic acids (branched chained fatty acids with a chain length of C_{30}–C_{54} in *Rhodococcus*). The capsules are polysaccharide and form the basis of type specificity within the species.

Cellular Products of Medical Interest

Capsule. In most species of gram-positive bacteria, the role of the capsule is to inhibit attachment to, and ingestion by, phagocytic host cells. *Rhodococcus equi* is a facultative intracellular parasite of macrophages, which implies that either the capsule is not expressed in vivo, or it has a different role than the one mentioned above.

Cell Walls. The gram-positive cell wall contains polysaccharides and lipids that are of medical interest. The lipoteichoic acids and peptidoglycan of the gram-positive cell wall interact with macrophage cells resulting in the release of proinflammatory cytokines.

Virulence-Associated Proteins (Vaps). Virulent strains of *R. equi* possess a large plasmid (85–90 kb) that contains 64 open reading frames. Within this plasmid is a Pathogenicity Island (a cluster of genes encoding virulence determinant(s), an integrase protein, a specific insertion site, and mobility) that contains genes encoding the seven known

Vaps (A–G). Vaps are responsible for the microorganism's ability to survive within phagolysosomes (resistance to acid and reactive oxygen intermediates) of macrophages. Whether Vaps are also responsible for interference with phagolysosome fusion is likely, but unproven. In addition, Vaps down regulate expression of gamma interferon by CD4 and CD8 lymphocytes of foals (but not of adult horses). With increasing age, there is a gradual increase in the ability of CD4 and CD8 lymphocytes to respond and secrete effective levels of gamma interferon in order to mount an effective immune response. Gamma-interferon is responsible for activating macrophages needed to destroy phagocytosed *R. equi*.

Miscellaneous Products. *Rhodococcus equi* produces diffusible "*R. equi* factors" (a phospholipase C and cholesterol oxidase) which lyse erythrocytes in synergy with phospholipase D of *C. pseudotuberculosis* (see Fig 31.3). These factors probably play little if any role in the pathogenesis of disease.

Growth Characteristics

Rhodococcus equi grows aerobically over a wide temperature range (starting at 10°C) on most media. Mucoid colonies ("spit-like") develop in about 48 hours, may reach large sizes (>70 mm), and may acquire a pink pigmentation.

Biochemical Activities

The agent is catalase, urease, and nitrate-positive but does not acidify routine fermentation media.

Resistance

The organism withstands up to 2.5% oxalic acid and 5% sulfuric acid for 60 and 45 minutes, respectively, a feature utilized in attempts at isolation from soil and feces. It is killed at 60°C within an hour.

Rhodococcus equi is susceptible to rifampin, erythromycin, gentamicin, and usually to chloramphenicol, tetracycline, and trimethoprim-sulfonamides, but not to beta-lactam antibiotics. The combination of rifampin and erythromycin is synergistic in vitro, forming the basis for the use of this combination for treating affected animals.

Variability

Twenty-seven capsular types are described. Their prevalence varies somewhat geographically.

Ecology

Reservoir

Rhodococcus equi occurs in soil and animal manure and, perhaps secondarily, the intestine of mammals and birds.

Disease is seen most frequently in horses, less frequently in swine, and rarely in cattle, sheep, goats, cats, humans, crocodilians, koalas, buffalo, and llamas.

Transmission

Infection is acquired by inhalation, ingestion, or congenitally via umbilical or mucous membrane exposure.

Pathogenesis

Mechanisms. After infection, *R. equi* is opsonized by complement components (C3b) generated by the alternate pathway. Opsonized *R. equi* associates with macrophages by way of the Mac-1 complement receptor, and is phagocytosed. *Rhodococcus equi* is a facultative intracellular parasite, surviving in macrophages through suppression of phagolysosomal fusion, and if fusion occurs, survival within the phagolysosome (Vap directed). In adult horses, antibodies to Vaps (from constant subclinical exposure) which presumably "blocks" these proteins from interacting with their targets (CD4 and CD8 lymphocytes), along with CD4 and CD8 lymphocytes that secrete effective levels of gamma interferon, result in activation of macrophages resulting in the elimination of the microorganism. In foals, not only is the level of antibodies to Vaps low during the time of susceptibility (see below), but also the secretion of gamma-interferon is down regulated (by Vaps). The prognosis in foals is related to the amount circulating anti-Vaps antibody (passively acquired from the dam), the number of *R. equi* that reach the lung, and the virulence of the microorganism. The numbers that reach the lung are related to the concentration of the microorganism in the environment, as well as the degree in which the defenses of the lung are compromised (see "Epidemiology," below).

Pathology. The organism is a parasite of macrophages. The lesions of *R. equi* infection are abscesses and granulomas. Elements of granulomatous inflammation include macrophages and giant cells, with neutrophils predominating in the caseopurulent portions.

Disease Patterns

Equine. Pneumonia in foals is the most significant manifestation of infection with *R. equi*. The agent affects mainly foals aged 1 to 6 months and causes a suppurative bronchopneumonia, producing large abscesses in the lungs and hilar lymph nodes. Occasionally there is localization in joints, skin, and spleen. Ulcerative intestinal lesions (gaining entrance via M cells overlying lymphoid nodules) with abscesses in mesenteric lymph nodes are common.

The prognosis varies indirectly with the age of the foal at the time of onset and is poorest for those affected at less than 2 months of age. The case fatality rate exceeds 50%.

Extrapulmonary disease occurs in foals and older horses. Rare uterine infections in mares are possibly related to perinatal exposure of foals.

Swine. *Rhodococcus equi* is recovered from both tuberculosis-like lesions in cervical lymph nodes of swine and normal nodes. Its pathogenic role is disputed.

Humans. *Rhodococcus equi* pneumonia is seen in immunosuppressed individuals. Affected foals are an uncommon source for humans.

Miscellaneous. Sporadic suppurative diseases have been described in diverse mammals. They are commonly localized in lymph nodes, lungs, and uterus. Fulminating bacteremias are observed in crocodiles and American alligators.

Epidemiology

Rhodococcus equi is part of the equine environment. Its concentration varies with the history of equine use of the premises. On problem farms, it is highest in the foaling and rearing areas. Susceptibility coincides with the fading of maternally transmitted immunity and precedes natural immunization by subclinical exposures. Gamma interferon production by CD4 and CD8 lymphocytes from young foals is repressed upon contact with Vaps.

The seasonal peak in summer is attributed to the abundance of 1) susceptible foals and 2) heat and dust, which impose added burdens on respiratory tract defenses.

Human infections are not uniformly linked to animal contact.

Immunologic Aspects

Functional CD4 (T_{H1}) and CD8 T lymphocytes (see Chapter 2) are necessary for protective immunity by "activating" macrophages by way of gamma interferon. Antibody, perhaps to the virulence-associated proteins (Vaps), is needed since maternally derived antibodies as well as passively administered antibody appear to be protective. Thus, both cell-mediated and humoral immunity are important.

Horses past infancy show signs of immunizing exposures to *R. equi,* resulting in humoral and cell-mediated responses. Both appear to be involved in enabling macrophages to kill infecting microorganisms. Antibody, detectable by enzyme-linked immunoadsorbent assay (ELISA), appears at 5 months and is passed by colostrum from mare to foal. Such passively acquired antibody declines by age 6 to 12 weeks, which is roughly the time of the highest prevalence of this disease.

No immunizing products are commercially obtainable. Attempts at immunization with Vap have been disappointing.

Laboratory Diagnosis

Demonstration of *R. equi* in samples from respiratory tracts of pneumonic foals constitutes a diagnosis of *R. equi* pneu-

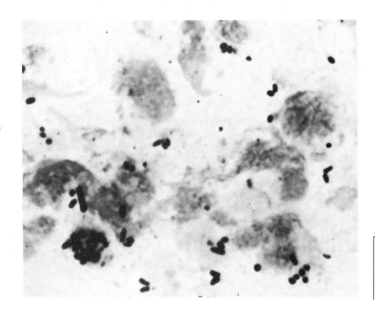

FIGURE 34.1.   Rhodococcus equi *in transtracheal aspirate from a pneumonic foal. Note coccal and bacillary shapes. Cluster on lower left is suggestive of intracellular colonization. Gram stain, 1000X.*

monia. In smears, organisms appear as intracellular and extracellular clusters of gram-positive cocci or rods (Fig 34.1). The identity of typical growth on blood agar (35–37°C) is confirmed morphologically, biochemically, and by synergistic hemolysis (see Fig 31.3). Specific primers are available enabling amplification of DNA by means of the polymerase chain reaction. Such techniques have shown to be useful in diagnosis, as well as detection of the microorganism in the environment.

Treatment and Control

The prognosis in *R. equi* foal pneumonia is always guarded. Chest radiographs give valuable prognostic clues. Animals with nodular or cavitary lung patterns and hilar lymph node enlargement respond less frequently to therapy than those with diffuse alveolar or interstitial reactions. The preferred treatment is erythromycin combined with rifampin.

Preventive measures include colostrum intake, dust control, and removal of foals from contaminated grounds. Prophylactic antimicrobic treatment is justifiable in epidemic situations.

35 Non–Spore-Forming Obligate Anaerobes

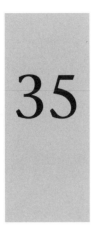

DWIGHT C. HIRSH

Non–spore-forming obligate anaerobes are a component of approximately 33% of bacteriologically positive samples of pyonecrotic material obtained from normally sterile sites of animals. On average, there will be two species of obligate anaerobes admixed with facultative species in samples of such material.

The gram-negative, non–spore-forming obligate anaerobe *Dichelobacter nodosus*, an important contributor to "footrot" of small ruminents, will be discussed separately.

Descriptive Features

Morphology and Staining

The non–spore-forming obligate anaerobes comprise a wide variety of gram-positive and gram-negative bacteria and include rods, cocci, filaments, and spiral organisms.

Cellular Anatomy and Composition

Capsules, flagella, and adhesins (also known as fimbriae or pili) are expressed by some. The cell wall composition is the same as that of their facultative and aerobic counterparts.

Cellular Products of Medical Interest

Capsule. Capsular polysaccharides, if produced, are important for those microorganisms that come in contact with the products and cells of the host. Capsular substances protect the outer membrane from the membrane attack complex of the complement cascade (in the case of gram-negative anaerobes), and inhibit the microbe from attachment to, and ingestion by, phagocytic host cells. The capsule is thought to endow a degree of hydrophilicity relative to the membrane of phagocytic cells. Most capsules are negatively charged, as are the membranes of phagocytic cells. The capsule of the gram-negative anaerobes *Bacteroides fragilis*, pigmented *Prevotella*, and *Porphyromonas* incite an intense inflammatory response.

Cell Wall. The cell walls of the obligate anaerobes are the same as their facultative counterparts. Gram-negative anaerobes produce a typical wall composed of lipopolysaccharide (LPS) and protein. The LPS in the outer membrane

is an important virulence determinant. Not only is the lipid A component toxic (endotoxin), but the length of the side chain in the O-repeat unit hinders the attachment of the membrane attack complex of the complement system to the outer membrane. LPS binds to lipopolysaccharide-binding protein (a serum protein), which in turn transfers it to the blood phase of CD14. The CD14-LPS complex binds to Toll-like receptor proteins (see Chapter 2) on the surface of macrophage cells triggering the release of proinflammatory cytokines. Gram-positive anaerobes produce a cell wall containing lipoteichoic acids and peptidoglycan, which interact with macrophage cells, resulting in the release of proinflammatory cytokines.

Miscellaneous Products. Toxins and metabolic by-products with toxic activity have been demonstrated. These include a cytotoxin produced by *Fusobacterium necrophorum*, an enterotoxin-like entity secreted by *Bacteroides fragilis*, and succinic acid, which is inhibitory to polymorphonuclear neutrophil leukocytes (PMNs). Many produce proteolytic and other enzymes that may play a role in their pathogenic activities.

Growth Characteristics

Obligate anaerobes do not use oxygen as a final electron acceptor; in fact, molecular oxygen is toxic to this group of microbes. When exposed to molecular oxygen, obligate anaerobes form hydrogen peroxide and superoxide anions. These toxic molecules are formed from the interaction of oxygen with various flavoproteins within the bacterial cell. Unlike aerotolerant bacteria, obligate anaerobes do not produce superoxide dismutase, nor do they usually produce catalase enzymes that break down superoxide to oxygen and hydrogen peroxide, or break down hydrogen peroxide to oxygen and water.

Ecology

Reservoir and Transmission

The non–spore-forming obligate anaerobes implicated in pyonecrotic processes are usually part of the normal flora, but they are sometimes transmitted by bites or other trauma involving contaminated fomites.

Pathogenesis

Disease results from the extension of the normal flora (both obligate and facultative anaerobic microorganisms) into a compromised site, either by contamination of a wound with nearby normal flora or from inoculation into tissue with contaminated instruments or teeth. The kinds of microbes found in samples of such material reflect the site of injury or the microbial population of the inoculating agency. Proliferation of anaerobes depends on the establishment of anaerobic conditions by trauma, vascular breakdown, or concurrent infection with (facultative) aerobes.

Anaerobic bacteria cannot live in healthy tissue because they cannot survive in the presence of oxygen. In compromised tissue, inflammatory cells and co-inoculated facultative microorganisms lower the Eh (a measure of oxygen concentration) sufficiently for anaerobes to grow.

Anaerobes elicit inflammatory responses due to components of their cell wall (lipopolysaccharide, gram-negative species; peptidoglycan, gram-positive and gram-negative species). Some anaerobes produce capsules that, due to their chemistry, are potent inducers of abscess formation. There is some evidence that co-inoculated facultative microorganisms induce capsule production by anaerobes.

Synergy occurs between facultative aerobic and anaerobic microorganisms. Aside from triggering capsule formation, facultative species scavenge oxygen, curtail phagocytosis of the anaerobic component, and may produce enzymes (beta-lactamase, for example) that might protect a penicillin-susceptible facultative or obligate anaerobic partner (and vice versa).

The most commonly isolated species of obligate anaerobes are shown in Table 35.1. The most common sites or processes that contain obligate anaerobes are shown in Table 35.2.

Table 35.1.   Most Commonly Isolated Obligate Anaerobes

Gram-Negative Rods	Gram-Positive Cocci	Gram-Positive Rods
Bacteroides	Peptostreptococcus	Clostridium
Prevotella		
Porphyromonas		
Fusobacterium		
Dichelobacter		

Table 35.2.   Relative Frequency of Obligate Anaerobic Bacteria with Respect to Disease Processes

Process	Percentage with Anaerobe
Draining tract	40–50
Abscess	30–40
Pleural effusion	30–40
Pericardial effusion	30–40
Peritoneal effusion	20–30

Association of enterotoxin-secreting strains of *Bacteroides fragilis* with diarrhea in calves, lambs, piglets, and infant rabbits has been described.

Immunologic Aspects

Immune responses play a minor part in resolving the pyonecrotic processes involving obligate anaerobes.

Laboratory Diagnosis

Sample Collection

Anaerobic culture is time-consuming and expensive and should be used only when it holds a reasonable promise of supplying useful information. Material obtained from sites that possess a normal anaerobic flora (feces, oral cavity, vagina) is not usually cultured anaerobically. Routine anaerobic culture of urine specimens or ear, conjunctival, or nasal swabs is very rarely justified. Suppurative and necrotic processes are the most promising sources of clinically significant anaerobic bacteria.

Samples of fluids for anaerobic culture are collected in vessels containing little if any molecular oxygen. The easiest way is to collect the sample directly into a syringe and expel all the air. Materials collected onto swabs or bronchial brushes must be placed in culture immediately or into an anaerobic environment (anaerobic transport medium). Refrigeration is detrimental to recovery of anaerobic bacteria; thus, samples should not be placed at temperatures less than 4°C. However, most samples that contain obligate anaerobes contain facultative species as well. Most facultative microorganisms grow in samples held at 25°C but poorly at 15°C (a temperature harmless to obligate anaerobes).

Direct Examination

Examination of stained smears prepared directly from the collected material may give valuable clues regarding the presence of anaerobic bacteria. Many obligate anaerobes have typical, unique morphologies: rods are usually narrow and thread-like in appearance; some having pointed ends or bulges. Most of the gram-negative species stain poorly with the saffranine used in the gram stain (thus will be pale staining in gram-stained smears). The material may have a very repugnant odor if anaerobes are present, whereas material without obligate anaerobes is usually not especially malodorous.

Isolation

Successful isolation depends on the care taken by the laboratory in shielding the bacteria from oxygen. If the sample is not processed immediately after collection, it must be held in a container free from oxygen, usually a container into which oxygen-free gas (e.g., O_2-free carbon dioxide) is flowing. The sample is plated onto a blood-containing medium (usually one with a brucella agar base) that has been freshly made and stored in an anaerobic environment (a special selective medium for isolating *B. fragilis* from feces contains polymyxin B, trichlosan, novobiocin, and nalidixic acid). After the plate has been inoculated, it is placed into an anaerobic environment and incubated at 37°C. The anaerobic environment is conveniently established by the interaction of a hydrogen-containing gas with the oxygen found in air in the presence of a palladium catalyst in a closed container, such as in an anaerobic jar or in a glove box. A major advantage of an anaerobic glove box with a built-in incubator is that inoculated plates can be examined at any time without being exposed to oxygen.

Most obligate anaerobes grow slowly, especially during the early stages, and plates are not examined for the first 48 hours unless they can be examined in an O_2-free environment (e.g., in a glove box). Since facultative species will grow anaerobically, colonies growing in an anaerobic environment must be tested for aerotolerance.

Identification

After an isolate has been shown to be an obligate anaerobe, the genus to which it belongs is determined by shape, gram-staining characteristics, growth in the presence of various antibiotics, and metabolic by-products formed from an assortment of substrates, as determined by liquid-gas chromatography. Reactions in prereduced anaerobically sterilized media containing different substrates help determine the species. Miniaturized identification systems are commercially available. Gas chromatographic analysis of cell fatty acids is sometimes used to identify an isolate.

Treatment, Control, and Prevention

Treatment of infectious processes that contain an anaerobic component most importantly involve drainage and the use of antimicrobial agents.

Susceptibility data are usually not available for at least 48 to 72 hours after the sample is collected. Prior to this time, if the presence of obligate anaerobes is suggested by the clinical presentation, direct smear, and other circumstances (odor), one of the following can be used: penicillin (ampicillin, amoxicillin), chloramphenicoll, tetracycline, metronidazole, and clindamycin. Though most anaerobes will test "susceptible" to trimethoprim-sulfonamides in vitro, this combination has unpredictable activity in vivo due to the presence of thymidine in necrotic material. The obligate anaerobes are resistant to all of the aminoglycoside antimicrobial agents as well as to most of the fluoroquinolones (trovafloxacin is the exception). Approximately 10% to 20% of the isolates, usually members of the *B. fragilis* group, will be resistant to the penicillins (penicillin G, ampicillin, amoxicillin) and first- and second-generation cephalosporins due to the production of a cephalosporinase, and often to tetracycline as well. Resistant isolates are susceptible to clavulanic acid-amoxicillin, clindamycin, metronidazole, and chloramphenicoll. Antimicrobial therapy should be aimed at both the facultative and the obligate anaerobic microorganisms. Between 70% and 80% of pyonecrotic processes containing an obligate

Table 35.3.   Facultative Microorganisms Found in Infectious Processes Containing Obligate Anaerobes

Animal Species	Facultative Microorganism
Dogs/cats	*Pasteurella*, enterics[a]
Horse	Beta-hemolytic *Streptococcus*, enterics[a]
Ruminant	*Arcanobacterium pyogenes*, enterics[a]

[a]*Escherichia coli* is the most common isolate.

anaerobe will also contain a facultative one. The most common are shown in Table 35.3.

DICHELOBACTER NODOSUS

Descriptive Features

Structure

Footrot is a contagious infectious disease affecting the epidermal portions of the foot of sheep and goats. The fully developed lesions cause a crippling lameness. Two gram-negative non–spore-forming anaerobes are primarily implicated: *Dichelobacter nodosus* and *Fusobacterium necrophorum*.

Dichelobacter nodosus, the specific cause, is a nonmotile rod measuring 2 to 10 μm by 0.5 to 1.0 μm. In smears from lesions, its ends are commonly swollen (Fig 35.1). Pili (Type 4, as are those of *Moraxella bovis*, *Neisseria gonorrheae*, *Pasteurella multocida*, and *Pseudomonas aeruginosa*) act as adhesins and confer twitching motility.

Cellular Products of Medical Interest

Adhesins (Pili, Fimbria). Adhesins (pili or fimbria) are involved with adherence of *D. nodosus* to interdigital epidermis that has been damaged by the proteases secreted by *Fusobacterium necrophorum*.

Cell Wall. The cell wall of the members of this genus is one typical of gram negatives. The lipopolysaccharide (LPS) in the outer membrane is an important virulence determinant. Not only is the lipid A component toxic (endotoxin), but the length of the side chain in the O-repeat unit hinders the attachment of the membrane attack complex of the complement system to the outer membrane. LPS binds to lipopolysaccharide-binding protein (a serum protein), which in turn transfers it to the blood phase of CD14. The CD14-LPS complex binds to Toll-like receptor proteins (see Chapter 2) on the surface of macrophage cells triggering the release of proinflammatory cytokines.

Proteases. Several proteolytic enzymes (serine and basic proteases) are secreted by *D. nodosus*. The proteases are regulated by the products of two Pathogenicity Islands (a cluster of genes encoding virulence determinant(s), an integrase protein, a specific insertion site, and mobility) named Vap (for *v*irulence-*a*ssociated *p*roteins), and Vrl (for *v*irulence-*r*elated *l*ocus).

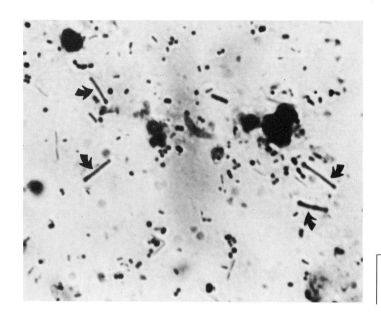

FIGURE 35.1.   *Exudate from ovine footrot. Mixture of bacterial species, with* Dichelobacter nodosus *recognizable as large rods with swollen ends: "dumbbells" (arrows). Gram stain, 1000X.*

Growth Characteristics

Dichelobacter nodosus is a strict anaerobe requiring added carbon dioxide and a rich medium, preferably containing protein. After several days, smooth colonies about 1 mm in diameter are produced.

Resistance

Dichelobacter nodosus survives in the environment 2 to 3 days and is killed by disinfectants and many antibiotics.

Variability

Colonial variation and virulence are related to abundance of piliation. Virulence also varies with proteolytic activities of strains. Ten major serogroups (A–I, M) are recognized, and are based upon differences in the antigenic constitution of the fimbrial adhesins. Examination of the organization of the genes encoding these adhesins reveals that adhesins belonging to serogroups A, B, C, E, F, G, I, and M are organized differently than those encoding adhesins belonging to serogroups D and H. Strains expressing adhesins of the former are termed "class I" and the later, "class II."

Ecology

Reservoir

The significant reservoir is the infected foot of sheep or goats. Cattle and swine strains are of low virulence.

Transmission

Transmission is by direct or indirect contact. The brief environmental survival time of the agent requires prompt colonization of new hosts.

Pathogenesis

Pathogenic mechanisms include the pili-mediated attachment to host cells, proteolytic activity, and synergy with *F. necrophorum*, to which *D. nodosus* supplies growth factors.

Disease Patterns

The sequence of events is typically as follows:

1. The interdigital epidermis is damaged, most commonly by maceration due to persistent soaking.
2. *Fusobacterium necrophorum*, a constituent of the fecal flora, infects the macerated skin and produces superficial inflammation, hyperkeratosis, parakeratosis, and necrosis (ovine interdigital dermatitis [OID]).
3. *Dichelobacter nodosus* from a footrot lesion colonizes (with the aid of its pili) and proliferates in the lesion initiated by *F. necrophorum*, producing interdigital swelling. Invasion of epidermal structures begins at the medial aspect of the claw and, probably with the help of bacterial proteases, advances to the epidermal matrix of the hoof, eventually separating it from the underlying dermal tissues ("underrunning").

Secondary invaders help maintain or aggravate the process. The result is extreme lameness, which becomes immobilizing when two or more feet are involved. Affected animals may starve.

Epidemiology

Footrot occurs on all continents. It is most serious in regions with a mild climate and periods of abundant rainfall (>20 inches [500 mm]). Dissemination of *D. nodosus* essentially ceases at ambient mean temperatures of less than 50°F (10°C), and footrot does not occur in arid regions and improves during dry periods in endemic areas. All ages of animals beyond nursing stages are susceptible, but genetic differences in susceptibility exist. Fine wool breeds are most severely affected. The agent is eliminated from contaminated pastures within 2 weeks.

Immunologic Aspects

Resistance is related to circulating antifimbrial antibody; it is serogroup-specific. Natural infection produces no immunity, but oil-adjuvant vaccines of appropriate specificity induce temporary protection and improve existing cases.

Laboratory Diagnosis

Diagnosis is usually clinical. Direct smears from the lesion reveal stout rods with terminal swellings (see Fig 35.1). Other microorganisms are usually also present, some of which—small gram-negative rods—often coaggregate around *D. nodosus.* Immunofluorescence confirms identification.

Culture (on selective media) is not routinely done.

Molecular techniques utilizing the polymerase chain reaction together with DNA primers specific for *D. nodosus* (e.g., the genes encoding the fimbrial adhesins) have been described for demonstration of the bacterium in samples obtained from infected feet as well as identification of isolates grown on artificial media.

Treatment and Control

Treatment begins with removal and exposure of diseased tissue by hoof trimming, followed by topical application of disinfectants or antibiotics, such as repeated treatment with 5% to 10% formalin, 5% copper sulfate, 10% to 20% zinc sulfate, or 5% tetracycline tincture. Use of chloramphenicoll (10%) is not permissible in the United States. Formalin, copper sulfate, and zinc sulfate are used in foot baths. Three 1-hour 20% zinc sulfate soaks at weekly intervals have proven effective without foot paring.

Systemic treatment with large doses of penicillin and streptomycin has been successful in the absence of topical therapy.

Control is achieved by a combination of repeated examination, vaccination, treatment of active cases, and segregation of active cases from the healthy flock. Care must be taken not to add infected animals to the flock. Contaminated lots should not be restocked for 2 weeks. Control programs should be instituted during dry weather.

Footrot of Cattle (Infectious Pododermatitis: Fouls)

Dichelobacter nodosus combined with *Fusobacterium necrophorum* can cause a coronary and interdigital dermatitis in cattle.

What is often called *bovine footrot* is etiologically and pathologically distinct from the ovine disease. The chief agent is *F. necrophorum.* Other bacteria, particularly pigmented anaerobic rods (*Prevotella*) are implicated. The process involves the dermis and subcutis, and produces a diffuse, often febrile necrotizing cellulitis, which may extend to joints or spread hematogenously. Sinus tracts develop in the foot region.

Injury, irritation, and maceration are likely predisposing factors. Their presence, rather than transmissibility, probably determines disease prevalence.

Cases are treated topically and by hoof trimming. Uncomplicated cases respond to systemic sulfonamides or tetracycline.

36 | *Clostridium*

DWIGHT C. HIRSH   ERNST L. BIBERSTEIN

Members of the genus *Clostridium* are gram-positive, spore-forming, anaerobic rods. In this chapter the diseases produced by members of this genus (Table 36.1) will be discussed under two categories: the invasive diseases (including the enterotoxemias and diarrheas) produced by *C. perfringens, C. novyi, C. haemolyticum, C. septicum, C. chauvoei, C. difficile,* and *C. piliforme*; and the noninvasive diseases produced by *C. botulinum,* and *C. tetani.* Briefly discussed will be *C. sordellii, C. colinum*, and *C. spiroforme*.

Descriptive Features

Morphology and Staining

Members of the genus *Clostridium* are gram-positive rods measuring 0.2 to 4 μm by up to 20 μm. Location and shape of endospores are consistent within a species.

Structure and Composition

Little of medical relevance is known of the ultrastructure and composition of clostridia. A surface-associated structure characterized by orderly paracrystalline protein arrays (S layer) is found in the cell wall of *C. difficile*. The role played by the S layer proteins is unknown. Some clostridia have been shown to produce pili or fimbriae (*C. difficile*), and others produce adhesive structures, presumably cell wall proteins. Considerable cellular intraspecific antigenic diversity and interspecific cross-reactivity exist but are of less interest than the serologic properties of toxins (see under respective species). Those that are motile have peritrichous flagella. Of pathogenic species, *C. perfringens* and *C. difficile* are encapsulated.

Growth Characteristics

Strictness of anaerobic requirements varies among clostridial species. In addition to an anaerobic environment, clostridia prefer 2% to 10% CO_2 in their atmosphere.

Most pathogenic clostridia require complex media including amino acids, carbohydrates, and vitamins. Blood or serum is beneficial. A near-neutral pH and temperature of 37°C are optimal.

Growth is usually visible within 1 or 2 days. Colonies are often irregular in shape and contour. Several clostridia swarm across moist agar media without forming colonies. Most clostridia produce hemolysis when grown on blood agar.

In liquid media, clostridia often grow in air provided a reducing agent is present (cooked meat pieces, thioglycolate), though growth occurs only in reduced portions of the medium.

Biochemical Activities

Clostridial cultures typically emit putrid odors due to products of peptide catabolism, which is a common mode of energy production.

Most clostridia attack carbohydrates, proteins, lipids, or nucleic acids. Biochemical reactions and their end products furnish a basis for species identification.

Resistance

The vegetative form is as susceptible to environmental stresses and disinfectants as other bacteria. Endospores impart resistance to drying, heat, irradiation, and disinfectants.

THE INVASIVE CLOSTRIDIA

CLOSTRIDIUM PERFRINGENS

Descriptive Features

Clostridium perfringens is a gram-positive, spore-forming, nonmotile, encapsulated obligately anaerobic rod that produces a variety of toxins (see below, "Cellular Products of Medical Interest"). Four of these toxins are used to "type" members of this species. There are five types designated A through E (Table 36.2).

Clostridium perfringens is associated with wound infections (gas gangrene), enterotoxemias in ruminants, and diarrhea in a variety of species.

Cellular Products of Medical Interest

Adhesins. *Clostridium perfringens* possesses a number of chromosomal genes whose sequences are similar to those encoding adhesins in other bacteria. These include genes encoding two fibronectin-binding proteins, and a protein responsible for binding collagen. Whether these sequences truly encode functional adhesins remains to be demonstrated.

Table 36.1.   Selected Members of the Genus *Clostridium* and Their Usual Source or Associated Condition

Species	Usual Source or Associated Condition
Clostridium botulinum	Botulism
C. chauvoei	Blackleg in ruminants, pigs
C. colinum	Enteritis and hepatitis in birds
C. difficile	Antibiotic/stress-induced diarrhea in horses, dogs, cats
C. haemolyticum	Bacillary hemoglobinuria in ruminants
C. novyi	Gas gangrene; big head in rams; black disease in ruminants
C. perfringens	Gas gangrene; enterotoxemia in ruminants, pigs, horses; necrotic enteritis in chickens; lamb dysentery; struck in sheep; pulpy kidney disease in ruminants; diarrhea in dogs, cats, and human patients
C. piliforme	Tyzzer's disease
C. septicum	Malignant edema in ruminants, pigs; braxy in sheep; necrotic enteritis in chickens
C. sordellii	Myositis and hepatitis in ruminants, horses
C. spiroforme	Mucoid enteritis of rabbits; antibiotic-induced enteritis in rabbits, guinea pigs, foals; enterocolitis in foals
C. tetani	Tetanus

Table 36.2.   *Clostridium perfringens* Types in Animal Disease

Type	Major Toxin Present			
	Alpha	Beta	Epsilon	Iota
A	+	−	−	−
B	+	+	+	−
C	+	+	−	−
D	+	−	+	−
E	+	−	−	+

Type E strains often present in cattle and sheep intestines, but are rarely implicated in enterotoxemia.

Capsule. The role of the capsule in disease produced by *C. perfringens* is undefined, but it probably acts as a deterrent to phagocytosis. Encapsulation is an important virulence determinant in wounds (e.g., gas gangrene), but probably not in the intestinal canal (e.g., enterotoxemias, diarrheal diseases).

Toxins. Clostridium perfringens produces a variety of protein toxins. Most, if not all are regulated by a global regulatory system ("VirR/VirS," see below):

1. Alpha toxin. Alpha toxin (Cpa or Plc for *C. perfringens* *a*lpha toxin or *p*hospholipase *C*, respectively) is produced by all *C. perfringens*. It is a phospholipase C (a lecithinase) that hydrolyzes phosphatidylcholine and sphingomyelin, both of which are constituents of host cell membranes. Alpha toxin also displays the "hot-cold" lysis phenomenon (see staphylococcal beta toxin, Chapter 27).

2. Beta toxin. The genes encoding beta toxin (Cpb for *C. perfringens* *b*eta toxin) are located on a plasmid. Beta toxin is a pore-forming toxin, which damages host target cells (intestinal epithelial cells, endothelial cells). In addition, beta toxin affects nervous tissue by influencing the distribution of calcium ions across their membranes thereby disrupting normal nerve conduction. It is susceptible to the proteolytic activity of trypsin.

3. Beta$_2$ toxin. The beta$_2$ toxin (Cpb2 for *C. perfringens* *b*eta$_2$ toxin) is newly described, but the role this toxin plays in associated disease is not well characterized. The gene encoding this toxin is sometimes located on a plasmid. Its mechanism of action is unknown. It is produced by *C. perfringens* isolated from the intestinal contents of pigs with necrotic enteritis, horses with enterocolitis, and dogs with diarrhea (beta$_2$ toxin-producing strains are isolated less often from clinically normal animals).

4. Epsilon toxin. The gene encoding epsilon toxin (Etx for *e*psilon *t*oxin) is located on a plasmid. Epsilon toxin "targets" lipid (cholesterol and sphingolipids) rafts found in eukaryotic cell membranes, though the toxin concentrates in brain and kidney. It is a permease that acts by affecting the cellular cytoskeleton resulting in an increase in the permeability of epithelial and endothelial cells (especially the microvasculature of the brain, leading to leakage of toxin into that organ). Etx is secreted as a protoxin that is activated by proteolytic enzymes.

5. Iota toxin. Iota toxin (Itx for *i*ota *t*oxin) is a binary toxin composed of a binding portion (Ib) that binds the toxin to target epithelial cells, and an enzymatically active portion (Ia). After the toxin binds to specific receptors on the cell surface, Ia gains entry into the cytoplasm. Though it is not clear precisely how entry occurs, it seems that a pore (composed of Ib) is formed in the cell membrane through which Ia traverses. Ia is an ADP-ribosylating toxin that ribosylates actin within the

host cell, resulting in disorganization of the cellular cytoskeleton and death of the affected cell.

6. Kappa toxin. Kappa toxin (Col for *col*lagenase) is a collagenase. Col is thought to aid spread of clostridial cells through the tissue.
7. Mu toxin. Mu toxin (Nag for *N-a*cetylgalactosaminidase) is a hyaluronidase. Nag is thought to aid spread of clostridial cells through the tissue.
8. Theta toxin. See perfringolysin O, below.
9. Sialidase. Sialidase (*neurami*nidase, or Nan) removes sialic acid residues from glycoconjugates on cell walls of eukaryotic cells resulting in disruptions of the intercellular matrix.
10. Hemolysins. A number of hemolysins are produced by *C. perfringens*. Their role in disease is unknown.
11. Enterotoxin. The genes encoding *C. perfringens* enterotoxin (Cpe for *C. perfringens enterotoxin*) are either chromosome- (isolates from human cases of food-related gastrointestinal disease), or plasmid-based (isolates from dogs with diarrhea, or from human patients with non–food-related gastrointestinal disease). Enterotoxin is produced during sporulation of *cpe*-containing *C. perfringens* (less than 10% of Type A strains, the strains in which Cpe is most commonly found). When the endospore is released, enterotoxin is also released into the surrounding milieu. Enterotoxin is a bifunctional toxin, first forming a pore in the apical portion of small intestinal epithelial cells resulting in fluid and electrolyte abnormalities, as well as providing access to tight junction proteins (specifically claudins and occuldins). Interactions of Cpe with tight junction proteins result in further losses in control of fluid and electrolytes.
12. Perfringolysin O (also known as theta toxin). Perfringolysin O (Pfo for *perfringolysin O*) is a cholesterol-binding cytolysin (see also novyilysin and chauveolysin, below; streptococcal streptolysin O, Chapter 28; listerial listeriolysin O, Chapter 33; and arcanobacterial pyolysin, Chapter 29). Pfo binds to cholesterol-containing rafts in the eukaryotic cell membrane, and forms a pore, which results in the death of the cell. In addition, Pfo is responsible for the lysis of membranes enclosing *C. perfringens*-inside of phagolysosomes, resulting in their escape into the cytoplasm of the phagocytic cell.

Regulation of Toxin Genes. Clostridium perfringens globally regulates its toxin production by the two-component regulatory system, VirR/VirS. VirS is a histidine kinase that acts as a "sensor" of environmental cues resulting in autophosphorylation of one of its histidine residues. This phosphate is then serially transferred to an aspartate residue, then to another histidine before being used to phosphorylate VirR, the "regulator." Phosphorylated VirR is a trascriptional activator of the genes encoding the products mentioned above. What environmental cues are "sensed" by *C. perfringens,* is unknown, but the composition of the intestinal contents appears to play an important role in the pathogenesis of the enterotoxemias (see below, "Epidemiology").

Ecology

Reservoir

Clostridium perfringens, Type A, occurs in intestinal tracts of humans and other animals and in most soils. Types B, C, D, and E are found mostly in the intestinal tracts of animals, and their survival in soil is variable.

Transmission

Transmission is by ingestion and wound infection.

Pathogenesis and Disease Patterns

Clostridium perfringens has the following disease patterns:

1. *Wound Infections (Gas Gangrene). Clostridium perfringens* Type A, alone or with other bacteria, causes anaerobic cellulitis and gas gangrene following inoculation into a normally sterile site. The membrane active toxins (alpha and perfringolysin O) account for the tissue destruction. Spread of the process is aided by collagenase (kappa toxin or Col), sialidase (Nan), and hyaluronidase (Mu toxin or Nag). Encapsulated *C. perfringens* resist phagocytosis. Those that are phagocytosed escape the phagolysosome by secretion of perfringolysin O. The process is a necrotizing cellulitis or myonecrosis with edema, hemorrhage, emphysema, and a febrile, often fatal, toxemia. This type of *C. perfringens* infection in animals is rare, but when it occurs it is associated most often with injection sites deep in muscle (mainly horses).
2. *Enterotoxemias.* Most animal diseases due to *C. perfringens* are intestinal and involve Types A, B, C, or D (rarely E):
   a. *Clostridium perfringens* Type A enterotoxemia has been implicated in outbreaks of gastritis and hemolytic disease of ruminants (enterotoxemic jaundice, the "yellows," "yellow lamb disease"); in hemorrhagic enteritis in cattle, horses, and infant alpacas; necrotic enteritis in poultry; food poisoning in humans; and antibiotic-associated diarrhea in humans; and is associated with diarrhea in dogs and cats (see below). Tissue destruction is probably due to the membrane active toxins (alpha and perfringolysin O), and the toxins that affect connective tissue (collagenase, hyaluronidase, and sialidase). Diarrheal disease in human patients and in dogs and cats is associated with Type A strains that contain the gene encoding Cpe (enterotoxin).
   b. *Clostridium perfringens* Type B enterotoxemia is an "Old World" disease. *Clostridium perfringens* Type B causes "lamb dysentery" in newborn lambs. Occasionally foals, calves, and mature sheep and goats are affected. Beta toxin is considered the principal factor producing hemorrhagic enteritis affecting the small intestine. Its trypsin susceptibility explains in part the predilection of

the disease for the newborn (colostrum contains antitrypsin substances). The signs are depression, anorexia, abdominal pain, and diarrhea. The course is rapid, with mortality rates approaching 100%. A chronic form occurs in older animals. The characteristic intestinal lesion is hemorrhagic enteritis. Extraintestinal lesions include congestion, edema, serosal effusions, and hemorrhages in various organs. The signs and pathology associated with this disease are due to the action of the membrane active toxins (alpha, beta, epsilon, and perfringolysin O), as well as those products that destroy the connective tissue components. Epsilon toxin, being a permease, increases intestinal permeability, ensuring its absorption into the circulation where it affects vascular endothelium, leading to fluid loss and edema, as well as damage to kidney function. Beta and epsilon toxins also affect the nervous system, and the severe depression, lack of response to corrective therapy, and high mortality may be due in part to this activity. Since epsilon toxin requires "activation" by proteolytic enzymes, its role in disease caused by Type B strains is less important than that played by beta toxin.

c. *Clostridium perfringens* Type C enterotoxemia involves neonatal calves, foals, piglets, and lambs worldwide. *Clostridium perfringens* Type C causes hemorrhagic enteritis in these species. This type is associated with necrotic enteritides in humans and birds and an often rapidly fatal toxemia-bacteremia of older sheep called *struck*. Beta toxin is considered the principal factor producing hemorrhagic enteritis affecting the small intestine. Its trypsin susceptibility explains in part the predilection of the disease for the newborn (colostrum contains antitrypsin substances). The signs are depression, anorexia, abdominal pain, and diarrhea. The course is rapid, with mortality rates near 100%. The signs and pathology associated with this disease are due to the action of the membrane active toxins (alpha, beta, and perfringolysin O), as well as those products that destroy the connective tissue components.

d. *Clostridium perfringens*, Type D, produces an enterotoxemia ("overeating disease," "pulpy kidney disease") in older lambs (<1 year) and occasionally in goats and calves. The key epsilon toxin is secreted as protoxin activated by intestinal proteases (explaining predilections for older animals since colostrum contains antitrypsin activity). Epsilon toxin increases intestinal permeability, ensuring its absorption into the circulation where it damages vascular endothelium, leading to fluid loss and edema. When toxin levels are high, affected capillary endothelial cells in the brain are damaged, and the resultant edema greatly increases the intracranial pressure. When the amount of toxin is lower, however (as might be the case in a par-

tially immune animal, or when the amount of toxin produced in the intestinal canal is less) it damages the capillary endothelial cells in the brain so that toxin levels are increased in that organ. This results in a focal symmetrical encephalomalacia (see Fig 71.1). In addition to these changes (which are toxin-dose related), epsilon toxin triggers catecholamine release, resulting in adenylyl cyclase activation, cAMP-related hyperglycemia, and glycosuria, a frequent finding in enterotoxemia.

Gross lesions may be absent. Postmortem autolysis is rapid. Subserous and subendocardial hemorrhages and excess fluid in the body cavities are sometimes seen. Cerebral hemorrhage and degenerative lesions are common in less acute cases. Histopathology may reveal enteritis.

Lambs may die without premonitory signs. Convulsions occur in agonal stages and diarrhea in protracted cases. Cattle and older sheep show neural manifestations. In goats, diarrhea is common. Death rates are high in lambs. In calves and goats, nonfatal subacute and chronic cases occur.

e. *Clostridium perfringens* Type E produces a relatively rare form of enterotoxemia in calves, lambs, and rabbits. The membrane active toxins (alpha, iota, and perfringolysin O) together with those toxins affecting connective tissue substances combine to produce this disease. Hemorrhagic enteritis, and ulcerative abomasitis (gastritis) are the pathologic lesions.

3. *Nonenterotoxemic Diarrhea.* Nonenterotoxemic diarrhea occurs subsequent to the interaction of enterotoxin (Cpe) with epithelial cells of the small intestine following sporulation of the microorganism in that environment. Though any type of *C. perfringens* can harbor the genes encoding Cpe, Type A is the most common. This disease is one of the most commonly occurring food-related diseases in human patients. The disease also occurs in dogs and cats. Signs range from watery to hemorrhagic diarrhea. In addition to altering fluid and electrolyte flow of the epithelium, Cpe damages epithelial cells and tight junctions leading to sloughing with accompanying inflammatory changes.

Epidemiology

Some normal animals, especially adults, commonly carry *C. perfringens* in their intestinal tracts. During outbreaks of diarrheal disease, pathogenic strains survive in soil long enough to infect other animals.

The determinant of enterotoxemic disease is the intestinal environment, which is influenced by diet and age. Overeating, especially on protein and energy-rich food (milk, legume forage, grain) is almost a prerequisite. In young animals, the excess feed is often passed, inadequately digested, into the intestine, where it provides a rich medium for proliferation and toxigenesis (up regulation of the VirR/VirS system, see above) by ingested or resident bacteria. Overloading slows intestinal motility, thereby favoring retention of bacteria and absorption of their toxins.

The age predilection of these diseases is due to the diet and the infantile digestive tract, which often lacks enzymes to inactivate the toxins. Colostral antitrypsin activity exacerbates this aspect. *Clostridium perfringens* spores are destroyed in the functional rumen, an organ that is rudimentary at birth. Type D proliferation in older lambs appears to be favored by high-carbohydrate intake.

Seasonal prevalence relates to the seasonal abundance of susceptible populations and rich forage.

Type A–associated conditions occur worldwide. Type B lamb dysentery occurs in Europe and South Africa, while Type B enteritis of sheep or goats is reported from Iran. Type C occurs worldwide and also causes overeating-type enterotoxemia in humans ("pig bel"). Type D is prevalent wherever sheep are raised. Type E is found in Britain, the United States, and Australia, and has been implicated in enterotoxemia. A toxin similar to its iota toxin is also produced by *C. spiroforme* and *C. difficile* (see below).

Immunologic Aspects

Immunity is antibody-mediated and correlates with antitoxin levels. Immunizing preparations often include bacterial components as well.

Passive and active immunization is important in the control of the diseases (see under "Treatment and Control," below).

Laboratory Diagnosis

Clostridium perfringens is relatively aerotolerant. It is nonmotile and produces a polysaccharide capsule in tissue. Spores are rarely demonstrable in exudates obtained from normally sterile sites.

Isolation follows inoculation of blood containing agar media, and incubation in an anaerobic environment. If *C. perfringens* is to be isolated from a contaminated environment (e.g., intestinal contents), the sample can first be heated to 80°C for 15 minutes (endospores will resist this treatment, whereas vegetative forms will not), and then placed into or onto isolation media. Diagnostic features include 1) alpha toxin-associated hemolytic activity (hot-cold lysis), 2) the clotting of milk followed by gaseous disruption ("stormy fermentation"), and 3) neutralization of alpha toxin activity on egg yolk agar containing specific anti-alpha toxin antibody (Nagler reaction).

In cases of enterotoxemia, stained (e.g., Gram's, Wright's, Giemsa) contents of the small intestine often contain large numbers of gram-positive rods resembling *C. perfringens*. This test is of limited value due to rapid postmortem bacterial overgrowth in all parts of the gut.

DNA primers specific for the various genes encoding the toxins have been developed for detection in feces or cultures by using the polymerase chain reaction (multiplex PCR).

Demonstration of toxin in the contents of the small intestine is definitive. Small amounts (<0.5 ml) of clarified intestinal contents are injected into the tail vein of mice. Death after more than a few minutes postinjection constitutes presumptive evidence of enterotoxemia. A preferable procedure utilizes injections of mixtures of three parts test fluid to one part known antitoxin to the various *C. perfringens* toxins.

An intradermal test for necrotizing activity in guinea pigs is more specific. If used on broth cultures, tests must be performed on both trypsinized and untrypsinized supernatants, since some toxins are destroyed while others are activated by trypsin. Samples must be fresh or kept frozen until tested.

Antemortem tissue invasion occurs consistently only with "struck," the Type C enterotoxemia of mature sheep. In other forms, isolation and typing may furnish supportive but rarely definitive evidence.

Lambs with Type D enterotoxemia usually test positively for glycosuria.

Cpe is detected immunologically in feces of affected dogs or cats by an enzyme-linked immunosorbent assay (ELISA). Although sporulation and Cpe production are coregulated, there is disagreement regarding the usefulness of determining the presence of spores in stained smears of feces as a method of diagnosis.

Treatment and Control

Most cases of enterotoxemia are too acute for successful treatment. Antitoxin of appropriate type may be given to sick animals and those at risk. Protection lasts 2 to 3 weeks. Prophylactic dosages, given subcutaneously, can be doubled and given intravenously for therapy.

Active immunization of dams with two injections of bacterin-toxoid combinations prior to parturition ensures nurslings passive protection for the first weeks of life.

During outbreaks, antitoxin and toxoid are often given and a second dose of toxoid is administered some weeks later. Protection of lambs against Type D enterotoxemia requires two vaccinations at monthly intervals. The course should be completed 2 weeks before the lambs are placed on full feed.

Commercial immunizing products usually cover Types C and D.

Ensuring against overeating is a worthwhile preventive measure where practicable. Feeding broad-spectrum antibiotics reduces the prevalence of enterotoxemia of lambs, but creates other problems (see Chapter 4). Feeding antibiotics to poultry reduces mortality in chickens due to necrotizing enteritis caused by *C. perfringens*, Type A.

Diarrhea in dogs and cats associated with *C. perfringens*, Type A producing Cpe, responds to metronidazole, macrolides (tylosin), or ampicillin.

CLOSTRIDIUM NOVYI

Descriptive Features

Clostridium novyi is a nonencapsulated, motile, gram-positive, obligately anaerobic rod producing large, oval, highly heat-resistant spores. There are three types (A, B, and C), which differ biochemically, epidemiologically, and pathogenically. Some would add *C. haemolyticum* as Type D (see below)

Clostridium novyi produces gas gangrene, "big head," and "black disease" of ruminants.

Cellular Products of Medical Interest

Toxins. Clostridium novyi produces a number of protein exotoxins that are responsible for the diseases associated with it. Of these, the alpha and beta toxins, and the cholesterol-binding cytolysin novyilysin have proven roles in the diseases produced by this species. Toxins have not been associated with strains of *C. novyi* Type C:

1. Alpha toxin. The alpha toxin is produced by *C. novyi* Types A and B. It is a glycosyltransferase that glucosylates Rho GTPases rendering them ineffectual in interacting with their substrates (i.e., they become biologically inactive). In addition, glycosylation blocks interaction of Rho GDP with guanine exchange factor, and the interaction of Rho GTP with GTPase activating factor, thereby preventing membrane cycling. As a consequence, several signaling pathways are disrupted, resulting in a breakdown of the cytoskeletal components of the affected cell, followed by its death.
2. Beta toxin. The beta toxin is produced by *C. novyi* Type B. It is a phospholipase C (a lecithinase) that hydrolyzes phosphatidylcholine and sphingomyelin (both of which are constituents of host cell membranes), resulting in death of the cell. This toxin is also hemolytic.
3. Delta toxin (Novyilysin). Delta toxin or novyilysin is produced by *C. novyi* Type A, and is a cholesterol-binding cytolysin (see also perfringolysin O, above, chauveolysin, below; streptococcal streptolysin O, Chapter 28; listerial listeriolysin O, Chapter 33; and arcanobacterial pyolysin, Chapter 29). Novyilysin binds to cholesterol-containing rafts in the eukaryotic cell membrane. Once bound, it forms a pore resulting in the death of the cell.
4. Miscellaneous toxins. *Clostridium novyi* produces a number of other protein "exotoxins" with uncertain roles in the pathogenesis of disease. These include a lecithinase (gamma toxin) produced by Type A strains, a lipase (epsilon toxin) produced by Type A strains, hemolysin (zeta toxin) produced by Type B strains, and a myosinase (eta toxin) produced by Type B strains.

Ecology

Reservoir and Transmission

Type A is common in soil. Types A and B occur in the normal intestine and liver of herbivores. All enter their hosts by ingestion or wound infection.

Pathogenesis

Of several toxins produced by *C. novyi*, alpha, beta, and novyilysin, which are lethal and necrotizing, are of established pathogenic significance. The pathogenic roles of the other toxins—lecithinase, hemolysin, lipase, and myosinase—are uncertain:

1. *Clostridium novyi* Type A is implicated in gas gangrene of humans and wound infections in animals. One of these, "bighead" of rams, starts as a fight injury at the top of the head. Toxic endothelial damage (by alpha toxin and novyilysin) produces edema involving head, neck, and cranial thorax. Death occurs in 2 days. The yellow tinge of the edema fluid, which is clear and gelatinous with little hemorrhage, is a postmortem change.
2. *Clostridium novyi* Type B causes infectious necrotic hepatitis ("black disease") of sheep and cattle, rarely horses and swine. Spores originating in the intestine reach the liver and remain there dormant within Kupffer cells. When liver cells are injured, as by fluke migration, resulting anaerobic conditions allow the spores to germinate. Vegetative growth results in toxin production (alpha and beta toxins) and dissemination. Death may be sudden or within 2 days of clinical onset. Signs include depression, anorexia, and hypothermia. Necropsy reveals edema, serosal effusion, and one or more areas of liver necrosis, containing bacteria. Subcutaneous venous congestion secondary to pericardial edema darkens the underside of the skin, suggesting the name "black disease."
3. *Clostridium novyi* Type C, the reported cause of osteomyelitis of water buffalo in Southeast Asia, produces no toxins or experimental disease.

Epidemiology

The agent occurs worldwide. "Bighead" is recognized in Australia, South Africa, and North America. Distribution of "black disease" largely coincides with that of the liver fluke *Fasciola hepatica*. Both diseases occur mostly in adult sheep, during summer and fall. "Black disease" affects preferably well-nourished animals.

Immunologic Aspects

Circulating antitoxin (antibodies to alpha, beta, novyilysin toxins) and antibody to cellular components of the organism presumably are the basis of immunity to *C. novyi* infections. Whole culture bacterins and toxoids have prophylactic value.

Laboratory Diagnosis

Liver lesions contain large gram-positive to gram-variable rods with oval subterminal, large spores, identifiable by fluorescent anti–*C. novyi* conjugates.

Culture requires the strictest anaerobic conditions, especially for Type B, which is also nutritionally fastidious. *Clostridium novyi* may be demonstrable in normal livers of herbivores within hours after death.

Toxin, in serosal effusions, can be demonstrated by animal tests (see under *C. perfringens*, above), but antitoxins for use in protection tests are not as readily available.

Detection in tissue or identification in culture can be accomplished by using molecular techniques. DNA primers designed to amplify species-specific portions of the gene encoding the flagellar protein flagellin have been used successfully to differentiate *C. novyi* Types A, and B, *C. haemolyticum*, *C. chauvoei,* and *C. septicum.*

Treatment and Control

There is no effective treatment. Control is directed at eliminating flukes and other hepatopathic agents. Prophylactic vaccination (two injections a month apart) with a bacterin-toxoid combination is generally effective.

CLOSTRIDIUM HAEMOLYTICUM

Clostridium haemolyticum is a nonencapsulated, motile, strict anaerobe, producing large, oval, highly heat-resistant spores. *Clostridium haemolyticum* (*C. novyi*, Type D) resembles *C. novyi* Type B in practically all phenotypic traits. Its toxin, a phospholipase C, is identical to *C. novyi* Type B beta toxin (see above), but is produced in much larger amounts. Serologic and toxigenic variants of *C. haemolyticum* have been noted.

Clostridium haemolyticum produces bacillary hemoglobinuria or "red water" disease of ruminants.

Ecology

Reservoir and Transmission

Clostridium haemolyticum exists in the ruminant digestive tract, in the liver, and in soil. Appearance of the disease in new, widely separated regions suggests that movement of cattle plays a part in its dissemination. Transmission is by ingestion.

Pathogenesis

The pathogenesis of bacillary hemoglobinuria involves ingestion of spores, colonization of the liver, liver injury, spore germination, and toxigenesis (see *C. novyi* Type B "black disease," above). The toxin is a phospholipase C (beta toxin), which produces a hemolytic crisis and death within hours or days. Other effects include serosal effusions and widespread hemorrhages. The diagnostic lesions are circumscribed areas of liver necrosis ("infarcts"), which are the effects of beta toxin. Clinically there are fever, pale, icteric mucous membranes, anorexia, agalactia, abdominal pain, hemoglobinuria ("red water"), and hyperpnea. Pregnant cows may abort.

Epidemiology

Bacillary hemoglobinuria occurs in North America in the Rocky Mountain and Pacific Coast states and along the Gulf of Mexico, and in Latin America, parts of Europe, and New Zealand. Although swampy lowlands are associated with endemic disease and flooding with the spread of infection, little is known of the agent's persistence in soil. Shedder animals may have a role in dissemination.

Cases are clustered in the second half of the year, typically among well-nourished animals a year or more of age. Correlation with fluke infection is less consistent than in "black disease" (see *C. novyi* Type B, above).

Immunologic Aspects

Immunity is antitoxic. Animals in endemic areas develop some immunity. Whole culture bacterin-toxoids are effective prophylactically.

Laboratory Diagnosis

Liver lesions are the best source of positive smears for Gram stains and immunofluorescence tests. Cultivation requires freshly poured blood agar and strict anaerobic conditions.

Detection in tissue or identification in culture can be accomplished by using molecular techniques. DNA primers designed to amplify species-specific portions of the gene encoding the flagellar protein flagellin have been used successfully to differentiate *C. novyi* Types A, and B, *C. haemolyticum*, *C. chauvoei*, and *C. septicum.*

Treatment and Control

Early treatment of sick animals with a broad-spectrum antibiotic (e.g., tetracycline), antitoxin, and blood transfusion produces good results. Animals in endemic areas are vaccinated minimally every 6 months and preferably 3 to 4 weeks before anticipated exposure.

CLOSTRIDIUM SEPTICUM

Clostridium septicum is a short, stout, and pleomorphic gram-positive, motile, spore-forming obligately anaerobic rod. In some exudates, long filaments are found.

Clostridium septicum is the leading cause of wound infections (malignant edema) of farm animals.

Descriptive Features

Cellular Products of Medical Interest

Toxins. *Clostridium septicum* produces a number of protein exotoxins that are purportedly responsible for the diseases associated with it. However, alpha toxin has been definitively shown to be the only virulence factor produced by this species:

1. Alpha toxin. The alpha toxin produced by *C. septicum* is a pore-forming, lethal toxin. Following secretion, it is bound to glycosylphosphatidylinositol (GPI)-anchored proteins on the eukaryotic cell surface (mainly endothelial cells, though not exclusively). There, the cell bound proteolytic enzyme, furin, cleaves it, resulting in fragments that insert into the membrane forming pores leading to death of the cell.
2. Beta toxin. The beta toxin of *C. septicum* has DNase and leukocytotoxic activity. The role played by this toxin in the pathogenesis of disease is undefined.
3. Gamma toxin. The gamma toxin of *C. septicum* has hyaluronidase activity. The role played by this toxin in the pathogenesis of disease is undefined.
4. Delta toxin (septicolysin O). The delta toxin of *C. septicum*, also known as *septicolysin O,* is a cholesterol-binding cytolysin (see also perfringolysin O and novyilysin, above, chauveolysin, below; streptococcal streptolysin O, Chapter 28; listerial listeriolysin O, Chapter 33; and arcanobacterial pyolysin, Chapter 29). Septicolysin O binds to cholesterol-containing rafts in the eukaryotic cell membrane. Once bound, it forms a pore resulting in the death of the cell. The role played by this toxin in the pathogenesis of disease produced by *C. septicum* is undefined.
5. Miscellaneous products. *Clostridium septicum* produces a number of other products (chitinases, neuraminidases, lipases, sialidases, and hemagglutinins) with undefined roles in the pathogenesis of disease.

Ecology

Reservoir and Transmission

Clostridium septicum occurs in soils worldwide and in the animal and human intestine. It is acquired by wound infection and ingestion.

Pathogenesis

Wound infection produced by *C. septicum* is called "malignant edema." All of the toxic products outlined above probably play a role, but only the alpha toxin has been shown to be definitively involved. Systemic effects are thought to be the result of endothelial damage throughout the body (leading to severe fluid and electrolyte imbalances) as well as the edema seen locally. Membrane active toxins (alpha and delta), dissolution of connective tissue components (gamma toxin), along with destruction of polymorphonuclear leukocytes and release of their digestive enzymes (beta toxin) may account for the tissue destruction observed.

The infectious process radiates from the point of inoculation within hours to days of exposure. A hemorrhagic, edematous, necrotizing process frequently follows fascial planes as adjacent muscle is darkened.

With muscular involvement and emphysema, there may be close resemblance to "blackleg" (*C. chauvoei*, below) and "gas gangrene" (*C. perfringens*, above).

Crepitant swellings change from painful and hot to anesthetic and cold. Signs include fever, tachycardia, anorexia, and depression. The course may be rapid and fatal within a day.

"Braxy" (Scots) or "bradsot" (Danish) is a fatal *C. septicum* cold-weather disease of sheep. *Clostridium septicum* produces a lesion in the abomasal wall comparable to the subcutaneous one described above. Clinical signs are mostly toxemia and gastrointestinal distress.

Human wound infections due to *C. septicum* may develop into cellulitis or "gas gangrene."

Epidemiology

"Malignant edema" may follow such procedures as castration, docking, shearing, tagging, and injections. Postparturient genital infections are sometimes linked to dystocia and unskilled obstetrical assistance.

"Braxy" or "bradsot" is seen mostly in Scotland and Scandinavia.

Immunologic Aspects

Immunity is probably antitoxin-dependent.

Laboratory Diagnosis

Sporulated rods may be demonstrable in exudates by Gram stain or immunofluorescence.

Clostridium septicum grows on ruminant blood agar under reasonably good anaerobic conditions, producing within 48 hours hemolytic colonies up to 5 mm in diameter, with rhizoid contours and a frequent tendency to swarm.

Though recovery and identification of this agent by culture are not difficult, positive results should be interpreted with caution. *Clostridium septicum* is an aggressive postmortem invader. Its presence may be unrelated to the problem at hand and may obscure that of more significant pathogens, such as *C. haemolyticum* and *C. chauvoei*.

Demonstration in tissue or identification of isolates is possible by using DNA primers that have been designed to amplify the gene (or portions thereof) encoding the alpha toxin by means of the polymerase chain reaction. All strains of *C. septicum* contain the genes encoding this toxin. Detection in tissue or identification in culture can also be accomplished by using DNA primers designed to amplify species-specific portions of the gene encoding the flagellar protein flagellin, which have been used successfully to differentiate *C. novyi* Types A and B, *C. chauvoei*, *C. haemolyticum*, and *C. septicum*. Likewise, *C. septicum* can be differentiated from *C. chauvoei* by the use of primers to amplify the 16S–23S DNA spacer regions.

Treatment and Control

Prognosis should be guarded. Possible therapy includes penicillin or tetracycline given systemically, incision, drainage, and irrigation of lesions with antiseptics.

Calves are vaccinated at 3 to 4 months of age, sheep and goats at weaning. Annual revaccination is advisable. Hygienic precautions at times of likely exposure are helpful.

CLOSTRIDIUM CHAUVOEI

Clostridium chauvoei is a gram-positive, motile, obligately anaerobic rod that produces subterminal or subcentral spores.

Clostridium chauvoei produces an emphysematous necrotizing myositis ("blackleg") in cattle.

Descriptive Features

Cellular Products of Medical Interest

Clostridium chauvoei produces a number of protein exotoxins that are purportedly responsible for the diseases associated with it:

1. Alpha toxin. The alpha toxin of *C. chauvoei* is described as an oxygen-stable hemolysin. This toxin is most likely comparable to the pore-forming, lethal alpha toxin of *C. septicum* (see above).
2. Beta toxin. The beta toxin of *C. chauvoei* has DNase activity. The role played by this toxin in the pathogenesis of disease is undefined.
3. Gamma toxin. The gamma toxin of *C. chauvoei* has hyaluronidase activity. The role played by this toxin in the pathogenesis of disease is undefined.
4. Delta toxin (chauveolysin). The delta toxin of *C. chauvoei*, also known as *chauveolysin,* is a cholesterol-binding cytolysin (see also perfringolysin O, septicolysin O, novyilysin above; streptococcal streptolysin O, Chapter 28; listerial listeriolysin O, Chapter 33; and arcanobacterial pyolysin, Chapter 29). Chauveolysin binds to cholesterol-containing rafts in the eukaryotic cell membrane. Once bound, it forms a pore resulting in the death of the cell. The role played by this toxin in the pathogenesis of disease produced by *C. chauvoei* is undefined.
5. Neuraminidase (sialidase). The neuraminidase of *C. chauvoei* removes sialic acid residues from glycoconjugates on cell walls of eukaryotic cells resulting in disruptions of the intercellular matrix. The role played by this toxin in the pathogenesis of disease is undefined.

Ecology

Reservoir and Transmission

Clostridium chauvoei inhabits the intestine, liver, and other tissues of susceptible and resistant species. Evidence that soil transmits "blackleg" is circumstantial (see under "Epidemiology," below).

Routes of infection are not known. Endogenous and soil-acquired infection via ingestion or injury is assumed.

Pathogenesis

The alpha (necrotizing), gamma (hyaluronidase), delta (chauveolysin) toxins together with the neuraminidase, are believed to be responsible for the initial lesions. Bacterial metabolism, producing gas from fermentation, may be contributory.

Seeding of tissues, especially skeletal muscle, with spores from the intestine, presumably precedes disease in cattle. Conditions favoring spore germination, bacterial growth, and toxin production cause formation of local lesions marked by edema, hemorrhage, and myofibrillar necrosis. The centers of lesions become dry, dark, and emphysematous due to bacterial fermentation, while the periphery is edematous and hemorrhagic. A rancid-butter odor is typical.

Microscopically, one finds degenerative changes in muscle fibers disrupted by edema, emphysema, and hemorrhage. Leukocytic infiltration is minor.

Clinically, there is high fever, anorexia, and depression. Lameness is common. Superficial lesions cause visible swellings, which crepitate on being handled. Often lesions are entirely internal (diaphragm, myocardium, tongue). Some animals die suddenly, others within 1 or 2 days.

Epidemiology

"Blackleg" occurs worldwide at rates that differ between and within geographic areas, which suggests a soil reservoir or climatic or seasonal factors yet to be defined. Young, well-fed cattle (<3 years) are preferentially attacked.

Exertion, bruising, or acute indigestion are suspected triggering events.

In sheep and some other species, *C. chauvoei* typically causes wound infections resembling malignant edema or gas gangrene. Other clostridia (*C. septicum, C. novyi,* and *C. sordellii*) may be present.

Immunologic Aspects

Circulating antibody to toxins and cellular components apparently determines resistance to *C. chauvoei*. Commercial formalinized adjuvant vaccines include up to six other clostridial components.

Laboratory Diagnosis

Sporulated gram-positive rods can be demonstrated in smears of infected tissues and identified with immunofluorescent reagents (see Fig 70.4).

Clostridium chauvoei requires strict anaerobic conditions and media rich in cysteine and water-soluble vitamins. The agent resembles *C. septicum* and is frequently recovered with it. Unlike *C. septicum* it ferments sucrose but not salicin and will not grow at 44°C. The use of DNA primers to amplify the 16S–23S DNA spacer regions (by using the polymerase chain reaction) will differentiate *C. septicum* from *C. chauvoei*. This assay can be used to detect the microorganism in tissue.

Detection in tissue or identification in culture can also be accomplished by using DNA primers designed to amplify (by using the polymerase chain reaction) species-specific portions of the gene encoding the flagellar protein flagellin, which have been used successfully to differentiate *C. novyi* Types A, and B, *C. chauvoei*, *C. haemolyticum*, and *C. septicum*.

Treatment and Control

Treatment is often disappointing. Penicillin should be given intravenously at first, followed by repository forms intramuscularly.

Cattle are vaccinated at 3 to 6 months of age and annually thereafter. Vaccination should precede exposure by at least 2 weeks. During an outbreak, all cattle are vaccinated and given long-acting penicillin.

Pregnant ewes are vaccinated 3 weeks prior to parturition, when infection often occurs. Lambs may require vaccination during their first year.

Change of pasture is advisable when cases are first observed.

CLOSTRIDIUM DIFFICILE

Clostridium difficile is a gram-positive, motile, encapsulated, spore-forming anaerobic rod. This species produces adhesins (pili or fimbria), and its cell wall contains paracrystalline arrays (S-layer) visible with the electron microscope.

Clostridium difficile is a significant cause of diarrheal disease in human beings (antibiotic-associated diarrhea which may progress to pseudomembranous colitis), but its significance in other animals is less clear. The microorganism has been isolated from symptomatic as well as asymptomatic dogs and cats. Association with a "trigger event" such as use of antimicrobial agents has been suggested but not proven. *Clostridium difficile* has also been isolated from normal horses; however, it is more frequently isolated from horses with diarrhea and associated protein-losing enteropathy, implying a causal relationship. Pathological findings in horses from which *C. difficile* has been isolated include hemorrhagic necrotizing enterocolitis, typhlocolitis, and pseudomembranous colitis. As with dogs and cats, there is some suggestion of association with antimicrobial agents, though *C. difficile*-associated disease has been reported in previously normal, unmedicated foals.

Descriptive Features

Cellular Products of Medical Interest

Adhesins. Clostridium difficile produces pili or fimbrial adhesins that probably play a role in adhesion to target cells in the large intestine. *Clostridium difficile* also produces a cell wall protein (Cwp66 for *c*ell *w*all *p*rotein of *66* kDa in size) with affinity for intestinal epithelial cells.

Capsule. Clostridium difficile produces a carbohydrate capsule that protects it from phagocytic cells.

Toxins. Clostridium difficile produces three toxins that are responsible for enteritis observed with this microorganism: toxin A ("enterotoxin"), toxin B ("cytolysin"), and ADP-ribosyltransferase:

1. Toxin A. *Clostridium difficile* Toxin A (ToxA or TcdA for *t*oxin *C. d*ifficile) is a glycosyltransferase that glucosylates Rho GTPases, rendering them ineffectual in interacting with their substrates (i.e., they become biologically inactive). In addition, glycosylation blocks interaction of Rho GDP with guanine exchange factor, and the interaction of Rho GTP with GTPase activating factor, thereby preventing membrane cycling. Several signaling pathways are disrupted, resulting in a breakdown of the cytoskeletal components of the affected cell including disruption of the tight junctions between intestinal epithelial cells. These changes result in death of the cell. The enterotoxic property of ToxA, in addition to the cytotoxic effects just described, is due to its ability to stimulate influx of PMNs by way of the enteric nervous system (through the release of substance P and mast cell degranulation). Prostaglandin synthesis by the recruited PMNs (and perhaps by affected host cells), as well as activation of various inositol-signaling pathways within affected host cells, results in the secretion of chloride ions and water (diarrhea).
2. Toxin B. *Clostridium difficile* Toxin B (ToxB or TcdB for *t*oxin *C. d*ifficile), like ToxA, is a glycosyltransferase that glucosylates Rho GTPases (see above). However, ToxB has little enterotoxic activity.
3. ADP-ribosyltransferase. *Clostridium difficile* produces an ADP-ribosyltransferase (Cdt for *C. d*ifficile *t*ransferase). Cdt is a binary toxin (see *C. perfringens* iota toxin, above, and *C. spiroforme*, below), composed of a binding portion (Cdtb) that binds to the target intestinal epithelial cells and an enzymatically active portion (Cdta). After the toxin binds to specific receptors on the cell surface, Cdta gains entry into the cytoplasm. Though it is not clear precisely how entry occurs, it seems that a pore (composed of Cdtb) is formed in the cell membrane through which Cdta traverses. Cdta is an ADP-ribosylating toxin that ribosylates actin within the host cell resulting in disorganization of the cellular cytoskeleton and death of the affected cell.

Variability

Clostridium difficile is quite variable. There are 12 serogroups (A–I, K, X, and S), as well as substantial variability in the gene encoding the flagellar protein flagellin (9 different groups). Random amplification of polymorhic DNA (RAPD) analysis demonstrates numerous types.

These differences are useful in determining the epidemiology of this microorganism.

Ecology

Reservoir and Transmission

Clostridium difficile is found in the intestinal canal of normal as well as clinically affected animals. The spores are resistant to most environmental stresses, which results in their widespread distribution in locations where animals are housed. There does not seem to be an overlap between those strains that produce disease in human patients and those that are associated with animals.

Pathogenesis

Clostridium difficile adheres to mucus or epithelial cells of the large intestine by pili or fimbria as well as the surface protein Cwp66. Disease most often follows a "trigger" event (e.g., antibiotics, nonsteroidal drugs, chemotherapeutic agents) that results in relaxation of the control the normal flora has on the numbers of *C. difficile*. Toxins are produced (ToxA, ToxB, and Cdt), resulting in death of the epithelial cells, which follows disruption of their actin cytoskeleton and tight junctions. Prostaglandin along with the products of the inositol pathway stemming from the intense inflammatory response (ToxA) results in fluid and electrolyte secretion. Diarrhea, with or without blood, results.

Epidemiology

Clostridium difficile–associated diarrhea appears to be linked to administration of antibiotics, stress, chemotherapeutic agents, or nonsteroidal anti-inflammatory drugs, although newborn foals have been shown to develop disease without a recognizable "trigger" event. Whether this organism moves among hospitalized patients, as with human patients in human hospitals, is unknown.

Clostridium difficile isolated from dogs and cats with diarrhea do not commonly contain the genes encoding Cdt.

Immunologic Aspects

Immunity is probably antitoxic, although the role of antibodies to *C. difficile* is unknown. Orally administered antitoxin (made in bovines) is protective for human patients.

Laboratory Diagnosis

The genes encoding the toxin(s) can be detected in feces by assays based on polymerase chain reaction (PCR). Immunologically based tests are available for the detection of the toxin (ToxA) in fecal specimens. *Clostridium difficile* can be isolated from feces by using a selective medium, CCFA (cycloserine, cefoxitin, and fructose agar).

Treatment and Control

Diarrhea-associated *C. difficile* responds rapidly to metronidazole. Unfortunately, metronidazole-resistant strains exist. The alternative antibiotic is vancomycin. There are no vaccines available. However, the use of orally administered yeast, *Saccharomyces boulardii*, has been shown to be useful in preventing the disease in human patients. In human hospitals, hand washing by health care personnel is a very efficient mechanism for curtailing spread. Disinfectants are not effective against the spores.

CLOSTRIDIUM PILIFORME ("BACILLUS PILIFORMIS")

An acute fatal diarrheal disease of laboratory mice with focal liver necrosis (Tyzzer's disease) is associated with a spore-forming organism, *Clostridium piliforme*, which occurs in bundles within hepatocytes. It is unable to grow on cell-free media. *Clostridium piliforme* is linked to identical diseases in rabbits, hares, gerbils, rats, hamsters, muskrats, dogs, cats, snow leopards, foals, and rhesus monkeys. Tyzzer's disease has been reported in a human patient infected with the human immunodeficiency virus, but not in immunocompetent persons.

Descriptive Features

Clostridium piliforme is a large, gram-variable, spore-forming rod that is motile by peritrichous flagella. Giemsa and silver stains are preferable to hematoxylin-eosin and Gram stains.

Growth has been obtained in embryonated hen's eggs and on cultured mouse hepatocytes.

Vegetative cells die even when deep-frozen or freeze-dried. Spores survive moderate heating, freezing, and thawing. Litter remains infective for months. Strains are pathogenically and morphologically uniform.

Ecology

Reservoir and Transmission

The source of the agent is the infected animal. The agent spreads by the ano-oral route and transplacentally. Many infections are believed to be endogenous and stress-triggered.

Pathogenesis

Lesions suggest hepatic invasion from the intestine via lymphatics and blood vessels. Foci of coagulation necrosis are periportal. There may be dissemination to the myocardium. Parasitized cells include hepatocytes, myocardial cells, smooth muscle, and epithelial cells of the intestine, in which a dysentery-like condition may develop. Lymphadenitis, especially of hepatic nodes, is seen in foals.

The course is usually under 3 days.

Epidemiology

Outbreaks are often stress-related (crowding, irradiation, steroid administration). Morbidity is high in laboratory animal colonies. Case fatality rates reach 50% to 100%, especially among young stock. In many colonies, subclinically infected individuals are evidently present; these are often identifiable serologically.

Laboratory Diagnosis

Laboratory diagnosis rests on the demonstration of typical bundles of intracellular bacilli (0.5 µm by 8.0 to 10 µm), especially in hepatocytes surrounding lesions (see Fig 68.5). Fluorescent antibody aids diagnosis.

A complement fixation test that utilizes an infected mouse liver extract as antigen is used to determine the degree on infection in mouse colonies.

Treatment and Control

Treatment of clinical cases is usually unsuccessful. Prophylactically effective antimicrobic drugs include erythromycin and tetracycline.

Other Species of Veterinary Interest

Clostridium sordellii is associated with a fatal myositis and hepatic disease in ruminants and horses, although the precise pathogenic process is not known. The agent produces numerous toxins and is experimentally pathogenic for many species of animals. Mixed clostridial bacterintoxoids usually contain *C. sordellii*.

Clostridium colinum causes quail disease, ulcerative enteritis, and necrotizing hepatitis of several species of fowl (see Fig 68.6). The agent is fastidious nutritionally and forms spores sparingly. Its life cycle is unknown, and a toxin has not been identified. The untreated disease is usually fatal. Streptomycin has been effective in the field.

Clostridium spiroforme is isolated frequently from rabbits with juvenile enteritis ("mucoid enteritis"). It may be one of several microorganisms implicated. Its exotoxin is identical to the iota toxin of *C. perfringens* Type E and the ADP-ribosyltransferase of *C. difficile*. It acts by ADP-ribosylating cellular actin.

THE NONINVASIVE CLOSTRIDIA

Clostridium botulinum (the cause of botulism) and *C. tetani* (the cause of tetanus) produce disease strictly through the action of neurotoxins—botulinum and tetanus toxins, respectively. Though botulinum and tetanus toxins have the same mechanism of action, they produce different diseases with different manifestations because the two toxins affect different sites in the nervous system.

Botulinum toxin and tetanus toxin block neurotransmitter release. Both toxins are zinc endopeptidases that interfere with the fusion of vesicles containing neurotransmitter with the membrane lining the presynaptic cleft. Interference is due to hydrolysis of the proteins involved with "docking," which precedes fusion of neurotransmitter-containing vesicles with the membrane lining the cleft. Hydrolysis of these proteins leads to degeneration of the synapse and blockage of neurotransmission. Regeneration of the synapse takes several weeks to months.

CLOSTRIDIUM BOTULINUM

Clostridium botulinum is a gram-positive, spore-forming, obligately anaerobic rod, which produces the disease botulism, a neuroparalytic intoxication characterized by flaccid paralysis. The intoxication is caused by any of seven protein neurotoxins (A to G) that are identical in action but differ in potency, antigenic properties, and distribution. They are produced by a heterogeneous group of clostridia, called *C. botulinum* (*C. botulinum* Group G has been renamed *C. argentinense*) on the basis of the toxins, which in some types (C and D) are bacteriophage-encoded.

Botulinum is seen mainly in ruminants, horses, mink, and fowl, particularly waterfowl. Swine, carnivores, and fish are rarely affected.

Descriptive Features

Morphology

Clostridium botulinum is a gram-positive, spore-forming obligately anaerobic rod. At a pH near and above neutrality, it produces subterminal oval spores.

Cellular Products of Medical Interest

Toxin. *Clostridium botulinum* produces several proteins with "toxic" activity (botulinum toxin, C2 toxin, and C3 exoenzyme), but only botulinum toxin has a central role in the production of botulism:

1. Botulinum toxin. There are seven types of botulinum toxin (BoNT for *b*otulinum *n*euro*t*oxin), differentiated by antigenic differences. Letters A through G depict the types. The type of neurotoxin characterizes the strain of *C. botulinum* producing it. Thus, a strain of *C. botulinum* producing Type A BoNT would be described as *C. botulinum* Type A.

   All seven types of BoNT are zinc endopeptidases with identical activity, i.e., hydrolysis of the docking proteins required by neurotransmitter-containing vesicles to fuse with the presynaptic membrane. Though the end result is the same (blockage of the release of neurotransmitter), the various types of BoNT hydrolyze different docking proteins. Types A and E hydrolyze SNAP (*s*y*n*aptosomal-*a*ssociated *p*rotein), Types B, D, F, G hydrolyze VAMP (*v*esicle-*a*ssociated *m*embrane protein also known as *synaptobrevin*), and Type C, which hydrolyzes SNAP and syntaxin. Once hydrolyzed, the synapse degenerates, taking weeks to months to regenerate.

BoNT is a "di-chain" molecule consisting of a light chain (with zinc endopeptidase activity), a heavy chain composed of a translocation domain (responsible for forming a pore through which the light chain passes), and a binding domain (responsible for binding to nerve cells). Secreted with BoNT are several "accessory" proteins thought to aid the survival of the toxin in the gastrointestinal tract.

BoNT binds to cholinergic nerve cells, each type of BoNT binding to a different receptor. After binding, the toxin is internalized by way of receptor-mediated endocytosis. Vesicles containing BoNT remain at the neuromuscular junction. Following a cleaving event, the light chain (the zinc endopeptidase) translocates across the vesicle membrane into the cytosol of the nerve cell where it hydrolyzes the docking proteins.

2. C2 toxin and C3 exoenzyme. Both the C2 toxin and C3 exoenzyme are ADP-ribosyltransferases. C2 toxin and C3 exoenzyme ribosylates G-actin and Rho, respectively, resulting in disruptions in the cytoskeleton. Neither enzyme appears to play a role in the disease process.

Resistance

Although heat resistance of spores varies between culture groups (see below, "Variability"), toxin types, and strains, moist heat at 120°C for 5 minutes is generally lethal. Exceptions exist. Low pH and high salinity enhance heat sterilization. Heating to 80°C for 20 minutes inactivates the toxin.

Salt, nitrates, and nitrites suppress germination of spores in foods.

Variability

There are seven types of toxins; they differ in antigenicity, heat resistance, and lethality for different animal species (probably related to receptor density on the surface of the

motor neuron). Four culture groups are also recognized (Table 36.3).

Ecology

Reservoir

Reservoirs of *C. botulinum* are soil and aquatic sediments. Vehicles of intoxication are animal and plant material contaminated from these sources. When animals die, *C. botulinum* spores, which are common in gut and tissues, germinate and generate toxin. This may be ingested by carrion eaters or contaminate the environment. In rotting vegetation, a similar process occurs.

Transmission

Apart from toxin ingestion, spore ingestion and wound contamination may lead to botulism.

Spore ingestion is important in human infant botulism. Wound-infection botulism is seen rarely in humans and horses.

Pathogenesis

Ingested BoNT is absorbed from the glandular stomach and anterior small intestine and distributed via the bloodstream. It binds to receptors and enters the nerve cell after receptor-mediated endocytosis. How BoNT gets from the bloodstream to the surface of nerve cells is not understood. Vesicles containing toxin remain at the myoneural junction. A fragment of the toxin (light chain) translocates across the vesicle membrane into the cytosol of the nerve cell and subsequently hydrolyzes a "docking" protein (which protein depends upon which botulinum toxin). The synapse degenerates and flaccid paralysis results due to the lack of neurotransmitter (acetylcholine). When this affects muscles of respiration, death due to respiratory failure occurs. No primary lesions are produced.

Clinical signs include muscular incoordination leading to recumbency, extrusion of the tongue, and disturbances

Table 36.3.   Botulinum Toxin Types: Distribution, Origin, and Pathogenicity

Type	Cultural Types	Geographic Occurrence	Source	Affected Species	Toxins Present
A	I	Western U.S., Canada, ex-U.S.S.R.	Vegetables, fruits (meats, fish)[a]	Humans (chickens, mink)	A
B	I, II	Eastern U.S., Canada, Europe, ex-U.S.S.R.	Meat, pork products (vegetables, fish)	Humans (horses, cattle)	B
Cα	III	New Zealand, Japan, Europe	Vegetation, invertebrates, carrion	Waterfowl	C_1 (C_2)[b]
Cβ	III	Australia, S. Africa, Europe, U.S.	Spoiled feed, carrion	Horses, cattle, mink, dogs (humans)	C_2, D (C_1)
D	III	S. Africa, ex-U.S.S.R., Southwest U.S., France	Carrion	Cattle, sheep (horses, humans)	C_2, D
E	II	N. America, N. Europe, Japan, ex-U.S.S.R.	Raw fish, marine mammals	Humans (fish)	E
F	I, II	U.S., N. Europe, ex-U.S.S.R.	Meat, fish	Humans	F
G[c]	IV	Argentina	Soil	Humans	G

[a] Parentheses indicate infrequency or variability.
[b] C_2 is not a neurotoxin but an ADP-ribosylating toxin affecting fluid movement across membranes. Its effects are cardiopulmonary-enteric, and its role in animal botulism is poorly defined.
[c] Strains producing this toxin are part of the species *Clostridium argentinense*.

in food prehension, chewing, and swallowing (see Fig 71.5). No changes in consciousness occur. The temperature remains normal unless secondary infections such as aspiration pneumonia supervene. In nonfatal cases, recovery is slow and residual signs may persist for months. Equine grass sickness, a commonly fatal dysautonomia, affecting the enteric nervous system is associated with the ingestion of BoNT secreted by *C. botulinum* Type C living in association with blades of grass (as a biofilm).

In birds the disease has been named "limberneck" after the drooping head posture, which often causes waterfowl to drown.

Epidemiology

Types A and B are found in all soils, including virgin soils; C, D, E, and F are linked with wet environments—that is, muddy soils or aquatic sediment. In animals, Types C and D predominate. Type C living in biofilms on the surface of blades of grass is the source of BoNT seen in equine grass sickness.

Dead cats or rodents in feed can be sources of outbreaks, as can chicken manure when used as a cattle feed supplement. Outbreaks on mink ranches are usually due to tainted meat, and those in fish hatcheries to fish food containing *C. botulinum* Type E spores that germinate in bottom sludge. Decaying vegetation triggers outbreaks in waterfowl. As lakes recede in summer leaving muddy shores or shallow pools, rotting plant material becomes accessible. *Clostridium botulinum* and its toxin are ingested and after death permeate the carcass, which is fed upon by blowfly larvae which absorb the toxin. Waterfowl ingesting these larvae become intoxicated.

Type D botulism is classically linked to phosphorus-deficient ranges, where grazing animals feed on carcasses and bones that often contain botulinum toxin. In South African cattle, the condition is called *lamziekte* ("lame disease").

Type B botulism has been seen in cattle and mules. In "toxo-infectious botulism" of foals ("shaker foal syndrome") and adult horses, no toxin has been demonstrated, but the agent has been isolated consistently from tissue.

Human botulism is usually traced to improperly processed meat, seafood, or canned vegetables. Infant botulism involves clostridial growth and toxinogenesis in the intestinal tract, producing the "floppy baby syndrome." Wound-infection botulism results from contaminated external injuries.

Immunologic Aspects

Resistance to botulism depends on circulating antitoxin. Some animals, such as turkey vultures, apparently acquire immunity through repeated sublethal exposure.

Laboratory Diagnosis

Diagnosis of botulism requires demonstration of toxin in plasma or tissue before death or from a fresh carcass. Isola-

tion of the organism, especially from intestinal contents, or postmortem demonstration of toxin is not definitive. Demonstration of toxin in feedstuffs, fresh stomach contents, or vomitus supports a diagnosis of botulism.

Toxin is extracted from suspect material (unless fluids) overnight with saline. The mixture is centrifuged and the clear portion filter-sterilized and trypsinized (1% at 37°C for 45 minutes). Guinea pigs or mice are injected intraperitoneally with the extract, mixtures of extract and antitoxins, and extract heated to 100°C for 10 minutes. Death due to botulism occurs within 10 hours to 3 weeks (average is 4 days) preceded by muscular weakness, limb paralysis, and respiratory difficulties. Any toxin must be neutralizable by one of the *C. botulinum* antitoxins.

Isolation of *C. botulinum* from suspect feeds or tissue begins with heating suspect material for 30 minutes at 65°C to 80°C to induce germination. Type E spores require, in addition, treatment with lysozyme (5 mg/ml of medium). Culture anaerobically on blood agar plates. Identification is by biochemical reactions and toxin production. Immunofluorescence is used to identify some cultural groups. Primers designed to amplify the genes encoding the various toxins (by the polymerase chain reaction) can be used to support the demonstration that *C. botulinum* has been isolated.

Treatment and Control

If recent ingestion is suspected, evacuation of the stomach and purging are helpful. Antitoxin treatment following onset of signs is sometimes beneficial, especially for mink and ducks. Mink and other animals at risk should be vaccinated with toxoid (Types A, B, C, D).

Removal of affected waterfowl to dry land saves many from exposure and drowning. Placing feed on dry ground lures birds from contaminated areas.

Guanidine and aminopyridine stimulate acetylcholine release, and germine intensifies neural impulses. Clinical reports on their use are few and mixed.

CLOSTRIDIUM TETANI

Clostridium tetani is a gram-positive, spore-forming, obligately anaerobic rod, which produces the disease tetanus, a neuroparalytic intoxication characterized by tonic-clonic convulsions. The intoxication is due to a protein neurotoxin.

All mammals are susceptible to varying degrees to tetanus, with horses, ruminants, and swine more susceptible than carnivores and poultry. In all animals, the mortality rate is high.

Descriptive Features

Morphology

Clostridium tetani is a gram-positive, spore-forming, obligately anaerobic rod. A distinguishing morphologic feature

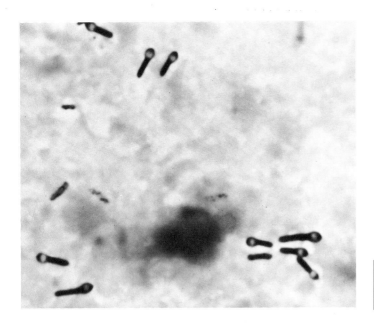

FIGURE 36.1.   Clostridium tetani *in tissues of a lamb recently castrated by the "elastrator" (rubber band) method. Scrotal impression, Gram stain, 1000X.*

of *C. tetani* is the spherical shape and terminal position of its spores ("drumstick," "racket," Fig 36.1).

Cellular Products of Medical Interest

Toxins. Clostridium tetani produces two toxins (tetanolysin and tetanus toxin), but only tetanus toxin is of clinical significance:

1. Tetanus toxin (tetanospasmin). The genes encoding tetanus toxin (TeNT for *te*tanus *n*eurotoxin) are located on a large plasmid. TeNT is released upon lysis of the clostridial cell.

    There is only one type of TeNT, a zinc endopeptidase, which hydrolyzes the docking proteins required by neurotransmitter-containing vesicles to fuse with the presynaptic membrane. TeNT hydrolyzes the docking protein VAMP (*v*esicle-*a*ssociated *m*embrane *p*rotein, also known as synaptobrevin). Once the docking proteins are hydrolyzed, the synapse degenerates, taking weeks to months to regenerate.

    TeNT is a "di-chain" molecule consisting of a light chain (with zinc endopeptidase activity), a heavy chain composed of a translocation domain (responsible for forming a pore through which the light chain passes), and a binding domain (responsible for binding to nerve cells).

    TeNT binds to cholinergic nerve cells by virtue of receptors that are different from those recognized by BoNT. These receptors are composed of lipid containing rafts and glycosylphosphatidylinositol (GPI)-anchored proteins. After binding, the toxin is internalized by way of receptor-mediated endocytosis. Vesicles containing TeNT travel by retrograde axonal transport to the inhibitory interneurons in

the ventral horn of the spinal cord. Following a cleaving event, the light chain (the zinc endopeptidase) translocates across the vesicle membrane into the cytosol of the nerve cell where it hydrolyzes the "docking" proteins involved with vesicles containing the neurotransmitters gamma aminobutyric acid (GABA) and glycine.

2. Tetanolysin. Tetanolysin is a cholesterol-binding cytolysin (see also clostridial perfringolysin O, septicolysin O, novyilysin, chauveolysin, above; streptococcal streptolysin O, Chapter 28; listerial listeriolysin O, Chapter 33; and arcanobacterial pyolysin, Chapter 29). Tetanolysin binds to cholesterol-containing rafts in the eukaryotic cell membrane. Once bound, it forms a pore resulting in the death of the cell. Tetanolysin has no known pathogenic significance in the production of tetanus.

Growth Characteristics

Clostridium tetani grows on blood agar under routine anaerobic conditions. There may be swarming. Its differential reactions (carbohydrate fermentation, proteolysis, indole production) vary with the medium used.

Spores resist boiling up to 1.5 hours, but not autoclaving (121°C/10 min). Disinfection by some halogen compounds (3% iodine) can be effective within several hours, but phenol, lysol, and formalin in the usual concentrations are ineffective.

Variability

Ten serologic types, based on flagellar antigens, are somewhat related to geographic strain origin. TeNT is antigenically uniform.

Ecology

Reservoir and Transmission

Clostridium tetani is widely distributed in soil and is often a transient in the intestine. Spores are introduced into wounds.

Pathogenesis

Spore germination requires an anaerobic environment as found in tissues devitalized by crushing, burning, laceration, breakdown of blood supply (e.g., umbilical stump or placental remnants), or bacterial infection. Under these circumstances, *C. tetani* proliferates and its toxin diffuses via vascular channels or peripheral nerve trunks. The toxin attaches to receptors on the nearest cholinergic nerve and is internalized within a vesicle, which travels retrograde inside the axons to the cell bodies in the ventral horns of the spinal cord. The light chain of the toxin translocates across the vesicle membrane into the cytosol where it hydrolyzes "docking" proteins and suppresses release of afferent inhibitory messenger substances (glycine, gamma aminobutyric acid) causing the innervated muscles to remain in sustained clonic or tonic spasms. The toxin also travels within the cord to other levels affecting additional muscle groups. Synapses degenerate following hydrolysis of the "docking" proteins, taking several weeks to regenerate.

The process described ("ascending tetanus") is typical of animals not highly susceptible to tetanus toxin (e.g., dogs and cats). Only nerve trunks near the toxigenic site absorb sufficient toxin to produce overt signs.

"Descending tetanus" is typical of highly susceptible species (horses, humans) in which effective toxin quantities are disseminated via vascular channels to nerve endings in areas remote from the toxigenic site. Toxin enters the central nervous system at many levels producing generalized tetanus, frequently beginning cranially. The sequence reflects susceptibility of various neurons.

Disease Patterns. Early signs, following an incubation period of a few days to several weeks, are stiffness, muscular tremor, and increased responsiveness to stimuli:

1. In horses, ruminants, and swine , which usually develop descending tetanus, retraction of the third eyelid, erectness of ears, grinding of teeth, and stiffness of the tail are observed. Bloat is common in ruminants. Feeding becomes impossible ("lockjaw"). Rigidity of extremities causes "sawhorse" attitudes and, eventually, recumbency. Tetanic spasms occur first in response to stimuli, but later become permanent. There is fecal and urinary retention, sweating, and high fever. Consciousness persists. Death, due to respiratory arrest, occurs in lambs and piglets within the first week, in adult animals in 1 to 2 weeks. Full recovery requires weeks to months.
2. In carnivores, the incubation period tends to be longer, and local (ascending) tetanus (stiffness, tremors) is frequently seen near the original wound. Progression may be slower than in ungulates, but signs and course are comparable.

Mortality is at least 50% and highest in the young.

Epidemiology

Occurrence of tetanus is linked to the introduction of *C. tetani* spores into traumatized tissue (see under "Pathogenesis," above): penetrating nail wounds of the foot, barnyard surgery, the use of rubber bands for castrating and docking sheep, ear tagging, injections, shearing wounds, postpartum uterine infections, perinatal umbilical infections, and small animal fights and leghold traps.

Immunologic Aspects

Acquired resistance to tetanus depends on circulating antitoxin. Small amounts have been demonstrated in normal ruminants. Survivors of tetanus with the possible exception of dogs and cats are susceptible to reinfection. The amount of toxin needed to result in tetanus in dogs and cats is sometimes large enough to elicit an antitoxin response.

Passive and active protection is provided by administration of antitoxin or immunization with toxoid, respectively (see under "Treatment and Control," below).

Laboratory Diagnosis

A gram-stained smear from a suspect wound may reveal the typical "drumstick" type of bacteria (see Fig 36.1). Their absence does not exclude tetanus, and their presence is merely suggestive as the morphology is not unique.

Wound exudate is plated on blood agar for anaerobic culture. Increased agar content (up to 4%) inhibits swarming, and a drop of antitoxin will inhibit hemolysis on that portion of the plate.

Replicate cooked meat broth cultures are incubated and some are heated at 80°C for varying periods (up to 20 minutes). All are incubated at 37°C for 4 days and subcultured to blood agar periodically during that time. Previously unheated ones are heated before subculture. Suspect isolates are identified by differential tests and confirmed as tetanus toxin producers by intramuscular injection of a 48-hour broth culture into two mice, one of which has received antitoxin.

Primers designed to amplify the gene encoding tetanus toxin (by the polymerase chain reaction) can be used to support the demonstration that *C. tetani* has been isolated.

Treatment and Control

Therapy aims at 1) neutralization of circulating toxin, 2) suppression of toxin production, and 3) life support and symptomatic relief to the patient.

The first objective is pursued by injection of adequate doses of antitoxin: 10,000 to 300,000 units for horses. Some suggest intrathecal administration.

Wound care and large doses of parenteral penicillin or metronidazole are aimed at stopping toxin production. Supportive treatment includes use of sedatives and muscle relaxants and exclusion of external stimuli. Artificial feeding by stomach tube or intravenously may be necessary after the hyperesthetic phase. Nursing care is most important.

Prevention

Wounds should be properly cleaned and dressed. During surgical procedures, especially on a mass scale under farm conditions, appropriate hygienic precautions should be observed. Horses, unless actively immunized, are given antitoxin after injury or surgery, and depot penicillin.

Active immunization employs formalinized toxoid, given twice at 1-to-2-month intervals and annually thereafter.

Passive immunity passes from immunized mare to nursing foals and appears to provide protection for about 10 weeks, when toxoid can be given.

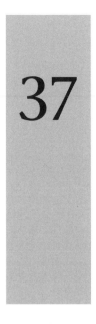

37

Filamentous Bacteria: *Actinomyces, Nocardia, Dermatophilus,* and *Streptobacillus*

Ernst L. Biberstein   Dwight C. Hirsh

Members of the genera *Actinomyces, Nocardia, Dermatophilus,* and *Streptobacillus* produce filamentous forms at some time in their growth cycle.

Actinomyces and Nocardia

Members of the genera *Actinomyces* and *Nocardia* are grampositive bacteria that grow in branching filaments. Apart from this pattern, these two genera have little in common. However, their morphologic resemblance and similarities in pathogenic patterns (pyogranulomatous inflammation with fistulous tracts) justify their consideration under a common heading. Table 37.1 summarizes their differential characteristics.

Actinomyces spp.

Descriptive Features

Morphology and Staining

Members of the genus *Actinomyces* are gram-positive diphtheroid or filamentous rods, about 0.5 μm in width. Branching filaments, often beaded due to uneven staining, are most readily demonstrable in pathologic specimens (Fig 37.1). In culture, diphtheroid forms predominate (see Chapter 31 for a discussion of this morphotype). As of this writing, there are approximately 25 species of *Actinomyces*, most of which are associated with diseases of human patients. The few that are involved with pathologic conditions in animals are listed in Table 37.2.

Structure and Composition

Actinomyces spp. have distinctive cell wall constituents (see Table 37.1). Surface fibrils in *A. viscosus* may be adhesins for host cells or other bacteria ("coaggregation"). Surface antigens are related to chemotactic and mitogenic activities.

Each named species of *Actinomyces* has group antigens and several serologic subtypes.

Growth Characteristics

Animal *Actinomyces* spp. are capnophilic or facultative anaerobes. All require rich media, preferably containing serum or blood. No growth occurs on Sabouraud's agar or at room temperature. Development of macroscopic colonies may require several days of incubation at 37°C. Colonial morphology varies between and within species. Hemolysis is rare.

Biochemical Activities

Actinomyces spp. are catalase-negative, with some exceptions (e.g., *A. viscosus* and *A. canis*).

Resistance

Actinomyces spp. are readily killed by heat and disinfectants and require frequent passage to survive in culture.

Ecology

Reservoir

Members of the genus *Actinomyces* are found on oral mucous membranes and tooth surfaces, the mucous membranes of the urogenital tract, and secondarily (presumably) in the gastrointestinal tract.

Transmission

Most actinomycotic infections are endogenous, that is, they are caused by introduction of a commensal strain into susceptible tissue of its host. Bites are another means of transmission (rare).

Table 37.1.   Contrasting Characteristics of Actinomyces and Common Pathogenic Nocardia

Characteristic	Actinomyces	Nocardia
Source	Endogenous	Exogenous
Atmospheric requirements	Anaerobic/microaerophilic	Aerobic
Catalase	– or +	+
Growth on Sabouraud's agar	–	+
Acid-fastness	–	+
Penicillin	Susceptible	Resistant[a]
Cell wall contains meso DAP[b]	–	+
Lysine	+	–
Mycolic acid	–	+
Lymph node involvement	Rare	Common
Granules in exudate ("sulfur granules")	Common	Rare

[a] "*Nocardia nova*" are susceptible to penicillin.
[b] Diaminopimelic acid.

Pathogenesis

Pathology. Members of the genus *Actinomyces* evoke pyogranulomatous reactions by unknown mechanisms. Bacterial colonies form in tissue, triggering suppurative responses in the immediate vicinity. Peripheral to this, granulation, mononuclear infiltration, and fibrosis furnish the granulomatous elements. Sinus tracts carry exudate to the outside; the exudate often contains yellowish "sulfur granules," which are colonial masses surrounded by a microscopic fringe of "clubs" consisting of mineral and possibly antigen-antibody complexes. They are also called rosettes (Fig 37.2, and see Fig 69.2). Alternatively, *Actinomyces* spp. may be found, usually in mixed culture, in abscesses, empyemas, or suppurative serositis.

Disease Patterns

Ruminants.   *"Lumpy jaw."* In "lumpy jaw" of cattle (and occasionally other ruminants), *A. bovis* and (exceptionally) *A. israelii* are introduced from an oral reservoir by a traumatic event (e.g., poor quality feed) into the alveolar or paralveolar region of the jaw initiating a chronic rarefying osteomyelitis. This leads eventually to replacement of normal bone by porous bone, which is laid down irregularly and honeycombed with sinus tracts containing pus. There may be dislodgement of teeth, inability to chew, and mandibular fractures. The lesion expands but has little tendency for vascular dissemination. Similar infections occur in humans and marsupials.

Horses.   *"Poll Evil" and "Fistulous Withers."* Supra-atlantal ("poll evil") and supraspinous bursitis ("fistulous withers"), sometimes contain *Actinomyces*, usually alongside other bacteria (e.g., *Brucella abortus*).

Cervical Lymphadenitis. An unspeciated *Actinomyces* is sometimes isolated from cervical abscess, mimicking *Streptococcus equi* subspecies *equi* infections.

Dogs and Cats.   *Actinomyces* are common isolates from suppurative serositides of small carnivores. In dogs, actinomycosis may be associated (e.g., by licking) with foreign bodies, particularly migrating grass awns, especially of the genus *Hordeum* ("foxtails"), which sometimes lodge near vertebrae, causing actinomycotic discospondylitis. Cutaneous actinomycosis in dogs is a rare noduloulcerative lymphangitis.

Swine.   *Mastitis.* Mastitis in sows is sometimes associated with *Actinomyces*.

Pneumonia. *Actinomyces* is sometimes recovered, along with other bacteria, from lung lesions in swine.

Abortion. *Actinomyces* is sometimes recovered from aborted fetuses.

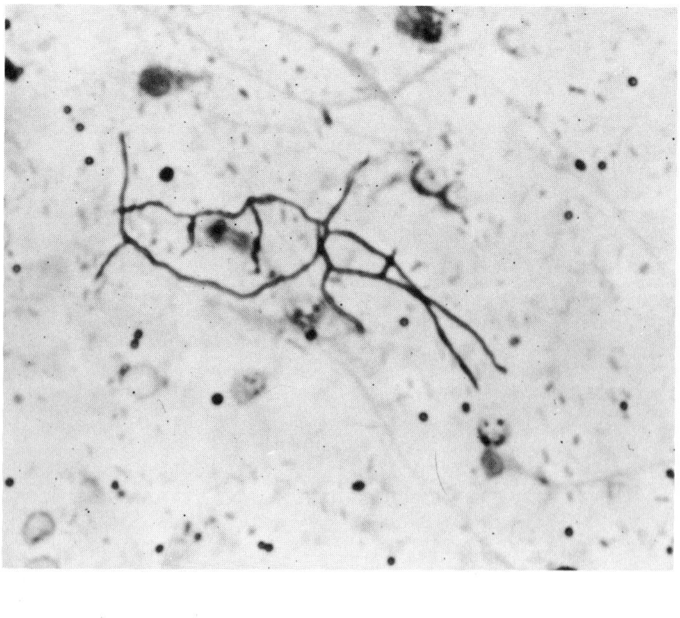

FIGURE 37.1.   Actinomyces *spp. in aspirate from retrobulbar abscess in a horse. Gram stain, 1000X.*

Table 37.2. Members of the Genus Actinomyces Affecting Animals and Their Usual Source or Associated Condition

Species	Usual Source or Associated Condition
Actinomyces bovis	Ruminant jaw ("lumpy jaw")
A. canis	Pyonecrotic processes of dogs; vagina of dogs
A. catuli	Pyonecrotic processes of dogs
A. coleocanis	Normal vagina of dogs
A. hordeovulneris	Plant awn-associated pyonecrotic conditions in dogs and cats
A. hyovaginalis	Abortion in swine; pneumonia in swine
A. israelii	Ruminant jaw ("lumpy jaw")—rare; pyonecrotic processes in dogs—rare
A. marimammalium	Disseminated disease in marine mammals
A. naeslundii	Abortion in swine—rare
A. suimastitidis	Mastitis in swine
A. vaccimaxillae	Ruminant jaw ("lumpy jaw")—rare
A. viscosus	Pyonecrotic processes of dogs and cats

Epidemiology

Actinomycosis is noncommunicable, except via bites (which is a rare form of transmission). Contamination of bursae or body cavities may be hematogenous or result from perforations of the alimentary tract, or body wall. Actinomycosis associated with plant awns ("foxtails") occurs in outdoor dogs in semiarid areas.

Actinomyces-associated diseases occur in goats, sheep, wild ruminants, monkeys, rabbits, squirrels, hamsters, marsupials, and birds. Except for occasional reported isolations of *A. israelii* in dogs and cattle, there is little to suggest interspecific transmission of *Actinomyces* spp.

Immunologic Factors

Infected humans show cell-mediated and humoral immune responses.

Circulating antibody, produced during infection, confers no protection. Specific resistance, if any, is probably cell-mediated. Phagocytes kill *Actinomyces*. No artificial immunization is available.

Laboratory Diagnosis

Sample Collection

Aspirates from unopened lesions or tissues, preferably including granules, are optimal.

Direct Examination

Suspected exudates are examined for "sulfur granules"—yellowish particles, varying in firmness, up to several millimeters in diameter. Granules are washed in saline and placed on a slide in a drop of saline. A cover slip is gently pressed down. The preparation is examined under subdued light (see Fig 37.2). Rosettes are suggestive of actinomycosis, especially if bacterial-sized filaments extend into the clubbed fringe.

Crushed granules, exudate, or tissue impressions are stained with Gram and acid-fast stains (Kinyoun's). Branching, gram-positive, beaded, non–acid-fast filaments suggest *Actinomyces* spp. (see Fig 37.1).

Isolation and Identification

Most strains obtained from animals do not require anaerobic incubation but benefit from increased carbon diox-

FIGURE 37.2. *"Sulfur granule" in bovine pleural fluid showing an amorphous center and clubbed fringe. Unstained wet mount, 400X.*

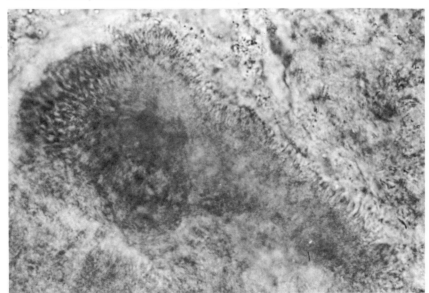

ide. Granules offer the best chance of isolation from the usually mixed flora. Colonies develop in 48 hours or more after incubation at 35–37°C. Organisms of suggestive morphology and staining characteristics are tested for catalase activity. Isolates grown on blood agar sometimes give false-positive catalase results.

Precise identification includes cell wall analysis (see Table 37.1) and biochemical tests. Many animal isolates cannot be assigned to existing species. DNA primers based upon the sequence of genes encoding the 16S ribosomal RNA have been designed for speciation of members of this genus by using the polymerase chain reaction.

Treatment and Control

In bovine actinomycosis, iodine compounds given orally (4 to 8 gm) daily or intravenously (75 mg/kg) weekly are used. Treatment must be interrupted when signs of toxicity appear (hypersalivation, anorexia, vomiting) but can be resumed some weeks later. Accessible soft tissue lesions can be drained or excised.

Penicillin and aminoglycoside combinations are often used on bovine actinomycosis. The contribution of aminoglycoside is uncertain. Isoniazid per os has been advocated. Bacteriologic cure of lumpy jaw will not restore normal bone structure, but the process can be arrested by systemic medication aided by drainage, lavage (iodine), and debridement of lesions.

In dogs and cats, surgery (drainage, lavage, excision, removal of foreign bodies) is required, supplemented by long-term antimicrobic therapy. A penicillin derivative (e.g., ampicillin) is the drug of choice. Alternatives are erythromycin, rifampin, cephaloridine, and minocycline. Aminoglycosides and fluoroquinolones are ineffective. Remnants of plant awns together with the propensity of

Actinomyces spp. to form cell wall–deficient variants (L-forms) make treatment of this condition difficult.

Where plant awns (foxtails) are prevalent, conscientious grooming is a critical preventive step.

NOCARDIA

Nocardiae are aerobic, saprophytic, gram-positive, partially acid-fast filamentous bacteria present in most environments. Diseases attributed to members of this genus occur in mammals, fish, mollusks, and birds (rarely). Generalized suppurative and pyogranulomatous processes occur in immunosuppressed and massively exposed individuals. Currently, there are 30 species included within the genus. *Nocardia asteroides*, the species most often associated in the literature with diseases of animals, has been shown to be composed of several species (*N. asteroides, N. abscessus, N. cyriacigeorgica, N. farcinica, N. nova,* and *N. transvalensis*). For this reason, in the discussion that follows, a species designation will not be given to the nocardial agents associated with the various diseases ascribed to members of this genus, unless isolates were identified by techniques (mostly DNA-based analyses) currently accepted for identification of this group of bacteria.

Descriptive Features

Morphology and Staining

Gram-stained *Nocardia* spp. are indistinguishable from *Actinomyces* spp. (Fig 37.3). Nocardiae alternate between the coccobacillary (resting phase) and the actively growing filamentous forms.

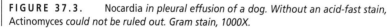

FIGURE 37.3. Nocardia *in pleural effusion of a dog. Without an acid-fast stain,* Actinomyces *could not be ruled out. Gram stain, 1000X.*

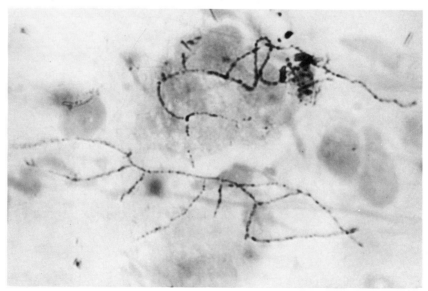

Structure and Composition

The cell wall is typical of gram-positive bacteria, with the addition of meso-diamino-pimelic acid (DAP), arabino-galactan, and mycolic acids (branched chained fatty acids with a chain length of C_{46}–C_{60} for *Nocardia*). The cell wall contains a high concentration of lipids. No exotoxins are known, but a superoxide dismutase acts as a virulence factor. Soluble antigens—largely protein—are type-specific.

Growth Characteristics

Pathogenic nocardiae are obligate aerobes growing on simple media (e.g., Sabouraud's) over a wide temperature range (10 to 50°C). Colonies, which appear after several days, are opaque and variously pigmented. The colony surface, waxy to powdery to velvety depending on the abundance of aerial growth, becomes wrinkled with age. Colonial diameters may reach several centimeters. In broth, a surface pellicle or sediment is produced, but little turbidity.

Biochemical activities include catalase production, acidification of various carbohydrates, and usually urea hydrolysis.

Resistance

Nocardiae thrive in the environment. All are susceptible to chlorine disinfectants (100 ppm/5 min) and benzalkonium chloride (100 ppm/10 min).

Variability

Colonial dissociation is seen in single strains. Serotypes are based on soluble antigens.

Ecology

Reservoir

Pathogenic nocardiae are saprophytes found in many climates in soils and water, either as indigenous flora or contaminants.

Transmission

Three main routes of infection are inhalation, trauma, and ingestion. Dust, soil, and plant material serve as vehicles. Nocardiae producing bovine mastitis are introduced and disseminated by equipment and personnel.

Pathogenesis

Mechanisms. Pathogenic nocardiae survive within phagocytic vacuoles by preventing phagolysosome formation. This is attributed to a surface lipid. Other cell wall lipids may trigger granulomatous reactions. Variations between strains and growth phases in cell envelope constituents are paralleled by changes in virulence and infectivity.

Superoxide dismutase and lysosomal enzyme inhibition protect against phagocytic killing.

Pathology. Nocardiosis is a predominantly suppurative process with variable granulomatous features. Lymph nodes are consistently involved. Hematogenous dissemination may result in osteomyelitis and widespread abscess formation. Central nervous involvement is rare in animals (though fairly common in human patients). In dogs, the common form is thoracic empyema with granulomatous serositis. Exudates are sanguinopurulent and sometimes contain small (<1 mm diameter), soft granules consisting of bacteria, neutrophils, and debris ("sulfur granule-like"). They usually lack the microstructure of sulfur granules sometimes seen with *Actinomyces* infections (see above, "Actinomyces").

Disease Patterns

Infections can be regional or disseminated. Local wound infections may extend to contiguous areas or regional lymph nodes.

Ruminants. *Mastitis.* Bovine nocardial mastitis is often initiated with "homemade" udder infusions (contaminated with *Nocardia*). Onset is sudden with fever, anorexia, and abnormal milk secretion. The affected gland is swollen, hot, and painful. Discharging fistulous tracts may develop. Lymphadenopathy is common, and there is occasional dissemination. The affected gland usually becomes nonfunctional. Fatalities (5% to 10%) may occur during the acute stage or upon rupture of the udder.

Bovine "Farcy." Bovine farcy is a chronic suppurative infection usually starting at the lower limbs. It involves the lymphatics of the extremities or head region and the associated lymph nodes. Ulcers and discharging sinuses form along the path of infection. Affected animals remain in general good health unless dissemination to internal organs occurs. The disease is restricted to the tropics and attributed to *N. farcinica* or *Mycobacterium farcinogenes* (see Chapter 38).

Miscellaneous. Pneumonia, abortion, and lymphadenitis are sometimes (rarely) encountered associated with *Nocardia*.

Horses. In horses, rare local or general infections with *Nocardia* are seen, the latter secondary to profound constitutional disturbances (equine Cushing's, combined immunodeficient foals).

"Norcardioform placentitis." "Norcardioform placentitis" is a relatively uncommon condition of mares. The agent, a gram-positive branching, filamentous bacteria, is associated with placentitis and abortion. Though similar to members of the genus *Nocardia* in morphology, the cause of this condition is the bacterium *Crossiella equi*, a microorganism unrelated to *Nocardia*.

Dogs and Cats. Dogs and cats develop debilitating, febrile illness. Pneumonia and suppurative pleuritis with empyema is the common finding. Dissemination occurs to liver, kidneys, bones, joints, and, rarely, the central nervous system. Case fatality rate exceeds 50%. *Nocardia nova* is the nocardial agent most commonly encountered.

Mycetoma. Nocardial mycetoma ("actinomycotic mycetoma" see Chapter 47) has been reported in dogs and cats.

Swine. Pneumonia, abortion, and lymphadenitis are sometimes (rarely) encountered associated with *Nocardia*.

Miscellaneous Species. Nocardiosis observed in birds (rare), whales, and dolphins are mostly respiratory with signs of dissemination.

Epidemiology

Pathogenic nocardiae occur worldwide, suggesting constant exposure. In humans, disease is associated largely with immunodeficiencies. This association is established in horses. In dogs disease may occur as a sequela to an immunosuppressive virus infection, e.g., canine distemper. Canine nocardiosis is most common in pups.

Bovine nocardial mastitis is most often traceable to unsatisfactory hygienic practices. Typically infection is introduced during the "dry period" with intramammary mastitis therapy. Acute mastitis is triggered when onset of lactation flushes the organism from limited foci through the lactiferous duct system. Alternatively, nocardiosis appears spontaneously in one animal and spreads in the course of milking operations.

Immunologic Aspects

Antibody and cell-mediated immune responses, including hypersensitivity, commonly develop during nocardial infections. Yet severe nocardiosis in several species is associated with immunosuppression, particularly of cell-mediated responses.

Antibody apparently confers little protection. Specific resistance is largely cell-mediated.

No practical immunization method is presently available.

Laboratory Diagnosis

Branching, gram-positive, acid-fast beaded filaments, along with shorter, coccobacillary forms, are found in smears made from nocardia-infected samples, impressions, and sections. Granules are sometimes observed.

Specimens for culture should not be chilled or frozen. Nocardial colonies on blood agar, incubated at 37°C, will be dull opaque, waxy to velvety, and hard to dislodge by loop or needle. Stains confirm nocardial morphology. Acid-fastness may be lost on culture. Catalase tests are positive, and the agent fails to grow serially under anaerobic conditions.

Serologic (immunodiffusion, complement fixation, enzyme-linked immunosorbent assays) and cutaneous hypersensitivity tests employing extracellular antigen to detect nocardial infection in cattle and dogs are of uncertain sensitivity and are not generally available.

Identification of isolates involves determination of cell wall constituents, as well as determination of restriction length polymorphism (RFLP) of DNA encoding the heat shock protein, GroEL. RFLP data combined with susceptibility to a battery of antimicrobial agents (piperacillin, ampicillin, erythromycin, imipenem, ciprofloxacin, cefo-

taxime, and tobramycin) aid in the identification of isolates. Determination of the sequence of the DNA encoding the 16S ribosomal RNA has also been used.

Treatment and Control

Antimicrobic therapy of nocardial mastitis may produce temporary clinical relief and cessation of shedding, but no permanent cures. Control involves removal of infected animals, thorough disinfection of premises and equipment, and scrupulous stabling and milking hygiene.

In other forms of nocardiosis, trimethoprim-sulfonamide therapy has produced impressive results, especially when combined with surgery.

Alternative drugs include minocycline and doxycycline. Nocardiae are fairly resistant to the fluoroquinolones. *Nocardia nova* responds to the penicillins and macrolides (erythromycin, clarithromycin), and the tetracyclines (doxycycline, minocycline).

Abscesses, empyemas, and serosal effusions are treated by drainage and lavage. Granulomatous proliferations require excision.

DERMATOPHILUS CONGOLENSIS

Dermatophilosis or streptothricosis (cattle and other species), rain scald or rain rot (horses), grease heal (horses), lumpy wool (sheep), and strawberry footrot (sheep) are infections due to *Dermatophilus congolensis*, a gram-positive, filamentous bacterium. In temperate climates, dermatophilosis is often a cosmetic problem controllable by management practices. In sheep and cattle, especially in tropical areas, it can severely affect productivity.

Descriptive Features

Morphology and Composition

The reproductive unit of *D. congolensis* is the motile coccoid "zoospore," about 2 μm in diameter. Upon germinating, zoospores sprout a germ tube, about 1 μm thick, which elongates and thickens, dividing both transversely and longitudinally, forming a strand several cell layers thick. Enclosed in a gelatinous sheath, constituent cells become coccoid as they differentiate into multiflagellated zoospores, which are liberated as the strand disintegrates, completing the life cycle.

Dermatophilus has a cell wall containing mesodiaminopimelic acid, but lacking glycine and arabinogalactan.

Growth Characteristics

Dermatophilus congolensis grows on blood and infusion media, but not on Sabouraud agar. It is aerobic and capnophilic. Hemolytic colonies, which develop in 48 hours, vary from mucoid to viscous and waxy, whitish-gray to yellow, and smooth to wrinkled. Glucose and some other carbohydrates are attacked nonfermentatively. Catalase, urease, and proteases are produced. The agent survives well in soil and on fomites.

There is colonial and antigenic variability, but all strains appear to share antigens.

Ecology

Reservoir

Dermatophilus congolensis does not multiply saprophytically. Its reservoir is infected animals. Cattle, sheep, goats, and horses are common hosts. It has been diagnosed in swine, dogs and cats, turkeys, primates (including humans), and wild mammals, including marine mammals. The distribution of *D. congolensis* is worldwide, but its greatest economic significance is in tropical Africa.

Transmission

Spread is by direct and indirect contact. Transmission occurs through flying and nonflying, biting and nonbiting arthropods. Injury by thorny range plants and shearing cuts may create portals of infection or inoculate the agent.

Pathogenesis

The disease is an exudative epidermitis. Its primary activity is confined to the living epidermis. As access to this is limited by hair, wool, sebaceous secretions, and the stratum corneum, infection depends on their disruption by soaking or trauma. Deposited zoospores, responding to a CO_2 gradient, "home" into deeper cell layers. Upon germination, germ tubes and filaments arborize within the epidermis and colonize hair follicles. A layer of inflammatory cells (largely neutrophils) forms under the infected epidermis, which keratinizes (see Fig 69.1). Beneath the neutrophils new epidermis forms, which in turn is invaded. The eventual result is a scab consisting of layers of neutrophilic exu-

date and infected keratinizing epidermis. The scabs are easily lifted by the hair, which protrudes from both surfaces.

The primary lesions are painless and nonpruritic. Wetting favors their expansion. Biting arthropods can infect areas protected from soaking rain (axilla, flank, ventral trunk). Soaking provides the preparatory step for lesions on the back (equine "rain scald"), feet, and legs (ovine "strawberry footrot," equine "grease heel"). The extent varies from a few scabby areas of roughened hair or "lumpy wool" to widespread loss of epidermis, causing secondary parasitisms or infections and eventual loss of the animal. This progressive form affects African cattle. Neglected cases of "lumpy wool" may lead to complete solidification of the fleece.

Dermatophilosis in nonepidermal tissue—tongue, the urinary bladder, lymph nodes, and subcutis—is reported in cats (rare).

Epidemiology

The prevalence of dermatophilosis depends on 1) infected animals; 2) dissemination, for example, by arthropods or thorny plants; and 3) susceptible hosts' epidermis rendered accessible by trauma or wetting.

Immunologic Aspects

Antibody is widespread among cattle in endemic areas. Its protective role, relative to that of cell-mediated resistance, is at present unsettled.

Attempts at artificial immunization have been inconclusive.

Laboratory Diagnosis

Gram or Giemsa stains of ground-up scabs usually show typical phases of the life cycle described (Fig 37.4). In suba-

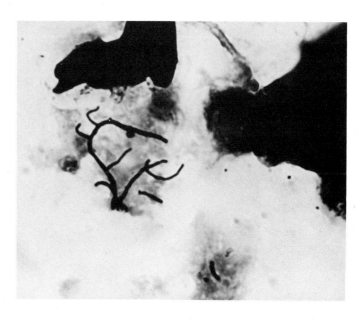

FIGURE 37.4.   Dermatophilus congolensis *in smear from a lesion of "rain scald" in a horse. Gram stain, 1000X.*

cute and chronic cases, bacterial elements may be rare and lack, for example, multicellular branching filaments. Zoospores resemble large cocci. They and other *Dermatophilus* fragments in skin debris may be identified by fluorescent antibody.

Dermatophilus congolensis is cultured on blood agar under 5% to 10% carbon dioxide at 35–37°C. Colonies appear within 48 hours and when gram-stained are seen to consist of branching filaments and zoospores. A wet mount reveals motile zoospores.

Treatment and Control

Acute cases are often self-limited. Mild cases respond to grooming and removal to shelter. Severe cases can be treated parenterally with penicillin G, tetracycline, chloramphenicol, or spiramycin.

Control should be aimed at minimizing skin trauma and exposure to rain and arthropods.

STREPTOBACILLUS MONILIFORMIS

The taxonomic position of *Streptobacillus moniliformis*, an agent of rat-bite fever, is uncertain. In rodents, it causes respiratory infections, and in rodents, turkeys, and humans, systemic infections that commonly localize in joints.

Descriptive Features

Streptobacillus moniliformis is a nonmotile, gram-negative, pleomorphic rod that often grows in long, beaded filaments bearing knobby irregularities. Its cellular proteins vary with geographic and pathologic sources. It requires blood or serum-enriched media and incubation for 48 hours or more at 35–37°C to produce visible gray, mucoid colonies. Dissociation into cell wall-deficient L-forms produces mycoplasma-like colonies that are recognizable among the conventional colonies. It is a facultative anaerobe, oxidase and catalase-negative, and ferments glucose and some other carbohydrates. Its resistance is not remarkable.

Ecology

The reservoir is the pharynx of rodents, particularly rats, and possibly small carnivores and swine. Infection is by bite or other contact with contaminated material, including ingestion, as in milk-borne "Haverhill fever" among humans.

Lesions are inflammatory and often purulent or necrotic. Rats and mice develop bronchopneumonia and guinea pigs cervical lymphadenitis. In turkeys and mice, septicemic infections lead to polyarthritis or synovitis and often death.

In humans, prostrating fever, accompanied by a rash on the extremities, precedes localization in joints, lymph nodes, lungs, or heart valves. Mortality rates may approximate 10% in untreated cases.

Immunologic Aspects

Little is known about immunity. Antibodies are produced during infection.

Laboratory Diagnosis

Diagnosis requires demonstration of the agent. It can be visualized directly by immunofluorescent reagents and cultivated in thioglycolate broth and blood agar or other rich media in a moist chamber. Identification is by morphologic and biochemical traits. The agent produces a unique array of cell wall fatty acids that can be determined chromatographically. Production of L-form colonies is favored by special media (e.g., Rogosa's).

Treatment and Control

The obvious preventive measure is avoidance of direct and indirect contact with likely carriers. Effective antimicrobics include penicillin G and tetracycline.

38 *Mycobacterium*

Dwight C. Hirsh   Ernst L. Biberstein

Members of the genus *Mycobacterium* are aerobic, acid-fast rods. There are approximately 100 members of this genus, and although most are saprophytic organisms that live in the environment, some are strict parasites inhabiting the mucous membranes of their host. Diseases produced by various species of mycobacteria include tuberculosis, leprosy (in human patients), and granulomatous diseases in previously normal or compromised mammals, birds, reptiles, and fish.

Descriptive Features

Morphology and Staining

Mycobacteria are predominantly rod-shaped, about 0.5 μm wide, and variable in length. Spores, flagella, and capsules are absent.

Mycobacteria, though cytochemically gram-positive, often resist staining with the Gram stain. Their most noted staining property is their acid fastness—i.e., once stained, they resist discoloration with 3% hydrochloric acid in ethanol. Mycobacteria can be stained with fluorescent dyes (e.g., auramine-rhodamine).

Structure and Composition

Mycobacterial cells abound in lipids, especially in their walls. Lipids account for acid fastness and some pathogenic and immunologic properties.

The surface mycosides (mostly glycolipids and peptidoglycolipids) determine colonial characteristics, serologic specificities, and bacteriophage susceptibilities.

Subsurface layers of long-chain branched mycolic acids and their esters make up the bulk of cell wall lipids. Acid fastness somehow depends upon these cell wall constituents. Mycolic acids are linked to the innermost peptidoglycan layer by way of arabinogalactans (see also *Corynebacterium*, Chapter 31; *Nocardia*, Chapter 37).

The presence of carotenoid pigments in some mycobacteria ("chromogens" vs. "nonchromogens") and their light dependence ("photochromogens" vs. "scotochromogens") is a basis for classifying nontuberculous mycobacteria.

Cellular Products of Medical Interest

Alkyl Hydroperoxidase Reductase. Ahp (for *alkyl hydroperoxidase reductase*) is responsible for resistance to superoxides and reactive nitrogen intermediates found within macrophage phagolysosomes.

Dimycolyl Trehalose (Cord Factor). Dimycolyl trehalose, among other effects, immobilizes neutrophils, acts as an adjuvant, evokes granulomatous responses, and causes mitochondrial disruption leading to disturbances in cellular respiration. Its relation to the "cord" pattern of mycobacterial growth is not proven.

Iron Acquisition. See next section, "Mycobactins and Exochelins."

Mycobactins and Exochelins. Mycobactins and exochelins are cell wall amines involved in iron acquisition. Exochelins are proteins that remove ferric iron from ferritin. Mycobactin is a complex lipid residing in the cell membrane of the microorganism and is responsible for transfer of iron from iron-exochelin complexes to the bacterium.

Sulfolipids (or Sulfatides) and Phosphatidyl Inositol Mannoside (PIM). Sulfolipids and phosphatidyl inositol mannoside (a phospholipid) aid in preventing the respiratory burst and phagolysosomal fusion, and interfere with function of reactive oxygen intermediates following ingestion by macrophages.

Surface Mycosides. Surface mycosides (mostly glycolipids and peptidoglycolipids) are considered helpful in ensuring bacterial survival within macrophages.

Waxes. Waxes of various kinds are contained within the cell wall, have adjuvant activity, and activate macrophages leading to granuloma formation.

Immunity to Members of the Genus Mycobacterium—General

Mycobacteria display a variety of surface proteins, carbohydrates, and lipids on their surfaces. These substances (mannose residues; lipoarabinomannan) or substances that are bound to them (e.g., opsonins such as complement proteins) react with receptors on the surface of macrophages (e.g., mannose receptors, complement receptors, Toll-like receptors).

A number of events occur following binding of mycobacteria to the surface of macrophages; the two most important are 1) direct activation, and 2) phagocytosis leading to activation. Direct activation is the result of components of the bacteria (mainly lipoarabinomannan) binding to macrophage cell surface receptors (e.g., the CD14/Toll-like receptor complex). Following phagocytosis, Toll-like receptors in the wall of the phagosome bind to cell wall–associated lipoproteins, resulting in the activation of the macrophage.

Activated macrophages secrete a variety of proinflammatory cytokines, the most important being interleukin 12 (IL-12). IL-12 induces the production of interferon γ (INF-gamma), granulocyte monocyte colony stimulating factor (GM-CSF), and migration inhibition factor (MIF), which attract and activate macrophages. Activated macrophages acquire the capacity to kill mycobacteria. INF-gamma up regulates macrophage expression of reactive oxygen (peroxidases, superoxides) and nitrogen (nitric oxide) intermediates that are responsible for killing ingested mycobacteria. In addition to the production of IL-12, activated macrophages produce IL-8 (a chemokine responsible for attraction of PMNs), monocyte chemoattractant protein (MCP) responsible for attraction of monocytes/macrophages, and monocyte inhibitory protein (MIP), which "holds" monocytes/macrophages, attracted to the infectious focus (formation of a granuloma).

In addition to killing by reactive oxygen and nitrogen intermediates, ingested mycobacteria are also a target for activated T_{H1} cells, gamma-delta T cells, and CD8 T cells, which kill both the macrophage and the mycobacteria within (granulysin is thought to be the material responsible). These T cells probably "recognize" stress proteins expressed by macrophages containing mycobacteria.

This cell-mediated response is characteristic of the infection, and is central to resolution of the infectious process.

THE AGENTS OF ANIMAL TUBERCULOSIS

Tuberculosis is a chronic granulomatous disease produced by *M. tuberculosis* (the agent of the disease in primates), *M. bovis* (in other mammals), and *M. avium* subspecies *avium* (birds, hereafter referred to as *M. avium*).

Descriptive Features

Growth Characteristics

Tubercle bacilli are strict aerobes that grow best on complex organic media such as Lowenstein-Jensen's, which contains, among other ingredients, whole eggs and potato flour. A dye, malachite green, inhibits contaminants. Oleic acid-albumin media, such as Middlebrook's 7H10 agar, are also used for isolation, often in combination with Lowenstein-Jensen's. Simple synthetic media containing ammonium salts, asparagine, citrate, glycerol, minerals and vitamins are unsuitable for isolation but support growth from large inocula.

The presence of glycerol favors growth of *M. tuberculosis* (eugonic) and *M. avium*, but not *M. bovis* (dysgonic).

Generation times of tubercle bacilli range from 12 hours upward, and it may take weeks before colonies are visible. A wetting agent, tween 80, expedites growth in liquid media, and transparent oleic acid-albumin agar media permits early discernment of colonies. *Mycobacterium avium* grows more rapidly than mammalian types.

The mammalian species grow at 33°C to 39°C, while avian and related mycobacteria (see below) grow at 25°C to 45°C, with the optimum being near the top of that range.

Colonial growth of mammalian tubercle bacilli is dry and crumbly. Avian forms grow in dome-shaped colonies.

Resistance

Tubercle bacilli survive exposure to 1N NaOH or HCl for 15 to 30 minutes, a circumstance utilized in decontaminating diagnostic specimens. Mycobacteria are resistant to many antimicrobial drugs, bacteriostatic dyes, and disinfectants. Phenolic disinfectants are the most effective.

Tubercle bacilli resist drying and survive for long periods in soil. They are killed by sunlight, ultraviolet irradiation, and pasteurization.

Variability

Genetically, the mammalian tubercle bacilli are variants of one species, *M. tuberculosis*: human, bovine, and murine. The vaccine strain BCG (bacille de Calmette et Guérin) is a modified *M. bovis*.

The avian tubercle bacilli constitute one species within the *M. intracellulare* group of saprophytic mycobacteria. Of the approximately 20 numbered serotypes in the *M. avium-intracellulare* complex, 1 through 3 are avian tubercle bacilli.

Ecology

Reservoir

The source of tubercle bacilli is tuberculous individuals. Humans perpetuate *M. tuberculosis*, cattle *M. bovis*, and chickens *M. avium*. The latter two can infect wild mammals and other species of birds, respectively, which occasionally become sources of infection for domestic animals.

Transmission

Tubercle bacilli are transmitted via the respiratory and alimentary routes through contaminated airborne droplet nuclei, feces, urine, genital discharges, milk from infected mammary glands, or contaminated feed and water. Percutaneous, transplacental, and transovarian (birds) infections are unusual. Intrauterine infection of calves occurred when bovine tuberculosis was common.

Pathogenesis

Mechanisms and Pathology. The infectious process begins with deposition of tubercle bacilli in the lung or on pharyngeal or intestinal mucous membranes. In previously unexposed animals, local multiplication occurs within. Resistance to phagocytic killing (cell wall chemistry and shunting to endosomal compartments rather than those that fuse with lysosomes) allows continued intracellular and extracellular multiplication. An inflammatory response (stemming from activation of macrophages, as well as stemming from the irritating nature of the mycobacterial cell wall) involving largely monocytes (with some PMNs) develops around the infectious focus. Infected host cells and bacteria reach draining lymph nodes, where proliferation and inflammatory responses continue.

After the first week, cell-mediated immune reactions begin to modify the host response from essentially a foreign body reaction (resulting from the irritating nature of the mycobacterial cell wall) to a reaction characteristic of infectious granulomas. Activated macrophages acquire the capacity to kill mycobacteria. Their efficiency in doing so depends on the adequacy of the immune response and the virulence of bacteria.

Epithelioid cells appear among the macrophages. They have oblong vesicular nuclei and pale, poorly delineated cytoplasm; they often become the predominant cells. A third, less common cell type is the Langhans giant cell, which is probably a cellular fusion product. It has a large amount of pale cytoplasm and, peripherally, many vesicular nuclei (Fig 38.1). Both cells are probably macrophage derivatives. They do not seem to be effective phagocytes. Their bacterial content presumably came from their macrophage precursors.

At the center of the lesion, caseation necrosis develops. A function of the hypersensitive state, it may proceed to calcification or liquefaction.

At the periphery of the lesion are unaltered macrophages mixed with lymphocytes. Fibrocytes appear, and a fibrous layer eventually invests the lesion, which is called a *tubercle* (Fig 38.2).

Tubercles may enlarge, coalesce, and eventually occupy sizable portions of organs. Such tubercles consist mostly of caseous material.

The process described is typical of human and ruminant tuberculosis caused by mammalian tubercle bacilli. It is chronic; the lesion is called *productive* or *proliferative*. Occasionally an acute exudative process takes place, marked by predominantly neutrophilic responses and fluid effusion. It is thought to be favored by such factors as a large infecting dose, focally delivered; high virulence of the infecting strain; constitutional predisposition of the host; a loose tissue architecture as in the lung, serous membranes, or meninges; and a high degree of tuberculous hypersensitivity. One such acute process is *tuberculous pneumonia*, which may cause extensive necrosis (largely due to an overly exuberant immune/inflammatory response) and be rapidly fatal ("galloping consumption"), resolve almost completely, or subside into the chronic pattern.

Cell-mediated responses influence the course of the disease in several ways. Primary infection is disseminated via lymphatics to lymph nodes and beyond these through the bloodstream, seeding many reticuloendothelial tissues. Cell-mediated immunity and macrophage activation eliminate these foci, except where they have developed furthest—that is, the point of primary exposure and the adjacent lymph node. Here primary lesions (Ghon or Ghon-Ranke complexes) persist. Sometimes, especially with alimentary tract exposure, they are "incomplete"— that is, only the lymph node lesion is discernible.

Once cell-mediated reactivity is established, subsequent reinfection follows a different course: antigen-specific T lymphocytes and activated macrophages promptly converge on the site, contain the infection, and prevent lymphatic spread.

Antigen-specific T lymphocyte responses, however, also mediate cytotoxic reactions and cause extensive tissue destruction, which is characteristic of progressive tuberculosis. While the lymphatic dissemination is limited by the immune response, tissue damage facilitates bacterial spread by contiguous extension, or erosion of bronchi, blood vessels, or viscera, introducing infection to new areas. Wherever microorganisms lodge, this reaction will

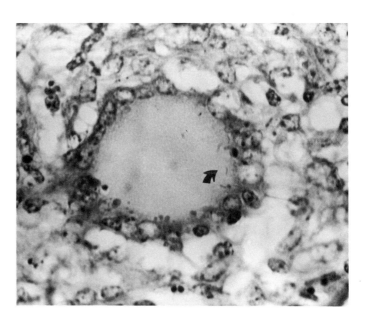

FIGURE 38.1. *Langhans giant cell with tubercle bacilli (arrow) among epithelioid cells in a bovine tuberculous lymph node. Ziehl-Neelsen stain, 1000X.*

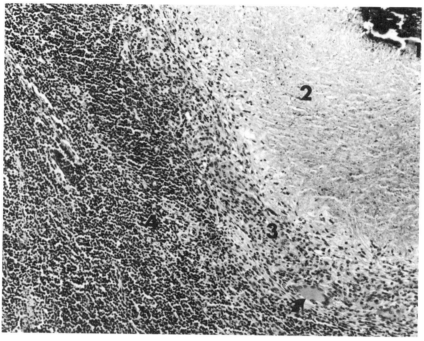

FIGURE 38.2. *Sector of tubercle showing a central area of calcification (1), surrounded by caseation necrosis (2). Adjoining is a zone of epithelioid (3) and giant cells (arrow). The outermost zone (4) contains other mononuclear cells, particularly lymphocytes, among which tracts of fibrous tissue are discernible. Hematoxylin-eosin stain, 100X.*

be repeated with cumulative consequences. Hematogenous dissemination may produce *miliary tuberculosis*: multifocal tubercle formation throughout an organ.

"Reinfection tuberculosis" is most often endogenous; that is, it results from reactivation of previously dormant foci.

Disease Patterns

Clinical tuberculosis is typically a debilitating illness characterized by progressive emaciation, erratic appetite, irregular low-grade fever, and occasionally by localizing signs such as enlarged lymph nodes, cough, and diarrhea. Many of these signs are the consequence of released cytokines.

Cattle. Cattle are usually infected with *M. bovis,* and the infection is centered on the respiratory tract and adjacent lymph nodes and serous cavities. The disease is commonly progressive via air spaces and passages. Hematogenous dissemination involving liver and kidney occurs. The uterus may serve as portal for fetal infection, a pattern virtually unknown in other domestic animals. Surviving calves commonly develop liver and spleen lesions. Udder infection is rare (<2% of cases) but has obvious public health implications.

Infection with *M. avium* is generally subclinical. Abortions resulting apparently from localization of *M. avium* in the uterine wall occur, in some instances repeatedly.

Mycobacterium tuberculosis causes minor, nonprogressive lesions in cattle.

Sheep and Goats. Sheep and goats are susceptible to *M. bovis* and perhaps slightly less so to *M. avium*, but they are resistant to progressive infection by *M. tuberculosis*. Disease patterns resemble those described in cattle.

Horses. Horses are rarely infected, but relatively more often with *M. avium* than with *M. bovis*. Infection enters usually by the alimentary tract, with primary complexes related to pharynx and intestine. Secondary lesions may be in lung, liver, spleen, and serous membranes. Lesions in cervical vertebrae may be due to a secondary, nonspecific hypertrophic periostitis.

Gross lesions are tumor-like. They lack caseation and gross calcification and contain few lymphocytes. There is fibroblast proliferation but usually no firm encapsulation.

Swine. Swine can be infected by tubercle bacilli, usually via the alimentary route, but only *M. bovis* causes progressive disease with classical lesions. *Mycobacterium tuberculosis* infections do not advance past regional lymph nodes. *Mycobacterium avium* infection, the predominant form in many countries, may disseminate to viscera, bone, and meninges. The lesions lack the organization of tubercles, but contain granulomatous elements. Caseation, calcification, or liquefaction is negligible. Bacteria may be abundant. Epidemiological studies as well as genetic analysis of *M. avium* isolates from swine have shown that "bird *M. avium*" is different from "swine *M. avium*" and "human *M. avium*." For this reason, it has been proposed that swine/human strains be designated as *M. avium* subspecies *hominissuis*.

Dogs and Cats. Dogs and cats are readily infected with *M. bovis* but rarely with *M. avium*. Dogs are also susceptible to *M. tuberculosis*. Intestinal and abdominal localization of infection is more common in cats than in dogs, reflecting a likely alimentary route of exposure.

Hypertrophic pulmonary osteoarthropathy (Marie's disease, acropachia), a nonspecific periostitis most noticeably affecting the long bones, sometimes affects tuberculous dogs (and horses). The etiology seems related to pulmonary incapacitation rather than to specific agents.

Ulcerative skin lesions are more common in cats than in other hosts, as is eye involvement, with tuberculous choroiditis leading to blindness.

Lesions, especially in dogs, often more closely resemble a foreign-body reaction than tubercles, since they may lack typical epithelioid and giant cells, and neither caseate, calcify, nor liquefy. The course is usually progressive.

Primates. Primates are susceptible to the two mammalian tubercle bacilli but resistant to *M. avium* unless severely compromised, as by human immunodeficiency virus (HIV) infection or preexisting bronchopulmonary disease. Such individuals also become infected with nontuberculous mycobacteria.

In humans, infection is usually contracted by inhalation of droplet nuclei originating from "open" human cases (that is, respiratory shedders). When tuberculosis was widespread, most cases did not develop beyond the primary complex in the respiratory tract. A minority became progressive clinical tuberculosis, resembling the bovine disease described above.

Infection with *M. bovis* typically occurred following ingestion of unpasteurized milk from a tuberculous cow. Primary invasion, through pharynx or intestine, resulted in lymphadenitis of adjacent nodes. Hematogenous dissemination to vertebrae could result in a hunchback, a condition now rare thanks to pasteurization of milk and eradication of bovine tuberculosis in industrial countries.

Mycobacterium tuberculosis and *M. bovis* cause progressive disease in captive nonhuman primates, which are resistant to *M. avium*, although intestinal infections resembling Johne's disease of ruminants (see below) are associated with members of the *M. avium-intracellulare* complex.

Immunosuppressed humans, especially those with acquired immunodeficiency syndrome (AIDS), appear susceptible to a variety of nontuberculous mycobacteria, for example, *M. genavense*, members of the *M. avium-intracellulare* complex (see above regarding *M. avium* from swine and humans, and the designation *M. avium* ssp. *hominissuis*), *M. simiae*, *M. marinum*, and *M. haemophilum*.

Birds. Birds are naturally susceptible primarily to *M. avium*. Most poultry infections occur via the alimentary canal and disseminate to liver and spleen. Bone marrow, lung, and peritoneum are often affected. Although the agent has been isolated from eggs, transovarian infection of chicks is rare. *Mycobacterium genavense* affects canaries and parrots.

Tubercle formation stops short of calcification.

Although *M. avium* affects many species of birds, psittacines are resistant but are susceptible to *M. tuberculo-sis*. Canaries also are more susceptible to mammalian than to avian bacilli.

Epidemiology

With eradication of cattle tuberculosis in industrial countries, the traditional reservoir in domestic mammals has disappeared. Game farms, animal parks, and zoos remain foci of *M. bovis* in technically advanced countries. Sporadic cases of canine tuberculosis often prove to be *M. tuberculosis* infections traceable to human contacts— "reverse zoonoses"—that are also found in nonhuman primates in laboratory colonies and zoos.

In commercial poultry establishments, rapid population turnover (<1 year) eliminating transgenerational transmission has eradicated *M. avium*. It remains a problem in barnyard flocks, however, particularly since the agent can survive in soil for several years.

Tuberculosis is typically a disease of captivity and domestication. When wild and captive infected populations are compared, clinical improvement and lack of spread in free-living animals contrasted with deterioration and high communicability in confined groups. Tuberculosis in wild populations seems to be a relative rarity. Nevertheless, *M. bovis*, probably originating from cattle, is endemic in badgers of southern England and in brush-tailed opossums of New Zealand, both of which are considered sources of infection for livestock.

Immature individuals often develop more severe lesions than older ones. Breed susceptibilities differ: zebu cattle are more resistant than European breeds, and fox terriers and Irish setters are more often infected than dachshunds and Doberman Pinscher dogs. The higher prevalence in dairy than beef cattle may reflect closer confinement, longer life spans, and greater productivity stress among dairy cows. Exemption from pregnancy and lactation may explain the lower disease prevalence in bulls than cows, although in dogs the reverse sex ratio is observed.

Immunologic Aspects

Immune Mechanisms of Disease

The key role of cell-mediated immune responses in the pathogenesis of tuberculosis has been discussed (see above, "Immunity to Members of the Genus Mycobacterium— General"). In their absence the disease may progress as a disseminating inflammatory disease (as it does in athymic mice) without the development of typical lesions.

Recovery and Resistance

Acquired resistance depends on cell-mediated responses. Under natural conditions this develops along with hypersensitivity, both of which are demonstrated in the *Koch phenomenon*: an already tuberculous guinea pig suffers a rapid, destructive, but limited reaction at the site of reexposure to tubercle bacilli, while a virgin animal develops persistent, progressive, disseminating, and eventually fatal disease when injected at the same anatomical site.

Immune-mediated hypersensitive reactivity and protective responses are separable: immunity can persist in experimentally desensitized animals and can be absent in sensitized subjects.

Antibody to tubercle bacilli does not protect against natural infection.

Artificial Immunization

Vaccination of humans with BCG produces temporary immunity and hypersensitivity. The benefits of vaccination have been greatest where exposure was most intense and negligible where prevalence was low. Vaccination in humans is focused on infants and tuberculin-negative individuals anticipating exposure.

BCG has been used in calves. This practice is inappropriate in countries attempting to eradicate tuberculosis because it interferes with the interpretation of the tuberculin test.

Mycobacterium microti, the vole bacillus, stimulates immunity to bovine and human tuberculosis. Its virulence is too variable to permit its use as a vaccine.

Among subcellular experimental immunogens, a ribosomal preparation is of interest because it produces protection without tuberculin hypersensitivity.

Laboratory Diagnosis

Sample Collection

Samples include tracheobronchial and gastric lavages; lymph node, thoracic, abdominal, and other aspirates; and urine, feces, and biopsy specimens. At necropsy, material is obtained from lesions.

Direct Examination

Fluids are concentrated by centrifugation in tightly capped containers. Samples intended for microscopy only are digested and disinfected with hypochlorite (bleach, Clorox). Smears of sediment or tissue are stained with an acid-fast stain, or with auramine-rhodamine where fluorescence microscopy is available. Histologic sections are stained with hematoxylin-eosin and acid-fast stains.

Positive results should be culturally confirmed.

Culture and Identification

Digestion and selective decontamination are advisable especially with specimens likely to contain a mixture of microorganisms.

Identification is based upon growth characteristics (fast versus slow), pigmentation (in the presence or absence of light), and biochemical reactions. These maneuvers are best left to a reference laboratory.

DNA probes, specific for the main groups, are commercially available. Amplification of mycobacteria-specific fragments of DNA by use of the polymerase chain reaction is an important way to demonstrate or identify members of this genus.

Animal inoculations are sometimes used.

Immunodiagnosis

Tuberculin Test. Cell-mediated hypersensitivity, acquired through infection, can be demonstrated systemically by fever, ophthalmically by conjunctivitis, or dermally by local swelling, when tuberculin or its purified protein derivative (PPD) is given by the subcutaneous, conjunctival, or intradermal route, respectively. Tuberculins are bacterial peptides liberated into culture media during growth. To some of them, or to their parent proteins, delayed-type hypersensitivity develops during infection.

In cattle, tuberculin, the equivalent of a 0.2 to 0.3 mg/dose of bovine PPD, is injected intradermally in the caudal, vulvar, or anal skin or, in some situations, the neck region. In positive cases, a swelling (>5 mm) develops within 72 hours. While tuberculin cannot induce the hypersensitive state, it may desensitize animals for weeks or months.

A positive test implies past or present infection, requiring the reacting animal to be slaughtered and necropsied. Where tuberculosis is rare, no lesions are often found in reactors (NVL, for *no visible lesion* reactors). Such apparently false-positive reactions are explained by hypersensitivity to nontuberculous, related agents such as other mycobacteria, or nocardiae. Simultaneous use of avian tuberculin, which detects hypersensitivity to several nontuberculous mycobacteria, often helps to decide, by comparative size assessment of the two reactions, whether sensitivity is due primarily to mammalian or a heterologous tuberculin. Other explanations for NVL are early states of infection, remote location of lesions, or microscopic sizes of lesions.

False-negatives occur in animals too recently infected and in advanced cases in which anergy develops due to antigen excess or immunosuppression. Nonspecific factors, such as malnutrition, stress, and impending or recent parturition, are alternative causes of anergy.

Rules governing the use of tuberculin tests in eradication programs vary from country to country.

Tuberculins of appropriate specificity are used on swine and poultry. In swine the ears are injected, in poultry the wattles (Fig 38.3). The reliability of tuberculin tests on horses, sheep, goats, dogs, and cats is not established.

Serology. Serologic tests have not been useful in diagnosis of mammalian tuberculosis. As a first step in poultry tuberculosis eradication, a whole-blood agglutination test is available. It is sensitive but lacks specificity.

Treatment and Control

First-line drugs for tuberculosis therapy are streptomycin, isoniazid (INH), ethambutol, and rifampin. Second-line drugs are pyrazinamide, para-aminosalicylic acid, kanamycin, cycloserine, capreomycin, and ethionamide. Because resistance often develops under a single-drug regimen, a combination is commonly used; a favored one in human medicine being INH-ethambutol-rifampin. Treatment is 9 months with rifampin included, 18 to 24 months without it.

Because of the public health hazards inherent in the

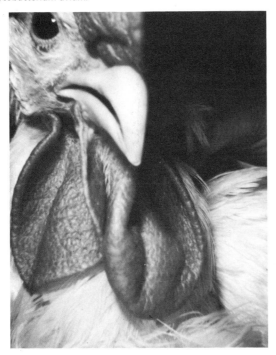

FIGURE 38.3. *Positive tuberculin reaction in the left wattle of a chicken experimentally infected three weeks earlier with* Mycobacterium avium.

retention of tuberculous animals, antituberculous chemotherapy of animals is discouraged. Prophylactic treatment with INH may be considered for pets recently exposed to tuberculosis. Some experimental successes with INH for prophylaxis and treatment of calves have been reported. In countries with eradication programs, treatment is generally discouraged or illegal.

Bovine tuberculosis is controlled by identification and elimination of infected animals. This approach has resulted in near-eradication of the infection in many countries. Continued surveillance is required to prevent resurgence.

In poultry, tuberculosis in backyard flocks is perpetuated by retention of birds and persistence of soil contamination.

Eradication of bovine, human, and avian tuberculosis will diminish infection hazards for other species.

THE AGENT OF JOHNE'S DISEASE

MYCOBACTERIUM AVIUM SSP. PARATUBERCULOSIS

Mycobacterium avium contains three subspecies, *avium*, *paratuberculosis*, and *silvaticum*. A fourth subspecies, *hominissuis* has been suggested to encompass strains that affect swine and humans. In general terms, subspecies *paratuberculosis* is differentiated from the other two by being mycobactin-dependent and possessing the DNA in-

sertion sequence IS900 (though neither trait is absolute). *Mycobacterium avium* subspecies *paratuberculosis*, hereafter referred to as *Mycobacterium paratuberculosis*, is the causative agent of a chronic, irreversible wasting disease of ruminants called *Johne's disease.*

Descriptive Features

Growth Characteristics

Like the rest of the genus *Mycobacterium*, *M. paratuberculosis* is an obligate aerobe. In the past, the growth dependency of *M. paratuberculosis* for mycobactin (an iron-binding lipid, see above, "Cellular Products of Medical Interest") has been used to differentiate it from other mycobacteria. This trait is shared, however, with other strains of *M. avium*. The medium of choice is Herrold's egg-yolk medium. Most strains are stimulated by pyruvate.

Growth is slow. Development of visible colonies requires 8 to 12 weeks of incubation at 37°C.

Mycobacterium paratuberculosis survives many months in soil or in organic matter when protected from direct sunlight and drying.

Ecology

Reservoir

The reservoir for *M. paratuberculosis* is the intestinal tract of infected animals, both the clinically affected and, more importantly, those infected but asymptomatic. In an affected herd, infected, asymptomatic fecal shedders may be 20 times more numerous than those showing clinical signs. An infected animal may also shed *M. paratuberculosis* into colostrum and milk, and may pass the organism to her fetus in utero. *Mycobacterium paratuberculosis* has been isolated from semen, seminiferous tubules, and the prostate glands of infected bulls.

Transmission

The infection is usually acquired through the ingestion or contact with fecally contaminated materials (food, fomites). In utero infection and ingestion of contaminated colostrum or milk are also possible routes.

Pathogenesis

The pathogenic mechanisms appear to involve cell-mediated immune phenomena. The granulomatous lesions associated with clinical disease are related to cell-mediated immunity. The organism is found within macrophages in the submucosa of the ileocecal area and the adjacent lymph nodes (ileocecal) following ingestion. Extraintestinal colonization suggests the existence of a blood phase, but this probably occurs after establishment of a primary focus of infection in the intestine. Whether this occurs soon after infection or later is not known. Initially the animal shows no signs of disease. The incubation period before overt clinical disease is 12 months or longer.

After ingestion, *M. paratuberculosis* enters M cells over lymphoid nodules of the ileocecal area. Shortly thereafter, macrophages within the nodule become infected, with *M. paratuberculosis* seen within phagosomes and phagolysosomes. Ingested microorganisms limit production of superoxides and discourage fusion of lysosomes with phagosomes. Those within phagolysosomes are relatively resistant to destruction (probably related to the chemistry of their cell wall), as well as the production of peroxidases such as Aph (see above, "Cellular Products of Medical Interest"). Intracellular *M. paratuberculosis* acquire iron for growth with the excretion of exochelins, which remove iron from macrophage ferritin. Iron is transported complexed with exochelin across the mycobacterial cell wall to the cytoplasmic membrane where mycobactin transports the iron into the cell. There is evidence that iron availability dictates the distribution of *M. paratuberculosis*, with most iron available within macrophages of nodules in the ileocecal area.

Release of cytokines by activated macrophages initiates the inflammatory and immune responses. The responses are initiated by the recruitment of specific T_{H1} lymphocytes and subsequent release of cytokines leading to the attraction of macrophages to the site of interaction of *M. paratuberculosis* and macrophage. Normally, gamma interferon (one of the released cytokines) would activate macrophages to deal effectively with ingested mycobacteria. Activation is compromised, however, by gamma delta T lymphocytes that are cytotoxic for the specific T_{H1} lymphocytes. This cytotoxicity is regulated by CD8 T lymphocytes. In addition, gamma interferon released by T lymphocytes is a poor activator of *M. paratuberculosis*-infected macrophages. The interaction between these cell types results in the formation of a slowly progressing granulomatous reaction as evidenced by the accumulation of macrophages in the submucosal region. Some macrophages die subsequent to the multiplication of mycobacteria within them, resulting in the release of microorganisms and phagocytosis by other macrophages. The granulomatous response and cellular infiltrate lead ultimately to sloughing of the mucosal epithelium and release of infected macrophages and mycobacteria into the lumen. Some have "staged" the progression of this disease in terminology that is used in describing leprosy (see below, "Feline Leprosy"): the early, localized granulomatous lesion being termed the "tuberculoid" stage, and the later-occurring diffuse infiltrative process being termed the "lepromatous" stage.

The disease in some affected animals progresses to malabsorption, protein-losing enteropathy, and overt clinical disease. However, only 3% to 5% percent of the animals in an infected herd progress to clinical disease. Other economic losses are traced to breeding problems (e.g., longer calving intervals), to reduced milk production due to an increased incidence of mastitis (not caused by *M. paratuberculosis*), and to general ill thrift.

Extraintestinal localization (e.g., mammary gland, fetus, sex organs of males) suggests a blood phase. There is a direct correlation between the degree of dissemination and the numbers of *M. paratuberculosis* in feces. Infected blood monocytes have been demonstrated and may be the manner in which sites outside of the intestinal tract become infected.

Disease Patterns

Cattle. Animals showing clinical signs present with chronic weight loss, diarrhea, but normal appetite and temperature. At this stage of the disease, the submucosa of the intestinal tract, extending both cranially as well as caudally from the ileocecal area is infiltrated with macrophages, epithelioid cells, and some giant cells that contain large numbers of *M. paratuberculosis*. The draining lymph nodes are almost always enlarged and filled with macrophages containing mycobacteria. The classical gross lesion in cattle is a permanent transverse corrugation of the intestinal mucosa caused by granulomatous inflammation within the lamina propria and submucosa (Fig 38.4). The extent of the infiltration is not always related to the severity of the clinical disease. The symptomatic disease usually progresses to a fatal outcome.

Sheep and Goats. Diarrhea is not a common clinical sign of the disease in these species. Herd unthriftiness, however, should prompt examination for *M. paratuberculosis*. Intestinal lesions in sheep and goats are less obvious than in cattle. Weight loss has been a consistent finding with affected goats.

Epidemiology

The young animal is the most susceptible to infection. Older animals can be infected, but only with very large inocula.

Many ruminant species are subject to infection. Clinical disease occurs mostly under conditions of domestica-

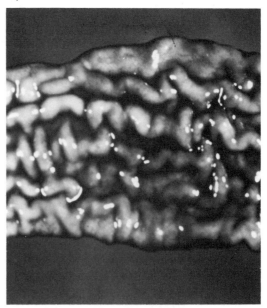

FIGURE 38.4. *Bovine intestine affected by Johne's disease showing permanent corrugation. (Photograph courtesy of Dr. Murray Fowler.)*

tion or captivity, especially in association with stress factors such as parturition, crowding, shipment, or faulty dietary regimes.

Genetics may play a part, as certain cattle breeds (Guernsey, Jersey, Shorthorn) seem to be preferentially affected.

High prevalence of inapparent shedders, chronicity of infection, and persistence in the environment favor dissemination of the agent. The overall prevalence in U.S. bovines is approximately 1% to 3% (the herd prevalence in Western Europe and North America has been estimated to be as high as 50%). The importance of transmission through milk and placenta is uncertain.

Bacteria resembling *M. paratuberculosis* have been isolated from humans with Crohn's disease (regional ileitis), a disease remarkably similar to Johne's disease.

Immunologic Aspects

The lesions and host responses are manifestations of cellular immunity. The cell-mediated immune response probably accounts for the low percentage of animals that progress to overt disease. Other problems, such as decreased milk production and increased calving intervals, may be indirectly due to the generalized immunosuppression observed in infected animals.

Artificial immunization is practiced in some areas of the world, and this practice seems to reduce the losses that occur due to this disease, but it does not eliminate the problem. In the United States, vaccination is not practiced because of its real or perceived interference with diagnostic tests (see below), since vaccinated animals will test positive for this disease and occasionally for tuberculosis as well.

Though cell-mediated immune responses are generated following infection, antibody responses are also observed mainly during the "lepromatous" stage of the disease.

Laboratory Diagnosis

Sample Collection

From cattle, samples from the ileocecal area (intestine or lymph nodes) are best, but mucosal scrapings from the rectum in the live animals are easier to obtain. Biopsies of ileocecal lymph nodes are performed on valuable cattle. In sheep and goats, examination of the ileocecal lymph nodes is the most rewarding. Samples of intestinal content or scrapings are least useful in these species.

Direct Examination

Impression smears of lymph nodes, or smears of rectal or intestinal scrapings, are stained by the Ziehl-Neelsen procedure. *Mycobacterium paratuberculosis* will stain acid-fast. They are short, slender rods, occurring in bunches (Fig 38.5). Other acid-fast staining structures in samples (saprophytic mycobacteria or bacterial endospores) will be solitary and quite large. Sections stained with hematoxylin-eosin reveal the typical granulomatous lesions. If stained by acid-fast procedure, masses of intra- and extracellular organisms can be demonstrated.

Isolation

Growth of the organism in vitro is a dependable way to make the diagnosis. Fecal samples or lymph node biopsies

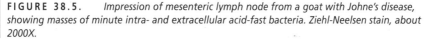

FIGURE 38.5. *Impression of mesenteric lymph node from a goat with Johne's disease, showing masses of minute intra- and extracellular acid-fast bacteria. Ziehl-Neelsen stain, about 2000X.*

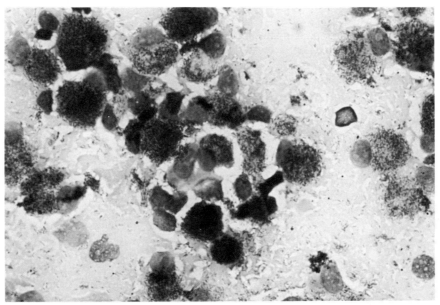

are first decontaminated with hexadecylpyridinium chloride. The decontaminated sample is placed in egg-yolk medium containing mycobactin (mycobactin J produced by *M. paratuberculosis* is preferred). Because some strains are inhibited by sodium pyruvate, egg-yolk medium with and without this substance should be inoculated, as should the same medium with and without mycobactin. The time required to develop visible colonies is about 8 weeks. Current techniques allow for the detection of one organism per gram of material.

A radiometric procedure (BACTEC-RCM) utilizing ^{14}C-palmitic acid followed by polymerase chain reaction amplification of the DNA insertion sequence IS900 (a *M. paratuberculosis*-specific sequence of DNA) has been described and allows detection in feces in 2 to 4 weeks.

Molecular Techniques

A number of DNA tests have been developed for the demonstration of the presence of *M. paratuberculosis*. All utilize a specific sequence for the development of probes or for the design of primers needed to amplify DNA by using the polymerase chain reaction. Specific sequences that have been exploited are those found in the gene encoding the 16S ribosomal RNA; the insertion sequence IS900 (proper primer selection is crucial since there are segments within this genetic element which are shared with IS1626, an insertion sequence found in subspecies *avium*; in addition, IS900 has 94% identity with a DNA sequence from *Mycobacterium cookii*, a saprophytic mycobacteria); *hspX*, a gene encoding a heat shock protein unique to *M. paratuberculosis*; and F57, a fragment of DNA that does not hybridize with DNA from any other bacteria.

Tests have been designed to determine the presence of *M. paratuberculosis* DNA in feces, tissue, and blood monocytes. Methods using feces, tissue, or milk suffer from a lack of sensitivity, which is due to inhibitors found in these substances. Steps taken to remove inhibitors found in feces, tissues, or milk greatly increases sensitivity. One means of doing this is to "capture" *M. paratuberculosis* with paramagnetic beads coated with antibody specific for the organism. Subsequent passage over a magnet removes the microorganisms, which are then analyzed by molecular (or other) means.

Immunodiagnosis

Immunodiagnostic procedures are run in parallel with cultures of the organism and examination of direct smears. Available tests rely either on the presence of antibody (formed during the lepromatous stage of the disease) or on delayed-type hypersensitivity to extracts of the organism (elicited throughout the disease process).

Delayed-Type Hypersensitivity Tests

There are three general types: an intradermal test, an IV johnin (johnins are bacterial peptides liberated into culture media during growth *M. paratuberculosis*), and a lym-

phocyte proliferation assay. The intradermal test requires the intradermal injection of johnin, followed by examination of the injection site for swelling 48 to 72 hours later. This test may result in as high as 75% false-positive reactors.

The IV johnin test is more specific. To some johnins, or to their parent proteins, delayed-type hypersensitivity develops during the infectious process. Reacting animals develop a fever of 1.5°F or higher following IV injection of johnin. This test detects about 80% of the cases showing clinical signs, but not many asymptomatic shedders.

The third type of test measures the cell-mediated immune status of the animal to *M. paratuberculosis*. Immunity can be measured by an in vitro lymphocyte-stimulation test. Peripheral blood lymphocytes are collected and exposed to johnin (or to its purified protein derivative). If the animal has developed cell-mediated immunity to the antigens of *M. paratuberculosis*, these lymphocytes will respond by proliferating and releasing cytokines. Proliferation can be measured by the addition of a radio-labeled nucleic acid precursor, or cytokines can be measured immunologically (e.g., commercial kits are available to measure interferon-gamma by an ELISA specific for this cytokine).

Serologic Tests

It is important to note that serologic tests are designed to detect antibody. Antibodies are formed during the lepromatous stage of the disease, i.e., during the later stages of the disease after shedding has commenced. The complement fixation test will result in about 75% false-positive reactors. The other serological tests, the agar gel immunodiffusion (AGID) test and the enzyme-linked immunosorbent assay (ELISA), are more specific. ELISA detects shedders before the AGID test, which becomes positive only after large numbers of *M. paratuberculosis* are in the feces.

Both the ELISA and AGID tests have been shown to be useful in diagnosing this disease in sheep and goats.

Treatment, Control, and Prevention

At present there are no economically useful antimicrobial agents that are effective against *M. paratuberculosis* in vivo. The newer macrolides, such as clarithromycin, and some experimental fluoroquinolones are effective in vitro, but are too expensive to use clinically. However, clofazamine, with or without either ethambutol or rifabutin are used when circumstances warrant (results have been disappointing with cure rarely, if ever, occurring). *Mycobacterium paratuberculosis* is resistant to isoniazid in vitro, and probably so in vivo.

Eliminating infected animals and preventing possible spread within the herd best attack the disease. Husbandry procedures that must be implemented include segregating the neonate from the dam and other adult animals, ensuring that parturition takes place in noncontaminated areas, and taking precautions against feeding neonates potentially infectious, unpasteurized colostrum or milk. Immunologic and cultural tests are applied to promptly identify those animals that are infected and shedding. Culture is used to confirm the results of the serological assays; it is also used in vaccinated herds where serological tests are not reliable. Molecular techniques that utilize nonfecal samples (such as peripheral blood) show great promise in speeding up the process of identifying affected animals.

Pasteurization is an important step in control on dairies, not only in assuring that calves receive milk or colostrum that is free of *M. paratuberculosis*, but also from a public health perspective since the relationship between *M. paratuberculosis* and Crohn's Disease is unclear. High-temperature, short-time pasteurization has been shown not to be 100% effective in killing *M. paratuberculosis* in naturally infected milk, but only if the numbers of microorganisms in the milk are large. This probably has little public health consequence in areas where large quantities of milk are mixed together from several dairies, thereby diluting any infected milk. However, this may be very important for producers that process milk from a single farm.

Prevention of the disease is difficult. Since there are few regulations governing the sale and shipment of possibly infected livestock, a producer has no way of ascertaining whether a purchased animal is uninfected except by testing. Until uniform tests and reporting procedures are established, the assurance that an animal is free of *M. tuberculosis* is not possible.

Parenteral vaccines, live and killed, are used in some countries but are not universally available.

MISCELLANEOUS MYCOBACTERIAL INFECTIONS

FELINE LEPROSY

There is no true leprosy in domestic animals. Since a disease of cats is called *feline leprosy*, key features of the prototype (human) condition are summarized:

1. *Mycobacterium leprae*, the acid-fast causative bacterium of human leprosy, has not been propagated in vitro. Limited infections can be produced in rodents. The nine-banded armadillo is susceptible to natural and experimental infection.
2. Leprosy affects superficial tissues, mainly skin and upper respiratory tract. Only in advanced cases are internal organs colonized.
3. Particular targets of infection are peripheral nerves.
4. The disease picture ranges between two extremes:
   a. In *lepromatous* leprosy, bacterial proliferation is profuse. Poorly circumscribed nondestructive lesions develop, dominated by a monocytic response but little other inflammatory reactivity. Cell-mediated immunity is suppressed, but circulating immunoglobulins are high.
   b. In *tuberculoid* leprosy, bacteria are scarce. Lesions are granulomatous, and cell-mediated

inflammatory responses are well developed. They cause neural damage, leading to anesthesia, paralysis, dystrophy, disfigurement, and mutilation.

5. The course extends over years and decades. Affected individuals die of complications traceable directly or indirectly to immune disorders or neural destruction.

Feline leprosy is a chronic noduloulcerative, nontuberculous mycobacterial infection of the skin.

Its acid-fast agent is believed by many to be *Mycobacterium lepraemurium*, a cause of leprosy-like disease in rodents. It is cultivable on a special medium, which also supports growth of the feline isolate. Known *M. lepraemurium* has failed to infect cats. However, sequence comparisons of DNA obtained from tissues of cats with feline leprosy show significant identity with *M. lepraemurium*.

Sources, mode of spread, and pathogenic mechanisms are unknown. Transmission by rodent bite or arthropod is suspected.

Judged from experimental infections, lesions of feline leprosy develop in 2 to 6 months. Nodules occur in cutis or subcutis in many sites, and are freely movable and painless. Ulceration and lymph node involvement are frequent. The general health is unaffected. Microscopically, the lesions are granulomas consisting largely of monocytic with variable neutrophilic, lymphocytic, plasma, and giant cell admixtures. Caseation necrosis and irregular neural involvement occur. Acid-fast bacteria abound within histiocytes.

Limited observations suggest the existence of lepromatous and tuberculoid forms.

Examination of stained (Ziehl-Neelsen) biopsies of affected sites reveals large numbers of acid-fast organisms. Routine culture for rapidly growing mycobacteria or for mycobacteria causing tuberculosis are negative. Use of DNA technology (polymerase chain reaction amplification of specific sequences; DNA probes) aid in making a definitive diagnosis.

Treatment includes surgical excision of affected sites (if possible). Antibiotics such as clofazimine have been tried with limited success. Postsurgical relapses are common.

CANINE LEPROID GRANULOMA SYNDROME

Canine Leproid Granuloma Syndrome is caused by an uncultured, saprophytic species of *Mycobacterium* (based on sequence comparisons of DNA obtained from infected tissue with other members of this genus as regards the gene encoding the 16S ribosomal RNA). Diagnosis is based upon demonstration of numerous acid-fast organisms in stained (Ziehl-Neelsen) biopsies or smears of affected tissue or sites. The condition affects the subcutis and skin of the pinnae, face, and body extremities. It is frequently self-limiting (though surgical excision or antibiotic therapy will hasten resolution). A combination of rifampicin and clarithromycin has been effective.

ULCERATIVE DERMATITIS OF CATS AND DOGS DUE TO RAPIDLY GROWING MYCOBACTERIA

The most common presenting complaints are chronic (months to years), nonhealing skin lesions. Histopathologic evaluation of biopsies of affected tissue reveals a pyogranulomatous inflammation. Microorganisms may stain poorly ("ghosts," or "speckled" structures, thought to represent nonstaining or poorly staining mycobacteria, respectively) when stained with Gram's or a Romanovsky-type stain (e.g., Wright's, Giemsa). When samples are stained with acid-fast stains (Ziehl-Neelsen), organisms are not often seen.

Culture on standard blood agar medium will result in the isolation of rapidly growing (48–72 hours incubation) colonies. Isolates are identified by biochemical traits, and by DNA tests. The most commonly isolated in western North America is *Mycobacterium fortuitum* (sporadically isolated are *M. chelonae-abscessus, M. flavescens, M. phlei, M. smegmatis, M. xenopi, M. ulcerans, M. thermoresistible*).

Percutaneous wound infection is the likely portal of entry. Treatment (surgical, antibiotics) has been disappointing. *Mycobacterium fortuitum* is susceptible in vitro to amikacin, cefoxitan, ciprofloxacin, clarithromycin, kanamycin, and minocycline, but resistant to doxycycline, erythromycin, gentamicin, tobramycin, trimethoprim/sulfonamides, and vancomycin.

BOVINE MYCOBACTERIAL ULCERATIVE LYMPHANGITIS

Nodulo-ulcerative skin lesions occur in cattle, particularly on the lower extremities and ventral trunk. They resemble tubercles and typically contain noncultivable acid-fast bacteria. They are of interest mainly because of their association with false-positive tuberculin reactivity.

39 *Chlamydiaceae*

Dwight C. Hirsh   Ernst L. Biberstein

Members of the family Chlamydiaceae ("chlamydiae") are obligate intracellular gram-negative bacteria incapable of obtaining energy by metabolic activities. Their life cycle alternates between noninfectious proliferative stages and infectious nonproliferative stages. The family contains two genera, *Chlamydia* and *Chlamydophila*. Chlamydiae are associated with a variety of diseases affecting an assortment of animal species (Table 39.1).

Descriptive Features

Morphology and Staining

Chlamydiae are coccobacilli 200 by up to 1500 nm in size. Though cytochemically gram-negative, they stain best with Gimenez, Macchiavello's, Castaneda, and Giemsa stains.

Life Cycle

Elementary bodies, 200 to 400 nm in size, enter susceptible cells by receptor-mediated endocytosis. The endosome "traffics" to pathways not involved with endosome-lysosome fusion. Elementary bodies change into noninfectious, metabolically active reticulate bodies, measuring 600 to 1500 nm, that generate, by binary fission, a new crop of elementary bodies that are released upon cell lysis (by lysosomal host enzymes). In vitro, the cycle requires 30 to 40 hours.

Elementary bodies appear red by Macchiavello's and Gimenez, blue by Castaneda, and reddish-purple by Giemsa stain, while reticulate bodies stain blue, green, reddish, and blue, respectively. Giemsa stain is best for the demonstration of both stages.

Structure and Composition

The cell envelope of elementary and reticulate bodies resembles a gram-negative cell wall but lacks peptidoglycan. A trilaminar outer membrane consists of protein and lipopolysaccharides. Proteins confer species and type-specificity, and may act as adhesins. Heparin-like derivates produced by chlamydiae are also proposed to act as adhesins by associating with heparin-binding receptors on host cells. The lipopolysaccharides, which have endotoxic properties (see Chapters 7 and 8, are specific to the family Chlamydiaceae.

The genome size, 6.6 by 10^8 Da, is among the smallest in prokaryotes. There is much RNA in the reticulate but little in the elementary bodies. In the reticulate body, electron-dense material is fairly uniformly dispersed throughout the cell interior, while in the developing elementary body it becomes increasingly concentrated into a compact nucleoid, which, in the mature elementary body, occupies most of the cell (Fig 39.1).

Cellular Products of Medical Interest

Adhesins. Heparin-like derivates act as adhesins by binding to heparin receptors on cells of the host.

Cell Wall. Though the cell walls of the members of this genus lack peptidoglycan, they do contain lipopolysaccharide (LPS). As in other gram-negative bacteria, LPS is an important virulence determinant. LPS binds to lipopolysaccharide-binding protein (a serum protein), which in turn transfers it to the blood phase of CD14. The CD14-LPS complex binds to Toll-like receptor proteins (see Chapter 2) on the surface of macrophage cells triggering the release of proinflammatory cytokines.

Miscellaneous Products. A soluble hemagglutinin and cell-bound heat-labile toxic effect, demonstrable in mice and on macrophages and neutralizable by type-specific antibody, is associated with elementary but not reticulate bodies.

Growth Characteristics

Chlamydiae do not grow on cell-free media. They grow well in the yolk sac of embryonated chicken eggs and in tissue culture (e.g., L-cells, McCoy cells), where they form intracytoplasmic colonies.

Reticulate bodies transport adenosine triphosphate (ATP) into cells and adenosine diphosphate (ADP) out of cells. In the presence of ATP, peptides are synthesized. The agents are "energy parasites." Elementary bodies show little biochemical activity.

Resistance

There is little resistance to common disinfectants, heat, and sunlight. Elementary bodies survive in water for sev-

Table 39.1.   Members of the Genera *Chlamydia* and *Chlamydophila* and Their Usual Source or Associated Condition

Species	Usual Source or Associated Condition	Obsolete Taxonomy
Chlamydia trachomatis	Trachoma, sexually transmitted disease, and lymphogranuloma venereum in human patients	
C. muridarum	Respiratory disease in mice and hamsters	*C. trachomatis* of mice
C. suis	Conjunctivitis, enteritis, and pneumonia in swine	*C. trachomatis* of swine
Chlamydophila abortus	Abortion in ruminants	*C. psittaci* abortion group
Cph. caviae	Conjunctivitis in guinea pigs	*C. psittaci* inclusion conjunctivitis agent
Cph. felis	Conjunctivitis and upper respiratory tract disease in cats	*C. psittaci* feline pneumonitis agent
Cph. pecorum	Abortion, conjunctivitis, enteritis, pneumonia, and arthritis in ruminants	*C. pecorum*
Cph. pneumoniae	Respiratory disease in human patients, koala bears, and horses	*C. pneumoniae*
Cph. psittaci	Ornithosis/psittacosis in birds, and human patients	*C. psittaci* avian group

FIGURE 39.1.   Chlamydophila psittaci *inclusion containing reticulate bodies (RB), condensing forms (CF), and elementary bodies (EB). The nucleoid of the elementary body has a polar eccentric location but occupies most of the cell. Transmission electron micrograph, 15,000X. (Reproduced by permission of Storz, J., Chlamydiales: Properties, cycle of development and effect on eukaryotic host cells. Curr Topics Microbiol Immunol 1977;76:167.)*

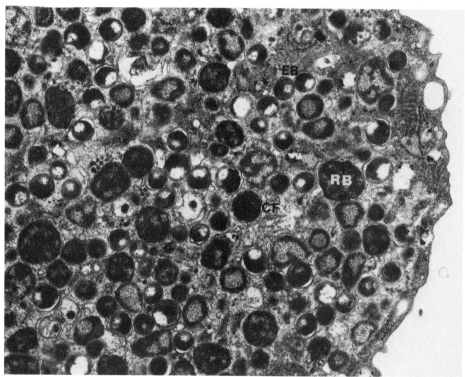

eral days at ambient temperatures and apparently persist in dried animal excretions for long periods.

Variability

Some of the chlamydiae show considerable variability as measured by the disease and host (biovariety or biovar), and by antigenicity of surface structures (serovariety or serovar). Below is a description of those chlamydiae that exhibit variability (serovars, biovars):

1. *Chlamydia trachomatis*. There are two biovarieties of *C. trachomatis*: the trachomatis biovar and the lymphogranuloma venereum biovar. The trachomatis biovar contains 14 serovarieties (A through K, Ba, Da, and Ia). Serovars A, B, and C are associated with trachoma, and serovars D through K are associated with sexually transmitted disease. The lymphogranuloma venereum biovar contains four serovars (L1, L2, L2a, and L3), which are associated with the sexually transmitted disease lymphogranuloma venereum.

2. *Chlamydophila pneumoniae.* There are three biovars of *Cph. pneumoniae*—biovar TWAR (named from the strain designations of the original isolates *TW*-183 and *Ar*-39), biovar Koala, and biovar Equine—that are associated, respectively, with respiratory tract disease in human patients; conjunctivae, urogenital tracts, and respiratory tracts of Koala bears: and respiratory tracts of horses.
3. *Chlamydophila psittaci.* There are eight serovars of *Cph. psittaci*, designated A through H. Serovar A affects psittacine birds and human patients in contact with them; serovar B is associated with pigeons, turkeys, and an unusual cause of bovine abortion; serovar C affects a variety of avian species and human patients in contact with them (mainly slaughterhouse contact); serovar D affects turkeys, parakeets, and human patients in contact with them (mainly slaughterhouse contact); serovar E affects mainly human patients; serovar F affects parakeets; serovar G is associated with hares and muskrats; and serovar H affects cattle.

Ecology

Reservoir

The respiratory, intestinal, and genital tracts of mammals and birds constitute the reservoir.

Transmission

Exposure is through inhalation or ingestion of infectious material. Egg transmission occurs in some birds.

Pathogenesis

Mechanisms. Elementary bodies attach to and are endocytosed by epithelial cells, where they multiply, having somehow averted phagolysosomal fusion by trafficking to endosomes that do not readily fuse to lysosomes. Synthesis of host DNA, RNA, and protein ceases and cells eventually disintegrate through host enzyme action. Microbial toxicity (LPS) and tissue damage elicit inflammatory responses.

Pathology. Pathologic changes vary with localization of infection. In pulmonary chlamydiosis, an exudative bronchiolitis and bronchopneumonia develop mostly in the anterior lobes as reddish-gray areas of consolidation with purulent exudate in the bronchioles. Microscopically, the smallest bronchioles contain predominantly neutrophilic exudates. In the acini, alveolar macrophages predominate. Edema may be marked. Epithelial damage in the bronchioles is variable. Mononuclear cells gradually replace neutrophils, and lymphoreticular cuffing is common in ruminants.

Ocular infections take the form of a catarrhal conjunctivitis.

Chlamydial arthritis involves all soft tissues near affected joints. Suppuration, edema, and hemorrhage are succeeded by granulomatous and fibrotic reactions.

Chlamydial abortions of ruminants are associated with a placentitis with cotyledonary necrosis and edematous or leathery intercotyledonary thickening. Lesions in the male genital tract of ruminants (epididymis, testicle, deferent duct) are granulomatous.

Chlamydial enteritis is associated with a granulomatous inflammation of the lamina propria and submucosa.

Chlamydiosis of birds is marked by fibrinous serositis of body cavities, air sacs, and organ surfaces. Lung, spleen, and liver are enlarged and congested. Microscopically, there is fibrinonecrotizing inflammation with mononuclear and heterophil leukocytes.

Disease Patterns

Ruminants. *Abortion.* Chlamydial abortion (almost always caused by *Cph. abortus*) occurs among previously unexposed ewes (enzootic abortion of ewes) and goats. Abortion occurs sporadically in cattle and rarely in other species. Ewes abort typically late in pregnancy without premonitory signs or after effects, except for a vulvar discharge and occasionally a retained placenta. Bovine abortions follow similar patterns.

Polyarthritis. Chlamydial polyarthritis (*Cph. pecorum*) affects mainly lambs and calves. In "stiff lamb disease" morbidity may be 80%, but the mortality rate is 1%. In calves, there may be systemic complications and high mortality.

Nervous System. Sporadic bovine encephalomyelitis (SBE) is a febrile disease predominantly of young cattle that is caused by *Cph. pecorum*. Clinical signs include locomotor, postural, and behavioral disturbances. There may be mild cough, nasal discharge, and diarrhea. The disease lasts from days to weeks, and morbidity and case fatality rates may reach 50%. Some outbreaks may continue for months, with new cases appearing irregularly.

Avian. Avian chlamydiosis (ornithosis, psittacosis) is caused by *Cph. psittaci*, and is most significant economically in turkeys. Onset is insidious and may occur weeks after exposure. Early signs are inappetence, weight loss, and the voiding of greenish-yellow, gelatinous droppings. Egg production is reduced. Severity varies with strain virulence (toxicity); morbidity may range from 5% to 80%, mortality from 1% to 30%. Geese and ducks are sometimes affected, chickens exceptionally so. Subclinical forms predominate in pigeons and psittacine birds.

Miscellaneous. *Pneumonia.* Chlamydial pneumonias, produced by a variety of chlamydiae (see Table 39.1) are seen particularly in pigs, cats, sheep, goats, and cattle, and are often subclinical or part of mixed infections (enzootic sheep pneumonia, shipping fever). The clinical importance of uncomplicated infections (e.g., "feline pneumonitis") is uncertain.

Conjunctivitis. Chlamydial conjunctivitis, although reported in cattle, dogs, pigs, guinea pigs, and koalas, is most noted in cats and lambs (see Table 39.1). It may pass through acute and prolonged chronic phases. In lambs, where it accompanies polyarthritis, secondary complications, keratitis, and corneal ulcerations are seen.

Epidemiology

The natural reservoirs for the various species of chlamydiae appear to be the animal species in which the natural disease occurs. Asymptomatic carriage is common.

Zoonotic acquisition of several species of chlamydiae occurs. Most importantly is *Cph. psittaci* from clinically affected or asymptomatic birds (slaughterhouse workers, pet owners). Unusual transmission for human patients includes *Cph. felis* from cats and *Cph. abortus* from affected sheep.

Immunologic Factors

Recovery and Resistance

Ewes that have aborted rarely abort again, and calves recovered from SBE resist reinfection. In other chlamydial diseases, which are often chronic and marked by remissions and relapses, there is little evidence of heightened resistance.

Cell-mediated and humoral immune responses are demonstrable by skin tests, lymphocyte stimulation tests, and serological reactions. Protective responses appear to be cell-mediated.

Artificial Immunization

Vaccination of animals against chlamydial infections often produces only short-lived partial protection, except against enzootic abortion of ewes (see under "Treatment and Control," below).

Laboratory Diagnosis

Diagnosis requires laboratory confirmation. Chlamydial inclusions are often demonstrable by appropriate stains (see "Life Cycle," above; Fig 39.2), including immunofluorescence within infected epithelium and macrophages. An enzyme-linked immunoadsorbent assay (ELISA) technique detects chlamydial antigen in vaginal discharges.

Isolation

Chlamydiae are isolated on tissue culture line cells (HeLa, McCoy for *Chlamydia spp.*; HEp-2, HL, BGM, McCoy for *Chlamydophila spp.*) or in fertile chicken eggs. Decontamination of suspect feces, placentas, urine, semen, and conjunctival fluids can be accomplished by treatment with combinations of gentamicin (50 µg/ml), vancomycin (75 µg/ml), and nystatin (500 units/ml). With tissue culture, centrifugation of the inoculum onto the monolayer on a cover slip is beneficial, and addition of cycloheximide (2 µg/ml) provides an added boost to chlamydiae. Growth occurs within 2 to 3 days of incubation.

Eggs are inoculated into the yolk sac and candled daily thereafter. Yolk sacs of embryos dying 3 or more days after inoculation are examined for chlamydial inclusions.

By either method serial subpassages are required to rule out chlamydiosis.

Presumptive isolates can be confirmed serologically by immunofluorescence, complement fixation tests, or by molecular means (see below).

Serologic Tests

Complement fixation and enzyme-linked immunosorbent assay (ELISA) tests are not generally available to veterinarians, although genus-specific antigens are marketed. The presence of antibody confirms a diagnosis only if its titer increased fourfold during the course of illness.

Molecular methods

Molecular techniques have been developed that utilize DNA primers designed to amplify genes (or portions thereof) encoding the 16S and 23S ribosomal RNA, and outer membrane protein 2 (*omp*2) by the polymerase chain reaction. These methods allow the means for detection of

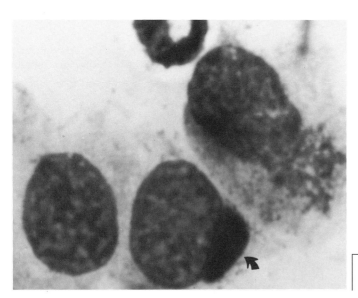

FIGURE 39.2.   *Chlamydial inclusion (arrow) in a conjunctival epithelial cell from a kitten. Wright stain, about 1000X.*

chlamydiae in tissues or exudates as well as identification of isolates.

Treatment and Control

Treatment

Tetracycline is the drug of choice in the treatment of chlamydial infections. In birds, flock treatment involves incorporating the drug in feed. Moderate doses (200 g/ton) are adequate for disease control in turkeys. Higher doses (2800 g/ton) are needed for tissue clearance. To limit outbreaks of abortion in ewes, intramuscular injections (20 mg/kg) of long-acting forms are given at 2-week intervals. Tetracycline is given orally to lambs (150 to 200 mg/kg) to prevent arthritis. For pet birds, tetracycline-containing millet (0.5 mg/g) is available.

Prevention

Vaccination against chlamydial infections has had variable success. Formalinized vaccines are beneficial in preventing enzootic ovine abortion (*Cph. abortus*). Feline chlamydial vaccines containing modified live or killed organisms attenuate clinical illness without curing or preventing infection (*Cph. felis*). A vaccine for avian chlamydiosis is not available (*Cph. psittaci*).

Prompt disposal of infected material and segregation of affected animals is helpful in control of ovine abortion. Young turkey poults should be placed in clean quarters, with no access to infected droppings and unexposed to potentially contaminated air currents.

Regulations governing import of exotic birds are designed to minimize introduction of psittacosis into household and resident bird populations.

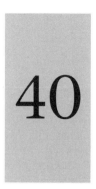

40 Mollicutes

Richard L. Walker

The mollicutes are members of the order *Mycoplasmatales* and class *Mollicutes* (soft skin). They are the smallest of the free-living prokaryotes and are devoid of cell walls. Only members belonging to the genera *Mycoplasma* and *Ureaplasma* are important in veterinary medicine. *Acholeplasma* are sometimes encountered, but usually as contaminants. *Mollicutes* is the correct term to use when collectively referring to members in this order; however, the trivial name "mycoplasma(s)" is also used for this purpose. Reclassification of haemotrophic rickettsial species of the genera *Haemobartonella* and *Eperythrozoon* to the genus *Mycoplasma* has been proposed based on 16S ribosomal RNA (rRNA) gene sequence analysis. These have collectively been given the trivial name "haemoplasmas."

The "nonhaemotrophic" mollicutes ("mycoplasmas") infect a wide range of animal species. Infections range from subclinical to severely debilitating and sometimes fatal diseases. Clinical manifestations include respiratory and urogenital tract infections, arthritis, mastitis, and septicemia. Most pathogenic species exhibit a high degree of host specificity. Infections in humans usually present as respiratory or urogenital tract disease.

The "haemotrophic" mollicutes ("haemoplasmas") also infect a wide range of animal species (especially the very young, or stressed). Hemolytic anemia is the most commonly encountered manifestation following infection with these bacteria.

Descriptive Features

Morphology and Staining

The cell morphology of the mollicutes is extremely pleomorphic. Cell shapes include spherical, ring-shaped, pear-shaped, spiral-shaped, and filamentous forms. Cells sometimes appear as chains of beads, the result of asynchronized genomic replication and cell division. The diameter of the spherical form ranges from 0.3 μm to 0.8 μm.

Mollicutes stain poorly by the Gram method. Giemsa, Castaneda, Dienes and new methylene blue stains are preferred.

Structure and Composition

The mollicutes are not only devoid of cell walls but lack the genetic capacity to produce one. They are bound by a single trilaminar membrane composed of proteins, glycoproteins, lipoproteins, phospholipids, and sterols. Cholesterol in the membrane provides for osmotic stability. A polar bleb has been demonstrated in some species and has a role in adherence to host cell surfaces. Capsules have also been described for some species.

The mollicutes have a small genome (600–1,400 kb) compared to other bacteria. The base composition is poor in guanine and cytosine with the mol% G + C of DNA ranging from 24 to 40% relating them most closely to the *Clostridium-Streptococcus-Lactobacillus* group. Sequence analysis of 16S rRNA indicates that mollicutes are most closely related to the genus *Clostridium*. The entire genome for some species has been sequenced. The mollicutes appear to have evolved by genome reduction. Transposons, plasmids, and bacteriophages have been demonstrated in some species.

THE NONHAEMOTROPHIC MOLLICUTES

The "nonhaemotrophic" mollicutes include members of the genus *Ureaplasma* and those of the genus *Mycoplasma* that are not associated with red blood cells. Unlike the "haemotrophic" mollicutes (see below), they can be grown in vitro on lifeless media. Clinical manifestations include respiratory and urogenital tract infections, arthritis, mastitis, and septicemia. Most pathogenic species exhibit a high degree of host specificity. Infections in humans usually present as respiratory or urogenital tract disease (Table 40.1).

Cellular Products of Medical Interest

Peroxide/Superoxide. Peroxides and superoxides are produced and may be important in disruption of host cell integrity.

Urease. Urease, produced by members of the genus *Ureaplasma*, may be involved in injury to host tissue as a result of the production of ammonia by urea hydrolysis.

Miscellaneous Products. Experimental inoculation of a 200kDa protein from the supernatant of *M. neurolyticum* cultures causes neurologic signs in mice. Vascular damage in the brain is evident but the mechanism of action is unclear. Poorly defined products, mostly lipoproteins, from some mollicutes induce interleukin-1, interleukin-6, and tumor necrosis factor production from activated macrophages. This may account for the endotoxic-like activity observed with some infections. Bovine ureaplasmas produce IgA protease, which cleaves IgA$_1$ and may aid

Table 40.1.   Animal Species, Agents, and Diseases Associated with Nonhaemotrophic Mycoplasma and Ureaplasma

Animal Species	Agent	Common Clinical Manifestations
Cats	*Mycoplasma felis*	Conjunctivitis
	M. gatae	Arthritis
Cattle	*M. alkalescens*	Arthritis, mastitis
	M. bovigenitalium	Infertility, mastitis, seminal vesiculitis
	M. bovis	Abscesses, arthritis, mastitis, otitis, pneumonia
	M. bovoculi	Keratoconjunctivitis
	M. californicum	Arthritis, mastitis
	M. canadense	Arthritis, mastitis
	M. dispar	Alveolitis, bronchiolitis
	M. mycoides subsp. *mycoides* (small colony variant)	Arthritis, pleuropneumonia (CBPP)[a]
	U. diversum	Infertility, pneumonia, vulvovaginitis
Chickens	*M. gallisepticum*	Respiratory disease
	M. synoviae	Airsacculitis, sternal bursitis, synovitis
Dogs	*M. canis*	Urogenital tract disease
	M. cynos	Pneumonia
	M. spumans	Arthritis
Goats	*M. agalactiae*	Agalactia, arthritis, conjunctivitis
	M. capricolum subsp. *capricolum*	Arthritis, mastitis, pneumonia, septicemia
	M. capricolum subsp. *capripneumoniae*	Pleuropneumonia (CCPP)[b]
	M. conjunctivae	Keratoconjunctivitis
	M. mycoides subsp. *mycoides* (large colony variant)	Abscesses, arthritis, mastitis, septicemia
	M. mycoides subsp. *capri*	Pneumonia, arthritis
	M. putrefaciens	Arthritis, mastitis
Horses	*M. felis*	Pleuritis
Mice	*M. neurolyticum*	Conjunctivitis, neurological disease
	M. pulmonis	Respiratory disease
Rats	*M. arthritidis*	Arthritis
	M. pulmonis	Respiratory disease, genital tract disease
Sheep	*M. agalactiae*	Agalactia
	M. conjunctivae	Keratoconjunctivitis
	M. ovipneumoniae	Pneumonia
Swine	*M. hyopneumoniae*	Enzootic pneumonia
	M. hyorhinis	Arthritis, pneumonia, polyserositis
	M. hyosynoviae	Arthritis
Turkeys	*M. gallisepticum*	Sinusitis, respiratory disease
	M. iowae	Embryo mortality, leg deformities
	M. meleagridis	Airsacculitis, decreased egg hatchability, perosis
	M. synoviae	Sternal bursitis, synovitis

[a]Contagious bovine pleuropneumonia.
[b]Contagious caprine pleuropneumonia.

in avoiding the host immune response on mucosal surfaces. Other proteases, hemolysins, and nucleases are also produced.

Growth Characteristics

The nonhaemotrophic mollicutes grow slowly and generally require 3 to 7 days' incubation before colonies are apparent. Growth is best at 37°C in an atmosphere of in-creased CO_2. Because of total or partial inability to synthesize fatty acids, exogenous sterols are required by *Ureaplasma* and *Mycoplasma*. They are not, however, required by *Acholeplasma*. Genera of veterinary importance are facultative anaerobes. Optimal pH for growth ranges from 6.0 for *Ureaplasma* up to 7.5 for other mollicutes. Mollicute colonies are small and difficult to visualize with the unaided eye. Colony sizes vary from 0.01 mm to 1.0 mm. When observed with a dissecting microscope,

FIGURE 40.1. *"Fried-egg" colony morphology that is typical of many* Mycoplasma *species.*

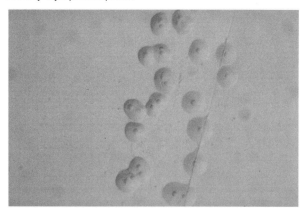

many species exhibit a "fried egg" morphology (Fig 40.1). This umbonate appearance is the result of the central portion of the colony embedding into the agar with a peripheral zone of surface growth. Some species produce film spots, which are composed of cholesterol and phospholipids and which appear as a wrinkled film on the media surface.

Resistance

The lack of a cell wall renders mollicutes resistant to the action of antimicrobial agents that affect the cell wall or its synthesis. They are sensitive to compounds that interfere with protein and nucleic acid synthesis. *Acholeplasma* species are resistant to 1.5% digitonin, whereas the growth of other mollicutes is inhibited by this concentration. In general, mollicutes survive outside the host for substantial periods in moist, cool environments. They are very susceptible to heat and most detergents (tween) and disinfectants (quaternary ammonium, iodine, and phenol-based compounds).

Variability

Variations in nutritional and atmospheric requirements account for some of the diversity among genera and species within genera. Differences in colony morphology and size can be used to distinguish some of the mollicutes. *Ureaplasma* species produce substantially smaller colonies than other mollicutes and often lack the fried-egg colony morphology. The colony size of *M. mycoides* subspecies *mycoides* isolates from goats is consistently larger than those isolated from cattle. This size difference is used to distinguish between the two variants. While some antigens are shared among the mollicutes, antigenic differences are sufficiently specific to allow for species identification. Animal host specificity is strongly exhibited by the pathogenic mollicutes and may be explained by specific host receptors necessary for attachment or the failure of the host to recognize host-adapted species as nonself.

Ecology

Reservoir

The major reservoir for the nonhaemotrophic mollicutes is the host they infect. Asymptomatically infected animals carry organisms on mucosal surfaces including nasal, conjunctival, oral, intestinal, and genital mucosa. The ear canal of goats has also been shown to be a reservoir for some of the pathogenic caprine mycoplasmas.

Transmission

Transmission occurs predominately by spread from animal to animal through direct contact and is mediated through aerosolization of respiratory secretions or through venereal transmission. Mechanical transmission is also important, especially with regard to bovine and caprine mycoplasma mastitis. In poultry, vertical transmission through hatching eggs is an important means of spread for many of the pathogenic avian species. Contaminated milk can be a source of infection for calves and goat kids. Little is known about the role of ectoparasites in transmission; however, pathogenic caprine species have been isolated from ear mites of goats.

Pathogenesis

Mechanisms. Attachment to host cells is the first step in establishing infection and is mediated through the anionic surface layer on most mycoplasmas. In some species, special attachment structures have been demonstrated, which appear to be encoded by a common ancestral adhesin gene. Host receptors for attachment are glycoconjugates and allow for colonization of mucosal surfaces. The ciliostatic capability of some *Mycoplasma* species further promotes establishment of infection. There is evidence that some *Mycoplasma* species can penetrate and exist inside non-phagocytic cells. Mycoplasmas have also been demonstrated to fuse with eukaryotic cell membranes.

Latent infections are common. Factors that allow for persistence include mechanisms to avoid the immune system such as antigenic variability of cell membrane lipoproteins or biological mimicry. Underlying factors such as age, crowding, concurrent infections, and transportation stresses lead to overt disease. Breaks in integrity of the epithelial barrier probably account for the initial step in breaching host defenses. Lipoproteins in the cell membrane, acting as modulins, play a major role in cytokine induction.

Acute, septicemic forms of disease result in a coagulopathy and widespread vascular thrombosis, which resembles a gram-negative septicemia and is, at least in part, mediated through induction of cytokines.

The pathogenesis of chronic infections is directly related to persistence of the organisms in the face of an intense inflammatory response. Peroxidation causes host tissue damage. Activation of complement and cytotoxic T lymphocytes further contributes to host injury.

Virulence varies among species and strains within species and accounts for some of the variations in disease manifestation. In some species, virulence is correlated with presence of an outer surface layer. A galactan polymer in *M. mycoides* ssp. *mycoides* has been shown to modulate the immune response and promote dissemination. Virulence is rapidly lost by in vitro passage. *Mycoplasma bovis* induces apoptosis in lymphocytes. *Mycoplasma dispar* can inhibit activation of macrophages.

In addition to specific effects related to mycoplasma, generalized effects on the immune system may increase susceptibility to secondary infections with other bacterial pathogens.

Pathology. The lesions associated with mycoplasma infections vary from acute to chronic and are dependent on the agent involved and the site affected. In acute infections, there is an inflammatory reaction with an infiltration of neutrophils and fibrin accumulation. Generalized infections lead to a fibrinopurulent exudate on serosal surfaces and synovial membranes. In persistent localized infections, tissue destruction can be substantial. Abscesses may develop at pressure sites in calves and are characterized by an eosinophilic coagulative necrosis with peripheral fibrosis. In cases of mycoplasma mastitis, pockets of purulent exudate may develop in affected mammary tissue. Eventually the affected gland becomes fibrosed. In the acute stage of mycoplasma infections of the joint, the joint becomes distended with fluid containing fibrin. As infections become chronic, there is villus hypertrophy of the synovia and a proliferative and erosive arthritis develops.

A marked pleural effusion develops in respiratory tract infections due to *M. mycoides* ssp. *mycoides* in cattle and *M. capricolum* ssp. *capripneumoniae* in goats. The subpleural tissue and interlobular septa become thickened and fluid filled. Affected areas of lung become hepatized with resulting sequestration of necrotic tissue.

An infiltration of lymphocytes and plasma cells is often observed in mycoplasma infections, particularly around vessels and in the submucosa. Peribronchial and peribronchiolar lymphoplasmacytic cuffing is a characteristic finding in respiratory tract infection. The profound lymphoplasmacytic proliferation observed in many infections is due to nonspecific mitogenic effects as well as to a specific antimycoplasmal immune response.

Disease Patterns

Infections can manifest in a variety of ways. Common manifestations include septicemias, disseminated infections involving multiple sites, or localized infections. Common manifestations caused by the different pathogenic species in major animal species are listed in Table 40.1.

Avian. Mycoplasmosis in poultry has important economic consequences. *Mycoplasma gallisepticum* causes a chronic respiratory disease in chickens, turkeys, and a number of other domestic avian species. Clinical signs include coughing, nasal discharge, and tracheal rales. Turkeys can develop sinusitis with production of a thick, mucoid exudate that results in severe swelling of the paranasal sinuses. Occasionally, clinical signs related to brain and joint involvement are recognized. Decrease in egg production also

occurs. *Mycoplasma synoviae* also infects a wide range of avian species. Synovitis resulting in lameness, swelling of joints and tendon sheaths, and retarded growth are common presentations. Sternal bursitis is also frequently observed. Airsacculitis, which is usually subclinical, is another manifestation. *Mycoplasma meleagridis* and *M. iowae* infections are mostly limited to turkeys. *Mycoplasma meleagridis* causes respiratory disease, predominately an airsacculitis, which is often clinically mild or inapparent. Skeletal deformities, including bowing or twisting of the tarsometatarsal bone and cervical vertebrae, are occasionally detected. Decreased egg hatchability is a serious consequence of *M. meleagridis* infections. Airsacculitis, leg deformities, and stunting in poults have been demonstrated experimentally with *M. iowae*. Decreased egg hatchability has also been noted with *M. iowae* infections. Natural outbreaks of conjunctivitis in finches caused by *M. gallisepticum* have caused substantial reductions in the finch population on the eastern coast of the United States.

Bovine. *Mycoplasma mycoides* ssp. *mycoides* (small colony variant) is considered the most virulent of the bovine mycoplasmas. It causes a respiratory disease, contagious bovine pleuropneumonia (CBPP), in cattle that ranges from a persistent, subclinical infection to an acute, sometimes fatal disease. Clinical signs include respiratory distress, coughing, nasal discharge, and reluctance to move. In severe cases, the animal will stand with its neck extended and mouth open to facilitate breathing. Subclinically affected animals serve as a source for maintaining and spreading infection in the herd. Most infections are limited to the respiratory tract, although arthritis occurs in calves.

Mycoplasma mastitis is caused by a number of species. *Mycoplasma bovis* is the most common cause and results in the most severe disease. *Mycoplasma californicum* and *M. canadense* are also frequently involved. *Mycoplasma alkalescens* and *M. bovigenitalium* have also been implicated as etiologic agents on occasion. Typically, there is a drop in milk production. The milk becomes thick and intermixed with a watery secretion and may progress to a purulent exudate (Fig 40.2). The udder is often swollen, although not painful. Sometimes all four quarters are involved. It is a destructive mastitis and often refractory to treatment. Most infections are limited to the mammary gland; however, arthritis subsequent to bacteremia occurs. In some cases disseminated infection results in periarticular involvement and fasciitis. Spread from cow to cow is directly related to inadequate management and sanitation practices.

Mycoplasma respiratory tract infections in calves often present as pneumonia in association with other bovine respiratory pathogens. *Mycoplasma bovis* is the predominant species recovered. *Mycoplasma dispar* causes a mild respiratory disease characterized by bronchiolitis and alveolitis and is usually precipitated by environmental stresses or a primary viral infection. Both *M. bovis* and *M. dispar* can be recovered as commensals from the upper respiratory tract.

Urogenital tract infections are caused by *M. bovigenitalium* and *Ureaplasma diversum*. Seminal vesiculitis in bulls and granular vulvitis, endometritis, and abortion in cows

FIGURE 40.2.   *Milk from a cow with severe mycoplasma mastitis. The milk is thickened with a watery component that contains small flakes of material.* Mycoplasma bovis *was recovered.*

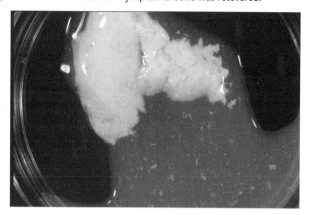

are associated with both of these organisms. Both are found as normal commensals in the lower urogenital tract.

Arthritis in calves occurs sporadically. While a number of different species can cause arthritis, *M. bovis* is most frequently recovered. Other less common presentations include otitis media and decubital abscesses (Fig 40.3). Otitis media usually occurs in conjunction with respiratory disease. Decubital abscesses have been associated with confined housing conditions. *Mycoplasma bovis*, again, is the usual agent.

Canine.   A number of *Mycoplasma* species have been isolated from dogs; however, little is known about the role they play in disease. Experimental and clinical evidence suggests *M. canis* can cause urogenital tract disease including prostatitis, cystitis, endometritis, orchitis, and epididymitis. The role of *Mycoplasma* in reproductive disorders of the bitch is uncertain. *Mycoplasma* spp. have been associated with pneumonia, often as secondary in-

vaders. *Mycoplasma spumans* has been reported to cause arthritis.

Caprine.   Mycoplasma infections in goats are economically important and can result in disease of epizootic proportion. *Mycoplasma mycoides* ssp. *mycoides* (large colony variant) infections present as a mastitis, pneumonia, bursitis or arthritis in adult animals. Some does develop a generalized toxic disease that can be fatal. A rapidly fatal septicemia is common in kids. Those that survive develop a chronic, destructive arthritis and/or bursitis (Fig 40.4). *Mycoplasma mycoides* ssp. *capri* causes a pleuropneumonia similar to that of goat strains of *M. mycoides* ssp. *mycoides*. It has been proposed that *M. mycoides* ssp. *mycoides* (large colony variant) be combined with *Mycoplasma mycoides* ssp. *capri* as a single subspecies *capri* based on the high DNA homology they share. Septicemia, arthritis, and mastitis occur with *M. capricolum* ssp. *capricolum* infections. *Mycoplasma capricolum* ssp. *capripneumoniae* (formerly *Mycoplasma* sp. F-38) causes contagious caprine pleuropneumonia (CCPP), which is similar to CBPP in cattle. Both *M. agalactiae* and *M. putrefaciens* cause mastitis. The mastitis due to *M. putrefaciens* is purulent in nature, while infections with *M. agalactiae* result in a decrease or total cessation in milk production. Both species can cause arthritis. *Mycoplasma conjunctivae* causes a keratoconjunctivitis that presents with lacrimation, conjunctival hyperemia, and keratitis. Pannus is sometimes evident.

Equine.   *Mycoplasma felis* is the only species that has been solidly associated with disease in the horse. It is recovered from the upper respiratory tract as a commensal but can cause a pleuritis, usually related to some exertional activity. The pleuritis is self-limiting and frequently resolves spontaneously.

Feline.   A variety of commensal mycoplasmas have been recovered from mucosal surfaces of cats. Relatively few are associated with disease. *Mycoplasma gatae* has been recov-

FIGURE 40.3.   *Abscess involving sternal area of calf. The abscess was related to pressure trauma.* Mycoplasma bovis *was recovered. (Courtesy Dr. H. Kinde.)*

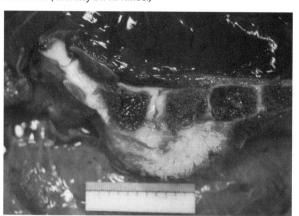

FIGURE 40.4.   *Bursitis in a 2-month-old goat kid. The bursa is distended with an amber-colored fluid and a white fibrinous material.* Mycoplasma mycoides subsp. mycoides *(large colony variant) was recovered. (Courtesy Dr. M. Anderson.)*

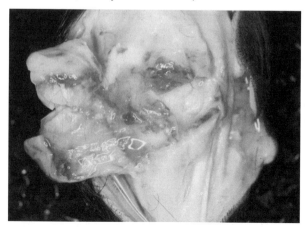

ered from cats with arthritis. *Mycoplasma felis* has been associated with a serous to mucoid conjunctivitis. Typically the conjunctiva is edematous; however, the cornea is not involved. A mycoplasma-like organism has been associated with subcutaneous abscesses, but neither the disease nor the organism has been well characterized. *Mycoplasma* spp. have been isolated as part of the polymicrobial component from pyothorax exudates.

Murine. *Mycoplasma pulmonis* causes a low-grade respiratory disease in rats. Infections involve the nasal cavity, middle ear, larynx, trachea, and lungs. The most common clinical sign is a low-pitched wheezing or snuffling resulting from the purulent nasal exudate. In mice, clinical signs are often inapparent, although a chattering sound and continued rubbing of the eyes and nose may suggest infection in the colony. Mortality is low and when it occurs is related to pneumonia. Genital tract infections with *M. pulmonis* are also recognized in rats. *Mycoplasma arthritidis* causes a polyarthritis in rats and mice, although many infections are subclinical. Experimental infections in mice result in joint swelling and, in some cases, posterior paralysis. Natural infections with *M. neurolyticum* generally do not cause disease, although conjunctivitis has been reported. Experimental inoculation with *M. neurolyticum* or cell-free filtrates causes a neurologic syndrome referred to as *rolling disease*.

Ovine. Compared to other ruminant species, mycoplasma infections in sheep are not as frequent or devastating. *Mycoplasma ovipneumoniae* is associated with pneumonia and usually in conjunction with other common bacterial pathogens of the ovine respiratory tract. Outbreaks of keratoconjunctivitis have been attributed to *M. conjunctivae*. Agalactic mastitis caused by *M. agalactiae* is similar to that observed in goats. Sheep can also be infected with many of the other species that affect goats.

Porcine. A number of important clinical entities are associated with mycoplasma infections in swine. Infections with *M. hyopneumoniae* present as a chronic respiratory disease, referred to as *enzootic pneumonia* (Fig 40.5). There is high morbidity but low mortality. The principal clinical sign is a chronic nonproductive cough. Affected pigs appear unthrifty and have retarded growth. *Mycoplasma hyorhinis* causes a systemic infection in pigs between 3 and 10 weeks of age. Initial signs include fever, inappetence, and listlessness. Swelling of the joints and lameness frequently follow. There is a characteristic polyserositis that involves pleural, peritoneal, and pericardial serosa. Synovial membranes are also affected. Chronic infections result in decreased weight gain. *Mycoplasma hyosynoviae* causes arthritis in growing pigs 12 to 24 weeks of age. Lameness and associated difficulty with mobility are the principal clinical signs.

Epidemiology

The primary source of most of the pathogenic mollicutes is the host that they infect. Introduction of an infected animal into an uninfected population accounts for dissemi-

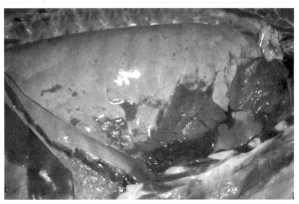

FIGURE 40.5. *Enzootic pneumonia in a pig caused by Mycoplasma hyopneumoniae. (Courtesy Dr. M. Anderson.)*

nation of infection. Asymptomatic carriers, usually colonized on mucosal surfaces, serve as the source for maintaining organisms in the population. Young animals are very susceptible to infection and generally develop more severe disease than adult animals. As a rule animal pathogens are not considered to have zoonotic potential.

Immunologic Aspects

Immune Mechanisms in Pathogenesis

The immune response of the host is intimately involved in the pathogenesis of disease. Consequences of both an active humoral and cellular immune response, as well as immunosuppressive effects of the pathogen itself, are involved in the pathogenic process.

Some mollicutes have been shown to possess nonspecific mitogenic properties and are able to induce a polyclonal B lymphocyte stimulation to a variety of antigens, including host antigens. *Mycoplasma arthritidis* possesses a small peptide that acts as a superantigen and stimulates a broad population of T lymphocytes. The resulting production of various cytokines and inflammatory reaction are detrimental to the host. Shared host and mycoplasma antigens, such as the galactans found in the lungs of cattle and in *M. mycoides* ssp. *mycoides*, can result in autoimmune disease. Mycoplasmas activate the complement cascade by the classical pathway, which contributes to the inflammatory response. While beneficial in controlling infections, the inflammatory response can result in damage to bystander host cells. Persistence of antigen in selected sites, such as joints, allows for further damage due to development of an immune complex–mediated inflammatory response. Induction of interleukin 1 (IL-1), IL-6, and tumor necrosis factor (TNF) from activated macrophages by many mycoplasmas leads to activation of cytotoxic T lymphocytes and results in an endotoxin-like effect.

Suppression or lack of the host immune response is important in allowing for persistence and avoidance of recognition by the host. A number of *Mycoplasma* species have been shown to decrease phagocytic activity of neutrophils and macrophages. Proposed mechanisms include decreasing the respiratory burst (*M. bovis*) or decreasing phagocytosis as a result of capsule production (*M. dispar*). Antigens shared between *Mycoplasma* species and the host tissues may result in a biological mimicry, whereby the host recognizes the mycoplasma as self, leading to persistent infections. Antigenic variability is another mechanism employed to evade host defenses. The pMGA gene family, which accounts for 16% of the entire genome of *M. gallisepticum,* generates antigenic variants of a major surface protein. Incorporation of host antigens by mycoplasmas, a condition referred to as *capping*, further aids some mollicutes in escaping detection by the immune system.

Mechanisms of Resistance and Recovery

Age, environmental conditions, genetic predisposition, crowding, and concurrent infections are all involved in contributing to resistance to infection or lack thereof. Minimizing predisposing stresses will minimize disease. Some of the innate host mechanisms for protection, such as the mucociliary escalator system in the respiratory tract, are important in preventing colonization.

The chronicity of mollicute infections suggests that the immune response is not very effective at controlling infection once established. Mycoplasmas stimulate a humoral response and specific antibodies can be demonstrated. Antibodies have been shown to enhance clearance. Cellular immunity is also recognized, although less is known about it. In the face of an intense inflammatory response, however, mycoplasmas generally appear able to avoid elimination.

Artificial Immunization

Vaccination is employed to control some mycoplasma diseases. An attenuated vaccine is used to protect cattle in areas where CBPP is enzootic. Protection lasts for approximately 18 months. Attenuated and killed, adjuvanted vaccines have been used with variable success to control some caprine infections, specifically those caused by *M. agalactiae*, *M. mycoides* ssp. *capri*, and *M. capricolum* ssp. *capripneumoniae*. Inactivated vaccines afford some protection for swine against infection with *M. hyopneumoniae* and *M. hyorhinis*. In poultry, live and inactivated vaccines are employed to control egg production losses and respiratory disease associated with *M. gallisepticum* infections.

Laboratory Diagnosis

Sample Collection

The appropriate sample for isolation attempt is determined by the clinical presentation and includes exudates, swabs from affected sites, affected tissues, and milk. The ear canals of goats can be sampled to detect inapparent carriers. Because of the mollicutes' fastidious nature, samples should be submitted to the laboratory as soon as possible after collection. During transportation, samples should be kept cool and moist. Various commercially available media

(Stuart's and Amies' without charcoal) are suitable for transporting swabs. If a prolonged transport time (greater than 24 hours) is expected, samples should be shipped frozen and preferably on dry ice or in liquid nitrogen.

Direct Examination

The variability in microscopic morphology and poor staining with the Gram method make direct examination for most mollicutes unrewarding. Direct fluorescent antibody tests and DNA fluorochrome staining have been described, particularly for diagnosing conjunctivitis and mastitis, but they are not widely used.

Isolation

No one media formulation is suitable for growth of all of the mollicutes. The media selected should be based on the specific species or group of species of interest. In general, a fairly complex media is required. Serum is the usual source of sterols and is required by most species. Different species, however, grow better with different sources of serum. The exception is the *Acholeplasma*, which have the ability to synthesize their own fatty acids and therefore do not require exogenous sterols. Yeast extract is also included as a source of growth factors. Growth of some species is enhanced or requires incorporation of specific substances such as vaginal mucus (*M. agalactiae*) and nicotinamide adenine dinucleotide (*M. synoviae*). Some goat mycoplasmas grow on sheep blood agar as small colonies and an alpha-type ("greening") hemolysis (Fig 40.6). Penicillin, thallium acetate, and amphotericin B are commonly added to media to inhibit contaminating bacteria and fungi. Specific immune sera directed against commensal mycoplasmas can be incorporated in media to allow for selective isolation for pathogenic species. For optimal recov-

FIGURE 40.6. *Growth of* Mycoplasma mycoides *subsp.* mycoides *(large colony variant) from a goat on a sheep blood agar/MacConkey agar biplate. The sheep blood agar is in the lower half of the plate. Tiny mycoplasma colonies are evident. No growth is present on the MacConkey agar (upper half). This is one of the few mycoplasmas that grows sufficiently on sheep blood agar to produce colonies that are small but are still visible to the naked eye.*

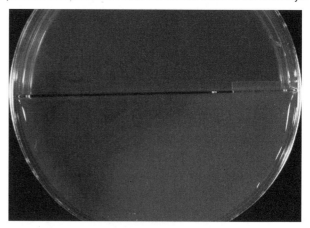

ery, samples are inoculated into both a liquid and solid media and incubated at 37°C in 5% to 10% CO_2 for at least 7 days. Some species require longer incubation times. Semen and joint fluids may contain inhibitory factors and should be diluted prior to culture to enhance recovery. Blind passages from broth to broth for up to three passages may enhance the recovery of poultry pathogens. *Ureaplasma* species are susceptible to pH changes as a result of hydrolysis of urea included in the media and must be subcultured frequently to maintain their viability when isolation attempts are made.

Identification

Plate media is examined with the aid of a dissecting microscope. Colonies with the typical umbonate morphology are stained directly with the Dienes stain to differentiate them from other bacteria (Fig 40.7). The mollicutes stain blue because of their inability to reduce methylene blue in the stain. Other bacteria reduce methylene blue by using it as a hydrogen acceptor in maltose oxidation and therefore appear colorless with the Dienes stain. The exceptions are L-form bacteria, which exhibit a similar colony morphology and staining reaction as the mollicutes. L-forms must be differentiated from mollicutes by demonstrating reversion of the L-form bacteria back to a walled form.

Digitonin sensitivity is used to distinguish *Mycoplasma* and *Ureaplasma* from *Acholeplasma*. A large zone of inhibition around paper disks saturated with 1.5% digitonin will be present with *Mycoplasma* and *Ureaplasma* but only a small or no zone is observed with *Acholeplasma*. Commonly used biochemical tests to further characterize isolates include detection of phosphatase activity, fermentation of glucose, and hydrolysis of arginine or urea.

Definitive identification is based on reactivity with specific antisera. A number of methods are employed based on either the ability of specific antisera to inhibit growth or metabolism or the demonstration of reactivity with a specific antisera using either a fluorescence or chromogen-based detection system. Growth inhibition tests employ

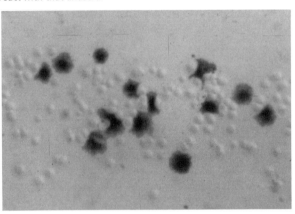

FIGURE 40.8. *Immunoperoxidase staining method used for typing mycoplasma isolates directly on agar media. Two different types of* Mycoplasma *are present in the sample. One type (M.* bovirhinis) *stains when anti-*Mycoplasma bovirhinis *antisera is used (darkly stained colonies); the other* Mycoplasma *isolate does not react with that antisera.*

antisera impregnated disks or antisera placed in wells in media and demonstrating a zone of inhibition. Metabolic inhibition tests use growth inhibition in liquid media and a color change based on pH as an indicator system. Other test procedures commonly used to demonstrate specific reactivity are direct or indirect immunofluorescence on colony impressions, colony epifluorescence, and immunoperoxidase staining of colonies on agar plates (Fig 40.8).

Nonserologic methods for species identification using polymerase chain reaction (PCR) have recently been described. Amplification of specific DNA sequences by PCR and restriction endonuclease analysis of PCR products have been used for identification and characterization of isolates. Randomly amplified polymorphic DNA analysis has been used for strain differentiation. Restriction endonuclease analysis, protein electrophoresis, and ribotyping have also been used to further characterize strains. DNA sequencing of selected genes, especially the gene encoding the 16S rRNA, is becoming more important as a tool for taxonomic placement of *Mycoplasma* species.

Antibiotics susceptibility testing of clinical isolates is not routinely performed. No standardized method or appropriate control organisms have been described.

Nonculture Detection Methods

Immunoperoxidase and immunofluorescent staining of histopathologic sections has been used successfully for identification of some species in tissues, including *M. bovis* in cattle tissues, *M. hyopneumoniae* in pig lungs, and some of the poultry mycoplasmas.

A number of PCR methods have been described for identification of pathogenic species directly from clinical material. Polymerase chain reaction tests for direct detection of some of the pathogenic poultry mycoplasmas are commercially available.

FIGURE 40.7. *Dienes-stained mycoplasma colonies with densely staining centers and lighter staining peripheries (75X).*

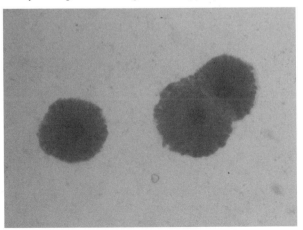

Immunodiagnosis

A number of immunodiagnostic tests have been developed for many of the important mycoplasma diseases. Many have not been standardized and are not in wide use. Problems with sensitivity, especially with asymptomatic carriers, are common. Lack of specificity as a result of cross-reacting antibodies is also a problem.

Enzyme-linked immunosorbent assays (ELISAs), plate agglutination, and hemagglutination inhibition tests are routinely used to detect flock infections with *M. gallisepticum*, *M. meleagridis*, and *M. synoviae* in poultry and are an important part of overall eradication programs used by commercial poultry operations. Commercially available tests are available for poultry.

Treatment, Control, and Prevention

Success of treatment varies depending on the species involved, the affected site, and time course of the disease. Although the mollicutes are susceptible to a number of antibiotics in vitro, treatment failures are common. Commonly used antibiotics include tetracyclines, tylosin, erythromycin, lincomycin, spectinomycin, and tilmicosin. Resistance to some of these antimicrobials, particularly of the macrolide class, has been noted. Animals that do respond to treatment often become carriers.

Control measures depend on the disease status of the country, specific disease, and animal species infected. Diseases such as CBPP and CCPP, which affect large populations of animals, are controlled by test and slaughter of affected herds in countries attempting to maintain a disease free status. Vaccination, culling of infected animals, and management changes to prevent dissemination are employed in countries where the disease is enzootic. In general, because of the poor success in treating infected animals, culling of clinically ill animals is often employed as a control measure in infected populations where test and slaughter is not feasible. Industry-driven efforts, particularly in the poultry industry, have outlined measures to eliminate or prevent infection. Attempts to eradicate infections, particularly in breeding flocks, include serologic testing and elimination of positive flocks and antibiotic treatment of hatching eggs to produce mycoplasma-free chicks. Treatment of eggs involves immersing warmed eggs in a chilled antibiotic solution, which promotes antibiotic penetration into the egg. Routine culturing of bulk tanks is used to monitor for mammary infections in cow and goat herds. Animals identified as shedding organisms in the milk are usually culled.

Preventing infection should be based on following strict biosecurity practices to preclude introduction of infected animals into a mycoplasma-free herd. New animals should be quarantined and tested before being mixed with the herd. Taking animals to shows and fairs and returning them to the herd may also serve as a source for introducing infection. This is an especially common scenario for outbreaks in goat herds. Good hygiene and management practices are important in preventing spread among animals where infections are enzootic. Because milk can be a source of infection, especially in goats, it should be pasteurized to prevent infecting young animals in the herd.

THE HAEMOTROPHIC MOLLICUTES

The haemotrophic mollicutes include microorganisms previously included in the genera *Haemobartonella* and *Eperythrozoon* (Table 40.2). All are parasites of red blood cells, and produce hemolytic anemia in the young, or stressed individuals (Fig 40.9). Subclinically infected animals are the source for haemoplasmas. Several members of this group are transmitted by ectoparasites. Unlike the nonhaemotrophic mollicutes, they have not been cultivated on lifeless media.

Infections with this group of microorganisms are usually asymptomatic. However, following a stressful event (e.g., concurrent infections with FIV or FeLV in cats infected with *M. haemofelis* or *M. haemominutum*) sometimes leads to the development of clinically apparent hemolytic anemia.

Infections with the haemoplasmas may cause icterus, splenomegaly, and bone-marrow hyperplasia.

Table 40.2.   Animal Species, Agents, and Diseases Associated with Haemotrophic Mycoplasma

Animal Species	Agent	Common Clinical Manifestations
Cat	*Mycoplasma haemofelis* *M. haemominutum*	Anemia (Feline Infectious Anemia)
Cattle	*M. wenyonii*	Anemia
Dog	*M. haemocanis*	Anemia
Llama	*M. haemolamae*	Anemia
Mice	*M. haemuris*	Anemia
Opossum	*M. haemodidelhidis*	Anemia
Sheep	*M. haemovis*	Anemia
Swine	*M. haemosuis*	Anemia

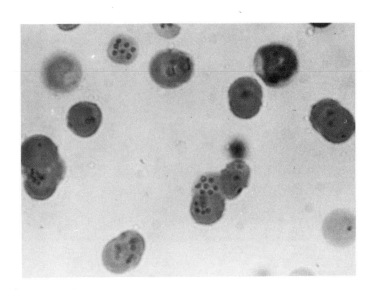

FIGURE 40.9. Mycoplasma haemofelis *on feline erythrocytes. Note coccal and ring forms. Wright's stain, 1000X.*

Diagnosis is based upon clinical signs, demonstration of the agent in stained (a Romanovsky-type stain, e.g., Wright's or Giemsa) smears of peripheral blood, or detection of genus and species-specific DNA following amplification using DNA primers and the polymerase chain reaction.

Treatment includes correction of the hemolytic anemia, and one of the tetracyclines.

41

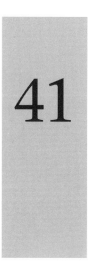

Rickettsiae: Rickettsia, Coxiella, and *Orientia*

JANET E. FOLEY   ERNST L. BIBERSTEIN

DWIGHT C. HIRSH

Members of the order *Rickettsiales* are minute obligate intracellular gram-negative bacteria. They are basically parasites of arthropods. Two families, *Rickettsiaceae* and *Anaplasmataceae,* within this order are of veterinary interest. The family *Rickettsiaceae,* which includes parasites of the vascular endothelium (*Rickettsia, Coxiella,* and *Orientia*), commonly referred to as "rickettsiae," and parasites of phagocytic cells (*Ehrlichia* and *Neorickettsia*), commonly referred to as "ehrlichiae." The family *Anaplasmataceae,* composed of the genus *Anaplasma,* parasitizes erythrocytes, phagocytes, and platelets.

The ehrlichiae (*Ehrlichia* and *Neorickettsia*) are discussed in Chapter 42, and members of the family Anaplasmataceae are discussed in Chapter 43. This chapter deals with the rickettsiae: *Rickettsia, Coxiella,* and *Orientia,* though only those associated with animal disease are discussed in detail (*Rickettsia rickettsii,* the cause of Rocky Mountain spotted fever in dogs and sheep, and *Coxiella burnetii,* the cause of Q fever in ruminants.

Descriptive Features

Rickettsiae measure up to 0.5 μm by 1.0 μm. Although structurally gram-negative, better visualization is achieved with Gimenez, Macchiavello, or Giemsa stains. The former two stain rickettsiae red, the latter purple. Electron microscopically and chemically, rickettsiae resemble other gram-negative bacteria. Endotoxin is present (see Chapters 7 and 8). Cells are nonmotile. The life cycle of *Coxiella burnetii* includes an endospore-like phase. Rickettsiae enter endothelial cells through endocytosis actively initiated by metabolizing rickettsial cells. They escape from the phagosome and multiply in the cytoplasm and, in some cases, the nucleus.

Rickettsiae are propagated in yolk sacs of chick embryos, cell cultures, and laboratory animals, notably guinea pigs or mice. The optimal temperature for growth is 33°C to 35°C, at which the generation time is about 9 hours. In cell culture, good growth may require incubation for several weeks, depending on the rickettsial species involved.

Glutamate is a key nutrient for rickettsiae, which utilize

it with the aid of transaminases, dehydrogenases, and enzymes of the citric acid cycle. There is little glycolytic activity. Rickettsial adenosine diphosphate (ADP) is readily exchanged for host adenosine triphosphate (ATP) across cell membranes. This "leakiness" of rickettsiae causes loss of critical metabolites, infectivity, and viability when agents are removed to extracellular sites, but is probably an adaptation to intracellular existence rather than its cause, which is unknown. Within hosts, *Coxiella burnetii* is an obligate intracellular bacterium, but it survives extracellularly in the environment for months, formalin, ultraviolet radiation, classical pasteurization at 63°C for 30 minutes, and occasionally even "flash" pasteurization (71.6°C for 10 to 20 seconds).

Many members of the rickettsiae are associated with invertebrate vectors, and some can be passed transovarially in ticks and mites. The pathogenic and ecologic relationships of important rickettsiae are shown in Table 41.1. There are three of veterinary interest: *R. rickettsii* belonging to the spotted fever group, *R. felis* in the typhus group, and *C. burnetii. Rickettsia felis* is included because preliminary research suggests that it is an important small-animal derived zoonosis, although it is not pathogenic for cats.

RICKETTSIA RICKETTSII

Ecology

Reservoir and Transmission

The agent of Rocky Mountain spotted fever (RMSF), *Rickettsia rickettsii* infects dogs (and people) in endemic areas. It is carried naturally by some 20 species of ixodid ticks, including *Dermacentor andersoni* (the wood tick) and *D. variabilis (*the American dog tick) in western North America and *D. variabilis* in the eastern portions of North America. It is passed transovarially in ticks. Serologic surveys suggest that most canine RMSF infections go unnoticed. Other tick-borne diseases (ehrlichiosis, babesiosis, borreliosis) should be considered along with RMSF in tick-infested dogs. RMSF is limited to the New World. Cases occur most commonly (and are increasing in prevalence)

Table 41.1. Some Diseases due to *Rickettsiae*: Agents, Reservoirs, Vectors, and Hosts

Disease	Causative Agent	Vertebrate Reservoir	Vectors	Transovarian Passage	Clinically Affected Hosts
Epidemic typhus					
Classical	*Rickettsia prowazekii*	Humans (recovered)	Lice	–	Humans
Sylvatic	*R. prowazekii*	Eastern flying squirrels	Fleas	–	Humans
Endemic (murine) typhus	*R. typhi*	Rats, opossums, cats	Fleas	–	Humans
Endemic typhus-like	*R. felis* (ELB agent)	Opossums, cats	Fleas	–	Humans
Scrub typhus	*Orientia tsutsugamushi*	Mice, rats	Mites	+	Humans
Rocky Mountain spotted fever,	*R. rickettsii*	Various feral mammals	Ticks	+	Humans (dogs, sheep)[a]
Q fever	*Coxiella burnetii*	Mammals, birds, fish?	Ticks, mites, insects[b]	?	Humans (ruminants)

[a] Occasionally affected.
[b] Airborne transmission commonly occurs in absence of vectors.

in eastern North America. Seasonal incidence parallels adult tick activity: *D. andersoni* is active in spring and early summer, while *D. variabilis* is active from midspring to late summer. The reservoir for RMSF is small mammals, which constitute a primary sylvatic cycle with immature ticks.

Pathogenesis

Rickettsia rickettsii replicates in the epithelium of the tick, and is transferred to salivary glands and ovarian tissue. After the tick bites a suitable host, *R. rickettsii* is injected and targets vascular endothelium, where they are endocytosed, escape the phagosome, and multiply in cell cytoplasm and nucleus. Rickettsial phospholipase and proteases damage endothelial cell membranes, leading to necrosis, vasculitis, hemorrhage, edema, perfusion inadequacies, thrombosis, and dyspnea. Clinically, the infection is rarely fatal, with affected dogs presenting with high fever (40°C), anorexia, vomiting, diarrhea, petecchiated or ecchymotic mucous membranes, and tenderness over lymph nodes, joints, and muscles. Purpuric and central nervous disturbances may occur later. These, and heart and kidney involvement, account for most fatalities. Unfortunately, severe necrosis of extremities may occur when the dog appears to be in convalescence.

Immunologic Aspects

Immune complexes are suspected in the pathogenesis of late vascular manifestations of RMSF. Humoral and cell-mediated responses occur. The latter especially are significant for removal of the agents by activated macrophages. No vaccine is available for RMSF.

Laboratory Diagnosis

Some rickettsial antigens, including those of *R. rickettsii*, cross-react with somatic antigens of certain *Proteus* (OX) strains, a phenomenon (Weil-Felix reaction) utilized in the diagnosis of rickettsial infections. This approach generally lacks species specificity. Indirect fluorescent antibody (FA)

and enzyme-linked immunosorbent assay (ELISA) are most commonly performed to detect IgG specific for rickettsial antigens. Negative or low titers may occur early in disease. Rickettsiae can be demonstrated in cells by direct immunofluorescence. Polymerase chain reaction-based tests are available to evaluate for *R. rickettsii* DNA in ticks and dogs.

Treatment and Control

Rickettsia rickettsii is susceptible to chloramphenicol, tetracyclines, and fluoroquinolones. Affected dogs must receive aggressive supportive therapy and possibly steroids. Prevention of RMSF in dogs requires tick control. Transmission depends on prolonged feeding by ticks and may be reduced by prompt tick removal.

Coxiella burnetii

Ecology

Reservoir and Transmission

The agent of Q fever, *Coxiella burnetii,* is distributed worldwide. It survives in the environment, unlike other rickettsiae, and can be disseminated by the airborne route. Survival may be related to the "small-cell-variant," an endospore-like growth phase. Natural hosts and vectors include some 125 mammalian species and many species of arthropods, including ticks, mites, fleas, lice, and flies, some of which support a sylvatic cycle of *C. burnetii*. Recent research suggests that the organism can occur in amoebae and crayfish, which may be an important mechanism of environmental persistence, and a source for infection of humans and other animals.

Most human cases of Q fever can be traced to exposure to infected sheep, cattle, and goats, either directly or via unpasteurized milk products. Outbreaks have occurred after wind currents carried infectious "spores" from infected dairies. Cattle and small ruminants can shed the bacteria in feces, sperm, and reproductive discharges.

Parturient cats and dogs have been implicated as sources of human infection.

Coxiella burnetii has been weaponized, and is considered an important agent of possible biological terrorism.

Pathogenesis

Coxiella burnetii is acquired through inhalation, ingestion, or arthropod bite and gains access to vascular endothelium and respiratory and renal epithelia. *Coxiella burnetii* multiplies within the phagosome, thanks to an enzyme system adapted to low pH (5.0). After hematogenous dissemination, 50% of humans are asymptomatic or have mild, self-limiting infection. Less than 10% develop severe disease with vasculitis, pneumonitis, splenomegaly, fever, and lymphocytosis. In animals, the pattern may be similar, although mildly affected animals may have latent infection, persisting particularly in the lactating mammary gland and the pregnant uterus. Latent infection is reactivated during parturition: sporadic abortion may result from placentitis or the delivery may be normal and produce viable young. In either case, rickettsiae are abundantly shed. The pathologic lesion in animals with mild or self-limited disease is a granuloma; people and animals with chronic active infection fail to contain the bacteria in a granuloma and there are abundant bacteria with severely vacuolated macrophages. Mortality in human cases is due to pneumonia, hepatic infection, or endocarditis.

In culture, *C. burnetii* transitions from a virulent phase I (resists macrophage killing and multiplies slowly) type to an avirulent phase II. Phase II bacteria have altered expression of cell wall lipopolysaccharide, do not occur in nature, and are killed by macrophages.

Immunologic Aspects

A phase II vaccine is available in some countries but has reported poor efficacy. A whole cell killed vaccine is given to researchers. There is considerable interest in the development of a phase I Q fever vaccine, which has proven effective experimentally in ruminants and humans.

Laboratory Diagnosis

Gimenez or other stains on suspect tissues will not differentiate between *C. burnetii* and *Chlamydophila psittaci*. *Coxiella burnetii* can be isolated following injection into guinea pigs and mice, embryonated eggs, or cell culture, but cells dissociate to phase II. In addition, the agent is considered dangerous to laboratory personnel. Paradoxically, even though animals are infected only with phase I bacteria, titers of antibodies to phase I antigen in acutely infected people are low, while antibodies to phase II antigens show a rapid fourfold increase. IgM antibodies against phase I do occur. If the infection becomes chronic, levels of antibodies to phase I become increased. This pattern may occur in animals, but long-term observations of acutely and chronically infected animals of various species are scarce. Indirect immunofluorescence, complement fixation, or ELISA tests are used to detect antibodies. In cell culture, eggs, and experimental animal tissues, direct immunofluorescent staining will identify an isolate. Polymerase chain reaction–based assays employing specific DNA primers are also used to document infections with this agent.

Treatment and Control

The major challenge for successful therapy is that the phagosome where *C. burnetii* persists is highly acidic, and most antimicrobial agents are not effective at such low pHs. Alkalinizing cells by using chloroquine has been shown to improve clinical efficacy of tetracycline. Drugs with moderate efficacy for *C. burnetii* infection include tetracycline, chloramphenicol, clarithromycin, enrofloxacin, and trimethoprim-sulfa. Long-term tetracycline feeding has been used in attempts to control mammary excretion of *C. burnetii,* which has met with mixed results. Pregnant sheep and goats may be treated with tetracycline to reduce the probability of abortion.

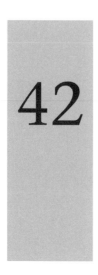

42

Ehrlichiae: Ehrlichia and *Neorickettsia*

Janet E. Foley   Ernst L. Biberstein

Dwight C. Hirsh

Descriptive Features

Members of the order *Rickettsiales* are minute obligate intracellular gram-negative bacteria. They are basically parasites of arthropods. Two families (*Rickettsiaceae* and *Anaplasmataceae*) within this order are of veterinary interest. The family *Rickettsiaceae*, which includes parasites of the vascular endothelium (*Rickettsia, Coxiella,* and *Orientia*), commonly referred to as "rickettsiae," and parasites of phagocytic cells (*Ehrlichia* and *Neorickettsia*), commonly referred to as "ehrlichiae." The family *Anaplasmataceae*, composed of the genus *Anaplasma*, parasitizes erythrocytes, phagocytes, and platelets.

The rickettsiae are discussed in Chapter 41, and members of the family *Anaplasmataceae* are discussed in Chapter 43. Discussed in this chapter are the ehrlichiae: *Ehrlichia* and *Neorickettsia*.

Ehrlichiae are white blood cell parasites that multiply within membrane-lined intracytoplasmic vesicles. Colonies (morulae) less than 4 µm in diameter that consist of "elementary bodies" smaller than 1 µm in diameter are demonstrable by examination of Giemsa-stained blood smears (Fig 42.1) or immunofluorescence. A cell wall is present.

The ehrlichiae are comprised of *E. canis, E. chaffeensis, E. ewingii, E.* (formerly *Cowdria*) *ruminantium, Neorickettsia helminthoeca, N.* (formerly *Ehrlichia*) *risticii,* and *N.* (formerly *Ehrlichia*) *sennetsu. Ehrlichia equi* has been reclassified as *Anaplasma phagocytophilum* (see Chapter 43). *Ehrlichia canis, E. chaffeensis, N. risticii, N. sennetsu,* and *E. ruminantium* have been propagated in cell culture, which simulates host conditions in vitro. The tick-transmitted species (*E. canis, E. chaffeensis, E. ewingii,* and *E. ruminantium*) are passed transstadially, but not transovarially, within the vectors. Blood may remain infectious for 10 days at room temperature, 14 days at refrigerator temperature, and 1.5 years if frozen.

EHRLICHIA CANIS, E. CHAFFEENSIS, AND E. EWINGII

Ecology

Reservoir and Transmission

The brown dog tick, *Rhipicephalus sanguineus,* is the vector of *E. canis,* the agent of canine monocytic ehrlichiosis. Although dogs and other canid hosts of *E. canis* may remain bacteremic for years, their blood is infectious for ticks generally for 2 weeks or less during the acute disease. Puppies and German shepherd dogs are most severely affected. The infection is concentrated in tropical and subtropical latitudes, but occurs on all continents except Australia. The vector of *E. ewingii,* the agent of one form of canine and human granulocytic ehrlichiosis (but distinct from granulocytic "ehrlichiosis" caused by *Anaplasma phagocytophilum*) is *Amblyomma americanum,* the lone star tick. *E. ewingii* appears most commonly in central North America although there are reports from coastal areas of North America as well. Although a few rare cases of human monocytic ehrlichiosis may be due to *E. canis* infection, most are due to infection with *E. chaffeensis,* which is closely related genetically and serologically to *E. canis.* Its vector is *Dermacentor variabilis,* the American dog tick, and its mammalian reservoir may be deer.

Pathogenesis

Each of these ehrlichiae is inoculated into its host by tick bite. Acute onset of disease follows an incubation period of 1 to 3 weeks, during which the agent proliferates by binary fission within monocytes (or granulocytes in the case of *E. ewingii*). In severe acute disease, lasting up to several weeks, there may be vasculitis and thrombocytopenia. Intravascular coagulation may occur, and leukopenia and anemia are common. Clinically, there may be fever, malaise, depression, inappetence, weight loss, pale mucous membranes, lymphadenopathy, and joint pain (the latter particularly in *E. ewingii* infection in dogs and people).

E. ewingii and *E. chaffeensis* occasionally progress to chronic or severe disease in humans, with polyarthritis, CNS disturbance, and pulmonary infiltrates. Canine monocytic ehrlichiosis appears unique in that affected

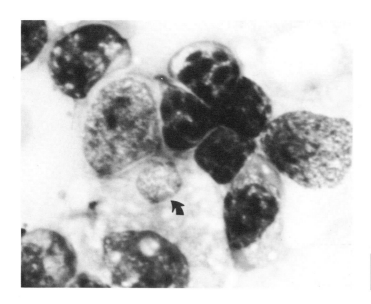

FIGURE 42.1.   Neorickettsia helminthoeca *colony (morula; arrow) in canine lymph node impression. Giemsa stain, 1000X.*

dogs may enter a latent stage and a final chronic phase. In the chronic phase, which may occur months to years after quiescent infection, reduction of all blood cell types may accompany hemorrhages (commonly epistaxis), edema, serosal effusions, dyspnea, interstitial pneumonia, anemia, secondary infections, and enlargement of spleen, liver, and lymph nodes. Hyperglobulinemia, glomerulonephritis, and widespread plasma cell infiltration suggest immunopathogenic mechanisms.

Immunologic Aspects

Progression to latent and chronic canine ehrlichiosis occurs more frequently in dogs with genetic predispositions and possibly impaired cell-mediated immunity. Latent infection appears to reside in the spleen. Although hypergammaglobulinemia usually is polyclonal, several cases of monoclonal gammopathy have been reported, suggesting almost malignant transformation of B lymphocyte clones and/or suppression of most other clones.

Cellular and humoral immune-mediated responses to infected mononuclear cells and platelets are suspected to contribute to blood cell destruction and bone marrow depression, polyarthritis, and uveitis; meningitis may be due to immune complex deposition. Resistance to reinfection is antibody and cell-mediated.

Laboratory Diagnosis

Giemsa-stained smears of buffy coat are examined for intracellular morulae. These are scarce and found mainly during the acute stage.

The agents of human and canine monocytic ehrlichiosis may be cultured in canine cell lines.

Serodiagnosis by indirect immunofluorescence may detect antibodies to these ehrlichiae, and polymerase chain reaction testing (utilizing specific DNA primers) is recommended to detect active infection in blood.

Treatment and Control

Tetracycline is effective in early monocytic ehrlichiosis but less so in advanced cases. Imidocarb dipropionate has also been recommended. Late-stage monocytic ehrlichiosis has a poor prognosis and is managed with doxycycline and steroids.

For prevention, tick control is imperative. People with recent tick bites receive doxycycline prophylactically for 10 days.

EHRLICHIA RUMINANTIUM AND *E. OVIS*

Ecology

Reservoir and Transmission

"African heartwater disease," caused by *E. ruminantium,* affects mostly ruminants. The disease is passed only by parenteral introduction of blood. Tick vectors are *Amblyomma* spp. Strains of *E. ruminantium,* though serologically uniform, vary in virulence. The infection is endemic in tropical Africa and parts of the Caribbean.

Ehrlichia ovis parasitizes bovine or ovine mononuclear cells, and *E. ondiri* also invades granulocytes. The latter causes bovine petechial fever (Ondiri disease) in the highlands of East Africa, a disease marked by fever, lowered milk yield, mucosal hemorrhages, and variable early mortality. Arthropod vectors are assumed.

Pathogenesis

Ehrlichia ruminantium multiplies in cells lining the sinusoids of lymph nodes, disseminates to the bloodstream, and colonizes endothelial cells, particularly cerebrocortical capillaries. Their presence induces little cellular inflammatory response, but does result in widespread vasculitis with effusion and epithelial and endothelial hemorrhage. Pericardial effusion, which gave the disease its name, is inconsistent. Affected animals also may develop encephalitis. Spleen, lymph nodes, and usually liver are grossly enlarged.

Clinical signs vary. In the peracute form, a fever of several hours' duration precedes collapse and death under convulsions. In the acute form, fever occurs followed within hours by disturbances including hyperexcitability, muscle tremors, ataxia, deficits in conscious proprioception, head pressing, coma, and seizures. Death within 2 to 10 days is the rule in sheep and likely in cattle. A subclinical form is also recognized. Mortality in sheep is from 6–80%.

Little is known about the pathogenesis of Ondiri disease.

Immunologic Aspects

Newborn animals and some cattle breeds are relatively resistant to *E. ruminantium.*

In surviving cattle, the agent disappears within 2 months after recovery, but cell-mediated immunity persists for up to 5 years.

Laboratory Diagnosis

Heartwater may be diagnosed by demonstration of the agent in a Giemsa-stained smear of cerebral cortex. Infected cerebral extracts will agglutinate with specific antibody. Polymerase chain reaction–based testing utilizing specific DNA primers can document the presence of *E. ruminantium* DNA in the sample.

Treatment and Control

Tetracycline treatment is effective if the disease is treated early. Tick control and vaccination are important preventive steps. Young calves and lambs (<4 weeks) or goats (<6 weeks) are vaccinated with virulent rickettsiae. Older animals may be infected and then treated with antimicrobial drugs, thus developing immunity. Heartwater is exotic in North America although common in the Caribbean. *Amblyomma* ticks have been introduced into North America a number of times on imported wildlife, including ungulates and reptiles. In 1999, leopard tortoises being imported through Florida were infested with *A. sparsum* that were test-positive for *E. ruminantium.*

NEORICKETTSIA RISTICII AND NEORICKETTSIA SENNETSU

Ecology

Reservoir and Transmission

Potomac horse fever (PHV), an acute equine diarrheal syndrome first noted in North American horses in Montgomery County, Maryland, is a monocytic ehrlichiosis

caused by *N. risticii. Neorickettsia risticii* is acquired orally probably in association with fluke metacercariae in water. The intermediate host of the fluke is a snail, although the full range of possible snail species associated with *N. risticii* has not been described. The geographic distribution of *N. risticii* includes most of North America. Dogs and cats can be experimentally infected with *N. risticii.* Sennetsu fever (*N. sennetsu*) is a disease in Malaysia and Japan that targets human monocytes. Little is known of its ecology.

Pathogenesis

The PHV agent infects equine monocytes, intestinal epithelium, and colonic mast cells. Clinically, PHV resembles ehrlichioses with fever, listlessness, anorexia, variable leukopenia, diarrhea, and, as a late complication, laminitis. Uterine infection has been observed. The fatality rate of cases with diarrhea is 20% to 30%. Ulcerative gastroenteritis is the most notable lesion at necropsy.

Immunologic Aspects

Immunologic factors are not fully understood. Antibodies to *N. risticii* cross-react with *N. sennetsu,* but not with *Anaplasma phagocytophilum* (formerly *E. equi*). Recovered horses are immune.

Laboratory Diagnosis

Microbiologic diagnosis involves demonstration of the agent in monocytes in Wright-stained blood smears. Serologic diagnosis is by an indirect fluorescent antibody test or by enzyme-linked immunosorbent assay (ELISA). *Neorickettsia risticii* DNA can be detected by the polymerase chain reaction.

Treatment and Control

Tetracycline, if given early, has been credited with reducing mortality to under 10%. Supportive care also is important. An effective bacterin is commercially available.

NEORICKETTSIA HELMINTHOECA AND ELOKIMIN FLUKE FEVER

Descriptive Features

The agent of salmon "poisoning," *Neorickettsia helminthoeca,* infects lymphoreticular tissues of canids. *Neorickettsia helminthoeca* multiplies in the cytoplasm of macrophages, frequently forming multiple morulae and filling the entire cell. Individual neorickettsiae may be dispersed through the cytoplasm. They are coccobacilli measuring usually less than 0.5 μm in any dimension and are demonstrable by Giemsa stain. *Neorickettsia helminthoeca* has been propagated in cell culture.

Ecology

Reservoir and Transmission

The reservoir of *N. helminthoeca* is the fluke, *Nanophyetus salmincola*, whose life cycle includes passage through a fish and a snail. The geographical distribution of salmon poisoning is limited by the range of the snail intermediate hosts of *N. salmincola (Oxytrema silicula)* and includes coastal areas of North America (northernmost California, Oregon, Washington, and British Columbia). Infections in nonendemic areas are due to planting of infected fish. Dogs (as well as bears, raccoons, and other animals) are the definitive hosts of the fluke, harboring the adults in their intestine, and are infected by *N. helminthoeca* by eating fluke-infected fish. Fluke eggs are shed in canine feces, embryonate, and hatch miracidia that invade the snail. Cercaria emerge from the snail and invade a fish, becoming sessile metacercaria encysted in the kidney. Upon being ingested by the definitive host, they become adults within 6 days. Uninfected flukes produce little disturbance in dogs.

Elokomin fluke fever, a mild form of salmon disease, attacks canids, ferrets, raccoons, and bears.

Pathogenesis

From the ingested fish kidney, metacercarial flukes emerge in the dog's intestine, develop into adults, attach, and release into the tissues *N. helminthoeca*, which colonizes lymphoreticular tissues throughout the body. Enlargement of lymphoid organs results from proliferation of reticuloendothelial components. A nonsuppurative meningoencephalitis is common.

Within 5 days to several weeks of exposure, dogs develop fever, anorexia, depression, weight loss, swollen lymph nodes, and often hemorrhagic enteritis. Vomiting and persistent, eventually hemorrhagic, diarrhea are typical. Death occurs in up to 90% of untreated cases within 2 weeks.

Immunologic Aspects

Dogs recovered from salmon disease are immune. The agent does not induce immunity to the closely related, epidemiologically identical Elokimin fluke fever agent.

Laboratory Diagnosis

Presence of eggs of *N. salmincola* in the feces of a dog showing pertinent clinical signs constitutes strong evidence of salmon disease, although many affected dogs do not shed fluke eggs in feces. Demonstration of rickettsiae in Wright-stained lymph node aspirates is definitive (see Fig 42.1).

Treatment and Control

Penicillin G, tetracycline, chloramphenicol, and sulfonamides given parenterally are usually effective. Supportive treatment is essential.

The best preventive measure is the exclusion of infected salmon from the canine diet. Flukes and *N. helminthoeca* are killed by cooking and by freezing for 24 hours.

43

Anaplasmataceae

JANET E. FOLEY ERNST L. BIBERSTEIN

Members of the order *Rickettsiales* are minute obligate intracellular gram-negative bacteria. They are basically parasites of arthropods. Two families within this order are of veterinary interest. The family Anaplasmataceae, composed of the genus *Anaplasma,* parasitizes erythrocytes, phagocytes- and platelets. The family *Rickettsiaceae,* which includes parasites of vascular endothelium (genera *Rickettsia, Coxiella,* and *Orientia*), commonly referred to as "rickettsiae," and parasites of phagocytic cells (genera *Ehrlichia* and *Neorickettsia*), commonly referred to as "ehrlichiae."

The ehrlichiae are discussed in Chapter 42 and the rickettsiae are discussed in Chapter 41. Discussed in this chapter are members of the genus *Anaplasma.*

The genus *Anaplasma* includes the species *Anaplasma marginale, A. centrale, A. ovis, A. caudatum, A.* (formerly *Ehrlichia*) *bovis, A.* (formerly *Ehrlichia*) *platys,* and *A.* (formerly *Ehrlichia*) *phagocytophilum. Anaplasmataceae* parasitize erythrocytes, platelets, and granulocytes in several classes of vertebrates and may cause anemias. The genera *Aegyptianella, Haemobartonella,* and *Eperythrozoon* have been reevaluated phygenetically and are classed currently with the family Mycoplasmataceae (Chapter 40).

Of the erythrocyte-infecting species, only *A. marginale* is a significant pathogen. *Anaplasma ovis* rarely causes anaplasmosis of sheep and is infective for goats and deer. *Anaplasma caudatum,* which has a tail-like appendage, has been seen in bovine infections alongside *A. marginale.* Its significance is uncertain. *Anaplasma centrale,* also found in cattle, is of interest as an immunizing agent against *A. marginale.*

The agents of human granulocytic ehrlichiosis (previously unnamed), equine ehrlichiosis (previously *Ehrlichia equi*), and ehrlichiosis of ruminants (previously *E. phagocytophila*) have been combined into a single species, *A. phagocytophilum.*

ANAPLASMA MARGINALE

Descriptive Features

In Giemsa-stained blood smears, *A. marginale* appears as purple structures (1 μm in diameter) near the periphery of erythrocytes (Fig 43.1). These marginal (inclusion) bodies are membrane-lined vacuoles containing up to 10 initial bodies (400 nm each) enclosed in a two-layered membrane. Initial bodies contain DNA and RNA but lack cell walls. The organism has been serially propagated in a tick cell culture. It requires an oxygenated atmosphere, is catalase-positive, and utilizes exogenous amino acids.

Ecology

Reservoir and Transmission

Infected ruminants are the reservoir of *A. marginale.* Although many species can be infected, few regularly develop disease. Some, such as deer, may be naturally infected and serve as a source of bovine anaplasmosis. The infection occurs on all continents. Transmission is by parenteral introduction of infected blood, in nature probably most often by ticks and blood-sucking flying insects, but also by contaminated instruments, transplacental, and conjunctival exposure.

Pathogenesis

Initial bodies enter erythrocytes by endocytosis after adhering to the cell surface by way of major surface protein-1 (Msp-1) and multiply by binary fission within the endosome. New initial bodies are released from the erythrocyte surface, possibly to contiguous cells, without discernible cell damage. Erythrocyte destruction occurs following an immune response to parasitized erythrocytes, resulting in indiscriminate erythrocyte removal by the macrophage system. Anemia, icterus, bile stasis, splenomegaly, and hepatomegaly follow. There is little intravascular hemolysis and no hemoglobinuria.

Illnesses, following incubation periods of up to 5 weeks, range from subclinical to peracutely fatal. Signs include anemia, fever, anorexia, depression, weakness, constipation, and abortion. Severity often varies directly with age and duration from hours to weeks. In mature cattle (>3 years), mortality may reach 50%. Disease is generally seen in cattle 1 year of age or older. Long-term carriage occurs in ticks.

Immunologic Factors

Humoral and cell-mediated responses develop after infection with *A. marginale. Anaplasma marginale* expresses at least five Msps, all of which display antigenic variation due

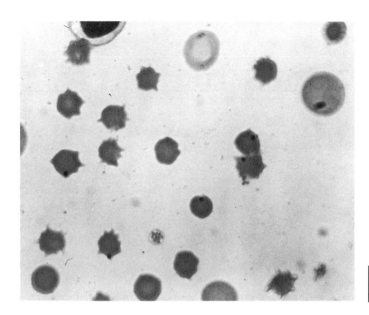

FIGURE 43.1.   Anaplasma marginale *in bovine erythrocytes.*
Wright's stain, 1000X.

in large part to the polymorphic nature of the encoding *msp* genes. The antigenic variation may explain the chronic nature of anaplasmosis. Antibody response is directed also to host antigens, and plays a role in pathogenesis. Immunity following recovery may not be permanent.

Natural infection in calves is subclinical and confers resistance to subsequent exposure. It may produce immediate or delayed clinical disease in the individual and may spread to other stock, requiring vector control. Resistance of calves outlasts maternal antibody and can be terminated by splenectomy.

Infection with *A. centrale*, resulting in mild disease, induces resistance to *A. marginale*. Two commercial vaccines are available for *A. marginale*. An inactivated *A. marginale* vaccine produces immunity of several months' duration subject to reinforcement through natural exposure. The erythrocyte constituents of the inactivated vaccine account for occasional immunohemolytic problems in neonatal calves nursing immunized animals. A modified live vaccine also is produced and induces lifelong immunity. However, this vaccine is contraindicated in pregnant cows and cattle older than 24 months.

Laboratory Diagnosis

Anaplasma marginale is demonstrable by routine blood stains, acridine orange, or immunofluorescence. The latter is most specific and sensitive. Acridine orange produces nonspecific staining of nucleic acids, whereas routine blood stains may not detect infection beyond the first few weeks. Molecular techniques such as the polymerase chain reaction utilizing specific DNA primers has been developed and are very sensitive.

Serologic methods include complement fixation, capillary agglutination, radioimmunoassay, enzyme-linked immunosorbent assay (ELISA), and a card agglutination test for field use. All are useful in detecting subclinical cases.

Treatment and Control

Tetracycline is effective against *A. marginale*. Clinical cases are treated by parenteral therapy, whereas the carrier state is treated by feed medication for up to 2 months. Vaccination and vector control are helpful.

ANAPLASMA PHAGOCYTOPHILUM AND A. PLATYS

Descriptive Features

In Giemsa-stained blood smears, *Anaplasma phagocytophilum* appears as membrane-bound morulae consisting of 1 to 10 bacteria within neutrophils and, less commonly, monocytes of ruminants, horses, dogs, and humans. *Anaplasma platys* occurs on the surface of canine platelets and causes a cyclic thrombocytopenia.

Anaplasma phagocytophilum has been serially propagated in a tick cell culture and human neutrophilic leukemia cells. It is aerobic, catalase-positive, and utilizes exogenous amino acids.

Ecology

Reservoir and Transmission

The reservoir hosts of *A. phagocytophilum* include rodents and possibly larger wildlife species such as coyotes and deer. Ecology varies significantly in different geographical regions, with the primary cycle in eastern North America involving the white-footed mouse (*Peromyscus leukopus*) and the deer tick (*Ixodes scapularis*). In Europe, the main vector is *I. ricinus,* and reservoirs include a variety of rodents. In western North America, the vector to humans and veterinary patients is the western black-legged tick (*I. pacificus),* although a rodent-specific tick, *I. spini-*

palpis, may be an important vector in the sylvatic cycle. Donkeys, sheep, goats, dogs, cats, and monkeys can be experimentally infected.

The reservoirs and vectors of *A. platys* are not known.

Pathogenesis

Anaplasma phagocytophilum occurs in granulocytes and, less commonly, monocytes primarily of ruminants in Europe (where it is called "tick-borne fever," TBF) and horses, dogs, and humans in North America. All hosts develop vasculitis associated with thromboses, thrombocytopenia, edema, and hemorrhage, especially in the distal limbs. Vascular changes are pronounced in testes and ovaries of ruminants. Leukopenia successively affects lymphocytes and neutrophils. Lesions include splenomegaly and hemorrhages along the intestinal tract. Histologically, a striking lack of lymphoid elements is observed.

Clinically, there is fever accompanied by depression, accelerated breathing, inappetence, hemorrhage, edema, anemia, icterus, and ataxia (especially in horses), and, in cows, a drop in milk yield. Ewes and cows may abort. The disease is mildest in young animals. A heightened susceptibility to secondary infections may be due to parasitization of neutrophils, leukopenia, and a lymphopenia affecting B lymphocytes. Tick pyemia (due to *Staphylococcus* infection) is commonly linked with TBF. Fatalities are due to rare secondary complications, such as respiratory infections or laminitis.

Dogs infected with *A. platys* develop cyclic thrombocytopenia via immune-mediated destruction, possibly accompanied by mild fever, and secondary immune-mediated disease such as uveitis.

Immunologic Aspects

As for *A. marginale,* there is antigenic strain variability involving mainly the major surface proteins, although the relevance in *A. phagocytophilum* infection is unknown. There is some serological cross-reactivity with *Ehrlichia* spp. although animals with *A. phagocytophilum* infection usually have higher specific, compared with cross-reacting, titers. Recovered animals are refractory to reinfection, although recurring illnesses have been reported in successive years. Recovery occurs after a peak in production in interferon gamma. No vaccines exist.

Splenectomy can reactivate or exacerbate *A. platys*-associated thrombocytopenia.

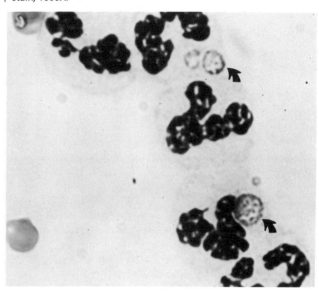

FIGURE 43.2. Anaplasma phagocytophilum *(formerly* Ehrlichia equi*) (arrows) in smear of buffy coat from horse. Wright's stain, 1000X.*

Laboratory Diagnosis

Morulae in neutrophils can be demonstrated in Wright-stained blood and buffy coat films most readily 48 hours after onset (Fig 43.2). Indirect immunofluorescent antibody (IFA) and ELISA tests have been developed using infected equine neutrophils and human leukemia cells for the IFA and recombinant antigens for the ELISA. The polymerase chain reaction (utilizing specifically designed DNA primers) is used to detect the microorganisms before antibodies are produced.

Individual *A. platys* organisms can be visualized on Wright-stained platelets of infected dogs. Previous exposure can be documented by IFA.

Treatment

Tetracycline is effective. The first dose can be given intravenously followed by daily doses intravenously or orally for 1 week. Reduction of exposure to ticks is desirable.

44 *Bartonellaceae*

Bruno B. Chomel   Rickie W. Kasten

Members of the Family *Bartonellaceae* are small gram-negative rods. Until recently, the genus *Bartonella* consisted of only one species, *B. bacilliformis*. The genus now contains all the species that were once included in the genera *Bartonella, Rochalimaea,* and *Grahamella.* The genus *Bartonella,* has been placed into the family *Bartonellaceae* (which has also been removed from the order *Rickettsiales*). Members of the genus *Bartonella* belong to the alpha-2 subgroup of the alpha-proteobacteria. Most of these bacteria are erythrocyte-adherent bacilli.

The present family consists of more than 20 species or subspecies, of which nine are human pathogens:

1. **Associated with disease in human patients.** *Bartonella bacilliformis* is the etiologic agent of Oroya fever, an acute bacteremic infection characterized by sepsis and hemolysis, and of verruga peruana, mainly a cutaneous nodular vascular eruption representing chronic infection.

   Bartonella quintana, the agent of trench fever, has also been found to be one of the agents of bacillary angiomatosis (BA), a vascular proliferative lesion observed in immunocompromised individuals, mainly with acquired immunodeficiency syndrome (AIDS). Bacillary angiomatosis can also be caused by *B. henselae.*

   Bartonella henselae causes cat scratch disease (CSD) in immunocompetent individuals.

   Bartonella elizabethae is associated with endocarditis in immunocompetent patients.

   Bartonella vinsonii subsp. *berkhoffii* and *B. washoensis* are associated with endocarditis or myocarditis.

   Bartonella grahamii has been associated with neuroretinitis.

   Bartonella vinsonii subsp. *arupensis* was isolated from the blood of a rancher with fever and mild neurological symptoms.

   Bartonella clarridgeiae is suspected to also be a minor agent of cat scratch disease.

2. **Associated with animal patients.** Some of the *Bartonella* species that are pathogenic to humans (*B. vinsonii* subsp. *berkhoffii, B. clarridgeiae, B. henselae, B. elizabethae* and *B. washoensis*) have recently been associated with various clinical entities, including endocarditis, in domestic dogs.

   Several other *Bartonella* species—such as *B. vinsonii* subsp. *vinsonii, B. doshiae, B. taylorii, B. peromysci, B. birtlesii, B. tribocorum, B. alsatica, B. talpae, B. koehlerae, B. bovis, B. schoenbuchensis,* and *B.*

capreoli—have only been isolated from the blood of various animal species, including various wild rodents, squirrels, rabbits, felids, canids, bovids, and cervids. At present, these species are not known to induce any specific disease in the infected animal.

Descriptive Features

Morphology and Staining

Bartonellaceae are fastidious, aerobic, short, pleomorphic gram-negative coccobacillary or bacillary rods (0.6 μm by 1.0 μm) that take from 5 to 15 days and up to 45 days on primary culture to form visible colonies on enriched blood-containing media, as they are highly hemindependent. In infected tissues, Warthin-Starry silver impregnation stain reveals small bacilli, which tend to appear as clumps of tightly compacted organisms. Similarly, small organisms can be identified in red blood cells by May-Grünwald Giemsa coloration. Bartonellae have a close evolutionary resemblance with members of the genera *Brucella, Agrobacterium,* and *Rhizobium.*

Cellular Composition

Bartonella bacilliformis and *B. clarridgeiae* are the only members of the genus that are motile by means of unipolar flagella. *Bartonella quintana* and *B. henselae* have a twitching motility associated to fimbriae or pili. Because of their slow growth, standard biochemical methods for identification are not as useful for identification. The bartonellae are oxidase and catalase-negative. Measurements of preformed enzymes and standard testing have revealed differences between species. Most species are biochemically inert except for the production of peptidases. The MicroScan Rapid Anaerobe Panel (Baxter Diagnostics, Deerfield, IL) has been reported to provide species identification. Whole cell fatty acid (CFA) analysis for the genus has proven useful for identification because *Bartonella* have a unique and characteristic whole cell fatty acid composition. The *Bartonella* have gas-liquid chromatography fatty acid profiles consisting mainly of $C_{18:09}$, $C_{18:19}$, and $C_{16:0}$. Molecular genetic methods such as restriction fragment length polymorphism (RFLP) of genes encoding citrate synthase, 16S ribosomal RNA (rRNA) or 16S-23S rRNA spacer region, and more recently analysis based on polymerase chain reaction (PCR) of random, repetitive extragenic palindromic sequences have been used to distinguish strains and species of

Table 44.1. Epidemiology of *Bartonella* Species or Subspecies Presently Described

Bartonella sp.	Reservoir	Vector or Potential Vector	Current Geographic Distribution
B. bacilliformis	Humans	Pheblotomines (*Lutzomyia verrucarum*) (sand flies)	Andes (Peru, Ecuador, Colombia, Bolivia, Chile, Guatemala)
B. quintana	Humans	Human body lice (*Pediculus humanis corporis*)	Worldwide
B. henselae	Cats (*Felis catus*)	Fleas (*Ctenocephalides felis*) Ticks?	Worldwide
B. clarridgeiae	Cats (*Felis catus*)	Fleas (*Ctenocephalides felis*)	Cosmopolite
B. koehlerae	Cats (*Felis catus*)	Fleas (*Ctenocephalides felis*)	California, France
B. vinsonii subsp vinsonii	Meadow voles (*Microtus pennsylvanicus*)	Ear mites (*Trombicula microti*)?	Canada
B. vinsonii subsp arupensis	White-footed mice (*Peromyscus leucopus*)	Fleas? ticks?	USA (Midwest)
B. vinsonii subsp berkhoffii	Coyotes (*Canis latrans*), dogs (*Canis familiaris*)	Ticks?	Cosmopolite
B. talpae	Moles (*Talpa europaea*)	?	United Kingdom
B. peromysci	Field mice (*Peromyscus* spp.)	?	United States
B. birtlesii	Wood mice (*Apodemus* spp.)	?	France, United Kingdom
B. grahamii	Bank voles (*Clethrionomys glareolus*)	?	United Kingdom
B. taylorii	Wood mice (*Apodemus* spp.)	?	United Kingdom
B. doshiae	Meadow voles (*Microtus agrestis*)	?	United Kingdom
B. elizabethae	Rats (*Rattus norvegicus*)	Fleas	Worldwide
B. tribocorum	Rats (*Rattus norvegicus*)	?	Cosmopolite
B. alsatica	Rabbits (*Oryctolagus cuniculus*)	Fleas? Ticks?	France
B. washoensis	California ground squirrel (*Spermophilus beecheyi*)	Fleas? Ticks?	Western USA
B. bovis	Domestic cattle (*Bos taurus*)	Biting flies? ticks?	Cosmopolite
B. capreoli	Roe deer (*capreolus capreolus*)	Biting flies? Ticks?	Europe
B. schoenbuchensis	Roe deer (*capreolus capreolus*)	Biting flies? Ticks?	Europe

Bartonella. RFLP or sequence analysis of DNA encoding 16S rRNA, citrate synthase genes after PCR amplification both directly from specimens or pure cultures have been largely used for detecting and characterizing *Bartonella*. More recently, identification has also been performed with the amplification of the DNA encoding the 16S-23S rRNA intergenic spacer region (ITS) or protein-encoding genes. The genes most widely used are those encoding the citrate synthase (*gltA*), the heat shock protein (*groEL*), the riboflavine (*ribC*), a cell division protein (*ftsZ*), and a 17kDa antigen.

Growth Characteristics

Traditionally, members of the genus *Bartonella* are cultivated in semisolid nutrient agar containing fresh rabbit blood (or sheep or horse blood) at 35°C (except for *B. bacilliformis*, which grows best at 28°C) in 5% CO_2. On primary isolation, some *Bartonella*, such as *B. henselae*, *B. clarridgeiae*, *B. vinsonii*, or *B. elizabethae* have colonies with a white, rough, dry, raised appearance and pit the medium. They are hard to break up or transfer. Other bartonellae such as *B. quintana* have colonies that are usually smaller, gray, translucent, and somewhat gummy or slightly mucoid.

Ecology

Reservoir, Transmission, and Geographic Distribution.

Most members of the genus *Bartonella* species are vectorborne organisms. The reservoirs, vectors, and geographic distribution are shown in Table 44.1.

Pathogenesis

Mechanisms. Bartonella quintana and *B. henselae* are clinically associated with proliferative neovascular lesions. The pathogenesis of bacillary angiomatosis involves injury and proliferation of the vascular endothelium both with *B. henselae* and *B. quintana*. These organisms induce endothelial cell proliferation and migration in vitro, and a protein fraction was identified as the angiogenic factor. *Bartonella* infection (in vitro) stimulated endothelial cell proliferation and induced obvious morphological changes due to modifications of the cytoskeleton. *Bartonella henselae* has been shown to induce infected cells to produce vascular endothelial growth factor, which in turn stimulated the proliferation of endothelial cells and the growth of *B. henselae*.

Bartonella henselae seems to share with *B. bacilliformis* a common mechanism for mediating pathogenesis. A bacteriophage-like particle similar to the bacteriophage observed in *B. bacilliformis* has been found in culture supernatant from *B. henselae*. This particle has at least three associated proteins and contains 14 kbp linear DNA segments that are heterogeneous in sequence. It has been speculated that an ancestor of *B. henselae* and *B. bacilliformis* acquired the ability to mediate angioproliferation as a means of enhancing its dissemination or its acquisition of nutrients within the host. It is possible that a common transducting phage may be the mechanism of genetic exchange by which the two organisms acquired this pathogenic trait.

All *Bartonella* species multiply and persist in red blood cells. *Bartonella bacilliformis* possess polar flagella that have been shown to mediate erythrocyte adhesion. For non-flagellated *Bartonella*, bundle-forming pili as well as surface proteins may play a role in erythrocyte adhesion. Until recently, mechanisms of persitence of *Bartonella* bacteremia in mammals were not well understood. Recent reports have revealed the intraerythrocytic localization of these bacteria, which is a unique strategy for bacterial persistence. Nonhemolytic intracellular colonization of erythrocytes would preserve the organisms for efficient vector transmission, protect *Bartonella* from the host immune response and contribute to decreased antimicrobial efficacy. Persistence of infection was recently demonstrated in a rat model using *B. tribocorum*. After a 5-day "hidden/silent" phase following experimental infection, the organism multiplied until there were an average of eight *Bartonella* per red blood cell. Thereafter, the organisms remained within the cell for the life of the erythrocyte. Nonhemolytic intracellular colonization of erythrocytes is likely a bacterial persistence strategy that preserves the *Bartonella* species for potential transmission by arthropods, because the reservoir host would serve as a source of infection for blood-feeding arthropods, which could then subsequently infect a new host.

Disease Patterns and Epidemiology

Human Patients. *Cat Scratch Disease.* Cat scratch disease (CSD) is caused by *Bartonella henselae*. In CSD, 1 to 3 weeks elapse between the scratch or bite of a cat and the appearance of clinical signs. In 50% of the cases, a small skin lesion, often resembling an insect bite, appears at the inoculation site, usually the hand or forearm, and evolves from a papule to a vesicle and partially healed ulcers. These lesions resolve within a few days to a few weeks. Lymphadenitis develops approximately 3 weeks after exposure and is generally unilateral. It commonly appears in the epitrochlear, axillary, or cervical lymph nodes. Swelling of the lymph node is usually painful and persists for several weeks to several months. In 25% of the cases, suppuration occurs. The large majority of the cases show signs of systemic infection: fever, chills, malaise, anorexia, headaches. In general, the disease is benign and heals spontaneously without sequelae. Atypical manifestations of CSD occur in 5% to 10% of the cases. The most common of these is Parinaud's oculoglandular syndrome (periauricular lymphadenopathy and palpebral conjunctivitis), but also meningitis, encephalitis, osteolytic lesions, and thrombocytopenic purpura may occur. Encephalopathy is one of the most serious complications of CSD, which usually occurs 2 to 6 weeks after the onset of lymphadenopathy. However, it usually resolves with complete recovery and few or no sequelae.

There were an estimated 22,000 human cases of CSD in the United States in 1992, some 2000 of whom were hospitalized. The estimated annual health cost of CSD was more than $12 million. From 55% to 80% of CSD patients are under the age of 20 years. There is a seasonal pattern, with most cases seen in autumn and winter.

New clinical presentations associated with *B. henselae* infection have been reported in immunocompetent persons, including neuroretinitis or bacteremia as a cause of

chronic fatigue syndrome, and a case of aggressive *B. henselae* endocarditis in a cat owner. *Bartonella henselae* was also recently determined as a frequent cause of prolonged fever and fever of unknown origin in children. Rheumatic manifestations of *Bartonella* infection have been recently described in children, including a case of myositis and a case of arthritis and skin nodules. Arthritis has also been described in a very limited number of cases. Other rheumatic manifestations related to *Bartonella* infection in humans include erythema nodosum, leukocytoclastic vasculitis, fever of unknown origin with myalgia, and arthralgia.

Endocarditis. Several *Bartonella* spp. have also been recognized as causative agents of blood culture–negative endocarditis or myocarditis in humans, including *B. henselae*, *B. quintana*, *B. elizabethae*, *B. vinsonii* subsp. *berkhoffii*, and *B. washoensis*. *Bartonella* spp. account for approximately 3% of all human cases of endocarditis, a percentage similar to endocarditis cases caused by *Coxiella burnetii*, the agent of Q fever (see Chapter 41).

Bacillary Angiomatosis. For bacillary angiomatosis in immunocompromised persons, the signs and symptoms are very different from CSD. Bacillary angiomatosis, also called *epithelioid angiomatosis*, is a vascular proliferative disease of the skin characterized by multiple, blood-filled, cystic tumors. It is usually characterized by violaceous or colorless papular and nodular skin lesions that clinically may suggest Kaposi's sarcoma, but histologically resemble epithelioid hemangiomas. When visceral parenchymal organs are involved, the condition is referred to as *bacillary peliosis hepatis*, *splenic peliosis*, or *systemic bacillary angiomatosis*. Fever, weight loss, malaise, and enlargement of affected organs may develop in people with disseminated bacillary angiomatosis. Endocarditis has also been reported in patients with bacillary angiomatosis.

Cats. No major clinical signs of CSD have been reported in cats under natural conditions, but infection is very common, especially in young kittens. It is estimated that about 10% of pet cats and up to 30–50% of stray cats are *Bartonella*-bacteremic at a given time. In western North America (California), a 40% prevalence of bacteremic cats was found in the San Francisco-Sacramento area. Minor clinical signs, including fever, enlarged lymph nodes, uveitis and mild neurological symptoms have been reported in experimentally infected cats. However, several cases of uveitis and a case of *Bartonella henselae* endocarditis were recently diagnosed in pet cats. Additionally, reproductive disorders (lack of pregnancy or pregnancy only after repeated breedings, stillbirths) have been observed in experimentally infected queens. Bacteremia usually lasts a few weeks to a few months. The organisms have been reported to be intraerythrocytic, and pili may be a pathogenic determinant for this *Bartonella* species. Cats can yield more than 1 million colony-forming units (CFU) per milliliter of blood. Direct transmission from cat to cat, as well as vertical transmission from bacteremic female cats to kittens, was unsuccessful in various experiments. Transmission from cat to cat was successfully achieved by depositing infected fleas collected from bacteremic cats onto noninfected kittens. Presence of *B. henselae* DNA was found in infected fleas. Epidemiological studies clearly demonstrate that antibody prevalence and bacteremia prevalence is the highest in stray cat populations living in warm and humid areas where flea infestation is usually higher.

Dogs. *Bartonella vinsonii* subsp. *berkhoffii* has been identified as an important cause of canine endocarditis, especially in large breed dogs. In a two-year prospective study of endocarditis cases, almost one-third of the 18 cases were caused by *Bartonella* species. *Bartonella clarridgeiae* and *B. washoensis* have recently been associated with dog endocarditis cases. The clinical spectrum of this infection in dogs has also been expanding, as it has been associated with cardiac arrhythmias, endocarditis and myocarditis, granulomatous lymphadenitis, and granulomatous rhinitis. In some dogs, intermittent lameness, bone pain, or fever of unknown origin can precede the diagnosis of endocarditis for several months. *Bartonella clarridgeiae* DNA was detected in a dog with lymphocytic hepatitis. *Bartonella henselae* DNA was initially detected in a dog with peliosis hepatis, and more recently in a dog with hepatopathy and in three dogs with various clinical entities. These three *B. henselae*–DNA-positive dogs presented nonspecific clinical abnormalities, such as severe weight loss, protracted lethargy, and anorexia. A fourth dog was diagnosed as being infected with *B. elizabethae* by PCR amplification and sequencing, increasing the number of *Bartonella* species identified in infected dogs. Serological studies in North America and Europe indicate that *Bartonella* infection in domestic dogs is quite rare (less than 5%), whereas high seroprevalence has been reported from dogs living in tropical countries (up to 65% of dogs tested from Sudan). In North America, especially in the Southeast, high seroprevalence has been reported in dogs also seropositive for various tick-borne pathogens (mainly *Erlichia*, *Babesia*, *Anaplasma*). A high seroprevalence (35%) has been reported in coyotes from California, and in one specific California county, 28% of the coyotes tested were bacteremic.

Rodents. Experimental infection of pregnant laboratory mice with *B. birtlesii* showed pathogenic effects on the reproductive function of these mice. Bacteremia was significantly higher in virgin females than in males. In mice infected before pregnancy, fetal loss and resorption was higher in infected mice than controls, and the weight of viable fetuses was significantly lower for infected than for uninfected mice. Transplacental transmission was also demonstrated, since 76% of the fetal resorptions were culture-positive for *B. birtlesii*. The histopathological analysis of the placentas of infected mice showed vascular lesions in the maternal placenta, which could explain the reproductive disorders observed. The isolation and characterization of the complete *vir*B homologue (*vir*B2–11) and a downstream located *vir*D4 gene in *B. tribocorum* has been recently described. An essential role for this VirB/VirD4 T4SS in establishing intraerythrocytic infection was demonstrated.

Immunologic Aspects

Infection by *Bartonella* organisms stimulates both the cellular and the humoral responses. *Bartonella henselae* and *B.* *quintana* induce proliferation and migration of endothelial cells. These effects are due to a trypsin-sensitive factor that appears to be associated with the bacterial cell wall or membrane or intracellular molecules. *Bartonella henselae* infects and activates endothelial cells. *Bartonella henselae* outer membrane proteins (OMPs) are sufficient to induce NFκß activation and adhesion molecule expression, followed by enhanced rolling and adhesion of leukocytes.

In infected individuals, specific antibodies can be detected a few days to a few weeks after infection. Most of the clinical cases of CSD or BA are associated with elevated titers against *B. henselae* or *B. quintana*. Immunity is usually long lasting in cases of CSD. Human cases of endocarditis are frequently associated with very high indirect fluorescent antibody (IFA) titers (>1:800).

In a murine model, spleen cells from infected C57BL/6 mice proliferated specifically upon stimulation with heat-killed *Bartonella* antigen, and CD4 T lymphocytes mainly mediate proliferative responses. These responses increased during the course of infection and peaked at 8 weeks post-infection. Gamma interferon, but not interleukin-4, was produced in vitro by spleen cells from infected animals upon stimulation with *Bartonella* antigens. As described also in humans, cats, and dogs, *Bartonella*-specific IgG antibodies were detectable in the serum of the infected mice by the second week, and the antibody concentration peaked at 12 weeks post-infection. IgG$_{2b}$ was the prominent isotype among the *Bartonella*-specific serum IgG antibodies. Therefore, *B. henselae* induces cell-mediated immune responses with a T$_{H1}$ phenotype in immunocompetent C57BL/6 mice.

In cats, *B. henselae* antibodies detected by IFA or enzyme-linked immunosorbent assay (ELISA) appear 2 to 3 weeks after experimental inoculation and usually persist for several months. Most infected cats are bacteremic for several weeks despite high antibody titers. Chronic bacteremia, despite a humoral immune response, is commonly observed among cats. There is no direct correlation between antibody titer and the magnitude of bacteremia; however, cats with IFA serologic titers of 512 or more are more likely to be bacteremic than cats with lower titers.

Dogs with endocarditis often show high antibody titers. In experimentally infected dogs, *B. vinsonii* subsp. *berkhoffii* establishes chronic infection, which may result in immune suppression, characterized by defects in monocytic phagocytosis, an impaired subset of CD8 T lymphocytes, and impaired antigen presentation within the lymph node.

Laboratory Diagnosis

For years, the diagnosis of CSD was based on clinical criteria, history of exposure to a cat, failure to isolate other bacteria, and/or histologic examination of biopsies of lymph nodes. A skin test using antigen prepared from pasteurized exudate from lymph nodes of patients with CSD was also used in diagnosing CSD, but this test was not standardized and elicited concerns about the safety of such a product.

Serologic tests, such as IFA or ELISA, and techniques to isolate the organism from human, dog, and cat specimens have been developed since the mid 1990s. Because *Bartonella* are intraerythrocytic bacteria, cell lysis using a lysis-centrifugation technique greatly facilitates bacterial isolation from the blood. However, blood isolation is seldom obtained from human cases of CSD and from domestic dogs. On the contrary, isolation is more commonly successful from human BA cases, for which serology is often negative. Isolation from the blood of natural reservoirs is also quite common with bacteremia prevalence ranging from 10 to 20 percent (such as for wild felids or coyotes) to up to 95% (beef cattle, deer).

For blood culture from cats, 1.5 ml of blood is drawn into lysis-centrifugation tubes (Isostat Microbial System, Wampole Laboratories). More recently, cat blood collection in EDTA tubes kept frozen at -70°C for a few days or weeks has been a preferred alternative because of easier handling and lower cost. For dogs or cattle a larger volume of blood can be collected (3–5 ml). The tubes are centrifuged and the pellet spread onto infusion agar plates containing 5% fresh rabbit blood, which are maintained at 35°C in a high humidity chamber with 5% CO_2 for 3 or 4 weeks. Colonies usually will develop in a few days from cat blood, although some strains may require a few weeks.

Other means of isolation of *Bartonella* have been by using Bactec blood-culture system or BacT/Alert blood-culture system. Identification of isolates as *Bartonella* can be performed by using enzyme-based identification systems, but is usually confirmed by DNA amplification using PCR-RFLP analysis. Several restriction endonucleases, such as *Taq*I and *Hha*I for citrate synthase gene, are used to digest the single product amplified by specific primers. PCR has also been used to identify *Bartonella* spp. in tissues, in absence of culture. Diagnosis of *Bartonella* endocarditis relies heavily on this method in humans and dogs in conjunction with high antibody titers.

Evidence of infection can be detected in humans or animals by detection of antibodies by IFA or ELISA. An IFA titer of at least 1:64 is considered positive. *Bartonella henselae* antibodies can be detected despite concurrent bacteremia in cats and sometimes in humans.

Treatment

In humans, antimicrobial treatment is generally indicated for patients with bacillary angiomatosis, bacillary peliosis, or relapsing bacteremia. Bacillary angiomatosis patients respond dramatically to macrolide antibiotics. Treatment with erythromycin, rifampicin, or doxycycline for at least 2 to 3 months in immunocompromised people is recommended, but relapses can occur. In such cases, patients should receive lifelong treatment with one of these antibiotics. For CSD, antimicrobial treatment is not generally indicated, because most typical cases do not respond to an-

timicrobial administration. Intravenous administration of gentamicin and doxycycline and oral administration of erythromycin have been used successfully in the treatment of disseminated CSD and therapy of patients with neuroretinitis. In cases of *Bartonella* endocarditis, patients receiving an aminoglycoside were more likely to fully recover, and those treated with aminoglycosides for at least 14 days were more likely to survive than those with shorter therapy duration.

In cats, antibiotic treatment (doxycycline, 25 mg to 50 mg twice daily; lincomycin, 100 mg twice a day for 3 weeks) may suppress bacteremia. Various antibiotics (doxycycline, erythromycin, enrofloxacin) have been shown to reduce the level of bacteremia in experimentally infected cats but do not eliminate infection, and the level of bacteremia may surpass the initial level a few weeks after the cessation of treatment. In dogs, macrolides (erythromycin, azithromycin) most probably represent the oral antibiotic class of choice for treating *Bartonella* infections, but to date no optimal protocol has been established.

Prevention

A large reservoir for *B. henselae* and possibly for *B. clarridgeiae* exists among the 68.9 million pet cats residing in one-third of homes in North America. Consequently, negative publicity about the perceived hazards of cat ownership is likely, especially for immunocompromised people. Seronegative cats are likely not to be bacteremic, but young kittens, especially impounded kittens and flea-infested kittens, are more likely to be bacteremic. Therefore, people who want to acquire a pet cat, especially if they are immunocompromised, should seek a cat raised in a cattery—if possible, an adult cat coming from a flea-controlled environment. Unfortunately, there is no correlation between seropositivity and bacteremia. Bacteremia can also be transient with relapses. Declawing cats has also been suggested but has a limited value, because fleas can transmit infection from cat to cat. Flea control, therefore, appears to be one of the major control measures to prevent cat infection and its spread from cat to cat. The most effective means of preventing *B. henselae* infection are common sense, hygiene, flea control, and, possibly, modification of behavior of the cat owners themselves. Wash hands after handling pets and clean any cuts, bites, or scratches promptly with soap and water.

For dog bartonellosis, where tick infestation could be a major risk factor for acquiring infection, tick and flea control measures should be used during the tick and flea season. Systematic inspection of the dog for the presence of ticks after a walk in infested areas is highly recommend.

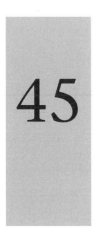

45

Yeasts—*Cryptococcus, Malassezia,* and *Candida*

Dwight C. Hirsh   Ernst L. Biberstein

Whether a fungus is categorized as mold or yeast is based upon the microscopic appearance in tissue or on routine culture media (the asexual stage). Microscopically, if hyphal structures are observed, the fungus is termed a *mold*; if single-celled, budding structures are observed, the fungus is termed a *yeast*. On routine culture media, molds will have a "fuzzy" or wooly appearance, and a yeast will be bacteria-like in its colonial morphology and consistency. Some pathogenic fungi will produce either hyphal-like structures or yeast-like structures, depending upon the conditions in which they are growing. Such fungi are called *dimorphic fungi* (Chapters 47, 48).

In this chapter, three yeast fungi will be discussed, *Cryptococcus, Malassezia,* and *Candida.*

CRYPTOCOCCUS NEOFORMANS

Cryptococcus neoformans is associated with ulcerative lesions affecting the mucous membranes of the upper respiratory tract (including nasal sinuses), the central nervous system (meninges), and eye (chorioretinitis) of cats (domestic animal most commonly affected) and dogs, and is an uncommon cause of mastitis in cattle. However, this yeast has the potential to affect all animals, including humans. In all species, there is the tendency for the central nervous system to become involved.

Descriptive Features

Morphology

Cryptococcus neoformans is a yeast. The spherical cells (3.5 μm to 7.0 μm diameter) produce single (usual) buds attached by slender stalks and surrounded by polysaccharide capsules (Fig 45.1).

Strains of *C. neoformans* have been experimentally converted to a mycelial, sexually reproducing phase, *Filobasidiella neoformans,* a basidiomycete.

Cellular Products of Medical Interest

Capsule. The polysaccharide capsule (composed primarily of a glucuronoxylomannan) prevents effective opsoniza-

tion, stimulates suppressor lymphocytes, is toxic to macrophages, and decreases inflammatory responses.

Melanin and Mannitol. Melanin and mannitol are free radical scavengers (reduce the toxicity of hydroxy radicals, superoxides, and singlet oxygen radicals found within the phagolysosome). Melanin is produced from phenols by phenoloxidase via the laccase pathway.

Phospholipase. Phospholipase is important for survival within macrophages, and is needed for the systemic spread of the yeast from the respiratory tract to the central nervous system. How this enzyme functions in this regard is not known.

Sialic Acids. Sialic acids found within the cell wall direct complement proteins toward the degradative pathway, rather than generating effective opsonizing fragments and anaphylotoxins.

Growth Characteristics

Cryptococcus neoformans grows on common laboratory media at ambient or body temperatures. Other members of this genus do not grow consistently at 37°C. Encapsulation is optimal on chocolate agar plates (see Chapter 14) incubated under 5% carbon dioxide at 37°C. Colonial growth may be apparent within 2 days or require several weeks. Colonies are grayish white to white and mucoid and can reach diameters of several centimeters.

Biochemical Reactions

Cryptococcus spp. hydrolyze urea. Their carbohydrate assimilation patterns are utilized in identification procedures. *Cryptococcus neoformans* (but few other *Cryptococcus* spp.) utilizes creatinine and produces melanin-pigmented colonies on media containing diphenolic and polyphenolic compounds. These substances are used in media for selective recovery of *C. neoformans.*

Resistance

Cycloheximide concentrations found in some fungal isolation media inhibit *C. neoformans.* Replication ceases above 40°C. Highly alkaline environments kill the agent.

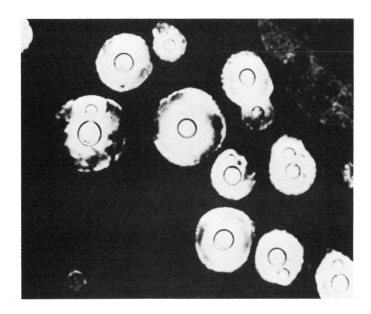

FIGURE 45.1.   Cryptococcus neoformans *in nasal granuloma of a mouflon. India ink wet mount showing encapsulated budding spherical yeast cells. 400X. (Photograph courtesy of Dr. Roy Henrickson.)*

Variability

Four antigenic types, A, B, C, and D based on the antigenic makeup of the capsular polysaccharides have been described. Phenotypic, genetic, and epidemiological differences between the antigenic types have resulted in the establishment of three varieties of *C. neoformans*: var. *grubii* (serotype A), var. *gattii* (serotypes B and C), and var. *neoformans* (serotype D). Varieties *grubii* and *neoformans* predominate in the temperate zone except for an area in Southern California, where variety *gattii* is prominent.

There are two mating types (sexual stages): MATa and MATα.

Ecology

Reservoir

Cryptococcus neoformans (var. *grubii* and *neoformans*) lives in surface dust and dirt. In soil it does not compete well with resident microbiota. *Acanthamoeba*, an amoeba, phagocytoses and destroys some strains of cryptococci. Interestingly, there are other strains that are capable of surviving within amoeba by using the same intracellular survival strategies that are used for their survival within macrophages. Thus, some strains are destroyed, while others are endosymbionts using amoebae as an environmental niche. In dried pigeon droppings (rich in creatinine, which inhibits other microorganisms), the fungus reaches high concentrations and survives for more than a year at much reduced capsular and cell size. *Cryptococcus neoformans* var. *gattii* lives mainly in association with decaying wood of the red river gum group of eucalyptus trees. Though eucalyptus trees are the main habitat for var. *gattii*, this variety has also been isolated from other tree types, bat guano, and a wasp nest. *Cryptococcus neoformans* var. *neoformans* and var. *grubii* are occasionally isolated from decaying wood in hollows of a variety of different species of trees.

Transmission

The route of infection is usually respiratory, rarely percutaneous. Cryptococcosis is noncontagious.

Pathogenesis

In an environment where moisture and nutrients are plentiful, *C. neoformans* makes little if any capsular material. In arid conditions, the capsule collapses and protects the yeast from dehydration. In either case, the size (approximately 3 μm) is small enough to make it to the lung alveoli. At physiologic concentrations of bicarbonate, CO_2, and free iron, a capsule is produced. The cryptococcal capsule is a very efficient activator of the alternate complement pathway resulting in the deposition of C3b on its surface. Thus opsonized, the yeast will adhere to the surface of phagocytic cells, but is poorly phagocytosed even in the presence of anticapsular antibody. Capsular polysaccharide increases participation of suppressor T lymphocytes and decreases antigen-processing, leading to a poor antibody response. Capsular polysaccharide also diminishes the chemoattractive effects of the anaphylotoxins C3a and C5a generated by activation of the alternate complement pathway. In the event phagocytosis occurs, the respiratory burst is diminished (capsule), and the production of melanin and mannitol by the yeast scavenge free radicals and reduce the hostile environment within the phagolysosome by inactivating superoxides, hydroxyl, and singlet oxygen radicals. In addition, phospholipase is produced, further diminishing the ability of phagocytic cells in eliminating the fungus. Thus, inflammatory responses are minimal and cryptococci grow into large space-occupying "myxomatous" masses, consisting of capsular slime, yeast cells, and few inflammatory cells. Eventually these masses acquire histiocytes, epithelioid cells, and some giant cells.

Development of pulmonary lesions is erratic. Infections often localize in the central nervous system (perhaps due to lower complement concentrations in the CNS and to high concentrations of catechols, a substrate for phenoloxidase, the enzyme the yeast uses to produce melanin) following dissemination from the lungs and are manifested by neurologic signs (see Fig 71.3). Eye involvement, leading to chorioretinitis and blindness, is relatively common.

Disease Patterns

Cats and Dogs. Cats and dogs are most often clinically affected. Signs include ulcerative lesions of the mucous membranes in nose, mouth, pharynx, and sinuses or myxomatous nasal masses. Central nervous system involvement is common. These lesions may arise from local infections. Most skin lesions are probably hematogenous.

Cattle. Cattle acquire cryptococcosis during administration of contaminated material of intramammary medication. There is gross swelling, hardening of the gland, and gradual changes in the secretions. Destruction of the lactiferous epithelium is extensive. Several glands may be irreversibly damaged. The disease rarely advances beyond regional lymph nodes.

Epidemiology

Cryptococcus can probably affect any mammal. Its occurrence is sporadic and worldwide. Birds, particularly pigeons, often carry the agent in their intestinal contents and contribute to its reservoir (see above). They are rarely affected clinically, and then mostly on mucosal surfaces.

Human cryptococcosis is often associated with immunosuppression (organ transplants, Hodgkin's disease, pregnancy, acquired immunodeficiency syndrome) or intensive exposure. Attempts to relate animal infections to similar circumstances have been speculative.

Bovine cryptococcal mastitis usually starts as an iatrogenically induced inoculation infection.

Cryptococcosis in koala bears is associated with contact with eucalyptus leaves contaminated with var. *gattii*.

Immunologic Aspects

Immunosuppression is a predisposing factor. The capsular polysaccharides produce immune paralysis, complement depletion, and antibody masking.

Humoral and cell-mediated phenomena (T_{H1} subset resulting in macrophage activation) evidently contribute to defense against cryptococcal infection. Macrophages participate in disposal of the agent. There is some evidence that T lymphocytes (CD4 and CD8) as well as natural killer cells kill or inhibit *C. neoformans* directly.

Results of experimental immunization have been equivocal. No vaccines are available.

Cryptococcosis does not appear to be a disease in cats infected with feline immunodeficiency virus (FIV) as it is in human patients infected with human immunodeficiency virus (HIV). FIV-positive cats respond to appropriate antifungal therapy; human HIV-positive patients respond poorly if at all.

Laboratory Diagnosis

Direct Examination

A small amount of sediment from exudates, tracheobronchial washes, and cerebrospinal fluids is mixed with an equal amount of India ink on a slide and a cover slip is added. Microscopically, the encapsulated organisms appear as bright circular lacunae in a dark field, containing the yeast cells in their centers (see Fig 45.1). Preparations stained with Romanovsky-type stains (Wright's, Giemsa) are also used to demonstrate the capsule (the body of the yeast will stain darker blue than the capsule). Fungal stains—e.g., periodic acid Schiff (PAS) and Gomori methenamine silver (GMS)—delineate the cell wall but not the capsule, which is stainable by mucicarmine. With Gram stain, cryptococcal cells often appear gram-positive.

In sections processed by the usual histologic methods, the capsules are unstained halos separating the yeast cells from tissue constituents or from each other.

Culture

Blood agar and Sabouraud's agar cultures (without cycloheximide) are incubated, respectively, at 37°C and room temperature (see Chapter 46). Suggestive colonies are examined by India ink wet mount. If found to consist of encapsulated yeasts, *C. neoformans* is confirmed by demonstration of urease activity, absence of lactose, melibiose and nitrate assimilation, and lethality for mice upon intracerebral or intraperitoneal injection.

Selective media incorporating antibacterial and antifungal drugs, creatinine and diphenyl, are used for environmental sampling.

Some normal dogs and cats harbor small numbers of *C. neoformans* in their nasal cavities. Therefore, care should be taken when interpreting culture results from samples obtained from this site. Examination of direct smears (the numbers of yeast in smears from clinically normal animals are too low to see) and/or analysis of serum for capsular antigen are helpful adjuncts to culture. Capsular antigen is not detectable in serum of normal dogs, regardless of whether they harbor *C. neoformans* in their nasal passages.

Immunodiagnosis

Antigen demonstration in serum and cerebrospinal fluid is attempted in diagnosis and assessment of patient progress. Latex particle suspensions coated with anticapsular antibody are marketed as slide agglutination test kits.

Antibody is irregularly demonstrable because of the "sponging" action of circulating capsular antigens. Its presence (demonstrated by indirect fluorescent antibody tests or by latex particles coated with capsular polysaccharide) is a favorable sign of decreasing antigen levels.

Treatment and Control

The treatment of choice for dogs and cats is fluconazole. Alternative therapy is 5-fluorocytosine, but its efficacy should be tested periodically as strains may be resistant or become resistant.

Therapy should be continued until clinical signs are resolved and antigen disappears from serum and cerebrospinal fluid.

Contaminated surfaces (pigeon lofts, attics) can be disinfected with lime solution (1 lb hydrated lime/3 gal water) prior to physical cleanup. Dirt removed is placed in containers and covered with hydrated lime powder, which can also be used on exposed floors and beams. Masks are worn during the operation.

MALASSEZIA PACHYDERMATIS

Members of the genus *Malassezia* are parasitic yeasts. There are seven species: *M. pachydermatis, M. restricta, M. globosa, M. obtusa, M. furfur, M. sympodialis,* and *M. sloof-fiae.* All, except *M. pachydermatis,* require lipids for growth (though *M. pachydermatis* is lipophilic). Only *M. pachydermatis* is commonly associated with animal disease, most often otitis externa, and dermatitis in dogs. However, each of the lipid-dependent species has been isolated from skin and external ear canals of normal and clinically affected dogs, cats, ruminants, and horses. Thus, the reason why *M. pachydermatis* is more commonly found may be due to the relative ease in which this species is demonstrated.

Descriptive Features

Morphology and Composition

Malassezia pachydermatis is an oval budding yeast (2 μm by 5 μm). In direct smears (and from colonies obtained from culture), there will be a single bud attached by a broad base (0.9 μm–1.1 μm) (Fig 45.2). Filaments are not usually observed, regardless of culture conditions. The cell wall is composed of glycoproteins (75–80%), lipids (15–20%), and chitin (1–2%).

Growth Characteristics

Though not requiring lipids for growth, *M. pachydermatis* is lipophilic, and growth is improved when lipids are added to the medium. Most strains of *M. pachydermatis* grow on blood agar plates, though the colonies will be very small (<1 mm in diameter, and sometimes only a "greenish" tint will be seen on the surface of the plate) after several days of incubation (optimum temperature is 37°C, although it will grow at temperature ranging from 25°C to 41°C). The yeast will grow in either an aerobic, or microaerophilic atmosphere (it does not grow well anaerobically).

Biochemical Reactions

Malassezia pachydermatis assimilates the carbon of glucose and D-mannitol, but does not ferment carbohydrates. Urea hydrolysis is strain-dependent.

Resistance

Malassezia pachydermatis is resistant to cycloheximide. It is sensitive to cold.

Variability

There are a number of biotypes of *M. pachydermatis* as reflected in variability in D-mannitol and sorbitol assimilation, hydrolysis of urea, and cell wall fatty acid concentration.

Seven genetic types (a through g) have been described

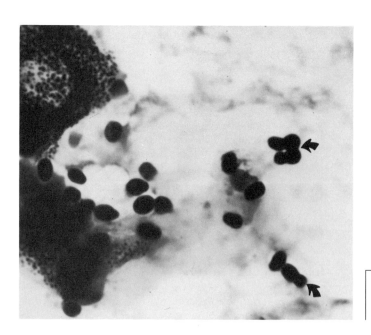

FIGURE 45.2.   *Exudate of canine otitis externa containing* Malassezia pachydermatis. *Note characteristic "shoe print" pattern of budding yeasts (arrows). Gram stain, 1000X.*

using the sequence of DNA encoding the large ribosomal subunit as the basis for comparison. Others have delineated four genetic types (A through D) after using the random amplification of polymorhic DNA method, together with sequence comparisons of the gene encoding chitin synthase.

Ecology

Reservoir

Malassezia pachydermatis lives on the skin and external ear canal of healthy animals, including dogs, cats, ferrets, pigs, and rhinoceros (from which it gets its name). The surface of *M. pachydermatis* has mannose-containing glycoproteins that are responsible for binding to mannose receptors on the surface of corneocytes, thus allowing adherence in this niche. It is rarely isolated from human skin, or the environment.

Transmission

Malassezia pachydermatis is an opportunistic fungus, contributing to disease processes already in progress (e.g., allergic dermatitis). The source of the yeast is endogenous (i.e., a member of the patient's normal flora). Iatrogenic disease has been reported for the transmission of the yeast from a dog with otitis externa to a human patient via the hands of a caregiver (the dog's owner) who handled a lipid-rich intravenous solution (for total parenteral nutrition) subsequently administered to the patient.

Pathogenesis

Malassezia pachydermatis plays a secondary, but significant role in otitis externa and dermatitis in a variety of animals, but most commonly in dogs, and to a lesser extent, cats (see Fig 69.4). The exact role played by *M. pachydermatis* remains unclear, and what causes the yeast to change from a harmless commensal to one that contributes to disease, is unknown. If its presence is ignored when formulating a treatment regimen, however, resolution of the disease process is problematic.

Epidemiology

Malassezia pachydermatis is a parasite of skin (including the external ear canal) of nonhuman animals. *Malassezia pachydermatis*–associated dermatitis is more commonly reported in Australian silky terriers, basset hounds, cocker spaniels, dachshunds, poodles, and West Highland white terriers. The yeast has worldwide distribution.

Immunologic Aspects

Malassezia pachydermatis is an opportunistic yeast, contributing to preexisting compromises of the skin and external ear. It is unknown how *M. pachydermatis* contributes to disease.

Laboratory Diagnosis

Direct Examination

The numbers of yeasts on normal skin or in the normal external ear canal are usually too low to visualize in samples taken from such sites. Thus, determining whether *M. pachydermatis* is a contributing factor to otitis externa or to a dermatological condition is relatively easy, because the numbers of yeasts will be high enough to be seen in samples taken from affected areas. However, some atopic dogs have been shown to have increased numbers of *M. pachydermatis* in normal as well as affected areas.

Samples taken with cotton-tipped swabs are the easiest to obtain from cases of otitis externa. Swabs are "rolled" over the surface of a microscope slide which are then stained with a Romanovsky-type stain (Wright's, Giemsa) or Gram's stain. Examination of smears will reveal yeasts with characteristic "bottle-shaped" or "shoe print" morphology (see Fig 45.2). If the swabs are also streaked onto the surface of a blood agar plate, small colonies (or a greenish coloration) will appear within 24–48 hours after incubation of the plate at 37°C in air.

Though *M. pachydermatis* can be demonstrated on affected areas of the skin, dermatologists recommend that some measure of numbers be made in order to gauge the success of treatment. Numbers are approximated by using adhesive tape to remove yeasts from the skin and then staining (Wright's, or Giemsa), followed by a microscopic examination of the tape. For example, the tape is placed "yeast-side" down on a microscope slide in a puddle of Wright's stain. The "preparation" is examined through a microscope with the tape acting as a coverslip. Less than two yeasts per 1000X field is about the maximum to expect from preparations made from the skin of a normal dog.

Molecular Techniques

Polymerase chain reaction amplification of DNA encoding either the large or the small ribosomal subunit together with the internal transcribed spacer region may be used to detect *Malassezia* spp. The same technology has been applied to speciation of the yeast.

Culture

As a means of determining whether *M. pachydermatis* is a contributor in otitis externa, culture is not worth the effort, because most samples taken from such conditions contain bacteria (e.g., *Pseudomonas*) that quickly overgrow the slower growing yeast. The determination that *M. pachydermatis* is involved can be made quicker by microscopic examination of samples.

Culture plays a role in assessing the microbiological makeup of dermatological conditions, as well as formulating a treatment regimen. Either tape preparations (press the tape on the surface of medium) or contact plates (petri plates with agar medium that "bulges" above the rim). Media that have proven useful include Dixon's (modified to contain lipid), Leeming Notman's, or Sabouraud's. Plates are incubated at 37°C in air or an atmosphere containing CO_2. Greater than two colonies per 0.5 square inch is considered abnormal.

Treatment and Control

Correction of the underlying condition is the most important aspect of treatment of *M. pachydermatis*–associated otitis externa or dermatitis. Almost all commercially available topical preparations that contain an antifungal agent (nystatin, clortrimazole, or miconazole) are effective in treating the fungal component of otitis externa. Medicated shampoos (e.g., miconazole + chlorhexidine), along with systemic antifungal administration (ketoconazole or itraconazole) are effective in reducing the influence of *M. pachydermatis* upon dermatological diseases. Griseofulvin is not effective.

CANDIDA

Candidiasis is usually due to the parasitic yeast *Candida albicans*, which inhabits mucous membranes of most mammals and birds. Of the more than 150 other species of *Candida* that are associated with many diverse habitats, few are associated with animal disease. Disease produced by members of the genus *Candida* usually occurs in an immunocompromised host.

The subsequent discussion deals with *C. albicans* unless otherwise indicated.

Descriptive Features

Cell Morphology, Anatomy, and Composition

On routine laboratory media and mucous membranes, *C. albicans* typically grows as oval budding yeast cells (blastoconidia), 3.5 μm to 6 μm by 6 μm to 10 μm in size. Under certain conditions of temperature, pH, nutrition, and atmosphere, yeast cells sprout germ tubes (Fig 45.3) that develop into septate-branching mycelium. "Pseudohyphae" is produced by elongation of the blastoconidia and their failure to

separate. In vivo, mycelial (a collection of hyphae) or pseudomycelial growth is associated with active proliferation and invasiveness.

The so-called chlamydospore (chlamydoconidium) is a thick-walled sphere of unknown function, attached by a suspensor cell to (pseudo)mycelium and essentially confined to in vitro growth (Fig 45.4) of *C. albicans* (rarely other *Candida* spp.).

The cell wall contains glycoproteins; the polysaccharide portions are glucans and especially mannans. Lipids and chitin are also present. Mannoproteins are found on the cell surface. Cellular products include peptidolytic enzymes, which may be virulence factors. Two major cross-reacting serogroups are recognized. These are termed *A* and *B*, and are identifiable with absorbed sera.

Candida can be stained with periodic acid Schiff (PAS), Gomori methenamine silver (GMS), and other fungal stains, but is usually studied in culture unstained. Polychrome stains (Wright's, Giemsa) are suitable for demonstrating it in tissue or exudate. With Gram stain, *Candida* cells often appear gram-positive.

Cellular Products of Medical Interest

Adhesins. Various cell wall components (chitin, mannoproteins, and lipids) have been associated with adherence to extracellular matrix proteins.

Miscellaneous Products. Proteases and neuraminidases have been proposed to play a role in pathogenesis. Cell wall glycoproteins have endotoxin-like activity (see Chapters 7 and 8).

Growth Characteristics

Candida albicans, an obligate aerobe, grows on ordinary media over a wide range of pH and temperature. At 25°C, creamy to pasty white colonies consisting predominantly of yeast cells appear in 24 to 48 hours. Production of (pseudo)mycelium is environmentally influenced, but the controlling factors are disputed. Incubation temperatures above 35°C, a slightly alkaline pH, and a rich, carbohydrate-free fluid medium are often recommended.

FIGURE 45.3.   *Germ tube production (arrows) by* Candida albicans *in serum. Unstained wet mount, 300X.*

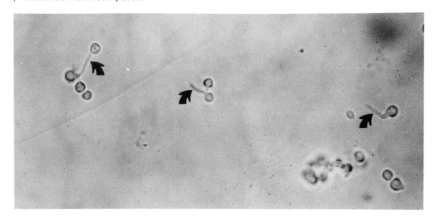

FIGURE 45.4. Candida albicans *culture on chlamydospore agar with trypan blue, showing pseudomycelium, yeast cells (blastoconidia) (right), and chlamydoconidia (left); 1200X.*

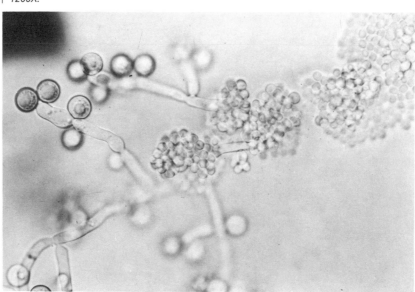

Differential ability to ferment or assimilate carbohydrates is the basis of species identification.

Candida species are killed by heat above 50°C, ultraviolet light, chlorine, and quaternary ammonium-type disinfectants. They withstand freezing and survive well in the inanimate environment. They are susceptible to polyene antimycotics, and usually to flucytosine and the azoles.

Reservoir

Candida albicans is associated with mucocutaneous areas, particularly of the alimentary and lower genital tract, of mammals and birds. Environmental sources are important especially for other *Candida* spp.

Transmission

Most *Candida* diseases arise from an endogenous source, that is, they are caused by a commensal strain. The bovine udder becomes infected via the teat canal by way of administered medication, during milking, by cow-to-cow spread, or from the environment.

Pathogenesis

Mechanisms. Chitin, mannoprotein, and lipids are possible adhesins, and in human candidiasis; several extracellular matrix proteins have been shown to be the receptor. Germ tube formation is correlated with experimental pathogenicity, but the role of mycelium formation in virulence is under dispute. Proteases and neuraminidase may be virulence factors. Cell wall glycoproteins have endotoxin-like activity.

Pathology. Candidiasis most frequently affects the mucous surfaces on which the agent is normally found, possibly the anterior digestive tract from mouth to stomach; it typically remains confined to areas of squamous epithelium. The genital tract, skin, and claws can be involved as well. Occasional respiratory, intestinal, and septicemic infections occur.

On epithelial surfaces, candidiasis forms whitish to yellow or gray plaques, marking areas of ulceration with varying degree of inflammation. Diphtheritic membranes may form in the gut or respiratory tract, and abscesses may form in the viscera. Granulomatous lesions are rare. Inflammatory responses are predominantly neutrophilic.

Disease Patterns

Birds. Avian candidiasis affects chickens, turkeys, pigeons, and other birds. It resembles thrush of humans involving the anterior digestive tract (see Fig 68.2). In the young, it can be a stunting disease and cause considerable mortality.

Swine. In the alimentary tract of pigs, candidiasis is seen as ulcerative lesions that may lead to rupture.

Equine. In the alimentary tract of foals, candidiasis is seen as ulcerative lesions that may lead to rupture. Equine genital infections cause infertility, metritis, and abortions.

Cattle. Pneumonic, enteric, and generalized candidiasis affects calves on intensive antibiotic regimens. *Candida* mastitis in dairy cows is typically mild and self-limiting, ending in spontaneous recovery within about a week. Bovine abortions have been reported.

Dogs and Cats. In dogs, candidiasis produces ulcerative lesions in the digestive and genital tract. Rarely, dogs develop septicemia with lesions in muscle, bones, skin, and

FIGURE 45.5.   Candida albicans *in nasal exudate from a dog. Note yeast cells (blastoconidia and pseudohypha. Gram stain, 1000X.*

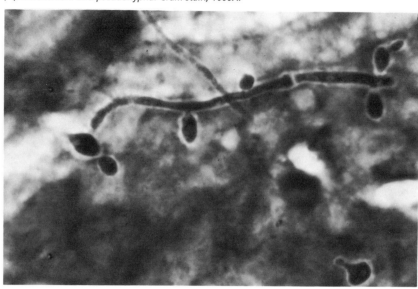

lower urinary tract (especially those with diabetes mellitus); feline pyothorax may rarely be due to *C. albicans*.

Other.   Lower primates and marine mammals may acquire mucocutaneous candidiasis.

Epidemiology

The common agents of candidiasis are commensal with most warm-blooded species. Disease is linked to immune and hormonal inadequacies, reduced colonization resistance (a measure of the "health" of the normal flora), or intensive exposure of weakened hosts or vulnerable tissues. These conditions account for susceptibility of infants, diabetics, subjects on antibiotic and steroid regimes, patients with indwelling catheters, and mammary glands of lactating cows.

Immunologic Aspects

Immunoincompetent individuals are preferred targets for infection.

Polymorphonuclear neutrophil leukocytes (PMNs) and activated macrophages form the chief defense against candidiases. The role played by opsonins (antibody; complement) is to facilitate phagocytosis. Macrophages are activated by gamma interferon secreted by T_{H1} cells stimulated by interleukin 12 from macrophages actively engaged in phagocytosis.

There is no artificial immunization.

Laboratory Diagnosis

In exudate, *Candida* appears as yeast cells (blastoconidia) or (pseudo)hyphae. All forms are demonstrable in un-

stained wet mounts, or in fixed smears stained with Gram's stain, Romanovsky-type stains (Wright's, Giemsa) or fungal stains—e.g., periodic acid Schiff (PAS) and Gomori methenamine silver (GMS) (Fig 45.5).

Candida albicans grows well on blood or Sabouraud's agar, with or without inhibitors (see Chapter 46). Other *Candida* spp. may be inhibited by cycloheximide. Yeast isolates producing (pseudo)mycelium can be considered *Candida* spp. Isolation of *Candida* spp. from mucous membranes (even in large numbers) suggests a diagnosis of candidiasis only in the presence of compatible lesions, and abundant (pseudo)hyphal forms in direct smears.

Incubation at 37°C for ≥2 hours of a lightly inoculated tube of serum will produce germ tubes if the isolate is *C. albicans* (see Fig 45.3), which also produced chlamydospores on cornmeal-tween 80 agar (see Fig 45.4). Yeast identification kits are commercially available.

DNA probes and tests for circulating antibody, antigen, and metabolites have had no adequate trial in veterinary medicine.

Treatment, Control, and Prevention

Correcting conditions underlying clinical candidiasis may in itself lead to recovery.

In poultry, copper sulfate in drinking water is a traditional treatment. Nystatin can be given in feed or water. It is also used topically in mucosal and cutaneous forms of candidiasis of mammals, as are amphotericin B and miconazole. Fluconazole (preferred) or flucytosine is useful for treating dogs or cats with lower urinary tract candidiasis.

In disseminated forms, oral fluconazole or flucytosine are drugs of choice. Susceptibility testing is advisable. Combined flucytosine-amphotericin B is sometimes used in humans and occasionally in animals.

46 Dermatophytes

ERNST L. BIBERSTEIN   DWIGHT C. HIRSH

Whether a fungus is categorized as mold or yeast is based upon the microscopic appearance in tissue or on routine culture media (the asexual stage). If hyphal structures are observed, the fungus is termed a *mold*; if a single-celled, budding structure is observed, the fungus is termed a *yeast*. On routine culture media, molds will have a "fuzzy" or wooly appearance, and a yeast will be bacteria-like in its colonial morphology and consistency. Some pathogenic fungi will produce either hyphal-like structures or yeast-like structures, depending upon the conditions in which they are growing. Such fungi are called *dimorphic fungi* (Chapters 47, 48).

Dermatophytes are molds capable of parasitizing only keratinized epidermal structures: superficial skin, hair, feathers, horn, hooves, claws, and nails. Those that have a sexual reproductive phase belong to the ascomycetes. Dermatophyte infections are called *ringworm (tinea)*.

Descriptive Features

Morphology

In their nonparasitic state, including culture, dermatophytes produce septate, branching hyphae collectively called *mycelium*. The asexual reproductive units (conidia) are found in the aerial mycelium. These units may be either *macroconidia:* pluricellular, podlike structures up to 100 μm long; or *microconidia:* unicellular spheres or rods less than 10 μm in any dimension. Shape, size, structure, arrangement, and abundance of conidia are diagnostic criteria. Hyphal peculiarities—spirals, nodules, "rackets," "chandeliers," and chlamydoconidia (chlamydospores)—are more common in some species than others, but they are rarely diagnostic. Pigmentation is useful in dermatophyte differentiation.

In the parasitic state, only hyphae and arthroconidia (arthrospores), another asexual reproductive unit, are seen. Except in size ranges, which overlap among dermatophyte species, arthroconidia are indistinguishable from species to species.

Sexual spores (ascospores) are absent in the parasitic phase.

The distinguishing features of the three genera of dermatophytes-*Microsporum, Trichophyton*, and *Epidermophyton*-are shown in Table 46.1. Only *Microsporum* and *Trichophyton* affect animals consistently.

Growth Characteristics

The traditional medium for propagating dermatophytes (and other pathogenic fungi) is Sabouraud's dextrose agar, a 2% agar containing 1% peptone and 4% glucose. Its acidity (pH 5.6) renders it mildly bacteriostatic and selective. The selectivity is enhanced by addition of cycloheximide (500 μg/ml), which inhibits other fungi, and gentamicin and tetracycline (100 μg/ml of each) or chloramphenicol (50 μg/ml), which inhibit bacteria. Dermatophytes are aerobes and nonfermenters. Some attack proteins and deaminate amino acids. They grow optimally at 25°C to 30°C and require several days to weeks of incubation.

Some dermatophytes in skin and hair (but not in culture) produce a green fluorescence due to a tryptophan metabolite that is visible under ultraviolet light (λ = 366 nm), sometimes referred to as a Wood's light. Of animal dermatophytes, only *Microsporum canis* produces this reaction.

Resistance

Dermatophytes are susceptible to common disinfectants, particularly those containing cresol, iodine, or chlorine. They survive for years in the inanimate environment.

Variability

There are a number of strains of each species of *Microsporum* and *Trichophyton*, making construction of effective immunizing products difficult.

Ecology

Reservoir

One speaks of geophilic, zoophilic, and anthropophilic dermatophytes when discussing dermatophytes having a soil, animal, or human reservoir, respectively. Table 46.2 shows the important dermatophytes affecting animals, with reservoirs and clinical hosts.

Rare causes of animal dermatophytosis are the anthropophilic, globally prevalent *M. audouinii, T. rubrum, T. tonsurans*, and *E. floccosum*, and the zoophilic *M. distortum*, which has been recovered from lesions of dogs, cats, horses, monkeys, and humans and appears to be restricted to Australia, New Zealand, and the Americas.

Transmission

Dermatophytes are disseminated by direct and, owing to their persistence on fomites and premises, indirect contact.

Pathogenesis

Mechanisms. Proteolytic enzymes (elastase, collagenase, keratinase) may determine virulence, particularly in severe inflammatory disease. Localization in the keratinized epidermis has been attributed to the lack of sufficient available iron elsewhere. This may account for the frequent arrest of dermatophytoses by inflammatory responses (through the influx of iron-binding proteins) and by enzyme inhibitors.

The infectious unit, a conidium, enters via a defect in the stratum corneum. Germination is triggered by unknown cues. The germ tube develops into hyphae branching among cornified epithelium. Portions of hyphae differentiate into arthroconidia. This growth pattern in the hairless skin predominates with some dermatophytes (*M. nanum, T. rubrum*). Hair invasion, which is prominent in most animal ringworm, begins with germination of a spore near a follicular orifice. Hyphal strands grow into hair follicles along outer root sheaths and invade growing hairs near the living root cells. Hyphae grow within the hair cortex, in the outer parts of which arthroconidia form and accumulate on the surface of the hair. This pattern (arthrospores on the outside of the hair shaft), called *ectothrix*, is characteristic of all significant animal dermatophytes. (*Endothrix* describes arthroconidial accumulation within the hair shaft.)

Pathology. The pathogenic process begins with colonization, during which the events just described occur but evoke little host response. There may be hypertrophy of the stratum corneum with accelerated keratinization and exfoliation, producing a scurfy appearance and hair loss. In dogs with *M. canis* infections, this is often the main effect. In adult cats there may be no signs.

The second phase begins at about the second week with inflammation at the margin of the parasitized area. Manifestations range from erythema to vesiculopustular reactions and suppuration. Mild forms are seen in *T. verrucosum* infection of calves. Severe reactions are typical in *T. mentagrophytes* infection of dogs and *M. gypseum* infection of horses. Local plaques ("kerion") may resemble certain skin tumors, especially in dogs. The inflammatory reaction may arrest the mycotic infection but become the primary problem through secondary suppurative bacterial infection.

The roughly circular pattern of the lesions and their inflamed margins suggested the terms *ringworm* and *tinea* (Latin for worm). Occasional cases of mycetoma are linked to dermatophyte infection, especially in Persian cats (see Chapter 47).

Disease Patterns. The patterns of dermatophytosis in domestic animals are summarized in Table 46.3.

Ringworm generally regresses spontaneously within a few weeks or months, unless complicated by secondary infections or constitutional factors. The agents may persist after clinical cure.

Epidemiology

Dermatophytoses often affect the young. Extent and severity are influenced by environmental factors. Crowding of animals or assembling of large numbers is often associated

Table 46.1.   Features of Dermatophyte Genera

	Microsporum	*Trichophyton*	*Epidermophyton*
Macroconidia	Usually present	Variable; often absent	Present
Walls	Thick	Thin	Thick
Surface	Rough	Smooth	Smooth
Shape	Spindle, cigar	Club (slender)	Club (broad)
Microconidia	Variable, often absent	Usual	Absent
Sexual form	Nannizzia	Arthroderma	None known

Table 46.2.   Important Dermatophytes of Animals and Their Reservoirs

Dermatophyte Species	Reservoir	Affected Animal Hosts	Humans Affected	Geographic Distribution
Microsporum canis	Cat	Cat, dog, horse[a] (goat, cattle, swine, others)[b]	++[c]	Worldwide
M. gallinae	Chicken, turkey	Poultry (cat, dog)	+[d]	Worldwide
M. gypseum	Soil	Dog, horse (cattle, cat, swine, others)	+	Worldwide
M. nanum	Soil	Swine	+	Africa, Australia, N. America
Trichophyton equinum	Horse	Horse	+	Worldwide
T. mentagrophytes	Rodent	Dog, horse, cattle, cat, swine, others	++	Worldwide
T. verrucosum	Cattle	Cattle	++	Worldwide
T. simii	Monkey	Monkey, poultry	+	India

[a] Equine isolates are usually sufficiently distinct to qualify for the recently validated species of M. equinum.
[b] ( ) = uncommon host.
[c] Important pathogen.
[d] Occurrence noted.

Table 46.3. Important Dermatophyte Infections in Domestic Animals

Host	Agent	Nature of Lesions
Horse	T. equinum	Dry, scaly usually noninflammatory (unless secondarily infected)
	M. gypseum	Often suppurative under alopecic thickened areas
	M. equinum	Not more than mildly inflammatory, resembling T. equinum lesions
Cattle	T. verrucosum	Painless, thick, white, "asbestos" plaques, local alopecia
Swine	M. nanum	Tannish, crusty, spreading centrifugally on trunk; painless, margins slightly inflamed. No hair loss.
Dog	M. canis	Typically noninflammatory, scaly, alopecic patches, occasional kerion
	T. mentagrophytes	Often spreading, extensively scaling to inflammatory lesions, secondary suppuration
	M. gypseum	As T. mentagrophytes
Cat	M. canis	Often subclinical in adults. Generally noninflammatory except in young kittens; may become generalized in debilitated kittens. Occasional mycetoma (Persian cats).
	T. mentagrophytes	As in dogs
Chicken	M. gallinae	Generally affects unfeathered portions. Whitish chalky scaling on comb and wattles, noninflammatory
	T. simii	Superficially similar to M. gallinae but often inflammatory and even necrotizing. A poultry problem only in India.

Ringworm is rare in sheep. Agents are *T. verrucosum, T. mentagrophytes,* and *M. canis.* The same species affect goats.

with increased prevalence. Improvement in calves often follows their release from damp, dark, crowded winter quarters to the outdoors.

Infected individuals of the same species perpetuate the important dermatophytoses of animals. Rodent sources of sporadic *T. mentagrophytes* infections in dogs and cats seem likely. Sporadic occurrence of the soil-derived *M. gypseum* infections contrasts with endemic to epidemic but bland infections of swine with geophilic *M. nanum.*

The major agents of animal ringworm are globally distributed.

Immunologic Aspects

Immune Mechanisms of Disease

The major antigens associated with dermatophyte infections are the keratinases (elicit cell-mediated responses) and glycoproteins (carbohydrate moieties stimulate anti-

body; protein moieties stimulate cell-mediated responses).

Antibody-mediated and cell-mediated hypersensitivities occur in the course of dermatophytoses. Their onset generally coincides with that of the inflammatory phase of infection and may contribute to its manifestations.

Sterile inflammatory skin lesions (phytids) occur in human ringworm infections. They are allergic reactions to circulating fungal antigens.

Recovery and Resistance

Antibodies play at best a limited role in resistance. Evidence favors cell-mediated mechanisms as decisive in protection and recovery.

Recovered individuals resist reinfection, although local reactions may be more acute and intense than on primary exposure. Acquired resistance varies in degree and duration with host, dermatophyte species, and possibly anatomical area.

Artificial Immunization

Mycelial *T. verrucosum* vaccines, inactivated and live avirulent, are used in Europe. They are credited with reducing the number of infected herds and new infections. Mixtures of *Microsporum* and *Trichophyton*—either as a live, attenuated vaccine or a killed product—have been disappointing in protecting cats from developing dermatophytosis, though they do appear to restrict spread upon individual cats. Although live vaccines appear to elicit a better immune (protective) response, the presence of numerous strains of *Microsporum* and *Trichophyton* make concocting such products difficult.

Laboratory Diagnosis

Direct Examination

In 50% to 70% of cases, hairs and skin scales infected with *M. canis* or *M. audouinii* may emit a bright greenish-yellow fluorescence under ultraviolet light, e.g., a Wood's light ($\lambda = 366$ nm).

Microscopic Examination

Skin scrapings and hair are examined microscopically for the presence of hyphae and arthroconidia. The scraping should include material from the margins of any lesion and the full thickness of the keratinized epidermis. The hair is plucked, so as to include the intrafollicular portion. The sample is placed on a slide, flooded with 10% to 20% potassium hydroxide, covered with a cover slip, and heated *gently*. The treatment clears the sample (makes it "transparent") while leaving fungal structures and enough of the hair and epidermis intact to reveal the agent in its relation to the parasitized structures.

Microscopic examination should begin under low power (100X) and subdued light. Infected hairs are encased in an irregular sheath of arthrospores that may double their normal thickness (Fig 46.1). At higher magnification

FIGURE 46.1.   *Cat hairs infected (center) and uninfected (right) with* Microsporum canis. *15% KOH mount. 100X.*

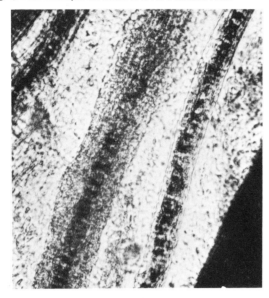

FIGURE 46.2.   *Cat hair infected with* Microsporum canis. *Focus is on arthroconidia surrounding the hair (ectothrix). 15% KOH mount. 400X.*

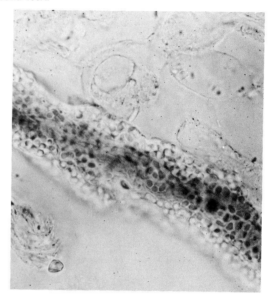

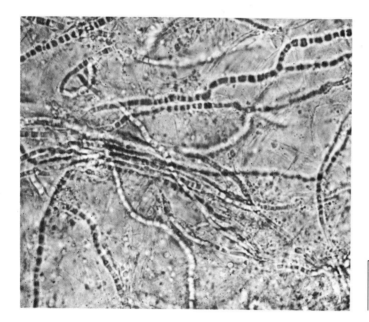

FIGURE 46.3.   *Dog skin scraping infected with* Tricophyton mentagrophytes *showing septate hyphae and chains of arthroconidia. 15% KOH mount. 400X.*

(400X) of such hairs, individual, spherical arthroconidia are recognizable (Fig 46.2). In hairless skin, branching hyphae and chains of arthroconidia occur (Fig 46.3).

Stains and penetrating and wetting agents (permanent ink, lactophenol cotton blue, dimethylsulfoxide) improve visualization. Calcofluor white reagent imparts fluorescence to fungal structures and facilitates diagnosis where a fluorescent microscope is available.

Culture

Scrapings are planted onto and into the surface of selective media (Sabouraud's agar with chloramphenicol and cycloheximide, Dermatophyte Test Medium [DTM], Rapid Sporulation Medium [RSM]), which are incubated at 25°C (room temperature) for up to 3 weeks. Samples suspected of containing *T. verrucosum* are incubated at 37°C. On DTM and RSM, an alkaline reaction suggests presence of a dermatophyte. (Dermatophytes, if given a choice of glucose and protein, will usually digest the protein first, leading to alkaline products; saprophytic fungi will most often utilize glucose, leading to acid byproducts. *Caution*: After the preferred substrate is utilized, the microorganism will make use of the other, shifting the pH in the other direction.)

Suspicious growth is examined microscopically. The ad-

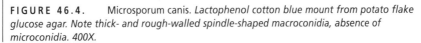

FIGURE 46.4. Microsporum canis. *Lactophenol cotton blue mount from potato flake glucose agar. Note thick- and rough-walled spindle-shaped macroconidia, absence of microconidia. 400X.*

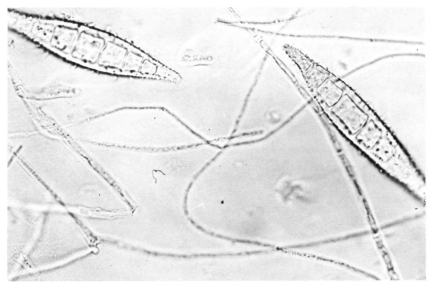

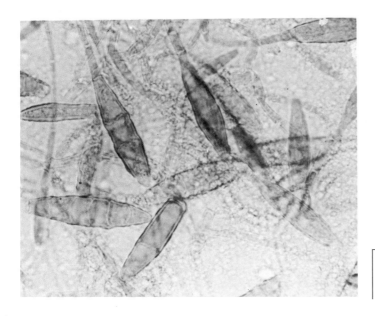

FIGURE 46.5. Microsporum gypseum. *Lactophenol cotton blue mount from Sabouraud's agar culture. Macroconidia are cigar-shaped and thin-walled; microconidia are absent. 400X.*

hesive side of a clear cellophane tape strip is pressed gently on the suspect colony (taken from RSM, or Sabouraud's agar with chloramphenicol and cycloheximide—dermatophytes do not sporulate well on DTM) and mounted in a drop of lactophenol cotton blue on a slide and examined microscopically (see Table 46.1, Figs 46.4–46.6). With *Trichophyton* spp., in the absence of diagnostic conidia, auxotrophic tests are used for speciation.

Knowledge of source (host species, type of lesion) aids significantly in provisional identification of animal dermatophytes.

Molecular Techniques

There are a number of DNA-based techniques that are available for direct examination of clinical samples, or for use in identification of an isolated dermatophyte. These techniques include determination of the sequence of DNA encoding specific products (e.g., chitin synthase 1 gene), determination of the sequence of the internal transcribed spacer region, determination of the sequence of the DNA encoding large ribosomal subunit (28S), and generation of unique DNA fragments following arbitrary or randomly primed polymerase chain reactions.

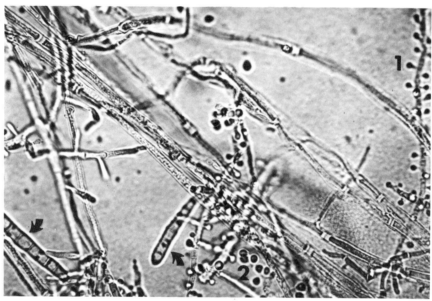

FIGURE 46.6. Trichophyton mentagrophytes. *Lactophenol cotton blue mount from potato flake glucose agar culture. Microconidia in single rows ("en thyrse," 1) and clusters ("en grappe," 2); thin-walled, long macroconidia (arrows). 400X.*

Treatment and Control

Combined topical and systemic treatment is often preferable. Of two systemic agents available, griseofulvin and ketoconazole, the latter is more costly and less proven. Both drugs are given orally and are relatively well tolerated. Griseofulvin in small carnivores is given for at least a month, or 2 weeks beyond clinical recovery. Use in large animals is inadequately documented. It is not approved for use in food animals. It is teratogenic in pregnant cats. Terbinafine (an allylamine antifungal that inhibits ergosterol biosynthesis, and concentrates in skin and nails) may be a useful alternative.

Antifungal orchard spray is effective on ringworm of large and small animals (Captan 45% powder, 2 tablespoons/gal). Affected areas are first clipped. In large animals, two applications at biweekly intervals are recommended. With dogs, weekly dips can be repeated to effect. Contact with human skin should be avoided. Thiabendazole (Tresaderm, Merck) is used on small and large animals.

Povidone-iodine (Betadine, Purdue Frederick) and chlorhexidine (Nolvasan, Fort Dodge), available as lotions and ointments, are general antiseptics with antifungal action.

A thorough cleanup of premises involving use of an iodine, chlorine, or phenol-containing disinfectant is essential. Utensils and equipment are disinfected with Captan or Bordeaux orchard spray.

Identification of carriers in kennels and catteries can be attempted by culture of brushings. The Wood's light (ultraviolet light) is useful in population screening of cat colonies where *M. canis* is the only concern. Infected individuals should be isolated and treated. Exposed animals are treated prophylactically.

Successful vaccination is widely practiced on European cattle. A live attenuated strain (*T. verrucosum*) appears to be most immunogenic. Neither live attenuated vaccines nor killed products have been effective in preventing dermatophytosis in cats.

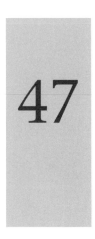

47

Agents of Subcutaneous Mycoses

Dwight C. Hirsh   Ernst L. Biberstein

Whether a fungus is categorized as mold or yeast is based upon the microscopic appearance in tissue or on routine culture media (the asexual stage). If hyphal structures are observed, the fungus is termed a *mold*; if a single-celled, budding structure is observed, the fungus is termed a *yeast*. On routine culture media, molds will have a "fuzzy" or wooly appearance, and a yeast will be bacteria-like in its colonial morphology and consistency. Some pathogenic fungi will produce either hyphal-like structures or yeast-like structures, depending upon the conditions in which they are growing. Such fungi are called *dimorphic fungi*, which are discussed below and in Chapter 48.

This chapter deals with dimorphic fungi and fungus-like microorganisms affecting skin and subcutis. To be discussed are *Sporothrix schenckii,* which is the cause of sporotrichosis in a variety of animal species, but more frequently in humans, horses, dogs, and cats; *Histoplasma capsulatum* var. *farciminosum,* the cause of epizootic lymphangitis in equids (horses, donkeys, mules); the agents of oomycosis (*Aphanomyces, Lagenidium, Pythium* and *Saprolegnia*), which cause a variety of diseases in fish and mammals; and miscellaneous conditions involving the skin and subcutis, including chromoblastomycosis, phaeohyphomycosis, and mycetoma. Systemic mycoses, of which skin lesions may be one manifestation, are described in Chapter 48.

SPOROTHRIX SCHENCKII

Sporotrichosis is a relatively rare disease caused by the saprophytic, dimorphic fungus, *Sporothrix schenckii*. This disease usually manifests as a chronic, ulcerative lymphangitis of skin and subcutis. Systemic (disseminated) disease occurs occasionally in immunocompromised human patients (e.g., alcoholics; individuals affected with the human immunodeficiency virus). Even though dissemination commonly occurs in cats, no association between underlying compromise and disseminated disease in veterinary species has been demonstrated.

Descriptive Features

Morphology and Staining

Sporothrix schenckii is a dimorphic fungus, i.e., it exhibits a different morphology depending upon the conditions of growth. At room temperature (25°C, on Sabouraud's agar), *S. schenckii* grows as a mold. This so-called saprophytic phase consists of septate hyphae, with oval or tear-shaped conidia (2 to 3 μm by 3 to 6 μm) in clusters on conidiophores and along hyphae (Fig 47.1). At 35–37°C (in tissue or on rich media, e.g., blood agar, incubated at that temperature), it exists as budding pleomorphic ("cigar-shaped") yeasts measuring up to 10 μm in the longest dimension (Fig 47.2). The yeast phase stains with the Gram's stain, and either phase accepts Giemsa or fungal stains (periodic acid-Schiff, Grocott methenamine silver, Gridley).

Cellular Constituents and Products

Sporothrix schenckii possesses a typical fungal cell wall containing chitin, and ergosterol. Various glycoconjugates found upon the wall have adhesive properties (see next section, "Cellular Products of Medical Interest").

Cellular Products of Medical Interest

Adhesins. The cell wall of *S. schenckii* contains glycoconjugates with affinity for extracellular matrix proteins (fibronectin, laminin, and Type II collagen). This interaction does not involve an "Arg-Gly-Asp" (RGD) sequence.

Cell Wall. The cell wall of *S. schenckii* contains several substances that may play a role in the virulence of this microorganism. These include lipid, melanin, peptide-rhamnomannan, and sialic acid:

1. Lipid. The lipid portion of the cell wall of *S. schenckii* inhibits phagocytosis by monocytes and macrophages.
2. Melanin. Melanin found in the cell wall protects *S. schenckii* from the effects of reactive oxygen intermediates within phagolysosomes of phagocytic cells. Melanin is a free radical scavenger (reduces the toxicity of hydroxy radicals, superoxides, and singlet oxygen radicals found within the phagolysosome).

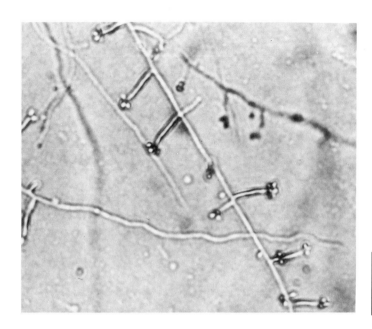

FIGURE 47.1. Sporothrix schenckii. *Hyphal strands on a plate of Sabouraud's agar incubated at 25°C. Hyphae bear conidiophores with daisy-like clusters of ovate conidia. Wet mount, about 400X.*

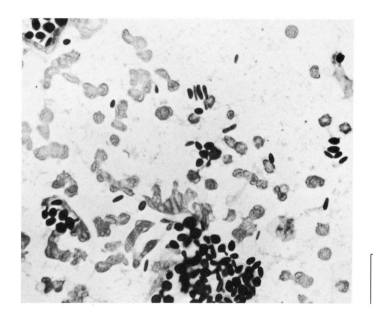

FIGURE 47.2. *Exudate from sporotrichosis lesion in a cat. Wright-Giemsa stain. Note pleomorphism of dark-staining yeast cells, some of which are budding. 1000X.*

3. Peptide-rhamnomannan. The peptide-rhamno-mannan fraction of the cell wall acts as an immuno-suppressive substance by suppressing the liberation of proinflammatory cytokines by phagocytic cells.
4. Sialic acids. Sialic acids found in the cell wall inhibit uptake of *S. schenckii* by phagocytic cells. Sialic acid directs complement proteins towards the degradative pathway, rather than generating effective opsonizing fragments and anaphylotoxins needed to generate an effective inflammatory response.

Proteases. Sporothrix schenckii produces two proteases, I and II. The significance of these enzymes in the pathogenesis of sporotrichosis is unclear.

Growth Characteristics

After several days on Sabouraud's agar at room temperature, initially moist, off-white to black colonies develop that become wrinkled and fuzzy. On blood agar at 35–37°C, whitish, smooth yeast colonies appear within a few days.

Variability

Examination of mitochondrial DNA (by restriction length polymorphism analysis) shows that there are at least 20 different types or strains of *S. schenckii* (1–20).

Ecology

Reservoir

Sporothrix schenckii is associated with plant material and soil worldwide. Occasionally it is isolated from mucous membranes of normal animals and animal products.

The disease occurs—rarely—in humans, horses, dogs, and cats, and has been reported in mice, pigs, rats, camels, dolphins, foxes, mules, goats, and chickens.

Transmission

The agent enters through skin contact, usually trauma. Rare cases of internal infection are due to inhalation or ingestion. Discharging lesions may be contagious, especially in cats where the numbers of microorganisms in exudates from this species are quite large. It has been isolated from nails of affected cats, and from clinically normal cats in contact with infected individuals.

Pathogenesis

Proteases are possible virulence factors and protease inhibitors have been shown to suppress nodule formation. Cell wall constituents and adhesins delay elimination of the microorganism. Typically the first lesion is an ulcerating cutaneous nodule. The infectious process follows subcutaneous lymph channels, producing suppurating ulcers at intervals. These heal slowly but often re-erupt. Lymphatics become thickened. Dissemination to viscera, joints, bones, and the central nervous system is common in cats.

Lesions are pyogranulomatous, having a purulent center surrounded by epithelioid cells, giant cells, and, peripherally, lymphocytes and plasma cells.

The course is protracted. Observations on humans suggest possible spontaneous recoveries.

Epidemiology

Sporotrichosis is acquired from the nonliving environment, but transmission from suppurating lesions is possible, particularly from cats. In humans, disseminated disease is seen in the immunosuppressed (e.g., alcoholics; individuals affected with the human immunodeficiency virus). Such an association has not been demonstrated in other animals.

Immunologic Aspects

Cell-mediated reactivity is significantly related to resistance. No artificial immunization procedures exist.

Laboratory Diagnosis

Direct examination of exudates is often unrewarding except with feline specimens, which generally contain abundant yeast cells (see Fig 47.2). With other hosts, fungal stains (see above) and immunofluorescence may help detect yeast cells.

The agent grows readily in culture. Identification requires demonstration of both phases.

Serologic tests (yeast cell and latex agglutination, agar gel diffusion) have had limited use in animals.

Molecular techniques utilizing the polymerase chain reaction with primers designed to amplify segments of the gene encoding the chitin synthase 1 have been used to demonstrate the fungus in clinical samples, as well as identification of isolates (useful when an isolate resists the mold-yeast conversion).

Treatment and Control

The cutaneous form responds generally to the oral administration of inorganic iodides. The azole drugs, especially itraconazole, are effective. Terbinafine (an allylamine antifungal agent which inhibits ergosterol biosynthesis) has shown some success in treating human patients with the cutaneous form of sporotrichosis. Amphotericin B and flucytosine are used on deep and disseminated forms.

HISTOPLASMA CAPSULATUM VAR. FARCIMINOSUM

Histoplasma capsulatum is a dimorphic fungus existing as a mold at 25–30°C (saprophytic phase) and as a yeast at 37°C (parasitic phase). This fungus has three varieties: *H. capsulatum* var. *capsulatum*, *H. capsulatum* var. *duboisii*, and *H. capsulatum* var. *farciminosum*. Varieties *capsulatum* and *duboisii* cause histoplasmosis, a systemic fungal disease that will be discussed in Chapter 48. Variety *farciminosum* causes epizootic lymphangitis (pseudoglanders), a chronic pyogranulomatous disease of equine (and rarely donkeys and mules) skin. Adjacent tissues, regional lymph nodes, and, rarely, internal organs may be involved. Epizootic lymphangitis is discussed below.

Descriptive Features

Morphology and Staining

Histoplasma capsulatum var. *farciminosum*, a dimorphic fungus, produces budding yeasts (2 to 3 μm by 3 to 4 μm) in tissue, and usually sterile hyphae in its mycelial form when grown at 25°C or room temperature. Exceptionally, arthroconidia, chlamydoconidia, and spherical, thick-walled macroconidia (spheroidal cells, 8 to 14 μm in diameter, studded with fingerlike projections, see Fig 48.4) are seen.

The yeast phase is best demonstrated with a Romanovsky-type stain (e.g., Wright's or Giemsa) or fungal stains (periodic acid-Schiff, Grocott methenamine silver, Gridley, see Fig 48.5).

Growth Characteristics

Histoplasma capsulatum var. *farciminosum* grows on common laboratory media (Sabouraud's glucose, infusion, and blood-supplemented media with or without cycloheximide and antibacterial agents) over a broad temperature range. The optimum for mycelial growth is 25° to 30°C, taking several weeks to form a cottony, white to brown colony. Pigmentation parallels abundance of macroconidia. The yeast phase requires rich media (e.g., glucose cysteine blood agar; brain heart infusion blood agar) and temperatures of 34° to 37°C, taking several days to form a cream to tan, yeast-like colony. Conversion of mold to yeast on blood-containing agar requires incubation at 37°C under 15% to 20% CO_2. Several passages may be needed to convert the mold to the yeast phase.

Resistance

Histoplasma capsulatum var. *farciminosum* is quite resistant to physical and chemical agents. It survives at ambient temperatures for months (several weeks in corrals and stables) and at refrigerator temperature or in a desiccated form for years.

Ecology

Reservoir

The reservoir is unknown; presumably infected equids (horses, donkeys, mules).

Transmission

Infection is thought to occur through skin wounds. Arthropods may play a part. Respiratory, conjunctival, and gastrointestinal infections are also reported.

Pathogenesis

A local skin nodule is found, which becomes abscessed and ulcerated. The ulcer may recur, enlarging each time, and ultimately heal by scarring. Typically, adjacent lymphatics develop nodules along their course, showing the same alternating activity. Adjacent lymph nodes develop abscesses draining by sinus tracts to the outside. Hematogenous spread and visceral involvement is possible. Histologically, the process evolves from suppurative to granulomatous (pyogranulomatous), marked by lymphocytes, macrophages, and giant cells, to eventual fibrosis. Yeast cells occur extracellularly and intracellularly, especially in macrophages.

Skin lesions, chiefly on head, neck, and limbs, are the predominant signs. The general condition is usually unaffected except in the primary respiratory tract or disseminated infections. Some mild cases do not progress beyond the local stage.

Epidemiology

Endemic areas include parts of Africa, much of Asia, and the Mediterranean littoral. The epidemiology of *H. capsulatum* var. *farciminosum* infection is unclear. Manifestations vary with geographic area. Seasonal peaks suggest arthropod transmission.

The disease mainly involves horses, but mules and donkeys may also be affected. Young horses (less than 6 years of age) are most susceptible.

Immunologic Factors

The role of immune mechanisms in pathogenesis or resistance is not known, but cell mediated immunity is probably the key host defense. Skin sensitivity develops following exposure, even in the absence of disease. Circulating antibodies, demonstrable by indirect fluorescent antibody, agar gel diffusion, or by the serum agglutination tests are indicative of infection.

Laboratory Diagnosis

Differential diagnosis includes sporotrichosis (see above, *Sporothrix schenckii*) and ulcerative lymphangitis produced by *Corynebacterium pseudotuberculosis* (see Chapter 31). The agent must be demonstrated. Direct examination of stained exudates (Wright's or Giemsa stained) or biopsy material (hematoxylin-eosin, periodic acid-Schiff, Grocott methenamine silver) may reveal intracellular (macrophages) or extracellular yeasts.

Histoplasma capsulatum var. *farciminosum* grows on Sabouraud's glucose agar with inhibitors (cycloheximide and chloramphenicol). Mycelial extracts contain genus-specific antigens demonstrable by agar gel diffusion or by the serum agglutination test. Growth patterns and microscopic morphology differentiate *H. capsulatum* var. *farciminosum* from *H. capsulatum* var. *capsulatum* (Chapter 48).

Treatment and Control

Intravenous iodides (with or without griseofulvin) have been relatively successful. Amphotericin B has been used with some success. In nonendemic areas, destruction of infected animals is advisable.

OOMYCOSIS

Oomycosis is caused by a member of a group of eukaryotic microorganisms belonging to the Kingdom Stramenopiles (which also contains the diatoms and brown algae). They are saprophytic microbes that usually live in water and moist soil. Though they are morphologically similar to fungi (they produce hyphae in tissue and grow as mold-like colonies on media in vitro), they are not members of the Kingdom Fungi. Members of this group are the agents of several plant and animal diseases. Historically, the most notorious is *Phytophthora,* the cause of the Irish potato famine, which at present is responsible for killing oak trees along the Pacific coast of North America. The following genera are associated with disease in animals: *Aphanomyces* (ulcerative disease of fish and crustaceans), *Lagenidium* (pyogranulomatous disease of dogs and cats identical clinically to pythiosis), *Pythium* (pyogranulomatous disease, called pythiosis, of a variety of animal species), and *Saprolegnia* (systemic disease of cultured salmonids). The discussion that follows is focused on *Pythium insidiosum*, the cause of pyogranulomatous conditions (pythiosis) of dogs ("swamp cancer"), horses ("Florida horse leeches"), cattle, cats, and humans.

Cutaneous Pythiosis ("Swamp Cancer"— "Florida Horse Leeches")

The genus *Pythium* contains about 85 species, and only *P. insidiosum* is associated with disease in animals. *Pythium insidiosum* causes ulcerative pyogranulomatous or fibrogranulomatous skin infections in horses, cattle, dogs, and cats, mainly in tropical or subtropical areas (in North America this disease is seen most frequently along the Gulf Coast). Dogs and horses are the species most commonly affected. The agent is an aquatic oomycete with wide (4 μm), sparsely septate hyphae. Lesions in horses are large (≤45 cm) discharging swellings, usually on extremities, ventral trunk, or head. The nasal mucosa may be involved. Hyphae are demonstrable within granulomatous coagula (termed "kunkers" or "leeches" in horses) consisting of necrotic macrophages, epithelioid cells, and giant cells, with eosinophilic admixtures.

Diagnostic methods include serology (an enzyme-linked immunosorbant assay), molecular techniques (utilizing primers designed to amplify *P. insidiosum*-specific DNA by means of the polymerase chain reaction [PCR]), immunohistochemical examination of exudates, and culture. Cultural techniques are tedious and time consuming and entail growth of a mold-like microorganism on Sabouraud dextrose agar or brain heart infusion agar after 24–48 hours at 30°C. Identification requires demonstration of motile zoospores and/or reaction of extracts of the isolate with reference antisera. The PCR-based assay mentioned is used to establish the presence of *P. insidiosum* in clinical samples as well as for identification of isolates. The PCR assay also successfully identifies members of the genus *Lagenidium* (another oomycete), which produces a similar clinical picture in dogs and cats.

Early diagnosis is the key to successful treatment. Treatments include surgery and antifungal therapy (amphotericin B). Immunotherapy utilizing killed whole organisms or extracts has shown promise.

CHROMOBLASTOMYCOSIS AND PHAEOHYPHOMYCOSIS

Chromoblastomycosis and phaeohyphomycosis are caused by dark-pigmented (dematiaceous) fungi. Most of the roughly 70 species implicated belong to the genera *Alternaria, Cladosporium, Cladophialophora, Curvularia, Exserohilum, Exophiala, Fonsecaea,* and *Phialophora.* In chromoblastomycosis, the fungal elements in tissue are large (<12 μm), pigmented, "sclerotic bodies" (Fig 47.3). Infections in which hyphae are present are called *phaeohyphomycosis.*

Chromoblastomycosis is rare in nonhuman mammals, but occurs in frogs and toads. Phaeohyphomycosis is seen sporadically in cats, dogs, horses, cattle, and goats and may be systemic. *Cladophialophora bantiana* is the fungus most commonly seen in dogs and cats, with central nervous system localization frequently observed.

The agents, soil- and plant-associated saprophytes, enter through skin and multiply subcutaneously, causing pyogranulomatous reactions. No tissue colonies or granules are seen. Nodular or larger swellings develop, which may ulcerate and discharge pus.

Diagnosis is by biopsy and culture. Sclerotic bodies (chromoblastomycosis) and hyphae (phaeohyphomycosis) are seen in stained (hematoxylin-eosin, periodic acid-Schiff, Grocott methenamine silver) biopsy sections. Culture, on Sabouraud's agar without inhibitors, often requires lengthy incubation. The resulting colonies range from olive to brown to black.

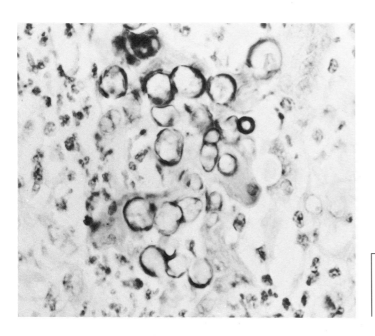

FIGURE 47.3.   *Chromoblastomycosis in the skin of a horse. Pigmented bodies suggestive of yeast cells (blastoconidia) are surrounded by inflammatory reaction. Hematoxylin-eosin stain, 400X.*

Lesions are excised, but may recur. Medical treatment (flucytosine, itraconazole, amphotericin B, ketoconazole) has given mixed results.

(EUMYCOTIC) MYCETOMAS

Swelling, granule formation, and discharging sinus tracts are characteristics of mycetoma. They may be associated with bacteria, most notably an actinomycete such as members of the genera *Nocardia* or *Actinomyces* (actinomycotic mycetoma, see Chapter 37) or a fungus (eumycotic mycetoma). Mycetomas are occasionally reported in cattle, horses, dogs, and cats. The cutaneous form is often nodular and is associated with similar nasal lesions.

Fungi associated with eumycotic mycetoma fungi include *Pseudallescheria boydii, Cochliobolus spiciferus* (the sexual forms of *Scedosporium apiospermum* and *Bipolaris spicifera*, respectively), and *Curvularia geniculata*. All are saprophytes that presumably enter via a wound. It is not clear what triggers this course of pathogenesis, because the same agents can cause other pathologic patterns.

Fungal colonies are surrounded by suppuration bordered by granulomatous reactions. Sinus tracts carry pus and granules, consisting of microorganisms and inflammatory components, to the surface. The processes are slowly progressive, involving adjacent tissues.

Treatment is excision if possible. Antifungal agents (azoles, amphotericin B) have been disappointing.

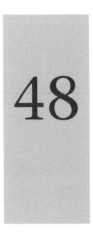

48

Agents of Systemic Mycoses

Dwight C. Hirsh   Ernst L. Biberstein

Whether a fungus is categorized as mold or yeast is based upon the microscopic appearance in tissue or on routine culture media (the asexual stage). Microscopically, if hyphal structures are observed, the fungus is termed a *mold*; if single-celled, budding structure is observed, the fungus is termed a *yeast*. On routine culture media, molds will have a "fuzzy" or wooly appearance, and a yeast will be bacteria-like in its colonial morphology and consistency. Some pathogenic fungi will produce either hyphal-like structures or yeast-like structures, depending upon the conditions in which they are growing. Such fungi are called *dimorphic fungi*. These fungi are discussed below and in Chapter 47.

The agents of most systemic (or "deep") mycoses are saprophytic fungi. Morphologically and ecologically diverse, they share disease-related features:

1. Many are dimorphic, that is, their saprophytic and parasitic phases differ morphologically. *Coccidioides, Histoplasma, Blastomyces,* and *Paracoccidioides* grow as molds in their inanimate habitat. In tissue, *Coccidioides* produces sporangia, whereas the others grow as budding yeasts.
2. Infection is usually by inhalation.
3. Host factors are often the decisive disease determinants. Some mycoses (aspergillosis, zygomycosis) are seen primarily in immunocompromised animals.
4. Lesions tend to be pyogranulomatous. After primary pulmonary infection, the course of disease is determined by the effectiveness of cell-mediated immune responses. If these are inadequate, dissemination may occur to bone, skin, central nervous system, or abdominal viscera.
5. Systemic mycoses are noncontagious. Although the agent is often demonstrably shed, it fails to infect individuals on contact.

This chapter discusses the dimorphic fungi *Coccidioides immitis, Histoplasma capsulatum,* and *Blastomyces dermatitidis,* together with the mold *Aspergillus*. The fungus *Pneumocystis* and the alga *Prototheca* are briefly mentioned.

COCCIDIOIDES

Members of the genus *Coccidioides* are dimorphic fungi, existing as a mold in soil (saprophytic phase) and as a spherical structure in tissue (parasitic phase). The genus *Coccidioides* contains two species, *immitis* and *posadasii*. The disease, coccidioidomycosis, is caused by both. *Coccidioides immitis* and *C. posadasii* differ in their preferred geographic habitats. Both species occur only in the western hemisphere in the Lower Sonoran Life Zone, apparently as a result of that area's peculiar soil properties and temperature and rainfall patterns. *Coccidioides immitis* is found in the Central Valley of California in the United States (mainly the San Joaquin Valley), whereas *C. posadasii* is found in non-California locations (Texas, New Mexico, Arizona in the United States, and in South America). Of domestic animals, dogs are most frequently affected, although horses are occasionally affected as well. Infections also occur in cats, swine, sheep, cattle, human and nonhuman primates, and some 30 species of nondomestic mammals.

Descriptive Features

Morphology, Structure, and Composition

In the soil, *Coccidioides* is a mold made up of slender septate hyphae that give rise, on thicker secondary branches, to chains of infectious arthroconidia (arthrospores, arthroaleuriospores, arthroaleurioconidia). These are bulging, thick-walled cells, 2.5 to 4.0 µm by 3.0 to 6.0 µm, separated by empty cells (disjunctors), through which breaks occur when arthroconidia are dispersed (Fig 48.1).

In tissue, arthroconidia grow into spherical sporangia with birefringent walls, "spherules" (10 µm to 80 µm diameter), which by internal cleavage produce several hundred "endospores" (2 µm to 5 µm diameter) (Fig 48.2). The walls disintegrate, allowing dissemination of endospores, each of which may repeat the cycle or, on a nonliving substrate, give rise to mycelial (a collection of hyphae) growth. Though only arthroconidia are naturally infectious, endospores can experimentally initiate disease. Sexual spores are not known.

"Coccidioidin" in supernatants of mycelial *Coccidioides* broth cultures is largely polysaccharide, but contains some amino acid nitrogen. It is used in cutaneous hypersensitivity and serologic tests. "Spherulin," a lysate of cultured spherules, is also used in skin tests.

FIGURE 48.1.   Coccidioides immitis. *Teased preparation from a 5-day-old culture on Sabouraud's agar. Lactophenol cotton blue mount. Thick-walled barrel- or brick-shaped arthroconidia alternate with empty cells. On lower left, an isolated arthroconidium with fragments of adjacent cells (disjunctors, hyaline pegs) attached. 400X.*

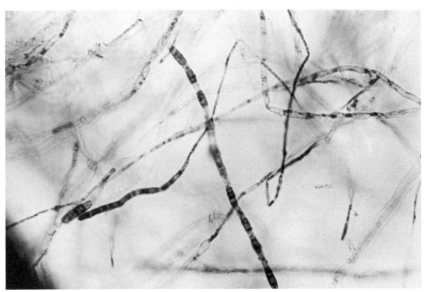

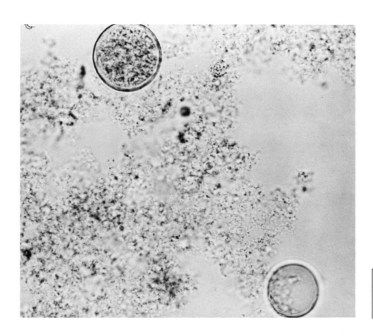

FIGURE 48.2.   Coccidioides immitis. *Transtracheal aspirate from a dog. Unstained. Top left: mature spherule (sporangium) with endospores. Bottom right: immature spherule. 400X.*

Cellular Products of Medical Interest

Adhesins. SOWgp (for *s*pherule *o*uter *w*all *g*lycoprotein) is a proline-rich glycoprotein adhesin on the surface of spherules. SOWgp has affinity for extracellular matrix proteins (laminin, fibronectin, collagen). SOWgp stimulates a strong T_{H2} lymphocyte response, resulting in elevated levels of antibody and suppression of the protective cell-mediated immune response. Mutants unable to produce SOWgp have greatly reduced virulence.

Miscellaneous Products:

1. Beta-glucosidase 2. Bgl2 (for *b*eta-*gl*ucosidase *2*) is an enzyme secreted by the endospores of *Coccidioides* that most likely plays a role in endospore morphology. Antibodies (IgM isotype) to Bgl2 are made early in the infectious process, and are useful diagnostically (detected by the precipitin test) to signal that a recent infection has occurred.
2. Chitinase 1. Cts1 (for *c*hi*t*inase *1*) is one of several chitinases that are involved with the formation of, and release of, endospores from the spherule. An

important target for the Cts enzymes is the "segregation apparatus" (a weblike mesh of chitin-containing structures within the spherule). Antibodies (IgG isotype) to Cts1 are made late in the infectious process (in disseminated disease), and are useful diagnostically (detected by the complement fixation test).

3. Beta-1, 3 glucanosyltransferase. Gel (for *glucan-elongating glucanosyltransferase*) is located on the surface of endospores. Gel elicits a strong T_{H1} lymhocyte response, resulting in elevated levels of gamma interferon followed by protection against disseminated disease (activates macrophages).

4. Serine proteases. These enzymes play a role in the stimulation of the inflammatory response elicited by *Coccidioides*. These enzymes digest elastin, collagen, and immunoglobulins

5. Urease. Though its role in virulence is unknown, the enzyme urease (Ure) elicits a strong protective immune response following stimulation of T_{H1} lymphocytes (activates macrophages).

Growth Characteristics

Coccidioides grows on simple media over a broad temperature range. On Sabouraud's or blood agar, growth is mycelial (mold). Over several days, initially dull gray colonies develop with sparse aerial mycelium, which gradually becomes more abundant. Arthroconidia are produced in 5 to 7 days. Bovine blood agar is hemolyzed. Much colonial variability exists.

Spherules (sporangia) can be demonstrated in vitro by growth at 40°C in media containing casein hydrolysate, glucose, biotin, glutathione, and a salt mixture (spherule medium).

Ecology

Reservoir

Coccidioides inhabits the soil in the Lower Sonoran Life Zone, including parts of California in North America (*C. immitis*) and the southwestern portion of the United States, Mexico, Central America, the northern and western rim states of South America, Argentina, and Paraguay (*C. posadasii*). High prevalence is associated with an annual rainfall of 5 to 20 inches and mean summer and winter temperatures of over 80°F and 45°F, respectively.

Arthroconidia resist drying and tolerate heat and salinity better than do competing soil organisms. In summer heat, *Coccidioides* survives in soil layers nearer the surface than its competitors. When conditions favor growth again after rains, *Coccidioides* repopulates the superficial soil layers first, ensuring its widespread dispersal.

Transmission

Infection is mainly by inhalation of arthroconidia. Primary cutaneous infections are rare.

Pathogenesis

Mechanisms and Pathology. Following inhalation, the barrel-shaped arthroconidia round into spherical-shaped endospores, which—following enlargement and internal cleavage—differentiate into multinucleate spherules containing hundreds of endospores, a process that takes several days. Spherules rupture, releasing endospores, and the cycle is repeated. Arthroconidia, endospores, and spherules trigger an inflammatory response in the lung (serine proteases are partly responsible). Arthroconidia and endospores are engulfed but not killed by phagocytes, and are conveyed to the hilar lymph node, where another inflammatory focus develops (as well as more spherules). Inflammation is stimulated in part by serine proteases, which are liberated during the growth of the fungus. Normally, cell-mediated immune responses arrest the process at this stage following stimulation of T_{H1} lymphocytes that activate macrophages (following specific response to Gel), permitting destruction of the endospores. Antibodies to Bgl2 are made during this phase of the infectious process. With inadequate cell-mediated immunity (caused by SOWgp-directed immunomodulation, genetic makeup, infectious dose), dissemination can occur to bones, skin, abdominal viscera, heart, genital tract, and eye (and rarely in animals to brain and meninges). Gross lesions are white granulomas varying from miliary nodules to irregular masses. Peritoneal, pleural, and pericardial effusions occur. Antibodies to Cts1 are made during this phase of the infectious process. Microscopically, the predominant response is pyogranulomatous: to arthroconidia and endospores, the response is suppurative; and to spherules, the response is proliferative, with epithelioid cells the chief component, admixed with giant cells, lymphocytes, and neutrophils (Fig 48.3).

Disease Patterns

Dogs. Disseminated disease of dogs is the pattern seen most commonly by veterinarians. The complaints are lassitude, anorexia, and loss of condition. There may be respiratory signs (including cough), fever, and lameness due to bone involvement or arthritis, or discharging sinuses from deep lesions.

Cats. Disseminated disease in cats presents with less osseous and more visceral involvement.

Horses. As with cats, there is usually less osseous and more visceral involvement.

Cattle, Sheep, and Swine. In these species, the disease is usually asymptomatic, limited to lungs and regional lymph nodes, and undiagnosed until slaughter.

Epidemiology

In all species, overt disease is the exception. Highest prevalence of canine systemic coccidioidomycosis is observed in male dogs, 4 to 7 years of age, with peak occurrence of illnesses January to March and May to July. These peaks may

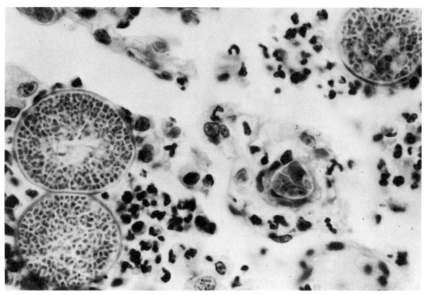

FIGURE 48.3.   Coccidioides immitis *in lung tissue of a Bengal tiger. Hematoxylin-eosin stain. Note prominence of neutrophils in exudate. 400X. (Photograph courtesy of Dr. Roy Henrickson.)*

represent seasonal stress and increased exposure, respectively. Geographic and climatic factors have been mentioned. Young Boxer dogs and Doberman pinschers appear particularly susceptible.

Immunologic Aspects

Cell-mediated hypersensitivity, as determined by skin tests, develops within one or more weeks of exposure and can persist indefinitely. Its presence is an indicator of resistance to progressive disease. Its absence is the rule in disseminated infections, and its return is a favorable sign.

IgM antibody (specific for Bgl2), demonstrable by tube precipitin or latex particle test, appears temporarily after infection and usually disappears again. IgG antibody titers (specific for Cts1), which are detectable by complement fixation and immunodiffusion tests, rise in disseminated disease and remain high (1:16) until the process is brought under control.

No vaccines are presently available.

Laboratory Diagnosis

Direct Examination of Specimens

Animal fluids and tissues are examined for spherules by wet mount in saline containing 10% KOH. Spherules are 10 to 80 μm in diameter, have a thick wall (<2 μm), and contain endospores when mature (see Fig 48.2). Free endospores look indistinct in wet mounts but are recognizable in fixed smears stained by a fungal stain (e.g., periodic acid-Schiff [PAS], Gridley, or Gomori methenamine silver stains).

Stained tissue sections (hematoxylin and eosin [H&E], Gomori methenamine silver, Gridley) show both the agent and the characteristic lesion (see Fig 48.3).

Culture

Blood agar and Sabouraud's agar with or without antibiotics are inoculated, tape-sealed, and incubated at 37°C and 25°C, respectively. All processing of cultures is done under a microbiological safety hood. Mycelial growth should be evident within a week and is examined for presence of arthroconidia in a lactophenol cotton blue wet mount. The isolate can be reconverted to the sporangial phase by animal inoculation or cultivation in a spherule medium (see above, "Growth Characteristics").

A commercially available "exoantigen" test kit furnishes prepared antisera to *Coccidioides, Histoplasma capsulatum*, and *Blastomyces dermatitidis* to be tested against extracts of suspect cultures in an immunodiffusion agar plate, where precipitation lines develop between extracts and their homologous antisera.

Immunodiagnosis

The complement fixation (CF) and immunodiffusion tests detect disseminated disease. Because it is quantifiable, the CF test gauges progress and cure of infection more accurately.

The coccidioidin skin test has been used in animal surveys.

Molecular Methods

Most molecular methods used to identify or detect *Coccidioides* make use of primers specific for sequences contained within the DNA encoding ribosomal RNA. These sequences are amplified using the polymerase chain reaction.

Treatment and Control

Amphotericin B has been the mainstay of anticoccidioidal therapy in human patients. Limitations are its toxicity and the intravenous route of administration, requiring hospitalization or frequent visits. Liposomal preparations of amphotericin B show promise because of lower toxicity, which makes possible higher doses. Ketoconazole and itraconazole are sometimes used in small animals. Given orally over a period of months, they have affected permanent cures. Toxic effects are relatively minor except during pregnancy, when fetal deaths may occur. The complement fixation titer is used to monitor the effect of treatment.

Vaccines are not available.

HISTOPLASMA CAPSULATUM VAR. *CAPSULATUM*

Histoplasma capsulatum is a dimorphic fungus existing as a mold at 25–30°C (saprophytic phase) and as a yeast at 37°C (parasitic phase). This fungus has three varieties: *H. capsulatum* var. *capsulatum*, *H. capsulatum* var. *duboisii*, and *H. capsulatum* var. *farciminosum*. Variety *farciminosum* causes epizootic lymphangitis (pseudoglanders), a chronic pyogranulomatous disease of equine skin and is discussed in Chapter 47. Varieties *capsulatum* and *duboisii* cause histoplasmosis, a systemic fungal disease of mammals. Variety *duboisii* is found only in Africa, whereas variety *capsulatum* is found worldwide, and is the most common cause of histoplasmosis. In this chapter, histoplasmosis will be discussed without regard to this varietal distinction, i.e., *H. capsulatum* var. *capsulatum*, and *H. capsulatum* var. *duboisii* will be regarded as *H. capsulatum*.

Descriptive Features

Morphology, Structure, and Composition

The free-living form of *H. capsulatum* consists of septate hyphae bearing spherical to pyriform microconidia 2 to 4 µm in diameter, and "tuberculate" macroconidia, thick-walled spheroidal cells, 8 to 14 µm in diameter, studded with fingerlike projections (Fig 48.4). In animal hosts or appropriate culture, the mold becomes a yeast consisting of oval, singly budding cells that measure 2 to 3 µm by 3 to 4 µm. A sexual, ascomycetous state, *Ajellomyces capsulatus*, has been described.

Histoplasmins, which are used in immunodiagnosis, are obtained from mycelial culture filtrates. They contain polysaccharides, with variable admixtures of glycoproteins and cellular breakdown products. Mycelial and yeast phases differ in cellular constituents, some of which (e.g., cell wall glucan) have been related to virulence.

Cellular Products of Medical Interest

Adhesins. Inhaled microconidia and yeast-phase parasitic forms are recognized by, and bind to, beta-2 integrins on the surface of neutrophils and macrophages. It is unknown what fungal structure is involved. Likewise, an unknown adhesin is responsible for the adherence of *H. capsulatum* to fibronectin receptors on dendritic cells. Adherence in this fashion to neutrophils, macrophages, or

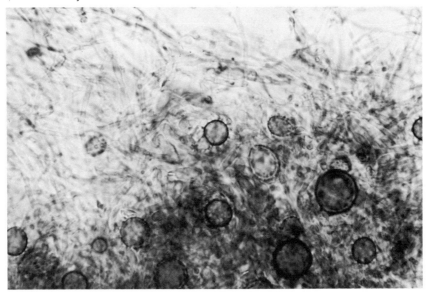

FIGURE 48.4. Histoplasma capsulatum, *mycelial phase. Teased preparation from a 7-day culture on Sabouraud's agar at 25°C. Lactophenol cotton blue mount. "Tuberculate" macroconidia and hyphae. The "tubercles" appear as projections from the thick cell walls, most obviously on the conidium in the center of the field. 400X.*

dendritic cells allows the fungus to enter the cell without triggering an effective oxidative burst and the generation of reactive oxygen and nitrogen intermediates.

Miscellaneous Products. *Histoplasma capsulatum* produces a variety of products that may play a role in histoplasmosis:

1. Calcium-binding protein (Cbp). The yeast (parasitic) phase of *H. capsulatum* produces a calcium-binding protein (Cbp) that permits the yeast phase to grow in low-calcium environments (the phagolysosome) by efficiently chelating calcium and delivering it to the fungus. In addition, since Cbp chelates available calcium within the phagolysosome, this impedes effectiveness of several calcium requiring lysosomal enzymes. Normal acidification of the phagolysosome is also a calcium-dependent event. *Histoplasma capsulatum* mutants unable to produce Cbp are avirulent.
2. H antigen. Host immune responses to H antigen were originally used as a diagnostic tool in the diagnosis of histoplasmosis. Subsequently, H antigen was found to be a beta-glucosidase that elicits a cell-mediated (protective) immune response to the yeast (parasitic) phase of *H. capsulatum*.
3. Iron acquisition. Iron is an absolute growth requirement for *H. capsulatum* (as it is for all life forms). *Histoplasma capsulatum* acquires iron in several ways: production of hydroxamate siderophores capable of removing iron from host iron-binding proteins (transferrin, lactoferrin); expression of a hemin-binding receptor on the surface of yeast (parasitic) forms; glutathione-dependent ferric reductase which reduces Fe(III) to Fe(II), thereby releasing it from host iron-binding proteins; and several poorly defined iron reductases on the surface of the yeast phase.
4. M antigen. Host immune response to M antigen was originally used as a diagnostic tool in the diagnosis of histoplasmosis. Subsequently, M antigen was found to be a catalase enzyme, which plays a role in the survival of the yeast phase within the phagolysosome.
5. Melanin. Melanin is produced by *H. capsulatum*. Melanin is a free radical scavenger (reducing the toxicity of hydroxy radicals, superoxides, and singlet oxygen radicals found within the phagolysosome).
6. Phagolysosome acidification. Normal phagolysosomes have a pH <5, a pH that optimizes the activity of many of the digestive enzymes found in this environment. *Histoplasma capsulatum* raises the pH of the phagolysosome to 6–6.5, thereby reducing the activity of these lysosomal enzymes. How the fungus does this is unknown.

Growth Characteristics

Histoplasma capsulatum grows on common laboratory media over a broad temperature range. The optimum for mycelial growth is 25° to 30°C. The cottony aerial mycelium is white, brown, or intermediate. Pigmentation parallels abundance of macroconidia. The yeast phase requires richer media (e.g., glucose cysteine blood agar) and temperatures of 34° to 37°C. Growth may take a week or more before characteristic colonies are seen.

Histoplasma capsulatum survives at ambient temperatures for months and at refrigerator temperature for years. It withstands freezing and thawing and tolerates heating for more than an hour at 45°C.

Variability

Histoplasma capsulatum exists as three varieties: *capsulatum*, *duboisii*, and *farciminosum*. Varieties *capsulatum* (worldwide) and *duboisii* (Africa) produce histoplasmosis, and variety *farciminosum* causes epizootic lymphangitis (pseudoglanders) of equids (see Chapter 47). Though *H. capsulatum var. capsulatum* is found worldwide, its central focus is in the Americas. Genetically, variety *capsulatum* is divided into 6 Classes: Class 1 and Class 2 are found in North America; Class 3 is found in Central and South America; Class 4 is found in Florida (North America); and Class 5 and Class 6 are found in human patients with acquired immunodeficiency syndrome (AIDS) from New York (North America) and Panama (Central America), respectively.

Ecology

Reservoir

Although most concentrated in the Mississippi and Ohio River watersheds of North America, *H. capsulatum* occurs sporadically worldwide. It is found in the topsoil layers, especially in the presence of bird (mainly starlings in North America, and chickens in South America) and bat guano, which provide both enrichment and inoculum. Birds are mainly passive carriers, whereas bats undergo intestinal infectious processes. *Histoplasma capsulatum* is favored by neutral to alkaline soil environments with annual rainfall between 35 and 50 inches and mean temperatures between 68°F and 90°F.

Transmission

Transmission is mostly by inhalation of microconidia or hyphal fragments, possibly by ingestion, and, rarely, by wound infection.

Pathogenesis

Mechanisms and Pathology. Microconidia, hyphal fragments (from the environment), or yeast cells (from an intraphagocytic cell environment) attach to macrophages in the lung by way of a beta-2 integrin. It is immediately phagocytosed, a minimal respiratory burst occurs, and a phagolysosome results following fusion with lysosomes. Microconidia and hyphal elements differentiate into yeast. Survival within the phagolysosome is related to

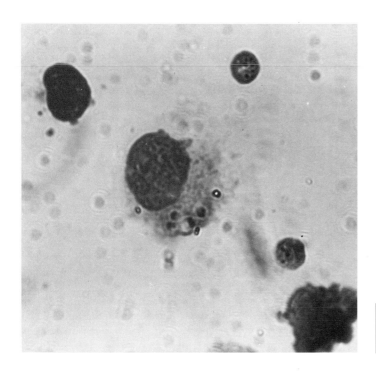

FIGURE 48.5. Histoplasma capsulatum, *yeast phase.*
Sediment of peritoneal exudate from a dog. Wright-Giemsa stain.
Four yeast cells within a macrophage. 1000X.

modulation of phagolysosome pH (around 6–6.5), secretion of M antigen (a catalase), secretion of Cbp, melanin, and successful acquisition of iron from intracellular iron stores. The yeast multiplies within the phagolysosome, ultimately killing the cell and the release of yeast cells (which continue the cycle). Intracellular multiplication continues until an effective cell-mediated immune response occurs resulting in activated macrophages, which effectively control the multiplication of the yeast.

Early events and lesions resemble those of tuberculosis. Thoracic lymph nodes become enlarged, and lungs may contain grayish-white nodules. The histologic response varies from suppurative to granulomatous inflammation. Caseation necrosis and calcification are common.

In disseminated disease, lymph nodes and parenchymatous organs are enlarged and may contain gross nodular lesions. There may be ulcerations of skin and mucous membranes, abdominal and pleural effusions, and involvement of the central nervous system (including eyes), skin, and bone marrow. The inflammatory exudate consists of macrophage elements colonized by yeast cells (Fig 48.5).

Disease Patterns. Histoplasmosis can occur in almost any animal species, but dogs are the most commonly affected. Dogs may develop a primary pulmonary form with coughing, fever, regional lymphadenopathy, and radiographic abnormalities. The more common form in dogs is disseminated disease, marked by lethargy, anorexia, weight loss, diarrhea, dehydration, and anemia. Hepatomegaly, splenomegaly, mesenteric lymphadenitis, and ascites may cause abdominal distension.

Comparable patterns have rarely been observed in cats.

Disease patterns in human patients parallel those described.

Epidemiology

Subclinical infections with histoplasmosis are common in dogs and cats—and humans—in endemic areas. Clinical disease is most prevalent in dogs aged 2 to 7 years, in early autumn (September to November) and later winter to early spring (February to April). No sex predilection is reported, but the pointing breeds, weimaraners, and Brittany spaniels have the greatest risk. Disseminated histoplasmosis in human patients and dogs is found in association with immunosuppression.

Immunologic Aspects

Recovery and resistance are governed by cell-mediated immune responses, while circulating antibodies have no apparent protective function. Recovery from histoplasmosis appears to confer immunity.

No vaccines are available.

Laboratory Diagnosis

Direct Examination

Smears of buffy coat, sediment of aspirates, and tissue impressions are stained with a Romanovsky-type (e.g., Giemsa, or Wright's) or a fungal stain (periodic acid-Schiff [PAS], Gridley, or Gomori methenamine silver) and examined for intraphagocytic yeast cells (see Fig 48.5).

In sections stained with hematoxylin-eosin, *H. capsulatum* appears as tiny dots surrounded by haloes. A duplicate fungal stain (e.g., periodic acid-Schiff [PAS], Gridley, or Gomori methenamine silver) can be helpful.

Immunofluorescence has been used to identify the yeast in tissue and exudates.

Culture

Specimens are inoculated onto blood agar and Sabouraud's agar (with inhibitors) and incubated in jars or plastic bags at room temperature for up to 3 months. Colonial growth may look reddish-wrinkled before the appearance of cottony brownish to white mycelium.

Microconidia and macroconidia are demonstrated in lactophenol cotton blue wet mounts. Dimorphism must be proven by conversion to the yeast phase in culture or by IV injection of mice. Mice will die within a few weeks. Their macrophages will contain the yeast forms.

A commercially available "exoantigen" test kit furnishes prepared antisera to *Coccidioides*, *Histoplasma capsulatum*, and *Blastomyces dermatitidis* to be tested against extracts of suspect cultures in an immunodiffusion agar plate, where precipitation lines develop between extracts and their homologous antisera.

Immunodiagnosis

Histoplasmin skin and CF tests using antigens of either mycelial or yeast origins have not been reliable diagnostic aids in animal infections. The position of the precipitin band in immunodiffusion tests differentiates early and recovered human cases (near serum well) from active and progressive ones (near antigen well). Limited use of these tests on animals has given erratic results.

A radioimmunoassay for antigen detection has been described.

Molecular Techniques

Molecular methods used to identify or detect *H. capsulatum* make use of primers for specific sequences contained within the DNA, e.g., genes encoding ribosomal RNA, or those encoding the M protein. These sequences are amplified using the polymerase chain reaction.

Treatment and Control

Azoles (ketoconazole, itraconazole, fluconazole) and amphotericin B have been used successfully in the treatment of some cases of canine histoplasmosis.

Relapses are common. The prognosis for disseminated cases is grave.

BLASTOMYCES DERMATITIDIS

Blastomyces dermatitidis is a dimorphic fungus existing as a mold in the soil (saprophytic stage), and as a yeast in tissue (parasitic stage). It causes the systemic fungal disease called "blastomycosis," which occurs most commonly in the eastern third of North America. Cases of the disease arise sporadically in Africa, Asia, and Europe. Affected hosts are human patients, dogs and, rarely, horses, cats, and wildlife species.

Descriptive Features

Morphology, Structure, and Composition

In the saprophytic phase (in soil or on artificial media at 25–30°C), the hyphae of *B. dermatitidis* produce conidiophores with spherical or oval smooth-walled conidia, 2µm to 10 µm in diameter. In tissue or on blood agar at 37°C, the agent is a thick-walled yeast, 8 µm to 15 µm in diameter that reproduces by single buds attached by a broad base (Fig 48.6). The fungus has a sexual form *Ajellomyces dermatitidis*.

Cell wall extracts contain 3 to 10 parts of polysaccharide to 1 part of protein. Protein is highest in the mycelial phase, while chitin is highest in the yeast phase. The lipid content

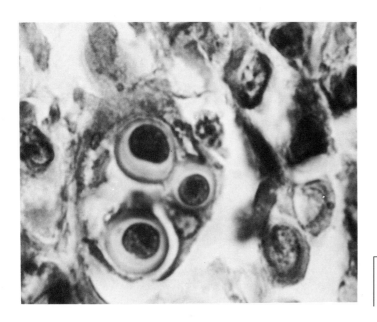

FIGURE 48.6.   Blastomyces dermatitidis, *yeast phase, in lung of dog. Hematoxylin-eosin stain. Note bud (lower right of upper yeast cell) attached by broad base to mother cell. 1000X.*

of *B. dermatitidis* is higher than in other fungi. Lipid, protein, and chitin levels vary directly with virulence.

Cellular Products of Medical Interest

Adhesin. The yeast phase of *B. dermatitidis* produces a protein adhesin termed Bad1 (for *Blastomyces adhesin 1*), formally called WI-1. Bad1 has two functions related to virulence of the fungus: 1) Bad1 adheres to beta-2 integrins on the surface of phagocytic cells, triggering uptake of the yeast, invoking a minimal respiratory burst, resulting in little generation of reactive oxygen and nitrogen intermediates; 2) Bad1 down regulates the production of proinflammatory cytokines (particularly tumor necrosis factor [TNF]) by affected macrophages. The amino acid sequence of Bad1 is homologous to the invasin protein produced by Yersinia (see Chapter 10). *Blastomyces dermatitidis* mutants that do not produce Bad1 are avirulent.

Miscellaneous Products. Blastomyces dermatitidis produces a variety of extracellular enzymes and products that may be involved with disease production. These include proteases, phosphatases, esterases, and glycosidases. Culture filtrates are leukotactic for human neutrophils. The role played by these products in the production of disease is unknown.

Growth Characteristics

Blastomyces dermatitidis grows on most media at room temperature and 37°C. Colonies develop from within 2 to over 7 days. Mold colonies, formed at ambient temperatures (25–30°C), are cottony white to tan depending on the abundance of conidia. Yeast colonies develop on blood agar at 37°C. They are opaque off-white to tan, with rough surface and a pasty consistency.

Variability

The two recognized serotypes are related to geographic origin of the strains. Similar geographic relationships are seen when polymerase chain reaction–based fingerprinting systems are used.

Ecology

Reservoir

There is limited evidence of natural reservoirs. Moisture, low pH, animal wastes, and decaying vegetation appear to favor colonization. Humidity promotes release of conidia.

Transmission

Blastomycosis most commonly begins by respiratory exposure. Percutaneous infection probably occurs in dogs.

Pathogenesis

Microconidia hyphal fragments are inhaled and convert to the yeast form within the alveolar spaces of the respiratory tract. The yeast expresses Bad1, which is followed by uptake (with minimal respiratory burst) by phagocytic cells. Down regulation of tumor necrosis factor production by affected macrophages delays stimulation of cell-mediated immunity (which is necessary to kill the yeast). In dogs, an inflammatory response involving macrophages and neutrophils and resulting in pyogranulomatous lesions occurs in the terminal bronchioles, followed by similar reactions in satellite lymph nodes. Blastomycosis is more often progressive than histoplasmosis and coccidioidomycosis. Dissemination involves superficial lymph nodes, skin, bones, bone marrow, eyes, viscera, mammary glands, and urogenital tract. The nodular lesions can be tubercle-like, with mononuclear cell types predominating, or there may be significant suppurative admixtures. Liquefaction and caseation occur, but calcification and encapsulation are exceptional.

Signs include skin lesions and respiratory distress with fever, depression, anorexia, and weight loss. Locomotor disturbances result from bone or joint infection or—rarely—central nervous system involvement. Ocular disease is common in disseminated blastomycosis. Most dogs with multiple organ system involvement die within months. Evidence for a benign form is uncertain. Blastomyces induce macrophages to produce elevated amounts of calcitriol resulting in hypercalcemia.

The disease in cats resembles that in dogs.

Epidemiology

Highest prevalence in dogs is from spring to fall. Male dogs less than 4 years of age are most often affected. Differential breed susceptibility has not been found. Though generally noncontagious, one human infection resulted from a dog bite. Risk factors for infection include proximity to waterways and excavation.

Immunologic Aspects

Impaired cell-mediated responsiveness may explain canine disseminated blastomycosis.

Humoral and cell-mediated responses occur as a result of infection. Cell-mediated immunity in mice is decisive in determining resistance. Artificial immunization is not available.

Laboratory Diagnosis

Direct Examination

Blastomyces dermatitidis can be demonstrated in wet mounts of exudates and tissue smears as thick-walled yeast cells with single buds attached by a broad base. In section, intracellular yeasts may be found (see Fig 48.6). Smears of aspirates, and tissue impressions are stained with a Romanovsky-type (e.g., Giemsa, or Wright's) or a fungal stain (periodic acid-Schiff [PAS], Gridley, or Gomori methenamine silver) and examined for yeast cells.

In sections stained with hematoxylin-eosin, *B dermatitidis* appears as thick-walled yeast cells with single buds attached by a broad base. A duplicate fungal stain (e.g., periodic acid-Schiff [PAS], Gridley, or Gomori methenamine silver) can be helpful (see Fig 48.6).

Culture

Cultures on Sabouraud's agar (with or without inhibitors) are incubated at ambient temperature (25–30°C) for up to 3 weeks. It is difficult to obtain the yeast form on primary isolation but it is relatively easy to convert the mold to the yeast phase by increasing the temperature to 37°C.

A commercially available "exoantigen" test kit furnishes prepared antisera to *Coccidioides, Histoplasma capsulatum,* and *Blastomyces dermatitidis* to be tested against extracts of suspect cultures in an immunodiffusion agar plate, where precipitation lines develop between extracts and their homologous antisera.

Immunodiagnosis

Blastomycin skin and complement fixation tests lack acceptable sensitivity and specificity. The commercially available agar gel double diffusion test (making use of antigens composed of a cell wall autolysate called "Antigen A") appears to be specific (96%) and sensitive (91%), but titers remain after successful treatment. Antibodies to Bad1 detected by various means (e.g., radioimmunoassay [RIA]) increase during disease, and decline with successful treatment, making detection of antibodies with specificity to Bad1 more useful clinically.

Molecular Methods

Molecular methods used to identify or detect *B. dermatitidis* make use of primers for specific sequences contained within DNA encoding ribosomal RNA (e.g., 28S RNA; the internally transcribed spacer region). These sequences are amplified using the polymerase chain reaction.

Treatment and Control

Blastomycosis responds to amphotericin B and ketoconazole (or both together), and to itraconazole. Fluconazole is moderately effective.

ASPERGILLUS SPP.

Members of the genus *Aspergillus* are ubiquitous saprophytic molds with opportunistic pathogenic patterns depending on impaired, overwhelmed, or bypassed host defenses. Of some 900 species, *A. fumigatus* is most frequent in animal and human infections.

Descriptive Features

Morphology and Composition

Aspergillus spp. are molds consisting of septate hyphae and characteristic asexual fruiting structures that are borne on

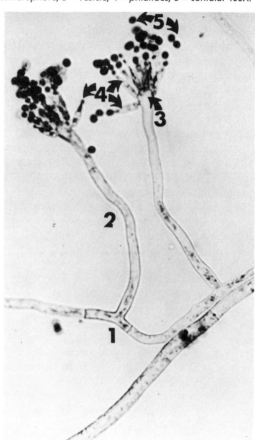

FIGURE 48.7.   *Anatomy of a member of the genus* Aspergillus (Aspergillus clavatus). *Lactophenol cotton blue mount from slide culture on Sabouraud's agar. 1 = foot cell, 2 = conidiophore, 3 = vesicle, 4 = phialides, 5 = conidia. 400X.*

conidiophores. Conidiophores are hyphal branches originating by a foot cell in the vegetative mycelium and ending in an expanded vesicle. The vesicle is covered by a layer or layers of flask-shaped phialides, from which chains of pigmented conidia (the asexual reproductive units) arise (Fig 48.7). They give the fungal colony its color.

In tissue, only hyphae are seen. In aerated cavities (e.g., nasal passages, air sacs, cavitary lesions), fruiting structures may be found (see Fig 73.8).

Fruiting bodies are important diagnostic features of *Aspergillus* spp. by which species are identified.

Cellular Products of Medical Interest

Adhesins. Members of the genus *Aspergillus* produce a number of surface proteins (conidial and hyphal) that bind to extracellular matrix proteins (collagen, fibronectin, fibrinogen, and laminin).

Cell Wall. The cell wall of *Aspergillus* displays a "pathogen-associated molecular pattern" that is recognized by Toll-like receptors (see Chapter 2) on the surface of host macrophages. Binding to these receptors leads to the secretion of proinflammatory cytokines.

Extracellular Enzymes. Aspergillus produces a number of

enzymes that have the potential to function in vivo to break down host tissue. These include elastase, proteases, and phospholipases. In addition, members of this genus produce catalases that reduce the effectiveness of peroxides generated by phagocytic cells.

Iron Acquisition. Aspergillus produces several hydroxamate siderophores (a ferrichrome and a fusarinine) needed to acquire iron from host iron-binding proteins (transferrin, lactoferrin).

Pigment (Melanin). Conidia of *Aspergillus* are pigmented. The pigment, melanin, is a free radical scavenger (reducing the toxicity of hydroxy radicals, superoxides, and singlet oxygen radicals found within the phagolysosome).

Growth Characteristics

Aspergilli grow on all common laboratory media over a wide range of temperatures (up to 50°C). Their biochemical activities have not been clearly related to virulence or utilized diagnostically.

Aspergilli thrive in the environment. Some are highly resistant to heat and drying. Most do not grow in cycloheximide-containing fungal media.

Ecology

Reservoir

Aspergilli are present in soil, vegetation, feed, and secondarily in air and water and objects exposed to them. *Aspergillus fumigatus* becomes predominant over competing microbiota in fermented plant material (e.g., hay, silage, compost). Animal disease outbreaks are often traced to such sources.

Transmission

Aspergillosis is acquired from environmental sources, generally by inhalation or ingestion. Most *Aspergillus* mastitis follows intramammary inoculation. Intrauterine infections in cattle result from dissemination of subclinical lung or intestinal infections. In poultry, egg transmission sometimes occurs (rare).

Pathogenesis

Mechanism. Following their deposition in tissue or on a surface (adhesins hinder removal) recognition (by way of "pathogen-associated molecular pattern") by phagocytic cells triggers an inflammatory response. Inflammation, along with release of fungal elastase, proteases, and phospholipases, results in tissue damage. Pigment and catalase delay destruction by phagocytic cells.

Allergenic factors, which are recognized in human aspergilloses, are insufficiently documented in animal disease.

Pathology. In pulmonary infection, suppurative exudate accumulates in bronchioles and adjacent parenchyma. It surrounds colonies of mycelial growth, which may extend into blood vessels and produce infected thrombi and vasculitis, leading to dissemination. Infection may also spread directly into adjacent air spaces. Granulomas develop; they are grossly visible as grayish white nodules and consist of mononuclear cells and fibroblasts. In older lesions, colonies are fringed by acidophilic clubs (asteroid bodies), which resemble actinomycosis (see Fig 37.2).

Lesions in avian lungs are caseous nodules. On serous membranes, caseous foci are covered by macroscopic mold colonies, accompanied by thickening of the membranes (e.g., air sacs) (Fig 48.8). The cellular response is acute suppurative to chronic granulomatous.

FIGURE 48.8.   *Aspergillosis in a waterfowl (grebe). The exposed air sac in the center contains one large mold colony (arrow) and a smaller one on the upper left. The air sac on the lower right (★) has had a portion removed (★), revealing luxuriant mold growth within. (Photograph courtesy of Dr. Murray Fowler.)*

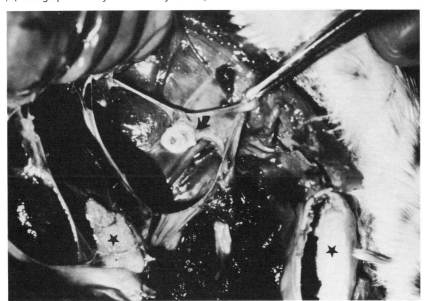

Bovine abortion results from hematogenous seeding of placentomes, which is possibly a response to a growth factor in placental tissue. There is hyphal invasion of blood vessels producing vasculitis and a necrotizing, hemorrhagic placentitis. The fetus undergoes disseminated infection with signs of emaciation and dehydration. Lymph nodes, viscera, and brain may be involved. Ringworm-like plaques on the fetal skin are often seen.

On mucosal surfaces (e.g., nasal passage, trachea), mold colonies form on top of necrotic tissue, which is surrounded by a hemorrhagic zone.

Disease Patterns

Pulmonary and disseminated infections, frequently involving kidneys and the central nervous system, occur in most species.

Avian. Avian aspergillosis, which affects many species of birds, sometimes in epidemics, reflects heavy exposure or severe stress on domestic flocks or pet bird operations, or the effects of oil spills on marine birds. The disease is usually a respiratory tract infection, sometimes with hematogenous dissemination. Signs are inappetence, listlessness, weight loss, dyspnea, sometimes diarrhea, and abnormal behavior and posture. The eyes are often affected. Mortality may approach 50%, especially in young birds. In mild cases, only gasping and hyperpnea may be seen. The course varies from a day to several weeks.

Ruminant. Bovine abortions usually occur late in pregnancy and resemble abortions due to other causes. Fetal skin plaques occur also in other mycotic abortions.

Mastitis due to *A. fumigatus* is reported at an increased rate, especially from Europe. It is usually chronic progressive, producing abscesses in the udder.

Dogs and Cats. Aspergillosis of mucous membranes occurs in dogs, rarely in cats, in nasal passages or paranasal sinuses. It is manifested by sneezing and unilateral or bilateral persistent nasal discharge that is unresponsive to medical treatment.

Aspergillus terreus and *A. deflectus* cause disseminated aspergillosis in dogs, particularly German shepherd dogs. Osteomyelitis is a common feature.

Horses. *Aspergillus* infection of the cornea is the leading cause of keratomycosis.

Vague upper respiratory signs may point to an aspergillosis of the equine guttural pouch.

Miscellaneous Species. Intestinal aspergillosis, presenting as diarrhea, occurs in calves, foals, and cats.

Epidemiology

Intensity of exposure is a significant feature in animal aspergillosis. Bovine abortion outbreaks are often related to moldy fodder. Aspergillosis in chicken flocks commonly coincides with the use of heavily contaminated litter.

Stress aspects are usually recognizable in outbreaks. Avian aspergillosis is seen under conditions of poor husbandry. In oiled seabirds, there is severely impaired thermal regulation. In pregnant cattle, advanced gestation combined with low-quality feed and poor weather and housing add up to severe challenge.

Canine nasal aspergillosis occurs especially in young dogs of dolichocephalic breeds. Some T lymphocyte deficiency may exist.

In keratomycosis of horses, the frequent history of topical antibacterial and steroid treatment suggests immunosuppression and impaired colonization resistance.

Immunologic Aspects

Circulating antibody with no demonstrably protective role may be present in dogs with nasal aspergillosis (see under "Treatment, Control, and Prevention"). Cell-mediated immunity may be related to resistance.

Immunization procedures are not available.

Laboratory Diagnosis

Direct Examination

Hyphae, fruiting heads, and conidia can often be demonstrated in samples either in wet mounts in 10% KOH or with calcofluor white. For fixed-stained smears, fungal stains (periodic acid-Schiff [PAS], Gridley, or Gomori methenamine silver) are best; Giemsa is satisfactory, and Gram of limited use. Septate branching hyphae constitute strong evidence of aspergillosis. Other fungi (*Penicillium, Pseudallescheria, Paecilomyces*) present a similar picture but rare. Conidia may occur in air passages or other exposed sites in the absence of infection (see Fig 73.8).

In stained tissue sections, septate hyphae dividing dichotomously at acute angles are the only structures seen.

Isolation and Identification

Aspergillus is readily cultured. Because it is a ubiquitous contaminant, interpretation of positive cultures is often problematic. Presence of the agent must always be correlated with pathologic and clinical findings. Identification of agents rests upon morphologic features and growth characteristics of isolates.

Immunodiagnosis

Serologic tests are useful adjuncts to the diagnosis of aspergillosis. Because the tests that are available are species specific, it is necessary to know which *Aspergillus* to expect. For example, *A. fumigatus* is most commonly seen in nasal aspergillosis of dogs, whereas disseminated aspergillosis in that species is either *A. deflectus* or *A. terreus*. An immunodiffusion kit for antibody detection is commercially available for detection of antibodies to *A. fumigatus*.

Molecular Methods

Primers designed to amplify DNA encoding ribosomal RNA (including the "internal transcribed spacer" region) are available for demonstration or identification of members of the genus. Amplification of DNA is by the polymerase chain reaction.

Treatment, Control, and Prevention

Aspergillosis in birds is generally not treated.

The nasal form in dogs is treated topically with instillation of clortrimazole or enilconazole into the nasal passages and sinuses. Itraconazole (given orally) has been successfully used to treat nasal aspergillosis when topical treatment was not possible.

Itraconazole has been beneficial in treating disseminated aspergillosis.

There is no established treatment for mammary aspergillosis.

For intestinal infections in pigs, foals, and calves, oral nystatin is recommended.

Keratomycosis is treated topically with antimycotic ointments and solutions.

Avoidance of massive exposure requires elimination of cattle feed, particularly hay and silage that has undergone noticeable deterioration. *Aspergillus fumigatus* only reaches high concentrations under conditions of "biologic heat" generation, after other microbiota are eliminated. With poultry litter, proper storage and frequent changes of litter can prevent such buildup.

OTHER SAPROPHYTIC FUNGAL PATHOGENS

Penicillium spp. are occasional causes of a nasal mycosis in dogs.

Scedosporium apiospermum is prominent as an agent of mycetoma (see Chapter 47).

Pseudallescheria boydii causes visceral mycetoma and pneumonia in dogs, ocular disease and abortion in horses, and mastitis and abortion in cattle.

Paecilomyces spp. is associated with disseminated canine and feline paecilomycosis with bone involvement and a respiratory epidemic in captive turtles have been reported.

Rhizopus spp, *Absidia* spp, *Mucor* spp, and *Mortierella* spp cause mycotic bovine abortion, gastrointestinal infections, marked by ulcerative lesions and mesenteric lymphadenitis, in ruminants, swine, and dogs, as well as respiratory and hematogenous infections affecting various viscera and the central nervous system. They are secondary to stress, such as dietary changes and inadequacies, antibiotic suppression of the gastrointestinal flora, concurrent infections, recent parturition, or trauma.

Rhinosporidium seeberi causes a granulomatous mucocutaneous infection affecting humans, horses, cattle, mules, dogs, goats, and some wild waterfowl.

Conidiobolus spp. and *Basidiobolus* spp. may cause nasal granulomas in horses.

Dematiaceous fungi (See Chapter 47, "Phaeohyphomycosis") have been associated with mycotic nasal granulomas in cattle.

PNEUMOCYSTIS

Members of the genus *Pneumocystis* are fungi capable of causing pneumonia in immunocompromised individuals. They have only been isolated from affected hosts (e.g., humans, dogs, cats, horses, pigs, goats, ferrets, mice, rats). At present there are two species, *jiroveci* (affecting human patients) and *carinii* (affecting all the rest). *Pneumocystis carinii* is composed of at least 30 varieties or "special forms," with each "special form" affecting a particular host. For example, *P. carinii* f. sp. *ratti*, affects rats, while *P. carinii* f. sp. *muris*, only mice. Thus, *Pneumocystis* is a host-specific fungus (and it is not zoonotic).

Spread is by way of aerosol. Affected hosts are almost always immunocompromised, though there are reports of animals (mainly foals) that have pneumocystis pneumonia without an obvious underlying condition.

The fungus has not been grown in a cell-free culture system. Diagnosis is made by examination of material containing alveolar macrophages (in whose cytoplasm spherical to crescent shaped cysts 4–7 μm in diameter are observed) stained with a Romanovsky-type stain (e.g., Giemsa, Wright's) or a silver stain (e.g., Gomori methenamine silver). DNA primers have also been designed to amplify specific segments of the fungal genome, so that detection and identification is possible using the polymerase chain reaction.

Treatment includes one or more of the following: trimethoprim-sulfonamides, dapsone, atovaquone, pentamidine, clindamycin, or trimetrexate/leucovorin.

PROTOTHECOSIS

Prototheca is an alga lacking chlorophyll. It multiplies by endosporulation, producing roughly spherical cells that are 8 μm to 25 μm in diameter (Fig 48.9). *Prototheca zopfii* and *P. wickerhamii* (which probably belongs to the genus *Auxenochlorella*) are occasionally pathogenic. They grow on fungal media (without cycloheximide) at 25°C and 37°C, respectively, into white to tannish dull colonies in less than a week and are differentiated serologically and by carbohydrate assimilation tests.

Prototheca spp. are widespread in nature. Exposure is by ingestion, percutaneously, or, in dairy cows, by intramammary injection.

Disease occurs in dogs, cats, cattle, deer, bats, snakes, fish, and humans. In dogs, it is usually disseminated and accompanied by hemorrhagic diarrhea. Central nervous system involvement and eye lesions are frequent. In cats and humans, cases to date have been cutaneous. Immuno-

FIGURE 48.9. *Prototheca sp. in bovine mastitis. Wright stain. The less intensely stained organisms show evidence of endosporulation. 1000X.*

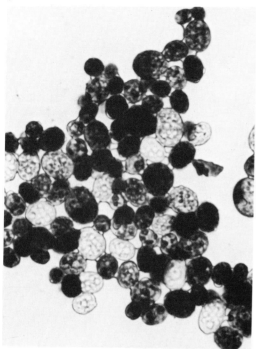

deficiency is suspected. In cattle, chronic progressive mastitis develops. Tissue reactions are pyogranulomatous.

The agent is easily cultured and can be demonstrated in unstained wet mounts from specimens or in fixed smears stained with a Romanovsky-type (Wright's or Giemsa) or fungal (periodic acid-Schiff [PAS], Gridley, or Gomori methenamine silver) stain (see Figs 48.9 and 69.7).

Amphotericin B and ketoconazole are used on humans. The agents are susceptible to the aminoglycosides in vitro. Treatment of animals has not been effective, although liposomal formulations of amphotericin B show promise.

PART III

Viruses

49

Pathogenesis of Viral Diseases

Yuan Chung Zee   N. James MacLachlan

Virus-Host Relationships

The outcome of any virus-host interaction can differ, depending on critical factors such as virus-cell interactions, species of animal host, route of exposure, mode of virus dissemination, and host resistance. Most virus-infected animals that present to veterinarians do so because they exhibit clinical signs of their infection. However, it is very important to recognize that microbial infections of animals often do not result in clinical disease. In fact, the majority of virus-animal interactions result in asymptomatic or subclinical infection, and viruses, however virulent, will not infect animals that are resistant to them. The potential consequences of virus-animal relationships are shown in Table 49.1.

There are several major routes of viral entry into a host: the respiratory, alimentary, and urogenital routes and direct transmission (such as by an insect or animal bite). Successful establishment of viral infection depends on the presence of susceptible cell receptors and the physicochemical nature of the viral agent. For example, viruses that infect animals through the alimentary tract typically are resistant to the low pH and potent enzymes that occur in the digestive tract.

Modes of Dissemination of Viruses Within the Hosts

Viruses cause two basic patterns of infection: localized and generalized (Fig 49.1). In localized infections, viral multiplication and cellular damage remain localized near the site of entry (e.g., the skin or the mucous membranes of the respiratory, gastrointestinal, or genital tract), so that the infecting virus spreads only to neighboring cells immediately adjacent to the original site of infection. For example, rhinovirus infections of animals are often restricted to the nasal epithelium and do not even spread to the lower respiratory tract. Other respiratory viruses, such as parainfluenza and respiratory syncytial viruses replicate within the lungs of infected animals, but tissue injury induced by these viruses typically remains restricted to the respiratory tract. Generalized infections develop through several sequential steps: 1) the virus undergoes primary replication at the site of entry and in regional lymph nodes, 2) progeny virus spreads through blood (primary viremia) and lymphatics to additional parenchymal organs, where 3) further viral replication takes place, 4) virus is disseminated to the other target organs via a secondary viremia, and 5) it multiplies further in these target organs where it causes cellular degeneration and/or necrosis, tissue injury, and clinical disease.

The incubation period is the asymptomatic period after infection and prior to expression of clinical disease. In generalized virus infections, overt disease begins only after the virus becomes widely disseminated in the body and has attained maximum titers. It is at this stage of the infection that the veterinarian usually is first alerted. Canine distemper illustrates a generalized virus infection of animals. The canine distemper virus initiates the infection at the site of entry, but then disseminates through the blood or the lymphatic system to produce generalized infection with involvement of a variety of target organs (Fig 49.2). The sequence of events during the incubation period and development of signs of disease in experimental canine distemper infections indicate that the different clinical signs that occur in individual animals depend on which of the various organ systems are infected by the virus. The virus is disseminated to these organs during viremia, which may be characterized by the presence of free virus particles in the blood or, as with canine distemper virus, blood cells also can serve as carriers to disseminate virus to target organs (cell-associated viremia). Cell-associated viremias typically involve blood leukocytes but some viruses, such as bluetongue virus, hog cholera virus, or parvovirus, can associate with red blood cells of the infected host. The dissemination of virus to the central nervous system (CNS) can occur by viremia or, in the case of rabies, by transmission along peripheral nerves.

Viral infections that occur without producing overt disease are very common and are potentially important in the dissemination of viruses. Significantly, inapparent infections can confer protective immunity against subsequent challenge with virulent strains of the same agent. Several factors are involved in producing inapparent infections: 1) the nature of the virus (e.g., virulent or attenuated strains), 2) degree of host immunity, 3) appearance of viral interference, and 4) failure of the virus to reach the target organ (e.g., due to the blood-brain barrier).

Table 49.1.　Potential Consequences of Virus–Animal Relationships

1. Animal is resistant to viral infection—no relationship established
2. Asymptomatic or subclinical infection—recovery or persistent infection
3. Acute viral infection—death, recovery, or persistent infection
4. Chronic viral infection—recurrent clinical disease, or persistent infection
5. Tumor formation

Host Responses to Viral Infections

The resistance of animals to virus infection is dependent in part on factors that act indiscriminately on most viruses and are therefore called *nonspecific* or *innate* resistance factors. These include hormonal factors, temperature, inhibitors other than antibody, and phagocytes. Phagocytosis is an important defense mechanism in bacterial infections. However, many viral agents are capable of infecting lymphcytes and/or monocytes/macrophages, and thus these cells actually can serve as a vehicle to spread virus through the host.

Interferon

Interferons are a group of cell proteins (cytokines) that can modulate the immune system, regulate the differentiation of certain cells, confer antiviral resistance on sensitive cells, and exert anticancer effects. Many viruses will induce interferon synthesis in infected cells, and many cell types have the ability to synthesize interferon after appropriate stimulation. At least three different types of interferon can be produced in the course of a viral infection:

alpha, beta, and gamma. Two distinct mechanisms have been identified in interferon-treated cells (Fig 49.3). The first involves the production in interferon-treated cells of a protein kinase (P1/eIF2alpha kinase), which in the presence of double-stranded RNA, blocks initiation of protein synthesis by phosphorylating the protein synthesis initiating factor eIF-2. The other mechanism involves an enzyme, 2–5A synthetase, which, in the presence of adenosine triphosphate (ATP) and dsRNA, synthesizes a group of oligoadenylates collectively known as 2–5A. 2–5A in turn activates a specific endonuclease that degrades viral and cellular RNA and so inhibits protein synthesis.

Besides its action on viral replication, interferon exerts other effects on cells, including effects on cell multiplication and regulation of such cellular functions as phagocytosis, production of antibodies and lymphokines by lymphocytes, expression of cell surface antigens, and cytotoxicity of cellular immunity. Interferon plays an important role in host resistance to viral infection.

Humoral and Cellular Immunity

Viruses are antigenic and typically induce a strong immune response after infection. Humoral immune responses lead to the production of antibodies that can be demonstrated by the usual serologic procedures, such as complement-fixation, agglutination, precipitation, and gel diffusion techniques. The basic principles governing these tests are identical with those used in bacteriology. Serological reactions like viral neutralization are unique to viruses and play an important role in terminating primary viral infection, limiting viremia, and preventing disease and reinfection. When preparations of virus are mixed with appropriate antisera and the mixtures are inoculated in susceptible hosts, infection will not occur if

FIGURE 49.1.　*Modes of viral dissemination within the host.*

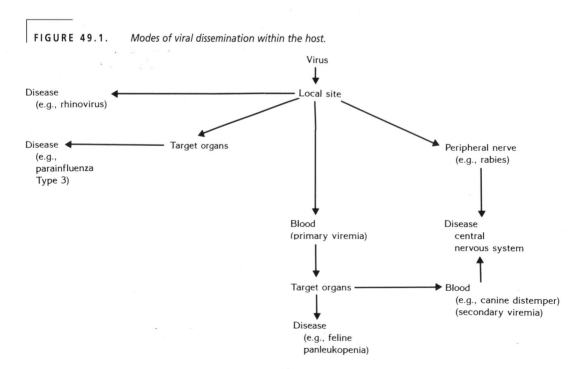

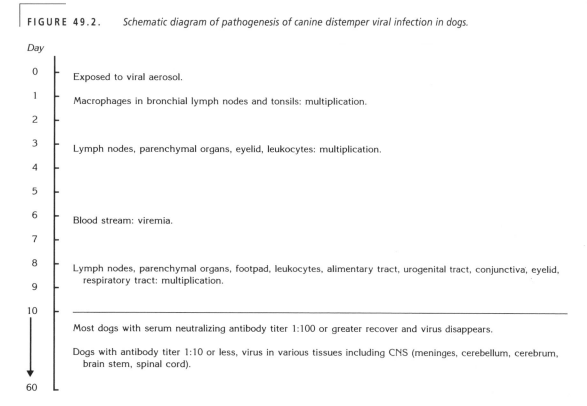

FIGURE 49.2. *Schematic diagram of pathogenesis of canine distemper viral infection in dogs.*

Figure 55.2. *Schematic diagram of pathogenesis of canine distemper viral infection in dogs.*

the antisera contain virus-neutralizing antibody. Three classes of immunoglobulins, IgG, IgM, and IgA, can serve as neutralizing antibodies. The interaction of virus and antibody, particularly antibodies specific to the viral antigens responsible for attachment to specific cell receptors, results in a virus-antibody complex formation that prevents attachment of virus to cell receptors, and to a lesser extent prevents the penetration of virus into the susceptible cell. It is possible to recover infectious virus from such apparently inert virus-antibody mixtures by simple dilution or centrifugation, suggesting that the virus and antibody may be linked in a loose combination in the initial stages of reaction. The interaction between virus and antibody does not physically alter viral structure; however, the complement system and antiviral antibody can induce lysis of enveloped viruses as well as destroy virus-infected cells.

Cellular immunity in viral infections, discussed in Chapter 2, is another important factor in host resistance to some viral infections. The destruction of virus-infected cells by immune lymphocytes can limit the dissemination of virus, particularly in instances where virus is transmitted from infected to noninfected cells through cell fusion. Recent evidence also indicates that macrophages play a role in host resistance to viral infections. Macrophages are key participants in the inflammatory response, and they can be activated either by interaction with viruses or by the soluble products produced by virus reacting with lymphocytes. Activated macrophages have been shown to participate in a wide range of host responses to viral infections, including phagocytosis of virus-antibody com-

plexes, production of interferon, cytotoxicity for virus-infected cells, and immunoregulatory functions.

Viral Immunosuppression

Several viruses of veterinary importance can infect lymphocytes, including canine distemper virus, feline panleukopenia virus, feline leukemia virus, bovine viral diarrhea virus, hog cholera virus, Newcastle disease virus, and infectious bursal disease virus of chickens. The destruction of lymphocytes and resultant atrophy of lymphoid tissues by the viruses can suppress or compromise immune response, predisposing the affected host to other opportunistic bacterial or viral infections.

A variety of spontaneous primary immune deficiency diseases occur in domestic animals (equine, bovine, ovine, porcine, canine, feline) that can predispose them to infectious diseases. A good example is the fatal respiratory tract infection of Arabian foals with combined immunodeficiency disorder (lack of production of functional T and B lymphocytes) by equine adenovirus.

Persistent Viral Infection

Persistent and latent virus infections are characterized by the fact that virus is not eliminated from the host. Disease may or may not occur in such chronically infected animals. Potential mechanisms of viral persistence include noncytocidal infection of host cells, destruction of im-

FIGURE 49.3. *Mechanisms of interferon action on protein synthesis.*

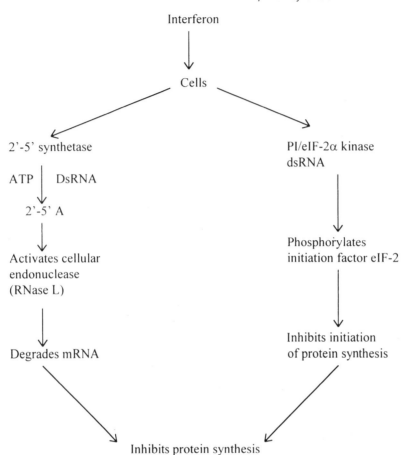

mune effector cells or growth within these cell types, evasion of protective host responses including cytokines and antibodies, and integration of the viral genome into that of the host cell. Persistent infections are those in which virus continuously is present, with or without expression of disease. Disease, when it does occur in persistently infected animals, often is a result of immunopathologic mechanisms. Latent infections are those in which virus is demonstrated only when reactivation (recrudescence) occurs; this is highly characteristic of herpesvirus infections.

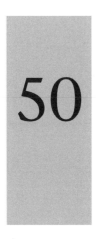

50

Parvoviridae and *Circoviridae*

YUAN CHUNG ZEE   N. JAMES MACLACHLAN

PARVOVIRIDAE

Parvoviruses are small (18–26 nm), nonenveloped icosahedral viruses that contain a linear single-stranded DNA genome (MW approximately 6×10^6 daltons). Members of the family *Parvoviridae*, genus *Parvovirus*, are the causative agents of specific diseases (Table 50.1). A variety of other animal parvoviruses have been identified, including chicken parvovirus, mink enteritis virus, mice minute virus, mouse parvovirus 1, and raccoon parvovirus.

FELINE PANLEUKOPENIA

Disease

Feline panleukopenia (syn. feline infectious enteritis) is a highly contagious, acute viral disease of cats characterized by high fever, anorexia, depression, vomiting followed by dehydration, diarrhea, and death. Leukopenia is characteristic of feline panleukopenia, and the severity of clinical disease often mirrors the severity of leukopenia. Cats of all ages are susceptible to infection, but mortality is highest among kittens. Cats can be infected by either the oral or respiratory routes, and the incubation period after infection is short. Intrauterine infection with feline panleukopenia virus may lead to neonatal death or congenital abnormalities of the central nervous system (CNS) manifested by cerebellar ataxia in kittens after birth; kittens up to 2 weeks of age are susceptible to the same teratogenic effects of feline panleukopenia virus infection.

Etiologic Agent

Physical, Chemical, and Antigenic Properties

Feline panleukopenia virus is a typical parvovirus. The virions are unenveloped (18–26 nm in diameter) with icosahedral symmetry. The genome is a single-stranded DNA molecule that includes two open reading frames, one of which encodes at least four proteins that mediate the functions required for transcription and DNA replication, and the other, which encodes the capsid proteins of the virus. VP3 constitutes the major capsid protein, and it appears to control tissue/cell tropism of the virus. Virus replication occurs within the nucleus of host cells and, because the virus lacks its own DNA polymerase, replication of parvoviruses requires cells that are cycling (late S phase or early G2 phase of the cell cycle) so that they can utilize host cell enzymes for their own replication.

Feline panleukopenia virus is closely related to canine parvovirus and to mink enteritis virus, although the three viruses can be distinguished by sequence analysis.

Resistance to Physical and Chemical Agents

Feline panleukopenia virus is very resistant to environmental factors and many commercial disinfectants. A 0.175% sodium hypochlorite solution (Clorox 1:30) is the most effective and practical virucidal disinfectant.

Infectivity for Other Species and Culture Systems

All members of the family *Felidae* are likely to be susceptible to infection with feline panleukopenia virus. A very closely related virus that is antigenically indistinguishable from feline panleukopenia virus causes enteritis in ranch mink, and the same virus can produce disease in raccoons and in coatimundi. Canine parvovirus Type 2 has emerged relatively recently, and it is ancestrally closely related to feline panleukopenia virus.

Feline panleukopenia virus grows in primary or continuous feline kidney cell cultures but not in canine cell cultures.

Host-Virus Relationship

Distribution, Reservoir, and Transmission

Feline panleukopenia occurs worldwide, and infected cats are the principal reservoir. Both infected cats suffering from acute disease and those having clinically inapparent infection excrete virus in their urine, feces, and various secretions. The infection spreads rapidly by contact with contaminated utensils, cages, and bedding, and the virus is highly stable in the environment.

Table 50.1.   Diseases Caused by Parvoviruses

Vernacular Name	Disease	Natural Host
Feline panleukopenia virus	Enteritis, ataxia	Cats
Mink enteritis virus	Enteritis	Mink
Canine parvovirus Type 2	Enteritis, myocarditis	Dogs
Porcine parvovirus	Stillbirth, mummification embryonic death, infertility	Swine
Bovine parvovirus	None	Cattle
Minute virus of canines[a]	None; diarrhea?	Dogs
Minute virus of mice	Developmental anomalies	Mice
Aleutian mink disease	Aleutian disease	Mink
Kilham rat virus	Developmental anomalies	Rats
Goose parvovirus	Hepatitis	Goose

[a] Also known as canine parvovirus Type 1.

Pathogenesis and Pathology

Cell-free viremia occurs for several days in kittens experimentally infected intranasally or orally with feline panleukopenia virus, during which the virus is disseminated throughout the body and infects cells with the necessary receptors. The virus then replicates in those cells that are in S phase of the cell cycle, particularly hematopoietic cells within the bone marrow and lymphoid tissues (thymus, spleen, and lymph nodes), leading to severe and protracted leukopenia that affects all white blood cell types and atrophy of lymphoid tissues. The rapidly dividing cells of the intestinal crypts also are highly susceptible to infection, which leads to marked destruction of the intestinal epithelium with resultant malabsorption diarrhea. Histologic lesions are characterized by necrosis of the epithelium of the intestinal crypts and marked destruction and depletion of lymphocytes in the lymph nodes, thymus, and spleen. Regenerative lymphoid hyperplasia may be present in the later phase of the disease.

In late term fetuses and very young kittens, the virus infects and destroys the cells within the external granular layer of the cerebellum, leading to cerebellar hypoplasia and atrophy as a consequence of failure of the internal granular layer to develop, and to degeneration and loss of Purkinje cells. Similar congenital lesions can be produced by in-utero infections of rats, hamsters, ferrets, and mice after infection at critical stages of gestation with the appropriate species of parvovirus.

Host Responses to Infection

Neutralizing antibodies first appear in cats at approximately 1 week after infection, and high titers of antibody generally are present after 10 to 12 days. Hemagglutination-inhibiting antibodies rise from the fourth day after infection, reaching a peak on the seventh day. These antibodies can persist in cats for several years. Maternal antibody with neutralizing titer of 30 or greater against feline panleukopenia virus protects kittens against viral infection, but it also interferes with active immunization by modified live or inactivated feline panleukopenia viral vaccines.

Laboratory Diagnosis

Clinical signs, the presence of leukopenia, and histopathological examination are useful for the presumptive diagnosis of feline panleukopenia. The diagnosis can be confirmed by one of the following laboratory methods: 1) isolation of feline panleukopenia virus from the feces or urine on feline kidney cells, 2) detection of viral antigen in infected tissues by capture ELISA or immunofluorescence staining with a feline panleukopenia virus-specific antisera conjugate, 3) polymerase chain reaction (PCR) amplification of viral nucleic acid, 4) serologic diagnosis is accomplished by enzyme-linked immunosorbent assay (ELISA) or indirect immunofluorescence, although paired sera are required to confirm the diagnosis.

Treatment and Control

There is no effective treatment for feline panleukopenia; thus control is achieved by vaccination, quarantine of cats that survive infection, and rigorous sterilization of premises that have housed affected cats. Highly effective inactivated and modified live feline panleukopenia viral vaccines are commercially available, although maternal antibodies can interfere with the immunization of young kittens.

CANINE PARVOVIRUS DISEASE

Disease

Parvoviral disease in dogs is characterized by the sudden onset of diarrhea, vomiting, anorexia, fever, depression, lymphopenia, and dehydration. Mortality is higher in puppies than adults. Very young puppies sometimes develop myocarditis without clinical signs of enteritis.

The disease occurs worldwide. It was first recognized in North America in 1978, but retrospective serological studies indicate that the virus rapidly spread around the world in the early 1970s to cause a subsequent global pandemic. Canine parvoviral disease is caused by canine parvovirus Type 2, which is a variant of feline panleukopenia virus. Canine parvovirus Type 2 has continued to evolve since it emerged in dogs, with the appearance of new variants that have been designated as canine parvovirus Type-2a and Type-2b. The minute virus of canines that does not produce disease in dogs has been designated as canine parvovirus Type 1.

Etiologic Agent

Physical, Chemical, and Antigenic Properties

Canine parvovirus Type 2 is very similar to feline panleukopenia virus.

Resistance to Physical and Chemical Agents

Parvovirus is very resistant to environmental factors, such as extremes of temperature, pH, and some disinfectants. The virus can persist for long periods in premises where infected dogs are kept and can be transmitted to other areas by fomites. It can be inactivated by common bleach such as Clorox (1:30).

Infectivity for Other Species and Culture Systems

Canine parvovirus Type 2 infects dogs of all breeds and other members of the family *Canidae*, such as wolves, foxes, and coyotes. Domestic cats without antibodies to the virus are susceptible to experimental infection but remain asymptomatic.

Canine parvovirus Type 2 can be propagated in primary cell cultures of canine or feline fetal lung and kidney, as well as continuous cell lines such as canine cell line A72 and feline cell lines NLFK and CRFK. The virus also grows in some cells from some other animal species.

Host-Virus Relationship

Distribution, Reservoir, and Transmission

Type 2 parvovirus infection of dogs and other members of the family *Canidae* is prevalent in many areas of the world. Parvovirus-infected dogs continue to excrete infectious virus in their feces for up to 10 days after the onset of infection, and the virus is readily transmitted between dogs by the feco-oral route.

Pathogenesis and Pathology

The pathogenesis of Type 2 parvovirus infection of dogs is similar to that of panleukopenia virus infection of cats, although cerebellar hypoplasia and atrophy is not recog-

nized as a consequence of in-utero infection of dogs with canine parvovirus. Similarly, myocarditis is a potential consequence of parvovirus infection of young pups, whereas it is not described in panleukopenia-virus infected kittens. Cell-free viremia precedes infection of the intestinal epithelium and lymphoid tissues, including thymus, tonsils, retropharyngeal and mesenteric lymph nodes, and spleen of infected puppies, and widespread infection of the intestinal mucosa occurs on about the sixth day after experimental inoculation. Fecal excretion of virus begins as soon as the third day after infection and peaks soon thereafter. Most infected dogs stop excreting virus by the twelfth day.

The most striking lesion of parvovirus enteritis in dogs is hemorrhage within the lumen of the small bowel and accompanying enlargement and edema of the mesenteric lymph nodes. Mottled white streaks within the myocardium are indicative of cardiac involvement in young puppies.

Microscopic lesions associated with canine parvoviral infection are confined to organs with large populations of rapidly proliferating cells, such as the small intestine, lymph nodes, and bone marrow. The most frequent findings in the small intestine are necrosis of crypt epithelium and atrophy of epithelial villi. Regeneration of intestinal epithelium occurs in dogs surviving the acute phase of enteric infection. Lymphocytolysis in the thymic cortex and germinal centers of lymph nodes is common and results in cellular depletion. In the myocardial form of parvoviral infection, the ventricular myocardium shows myofiber degeneration and necrosis that is accompanied by infiltration by mononuclear cells.

Host Response to Infection

Dogs infected with parvovirus rapidly develop high, long-lasting titers of virus neutralizing antibodies. The immunity that develops after natural infection appears to be lifelong in dogs that survive. Cellular immune responses also are generated during infection, and likely are important in limiting virus replication during acute infection.

Laboratory Diagnosis

Clinical signs, history, contrast radiography, and histopathological examinations are useful in a presumptive diagnosis of canine parvoviral disease. Laboratory procedures used to confirm the diagnosis include the following:

1. Isolation of canine parvovirus Type 2 from the feces or tissues of infected animals on susceptible cell cultures, or by identification of parvoviral nucleic acid in infected tissues by PCR.
2. Detection of parvoviral antigen in the histological sections of intestine by the immunofluorescent or immunohistochemical staining with virus-specific antibodies.
3. Demonstration of parvovirus in feces or infected tissue by electron microscopy or immunoelectron microscopy.
4. Identification of parvovirus in feces by hemagglutination test using swine or rhesus monkey red blood

cells and the specific hemagglutination-inhibition by anticanine parvovirus antiserum.

5. Detection of parvovirus in feces by ELISA using monoclonal antibodies to the canine parvovirus Type 2 hemagglutinating protein.

6. Demonstration of anticanine parvovirus antibody in serum by such serologic tests as hemagglutination inhibition, virus neutralization, or ELISA. The IgM-capture ELISA can be used to confirm recent infection of dogs.

Treatment and Control

Severe cases of canine parvoviral disease are characterized by marked dehydration and metabolic acidosis, thus supportive treatment relies on replacing lost body fluids and correcting disturbed electrolyte balance and acidosis. Broad-spectrum antibiotics are used to prevent secondary bacterial infections. Vaccination of susceptible canine populations remains the best prophylaxis for canine parvoviral infection. Antibody levels correlate directly with the degree of protection. Effective inactivated and modified live parvoviral vaccines are available, although the presence of maternal antibodies interferes with active immunization of puppies. Canine parvovirus is very resistant to environmental factors and can persist under adverse conditions for a long period, thus prompt disinfection of premises where infected animals are being kept and vaccination of puppies prior to their introduction to such premises are important in preventing this disease.

PORCINE PARVOVIRUS INFECTION

Disease

Infection of swine with porcine parvovirus occurs worldwide and sometimes leads to reproductive failure in swine and cutaneous lesions in piglets. Transplacental infection of fetuses leads to stillbirth, mummification, embryonic death and infertility, the so-called SMEDI syndrome. The porcine reproductive and respiratory syndrome virus is now considered to be a more important cause of SMEDI syndrome than porcine parvovirus.

Etiologic Agent

Physical, Chemical, and Antigenic Properties

Porcine parvovirus resembles feline and canine parvoviruses. There is only one serotype, and porcine parvovirus is antigenically different than other parvoviruses.

Resistance to Physical and Chemical Agents

Porcine parvovirus is very resistant to heat, enzymes, and most commercial disinfectants. The virus is inactivated by heat at 73°C for 30 minutes or at 70°C for 1 hour, or by exposure to 0.5% sodium hypochlorite for 5 minutes, to 0.06% potassium dichloroisocyanurate for 5 minutes, or to 3% formaldehyde for 1 hour.

Infectivity for Other Species and Culture Systems

Porcine parvovirus apparently infects only swine. The virus can be propagated on primary or secondary cultures of fetal porcine kidney cells and swine testicle cells.

Host-Virus Relationship

Distribution, Reservoir, and Transmission

Parvovirus infection is endemic in many herds, and infected swine serve as the reservoir of infection. Infected swine develop a viremia and shed virus in their oral secretions and feces. Since the porcine parvovirus can persist in the environment for long periods of time, contaminated premises serve as a major reservoir of virus that is responsible for its transmission to susceptible animals. Carrier boars also can disseminate the virus in their semen. Although rats may be infected experimentally with porcine parvovirus, they are unlikely to serve as natural reservoirs of the virus.

Pathogenesis and Pathology

Swine infected with porcine parvovirus produce antibodies without developing clinical disease or obvious lesions. Reproductive disease occurs when seronegative sows are exposed to the virus during gestation, and the consequences (fetal death with or without mummification, embryonic death, or infertility) of transplacental transmission of the virus are reflective of the gestational stage of the sow at infection. Lesions within stillborn fetuses are often nonspecific, but can include foci of necrosis and mononuclear cell infiltration in organs such as the liver, heart, kidney, and cerebrum.

Host Responses to Infection

Piglets and nonpregnant adult swine infected with porcine parvovirus develop viremia without obvious clinical disease. These animals develop a strong humoral immune response and are resistant to subsequent reinfection with the virus. Piglets acquire high titers of virus-specific antibodies through the colostrum of immune sows.

Laboratory Diagnosis

Parvovirus antigen can be detected in the tissues of affected fetuses by immunofluorescent or immunohistochemical staining or by capture ELISA. A PCR assay has also been developed for the detection of porcine parvovirus.

Treatment and Control

There is no treatment for reproductive failure produced by porcine parvovirus, and vaccination of breeding gilts remains the best method to ensure that gilts develop active immunity prior to being bred. Both inactivated and modified live vaccines are available, but vaccination must be carefully timed to ensure that animals are immunized after passive antibodies are lost and before the animals are bred.

ALEUTIAN DISEASE IN MINK

Disease

Aleutian disease (AD) in mink is a chronic progressive disease characterized by anorexia, polydipsia, severe anemia, and hemorrhages. The disease has a long incubation period. Characteristic features of the disease in adult minks are dissemianted plasmacytosis (aggregates of plasma cells in many tissues), uveitis, vascular damage, hypergamma-globulinemia, and glomerulonephritis, the last of which is caused by deposition of circulating immune complexes. In newborn mink kits, Aleutian disease virus (ADV) causes a fatal, acute interstitial pneumonitis. A genetic predisposition for the disease exists in Aleutian mink. It appears that mink homozygous for the recessive Aleutian gene have a genetic defect in preventing the clearance of circulating immune complexes.

Etiologic Agent

Physical, Chemical, and Antigenic Properties

Aleutian mink virus resembles the other parvoviruses that previously were described. The Aleutian disease virus is antigenically unrelated to mink enteritis virus, which is closely related to feline panleukopenia virus.

Resistance to Physical and Chemical Agents

Aleutian mink virus is inactivated by sodium hypochlorite, iodophor, glutaraldehyde, formalin, and phenols.

Infectivity for Other Species and Cell Systems

Aleutian disease virus infects mink of all types, although disease is more prevalent in the Aleutian mink. Ferrets can be infected with ADV, but they do not develop clinical signs of the disease. The virus can be propagated in fetal mink kidney cell cultures or in feline cell lines.

Host-Virus Relationship

Distribution, Reservoir, and Transmission

Aleutian disease of mink is present in many mink ranches worldwide. The virus is found in the blood, saliva, feces, and urine. Mink with overt clinical signs or with inapparent infection are the reservoirs of infection. The disease is transmitted by fecal-oral or respiratory routes.

Pathogenesis and Pathology

In mink experimentally infected with ADV, viral antigen is first detected in the intestine and kidney and subsequently in the spleen, liver, kidney, lymph nodes, and bone marrow. There is a significant increase in the amounts of gamma globulin and anti-DNA antibody in the sera of infected mink. The serum gamma globulin does not neutralize ADV, and immune complexes appear in circulation as early as 2 weeks after infection. The glomerular deposition of immune complexes results in glomerulonephritis.

Host Responses to Infection

Hypergammaglobulinemia (predominantly IgG) is the most prominent feature of mink infected with ADV, but the presence of this antibody does not facilitate virus clearance.

Laboratory Diagnosis

Solid-phase radioimmune assay, direct immunofluorescence, and immunoperoxidase staining techniques can be used to demonstrate AD viral antigen in tissues. The counterimmunoelectrophoresis (CIE) test for AD viral antibody can be used to identify infected mink.

Treatment and Control

No effective vaccines have been developed for the AD of mink. Control is achieved through the isolation and/or elimination of affected animals.

CIRCOVIRIDAE

Circoviruses recently have been shown to be important pathogens of animals. Like parvoviruses they are small nonenveloped icosahedral viruses (approximately 12–26 nm) with a genome of single-stranded DNA. Important viruses within the family *Circoviridae* include beak and feather disease virus, chicken infectious anemia virus, and porcine circovirus. A pathogenic circovirus also has been identified in pigeons, and similar viruses infect humans as well as other bird species.

BEAK AND FEATHER DISEASE

Disease

Beak and feather disease (BFD) is a disease of psitaccine birds. The severity of BFD varies with the age and species of the affected bird. The characteristic changes associated with BFD are the appearance of necrotic and abnormal feathers (feathers that are bent, contain hemorrhages, or are prematurely shed), although the pattern of abnormal feathering varies with the age of the bird at infection. Beak and nail deformities occur in some chronically affected birds. Severe, acute disease characterized by pneumonia, enteritis, rapid weight loss, and death is particularly common in neonatal cockatoos and African grey parrots, and death may occur in these birds before feather abnormalities occur.

Etiologic Agent

Physical, Chemical, and Antigenic Properties

Virions of BFD virus are approximately 19–26 nm, nonenveloped, with a genome of circular single-stranded DNA that is transcribed to produce a single, polycistronic mRNA that encodes at least three proteins.

Resistance to Physical and Chemical Agents

Although the specific properties of BFD virus remain to be determined, other circoviruses are resistant to low pH (pH 3), high temperature (>70°C), as well as many chemicals, such as chloroform, ether, and alcohol.

Infectivity for Other Species and Culture Systems

The BFD virus appears to infect only psittacine birds, and it has yet to be propagated in cell culture systems.

Host-Virus Relationship

Distribution, Reservoir, and Transmission

Psittacine BFD has been described among birds in North America, Europe, Asia, and Australia. The virus likely has been disseminated by the movement of infected Australian psittacine birds, because BFD virus is endemic in free-ranging populations of several psittacine species in Australia, notably cockatoos. A wide variety of cockatoos, parrots, lovebirds, and parakeets are susceptible to BFD. The virus is spread directly between infected and susceptible birds by aerosol or by fomites. The feather dust, excretions, and secretions from infected birds all contain BFD virus, and the virus is very stable and resistant in the environment. Vertical transmission of the virus from infected birds to their chicks also may contribute to dissemination of the virus.

Pathogenesis and Pathology

The majority of free-ranging and captive birds exposed to BFD virus develop only subclinical infections and are resistant to reinfection. The age of the bird at initial exposure, the presence and levels of protection provided by maternal antibody, and the route and titer of the infecting virus all likely influence the outcome. The incubation period of BFD virus infection is often prolonged, and signs of disease including death may not occur until long after initial infection. Acute or peracute death occurs in very young birds that lack maternal immunity. Affected young birds may exhibit inappetance, lethargy, crop-stasis, progressive feather abnormalities, and eventual death. Death in some birds likely is a consequence of secondary infections, perhaps associated with immune suppression. Histologic lesions are dependent on the duration and severity of the disease in individual birds, but characteristic intranuclear and intracytoplasmic inclusion bodies may be present in the epithelial cells lining the feather shaft, and in macrophages in the thymus, bursa, and other lymphoid tissues.

Host Responses to Infection

Birds that previously were exposed to BFD virus are resistant to reinfection. Maternal antibodies likely provide passive protection of chicks against BFD virus infection for several weeks after birth.

Laboratory Diagnosis

Diagnosis of BFD currently is dependent on identification of the clinical signs and characteristic gross and histologic changes in the tissues of affected birds. Both nucleic acid hybridization and immunohistochemical staining assays can be used to detect BFD virus in the tissues of affected birds.

Treatment and Control

Control of BFD currently is dependent on the elimination or quarantine of carrier birds to prevent transmission of BFD virus to susceptible cohorts. Several vaccines have been developed to prevent BFD virus infection, but they currently are not widely available.

CHICKEN INFECTIOUS ANEMIA

Chicken infectious anemia (CIA) is a disease of young chickens (2–4 weeks of age), characterized by aplastic anemia, generalized lymphoid atrophy, and profound immune suppression that leads to secondary (opportunistic) viral, bacterial, and fungal infections. Birds become resistant to CIA disease after approximately 3 weeks of age, but the disease causes serious economic losses to the poultry industry worldwide. Genetically distinct strains of CIA virus are recognized, although these are antigenically similar or identical and there is little difference in the virulence of individual strains. CIA virus is highly resistant to most treatments. The virus is infectious only to chickens, although related viruses may infect other bird species. The CIA virus can be propagated in chicken embryos, day-old chicks, and in avian T and B lymphocyte lines. Diagnosis is by virus isolation, PCR detection of the virus, or immunohistochemical staining of the tissues of affected birds, using CIA virus-specific antibodies. Serological assays (ELISA, indirect immunofluorecsence, and virus neutralization) have been developed for serological detection of CIA virus infection of birds. The virus is disseminated both horizontally and vertically, and vaccination of breeding flocks with modified live virus is used to prevent vertical transmission of the virus. No specific treatment is available for chickens infected with CIA virus.

PORCINE POSTWEANING MULTISYSTEMIC WASTING SYNDROME

Two distinct types of porcine circovirus (Types 1 and 2) have been identified in pigs. Type 1 porcine circovirus originally was identified as a cell culture contaminant and is not known to cause any disease in pigs. In contrast, Type 2 porcine circovirus recently was incriminated as the cause of postweaning multisystemic wasting syndrome (PMWS) in swine. PMWS is an economically important disease of young pigs that is characterized by generalized lymph node enlargement, chronic pneumonia, and weight loss. Characteristic histologic lesions include generalized lymphoid depletion and granulomatous inflammation. Macrophages in affected lymphoid tissues may contain basophilic inclusion bodies. Whereas Type 2 circovirus infection is ubiquitous in swine herds, PMWS occurs only sporadically in susceptible swine, suggesting that other factors may potentiate development of PWMS in circovirus-infected pigs. The porcine circovirus Type 2 may be detected in the tissues of pigs by immunohistochemistry, in situ hybridization, or by PCR assay. The virus can be propagated in cell culture, and ELISA assays have been developed for serological detection of Type 2 circovirus infection of swine.

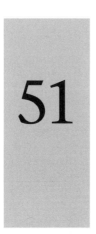

51

Asfarviridae and *Iridoviridae*

N. James MacLachlan   Jeffrey L. Stott

ASFARVIRIDAE

The *Asfarviridae* includes just one genus, the genus *Asfivirus,* of which African swine fever virus is the type species.

African Swine Fever Virus

Disease

African swine fever (ASF) is a highly contagious disease of domestic and some species of wild swine. Disease in ASF virus-infected pigs ranges from peracute to chronic and inapparent; incursions of the virus into native populations of domestic swine typically result in extensive outbreaks of acute ASF, and the subacute and chronic forms appear after the virus becomes established in the pig population. Acute, severe ASF has a high mortality, often approaching 100%, and death may occur prior to development of clinical signs. The disease is characterized by high fever and leukopenia, often followed by the appearance of erythema (red areas on the skin), weakness, accelerated respiration and pulse, vomiting, bloody diarrhea, and nasal and conjunctival discharges. Subacute ASF is characterized by less dramatic clinical signs and death or recovery in 3 to 4 weeks. Affected pigs typically experience a high fever; abortion is common and may be the only sign of illness. Pigs with chronic ASF fail to thrive (stunting and emaciation), and exhibit swollen joints and lameness, skin ulcerations, and pneumonia.

Etiologic Agent

Physical, Chemical, and Antigenic Properties

African swine fever virus is an enveloped DNA virus with a nucleoprotein core of 70–100 nm that is surrounded by lipid layers and an icosahedral capsid of 170–190 nm in diameter. The virion is surrounded by a lipid-containing envelope (Fig 51.1). The genome is a single large (170–190 kilo bases) molecule of double-stranded DNA that includes approximately 150 open reading frames. Virions contain more than 50 different proteins, including a large number

of enzymes and proteins required for replication. The viral genome also encodes proteins that appear to modulate the protective host antiviral response.

Several genetically distinct groups of ASF virus have been identified by restriction endonuclease analysis of the genomes of ASF viruses isolated in different regions of the world. Strains of ASF virus can vary markedly in their virulence in swine.

Resistance to Physical and Chemical Agents

African swine fever virus is stable in tissues and excretions. The virus can withstand a considerable range in pH (pH 4 to 13). The ASF virus is inactivated by heating to 60°C for 20 minutes and by lipid solvents and some disinfectants (paraphenylphenolic disinfectants are very effective against the virus).

Infectivity for Other Species and Culture Systems

African swine fever virus infects domestic and wild pigs (including European wild boars), warthogs, giant forest hogs and bush pigs. Soft ticks of the genus *Ornithodoros* transmit the virus as biological vectors. Only domestic and wild pigs (feral pigs and European wild boars) express clinical disease, whereas African wild pigs do not.

African swine fever virus replicates in pig macrophages, and can be propagated in vitro on cultures of swine bone marrow cells, monocytes, and alveolar macrophages. The virus can also be adapted to various established cell lines (pig kidney, VERO, and BHK).

Host-Virus Relationship

Distribution, Reservoir, and Transmission

African swine fever was first described in European domestic pigs in Kenya in the early 1900s, and the disease regularly has emerged into other regions of the world since that time. The disease spread outside of Africa for the first time in 1957 when it appeared on the Iberian Peninsula, and subsequently has occurred in Mediterranean Europe (Spain, France, Italy, Malta, Sardinia), northern Europe (Belgium and the Netherlands), the Caribbean (Cuba, the Dominican Republic, and Haiti), and South America

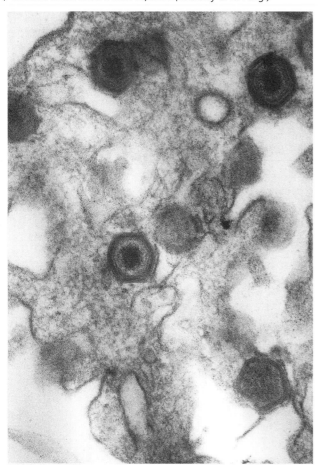

FIGURE 51.1. *African swine fever virus in thin section of infected tissue culture cells. 58,000X. (Courtesy of IC Pang.)*

Pathogenesis and Pathology

Following oral or nasal exposure of domestic pigs to ASF virus, virus replication initially occurs in the upper respiratory tract with subsequent dissemination to adjacent lymph nodes and then systemic spread via leukocytes, erythrocytes, or both in the lymph and blood; this occurs within 3 days postinfection and corresponds closely with the onset of pyrexia. The virus replicates in macrophages; thus highest titers of virus occur in those tissues in which macrophages are most abundant.

Acute severe ASF is characterized by edema and hemorrhage within internal organs, particularly the lymph nodes and spleen, which can be very large and intensely hemorrhagic. Pulmonary edema and intestinal congestion and hemorrhage also are common. The lesions of subacute ASF are similar but less pronounced, whereas animals with chronic ASF may show fibrinous pericarditis and pleuritis, lobular consolidation of the lungs, swollen joints, and patchy necrosis of the skin. Lesions in aborted piglets are relatively nonspecific, but may include disseminated petechial hemorrhages.

Microscopic lesions are most pronounced in the lymphoid tissues, and include extensive necrosis of both lymphocytes and mononuclear phagocytic cells. Endothelial cell necrosis and thrombosis of the pulmonary vasculature is common in fulminant cases of acute ASF.

Host Responses to Infection

Pigs that survive infection with ASF virus develop a strong humoral immune (antibody) response; however, this response is largely ineffectual in neutralizing the virus. Why the antibody response of swine to ASF is largely ineffectual remains uncertain, but it clearly is a reflection of the inherent properties of ASF virus itself. Nevertheless, efforts at developing an effective vaccine are complicated by the inability of swine to produce high titers of neutralizing antibodies to the virus.

Laboratory Diagnosis

Laboratory tests are required to distinguish between hog cholera and ASF, because the two diseases cause very similar signs and lesions in susceptible pigs, including fever, high mortality, and hemorrhages within internal organs. Tissues submitted should include spleen, liver, lymph nodes, and blood. Virus isolation can be used to identify ASF virus, and then confirmed with hemadsorption. Immunofluorescent or immunoperoxidase staining of sections of tissue from affected pigs using ASF virus-specific antisera provides a rapid method of diagnosis. Techniques based on polymerase chain reaction (PCR) can also be used to rapidly identify the presence of ASF virus genomic material.

Treatment and Control

There is no effective vaccine or treatment for ASF. Eradication of the disease is accomplished by slaughter and dis-

(Brazil). African swine fever has been described throughout much of Africa.

The ASF virus exists in two distinct cycles of infection: first, a sylvatic cycle in ticks and wild pigs in Africa; and, second, epidemic and endemic cycles in domestic swine. The reservoirs of the sylvatic cycle of ASF virus infection in Africa are persistent or inapparent infections in African wild pigs (warthogs in particular) and the soft tick vector. Vertical transmission of ASF virus in the tick vector makes them an especially efficient reservoir of the virus. The virus spreads into domestic swine through the bites of infected ticks, or by ingestion of tissues from carrier swine. The virus then is readily transmitted to susceptible pigs by direct contact, including aerosols and fomites. The virus is easily transmitted over long distances because of its stability in infected tissues, including uncooked and some cured pork products. Importantly, soft ticks become infected with the virus after they feed on viremic swine, and thus they can become reservoirs of the virus after it incurs into previously noninfected regions. Pigs that survive infection with ASF virus become carriers of the virus.

posal of all exposed pigs after the virus incurs into new areas. These drastic measures, however, may not prevent the virus from spreading to the local populations of soft ticks and wild pigs. Premises that undergo eradication procedures must not only slaughter all pigs but also must be treated with insecticides and disinfectant containing O-phenylphenol with surfactants and must remain free of livestock for at least a month. Prior to restocking, susceptible sentinel animals should be placed on the premises to confirm eradication of the virus.

IRIDOVIRIDAE

The family *Iridoviridae* includes four genera (genus *Iridovirus, Chloriridovirus, Ranavirus,* and *Lymphocystisvirus*) that are serologically distinct. Viruses in the genera *Ranavirus* and *Lymphocystisvirus* cause important diseases of fish.

Iridoviruses are enveloped viruses that have icosahedral symmetry with a virion diameter of 120–200 nm but occasionally up to 350 nm. The genome is a single molecule of double-stranded DNA of between 140 and 300 kilo base pairs. Iridoviruses, like asfarviruses, are structurally complex with large numbers of virus-specific proteins (at least 36) encoded by the genome. A single protein constitutes the majority of the outer capsid. The double-stranded DNA genome is circular and terminally redundant with many of the internal cytosine residues being highly methylated. Definitive diagnosis is best made by viral isolation and/or characterization of the genome by molecular biology techniques.

Lymphocystis virus infects a wide variety of fish and causes unsightly wart-like cutaneous lesions. These lesions consist of benign proliferations of hypertrophied, virus-infected cells (fibroblasts and osteoblasts) on the skin, peritoneum, and mesentery. The lesions typically resolve with minimal mortality. The virus spreads by direct contact through abrasions, especially when fish are crowded; thus disease caused by lymphocystis virus is especially important in fish raised in aquaria and in some commercial aquaculture operations. Two strains of lymphocystis disease virus (LCDV) have been described, with LCDV-1 being associated with flounder and LCDV-2 being associated with dabs. In contrast, the *Ranavirus* genus has been associated with high mortality in both farmed and free-ranging fish. These pathogenic iridoviruses causing fatal systemic disease are closely related to frog virus 3 (FV3), the latter serving as the prototype ranavirus. Members of this genus have been reported to cause epizootic hematopoietic necrosis and systemic hemorrhagic disease in fish.

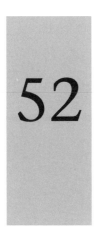

52

Papillomaviridae and *Polyomaviridae*

Yuan Chung Zee   N. James MacLachlan

PAPILLOMAVIRIDAE

The papillomaviruses are widespread among mammals, having been identified in cattle, sheep, goats, deer, elk, horses, rabbits, dogs, monkeys, pigs, opossums, mice, elephants, and several species of birds. Cottontail rabbit papillomavirus is the type species. Virus-induced papillomas (warts) are benign, hyperplastic epithelial proliferations of the skin or mucous membranes that may undergo malignant transformation in certain circumstances. Some papillomaviruses also cause proliferations of mesenchymal tissues in the skin, with or without associated epithelial proliferations. Those proliferations with exclusively epithelial proliferation are papillomas, whereas those with proliferation of both mesenchymal (fibrous tissue) and epithelial tissue are termed fibropapillomas. Papillomaviruses are highly species-specific, and thus are generally contagious only to the animal species in which they naturally occur. Virus-induced cutaneous papillomas (warts) are common in horses and cattle and infrequent in dogs, sheep, and goats. Not all papillomas are caused by viruses, and papillomaviruses have yet to be identified in cats.

Etiologic Agents

Papillomaviruses have naked icosahedral capsids approximately 55 nm in diameter (Fig 52.1). The viral genome is a single circular molecule of double-stranded DNA that encodes between 8 and 10 proteins; 2 are structural (L1 and L2) and the remainder are nonstructural proteins that are essential for virus replication.

Papilloma Types

Papillomaviruses are highly restricted in both their host specificity, tissue and cell tropism, and sequence relatedness. They are distinguished also on the basis of the lesions they induce, including skin papillomas (warts), proliferation of nonstratified squamous epithelium (polyps), and subcutaneous fibromas with or without associated cutaneous papillomas (fibropapillomas).

BOVINE PAPILLOMAVIRUSES

At least six types of bovine papilloma virus are distinguished on the basis of their antigenic and nucleotide sequence homologies. They can be further distinguished on the basis of the nature of the lesions that they cause in cattle. Cutaneous fibropapillomas (warts) caused by papillomaviruses Types 1, 2, and 5 occur commonly in calves less than two years old. They appear most frequently on the head, especially in the skin around the eyes. They may also appear on the sides of the neck and less commonly on other parts of the body. They begin as small, nodular growths that then grow rapidly into dry, horny, whitish, cauliflower-like masses that eventually regress spontaneously. The histological appearance is a variable mixture of proliferating dermal fibrous tissue and overlying epithelium. Infectious papillomas (without a fibrous tissue component) that occur on the skin and teats of dairy cattle are also associated with infection by bovine papillomaviruses, as are some epithelial proliferations (polyps) that occur in the bladder and gastrointestinal tract, particularly those that affect the esophagus, forestomachs, and intestines.

Fibropapilloma is a papillomavirus-induced tumor that occurs on the penis of young bulls and the vagina and vulva of young heifers. These are fleshy, raised multinodular proliferations that consist of abundant fibrous tissue covered by epithelium of variable thickness.

Host immune responses eventually control papillomavirus infections because most warts persist for variable periods and usually spontaneously regress. The host is then immune to reinfection with the same virus, but not to other types of bovine papillomavirus. Treatment of bovine papillomatosis with finely ground wart tissue suspended in a 0.4% formalin solution has been used for many years to combat outbreaks of the disease, but it is difficult to evaluate the efficacy of this procedure since the disease is self-limiting and its duration varies between individual animals. A significant proportion of vaccinated animals apparently fail to reject their warts after vaccination with autologous tumor preparations. Cattle vaccinated with the L2 structural protein of bovine papillomavirus Type 4 did not develop alimentary papillomas when challenged with that virus type.

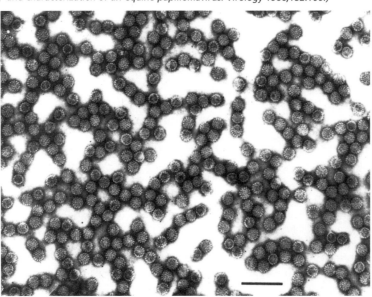

EQUINE PAPILLOMAVIRUS AND EQUINE SARCOIDS

Skin warts of horses are not as common as those affecting cattle. They develop most often on the nose and around the lips of young horses, appearing as small, elevated, papillary (horny) masses. They also occur in the inner aspects of ear (aural plaques). The causative virus is spread by direct contact of infectious material through wounds and cutaneous abrasions. The virus can be experimentally transmitted to horses by intradermal inoculation of a suspension of wart tissue, but not to other animal species. Equine papillomas are usually self-limiting and disappear spontaneously in 4 to 8 weeks, although they can progress to squamous cell carcinoma in rare instances. Natural infection provides solid immunity.

Sarcoids are common skin tumors of horses that grossly and histologically resemble fibropapillomas of cattle. Interestingly, the genome of bovine papillomavirus (Types 1 or 2) is present within some of these tumors, whereas that of equine papillomavirus is not. Sarcoids have been reproduced by direct inoculation of bovine papillomavirus into susceptible horses. The tumors range from being largely epithelial in nature to intensely fibroblastic, and the histological diagnosis is dependent on demonstrating both epithelial and mesenchymal components to the tumor. Sarcoids are frequently multiple in affected horses, and they commonly are ulcerated. Recurrence after surgical removal is common, but metastasis has not been described; thus they are not malignant tumors despite their locally aggressive behavior.

CANINE ORAL PAPILLOMAVIRUS

Canine papillomavirus induces warts in the mouths of dogs. The warts generally develop on the lips and spread to the buccal mucosa, tongue, palate, and pharynx. The warts are usually benign and disappear spontaneously after several months. Dogs recovered from the infection develop immunity to reinfection. The infection is highly contagious, often spreading through all the dogs in a kennel. Warts have been experimentally transmitted by rubbing pieces of wart tissue on scarified mucous membranes of susceptible dogs. Under such conditions the incubation period was from 4 to 6 weeks. Infectious venereal papillomas (warts) also have been described in dogs.

POLYOMAVIRIDAE

Polyomaviruses have not been associated with diseases of domestic animals with the notable exception of an avian polyomavirus that causes an acute generalized infection in fledgling budgerigars. Polyomaviruses are nonenveloped 40 nm in diameter, with an icosahedral capsid and a genome of a single molecule of circular double-stranded DNA. The genome encodes at least three structural and five nonstructural proteins.

53 *Adenoviridae*

Yuan Chung Zee   N. James MacLachlan

Adenoviruses have been isolated from many species of animals, but it is likely that additional animal adenoviruses exist that have not yet been identified. The host range of individual adenoviruses frequently is highly restricted. Although adenovirus infections of animals are often asymptomatic or subclinical, some adenoviruses are pathogenic and cause respiratory and/or systemic diseases. Table 53.1 lists the diseases of domestic animals caused by adenoviruses.

The family *Adenoviridae* is divided into two genera: *Mastadenovirus,* which includes adenoviruses that infect mammals, and *Aviadenovirus,* which includes adenoviruses that infect birds. Members of these two genera do not share a common group antigen. Adenovirus virions are nonenveloped icosahedrons that are 70 nm to 90 nm in diameter and are composed of 252 capsomers (Fig 53.1). Extended fibers project from the virion surface. The genome of adenoviruses is a large molecule (26–45 kilo bases) of double-stranded DNA. Approximately 40 different proteins are encoded by the adenovirus genome. Adenoviruses replicate in the nucleus of infected cells.

INFECTIOUS CANINE HEPATITIS (CANINE ADENOVIRUS 1)

Disease

Infectious canine hepatitis (ICH) is a disease of dogs caused by canine adenovirus 1 (CAV-1). Although once an important disease of dogs, ICH is increasingly rare in much of the world, perhaps as a result of widespread vaccination. The majority of infections are asymptomatic, but the disease in susceptible dogs is characterized by fever, hepatic necrosis, and widespread hemorrhage as a consequence of vascular injury. Affected dogs may exhibit increased thirst, anorexia, tonsillitis, petechial hemorrhages on the mucous membranes, and diarrhea, and be reluctant to move. During the acute phase of illness, dogs may also develop conjunctivitis and photophobia. Severe ICH is most likely to occur in pups that are not immune to the disease.

Most dogs that survive acute ICH recover uneventfully, but transient corneal edema may occur in some convalescent animals after acute signs disappear. The CAV-1 also has been implicated as a cause of chronic progressive hepatitis and interstitial nephritis, but its role in spontaneous occurrence of these disorders in dogs is highly conjectural (CAV-1 is most unlikely to be a significant cause of either of these two common diseases of dogs).

Etiologic Agent

Physical, Chemical, and Antigenic Properties

Canine adenovirus Type 1 (CAV-1) is antigenically related but distinct from canine adenovirus 2. Canine adenovirus 1 is morphologically similar to other adenoviruses, but antigenically distinct.

Resistance to Physical and Chemical Agents

CAV-1 is resistant to ether, alcohols, and chloroform. It is stable for at least 30 minutes at a wide range of pH (3 to 9), and is also stable in soiled material at room temperature for several days. Viral infectivity is lost after heating for 10 minutes at 50 to 60°C. Steam cleaning and treatment with iodine, phenol, sodium hydroxide, or lysol are effective means of disinfection.

Infectivity for Other Species and Culture Systems

Canine adenovirus 1 causes clinical disease in dogs and other Canids (wolves, foxes, and coyotes). Skunks and bears also are susceptible. Infection in foxes can manifest as encephalitis. Canine adenovirus 1 replicates well in canine kidney cells.

Although some strains of CAV-1 and CAV-2 are oncogenic in inoculated hamsters, these viruses have not been associated with neoplastic disease in dogs.

Host-Virus Relationship

Distribution, Reservoir, and Transmission

Infectious canine hepatitis has a worldwide distribution, although clinical disease is increasingly rare. The infection is spread through the urine of infected dogs. Dogs may retain virus in their kidneys and shed it in urine for months after infection.

Pathogenesis and Pathology

Following aerosol infection, the virus localizes in the tonsils and spreads to regional lymph nodes and then to the

Table 53.1.   Diseases of Domestic Animals Caused by Adenoviruses

Virus	Type of Disease
Mastadenovirus	
Bovine adenovirus, Types 1–10	Conjunctivitis, pneumonia, diarrhea, polyarthritis
Canine adenovirus Type 1 (CAV-1; infectious canine hepatitis)	Hemorrhagic and hepatic
Canine adenovirus Type 2	Respiratory
Equine adenovirus Types 1–2	Respiratory
Ovine adenoviruses Types 1–6	Respiratory and enteric
Porcine adenoviruses Types 1–4	Diarrhea or meningoencephalitis, or both
Deer adenovirus	Systemic vasculitis, with hemorrhage and pulmonary edema
Aviadenovirus	
Chicken adenoviruses Types 1–12	Respiratory disease, enteric disease, egg-drop syndrome, aplastic anemia, atrophy of the bursa of Fabricius
Turkey adenoviruses Types 1–4	Respiratory disease, enteritis, marble spleen disease

Deer adenovirus, egg-drop syndrome virus of poultry, bovine adenovirus 4, and duck adenovirus 1 are proposed to be members of a new genus *Atadenovirus*; similarly, hemorrhagic enteritis of turkeys virus and marble spleen disease of pheasants virus are proposed to be members of a new genus *Siadenovirus*.

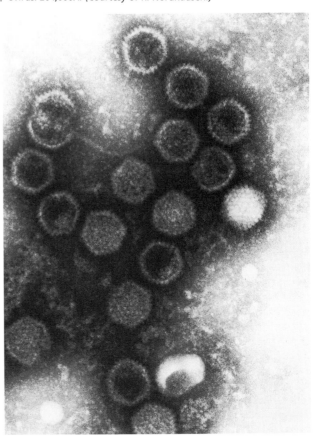

FIGURE 53.1.   *Negatively stained preparations of avian adenovirus. 204,000X. (Courtesy of R. Nordhausen.)*

systemic circulation. Viremia results in rapid dissemination of virus to all body tissues and secretions, including saliva, urine, and feces. The virus has a particular tropism for hepatocytes and endothelial cells, which produces the characteristic signs of the disease. Virus-induced injury to endothelial cells leads to consumptive coagulopathy (disseminated intravascular coagulation) and a generalized bleeding tendency (hemorrhagic diathesis) that is reflected by abnormal clotting parameters.

Dogs that die during the acute phase generally have edema and hemorrhage of superficial lymph nodes and cervical subcutaneous tissue. The abdominal cavity often contains fluid, which may vary in color from clear to bright red. Hemorrhages are present on all serosal surfaces. A fibrinous exudate may cover the liver, which can be swollen and congested. The gall bladder characteristically is edematous. Large characteristic intranuclear inclusion bodies may be present in hepatocytes, vascular endothelium, and macrophages.

The ocular lesions that develop in some dogs that recover from ICH are the result of deposition of immune complexes within the ciliary body of the eye.

Host Response to Infections

Recovery from ICH, regardless of the severity of illness, results in long-lasting immunity that likely is lifelong. Recovered animals have high titers of neutralizing antibody to CAV-1.

Laboratory Diagnosis

The diagnosis of ICH can be confirmed by serologic testing (complement fixation, hemagglutination inhibition, enzyme-linked immunosorbent assay [ELISA]) to demonstrate rising titers of antibody to CAV-1, polymerase chain reaction (PCR) detection of viral nucleic acid or virus isolation from affected tissues, or immunohistochemical staining of tissues with CAV-1–specific antibodies.

Treatment and Control

Therapy for dogs that develop ICH involves supportive and symptomatic treatment. Control is by vaccination and strict sanitation of affected premises with quarantine of exposed dogs. Available vaccines include both inactivated and modified live virus varieties, including CAV-2 vaccines that induce heterologous protection against CAV-1. CAV-2 vaccines do not induce immune complex uveitis in dogs as do some other modified live virus vaccines. Care must be exercised to ensure that maternal antibodies do not interfere with active immunization of pups, because vaccination success is directly related to the level of neutralizing antibody.

CANINE ADENOVIRUS TYPE 2

Canine adenovirus Type 2 (CAV-2) has been isolated from dogs with acute cough and is one of several infectious agents implicated in infectious tracheobronchitis (kennel cough). Experimental infection produces mild pharyngitis, tonsillitis, and tracheobronchitis, and virus persists in the respiratory tract for up to 28 days. Unlike CAV-1, CAV-2 does not produce generalized disease, is not excreted in the urine, and does not produce renal and ocular lesions. CAV-2 is antigenically related to CAV-1, and CAV-2 vaccines have been developed as ICH vaccine since they do not produce postvaccinal ocular lesions.

BOVINE ADENOVIRUSES

The bovine adenoviruses (BAV) are currently classified into ten serotypes (BAV 1–10), of which BAV 3 and BAV 5 appear to be more pathogenic than the other serotypes. Adenoviruses typically produce pneumonia or enteritis but only in very young or immunosupressed cattle. Adenoviruses are frequently isolated from apparently normal cattle, and serologic surveys indicate that asymptomatic or subclinical BAV infection of cattle occurs worldwide. Bovine adenovirus 3 can produce mild pneumonia in susceptible calves, with necrosis of the epithelium lining terminal airways in the lungs, causing necrotizing bronchiolitis with characteristic intranuclear inclusion bodies in the affected epithelial cells.

Immunocompetent calves inoculated with bovine adenoviruses develop neutralizing antibodies in 10 to 14 days, and immunity after natural infection is long-lasting. Diagnosis requires viral isolation or serology. Bovine adenoviruses can be isolated from rectal, nasal, or conjunctival swabs. Most types do not produce characteristic cytopathogenic effects until after several blind passages.

Although no vaccines are licensed for use in the United States, there is limited use of vaccines against BAV 1, 3, and 4 in Europe.

EQUINE ADENOVIRUS

Adenovirus infection rarely results in respiratory tract disease in healthy horses, and immunocompetent foals normally develop either subclinical or asymptomatic infections. However, Arabian foals with severe combined immunodeficiency (SCID) are highly susceptible to infection with equine adenovirus 1. The respiratory disease induced by equine adenovirus in SCID Arabian foals is protracted and characterized by coughing, dyspnea, and fever. These foals also develop generalized adenovirus infections, with involvement of a variety of organs and tissues.

There are two serotypes of equine adenovirus, as determined by serum neutralization. For laboratory diagnosis, virus may be isolated from infective tissue and nasal and ocular swab material in equine fetal kidney or equine fetal dermis cell cultures. The virus can be identified by electron microscopy or by immunofluorescent (IF) or immunohistochemical staining of infected tissues. Adenovirus nucleic acid also can be detected by PCR assay. Viral neutralization and hemagglutination-inhibition test are used to detect the presence and rise of antibody titers for serological diagnosis of adenovirus infections.

There is no commercially available vaccine.

OVINE ADENOVIRUSES

Adenoviruses have been isolated from the feces of apparently normal sheep and from lambs with respiratory disease. Six serotypes have been identified. The pathogenic role of most of the ovine adenoviruses is uncertain because they typically produce only mild or inapparent infection of the respiratory or gastrointestinal tracts. However, apparent outbreaks of adenovirus-induced pneumonia and enteritis have been described in lambs, as have sporadic cases of generalized (systemic) infections of very young lambs.

DEER ADENOVIRUS

A unique adenovirus recently was identified as the cause of a fatal systemic hemorrhagic disease of mule deer (including black-tailed deer). The virus originally was identified as the cause of extensive outbreaks of fatal disease in mule deer in North America (California), but subsequently has been recognized to have a much wider distribution. A similar disease has also been identified in moose. The causative adenovirus is genetically unique and is serologically related to some adenoviruses of cattle (BAV) and goats. It is proposed that deer adenovirus be included in a new genus *Atadenovirus,* along with BAV 4, duck adenovirus 1, and certain other adenoviruses. The virus causes either localized or systemic vascular injury as a consequence of infection of endothelial cells and subsequent thrombosis, leading to severe pulmonary edema, ulceration of the oral cavity and gastrointestinal tract, and widespread hemorrhages. The virus can be propagated in primary deer respiratory epithelial cell cultures, but diagnosis is based on the characteristic gross and histologic lesions, immunohistochemical staining with antisera to BAV, and electron microscopy.

AVIAN ADENOVIRUSES

Adenoviruses infect poultry and other bird species worldwide. Although adenoviruses are often isolated from apparently normal birds, specific diseases also are associated with adenovirus infections. These include egg-drop syndrome, a disease of both wild and domestic birds that is characterized by production of eggs that lack shells or have abnormally soft shells, and hemorrhagic enteritis of turkeys and marble-spleen disease of pheasants, which are similar diseases characterized by intestinal hemorrhage and enlargement of the spleen of affected birds.

54 *Herpesviridae*

Alex A. Ardans

The family *Herpesviridae* consists of viruses that have been isolated from a wide range of animal species, humans, fish, and invertebrates such as oysters. Herpesviruses have been found in virtually every species that has been investigated. Within this group of viruses, there is wide variation in biological properties including pathogenicity, a propensity to form latent infections, and oncogenic potential. Herpesviruses are morphologically similar, with a double-stranded DNA core and an icosahedral capsid consisting of 162 capsomeres, surrounded by a granular zone composed of globular proteins (tegument) and encompassed by a lipid envelope (Fig 54.1). The genome of herpesviruses is large, 125–135 kilobases, and encodes many different proteins; functions of the proteins encoded by the viral genome include virus replication, virus structural proteins, and a variety of proteins that regulate cell growth and modulate the host's antiviral response.

The family *Herpesviridae* consists of three major subfamilies, alpha-, beta-, and gammaherpesvirinae, which were initially distinguished by host range, duration of reproductive cycle, cytopathology, and latent infection characteristics. The alphaherpesvirinae have a variably-restricted host range, are generally highly cytopathic in cell culture, have a relatively short replicative cycle (24 hours), and frequently cause latent viral infections in sensory ganglia. Betaherpesvirinae have a variable host range and a long replicative cycle; infected cells often become enlarged (cytomeglia, thus their designation as cytomegaloviruses). Latency can be established in numerous tissues. Gammaherpesvirinae, with some exceptions, tend to be tropic for B or T lymphocytes (lymphotropic), replicate in lymphoblastoid cells, and may cause lytic infections in certain types of epithelial and fibroblastic cells. Infection is frequently arrested at a prelytic stage with persistent and minimum expression of viral genome in the cell. Latency frequently is established in lymphoid tissue. Host range is narrow with experimental hosts usually limited to the order of the natural host.

EQUINE HERPESVIRUSES

Disease

There are nine proposed equine herpesviruses, five that infect horses (EHV 1 through 5), three that infect donkeys (EHV 6-8; asinine herpesviruses 1-3), and one that likely is derived from zebras (EHV-9). EHV-1, EHV-3, EHV-4, EHV-6 (asinine herpesvirus 1), EHV-8 (asinine herpesvirus 3), and EHV-9 are typical alphaherpesviruses and EHV-2, EHV-5, and EHV-7 (asinine herpesvirus 2) are classified as gammaherpesviruses. EHV-1 has been associated with abortions, upper respiratory disease, and neurologic disease. EHV-2 has been isolated from cases of chronic pharyngitis, mild respiratory disease in young horses, severe respiratory disease in foals 3 to 4 months old, and from clinically normal horses, and its pathogenic significance remains uncertain. Venereal disease (coital exanthema) is a well-recognized clinical manifestation of EHV-3. EHV-4 shares a close antigenic relationship with EHV-1 and has been associated with respiratory disease and sporadic abortions. EHV-5, like EHV-2, has been isolated from horses with upper respiratory diseases, but its pathogenic significance still is uncertain.

Etiologic Agent

Physical, Chemical, and Antigen Properties

The equine herpesviruses have typical morphology and cannot be distinguished from each other based on their morphology. They are, however, antigenically distinct and can be distinguished by serological assays.

Resistance to Physical and Chemical Agents

The equine herpesviruses are inactivated by ether, acid (pH 3), and exposure to heat of 56°C for 30 minutes.

Infectivity for Other Species and Culture Systems

Equine herpesviruses 1–5 usually infect only horses. Ocular disease due to EHV-1 characterized by vitritis, retinitis, and optic neuritis leading to blindness has been described in new-world camelids (alpacas, llamas). Limited serologic surveys have not demonstrated widespread infection in these species. EHV-1 can be propagated in equine fetal kidney, rabbit kidney, and L (mouse fibroblast) cells, resulting in formation of cytopathic effect and intranuclear inclusion bodies.

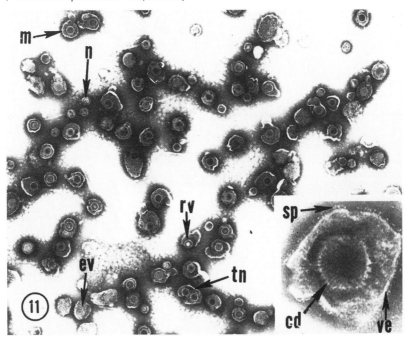

FIGURE 54.1. *Negatively stained preparation of infectious bovine rhinotracheitis virus. n = nucleocapsid, ev = envelope, rv = enveloped virus, tn = twin nucleocapsids. 17,000X. Inset: Minute projections on the envelope of a matured virus. sp = virus spikes, cd = virus core, ve = virus envelope. 100,000X. (Reproduced with permission from Talens LT, Zee YC. Purification and buoyant density of infectious bovine rhinotracheitis virus. Proc Exp Biol Med 1976;151:132.)*

EQUINE HERPESVIRUS-1

Disease

Equine herpesvirus-1 (EHV-1) causes abortion in mares, respiratory tract disease in young horses, and occasional neurologic disease. While abortion in mares may occur as early as 4 months of gestation, it most frequently occurs between the seventh and eleventh months of gestation and usually without any premonitory signs. Foals infected in utero may be born alive but are usually weak and die within 2 to 3 days. Myeloencephalitis with signs of ataxia and posterior paresis has been associated with certain strains of EHV-1.

Host-Virus Relationship

Distribution, Reservoir, and Transmission

EHV-1 is prevalent in horses worldwide. The virus appears to be maintained in the horse, but it is possible that dogs, foxes, and carrion birds may carry infection with fragments of aborted fetuses from one farm to another. Respiratory disease is transmitted by droplet infection. In addition, transmission may also occur by direct contact with virus-laden aborted fetuses or placentas. The annual occurrence of respiratory disease in young horses suggests the existence of carriers and latent infections.

Pathogenesis and Pathology

The pathogenesis of EHV-1 abortions remains an enigma. Viremia in the presence of neutralizing antibodies has been detected in experimentally induced abortions and virus cultured from the buffy coat, but not from the cell-free plasma or from washed red-cell suspensions. The cell-associated virus may escape neutralization by antibody, but the mechanism by which the virus reaches the fetus is unknown.

Macroscopically, the most prominent lesions of the fetus are jaundice, mucous membrane petechiation, subcutaneous and pleural edema, splenic enlargement with prominent lymphoid follicles, and focal hepatic necrosis. Histologically there is bronchiolitis, pneumonitis, severe necrosis of the splenic white pulp, and focal hepatic necrosis, all accompanied by intranuclear inclusion bodies. The early fetus (<3 months) shows little or no response to the viral infection. However, the fetus in its last 4 months of gestation shows a marked ability to react in a specific manner to the presence of the virus. Lesions in the fetus less than 7 months of age differ from those in older fetuses, suggesting that the lesions represent a fetal response to the virus.

Host Responses to Infection

Experimentally, within 24 hours after exposure to EHV-1, foals and mares demonstrate a leukopenia of 24 to 48 hours' duration. Virus persists in circulating leukocytes for as long as 9 days following infection. Abortion in mares may occur as long as 90 to 120 days following infection. Both complement-fixing and virus-neutralizing antibodies appear in the sera of infected horses. In general, complement-fixing antibodies are demonstrable for 6 months after infection, with virus-neutralizing antibodies persisting longer. IgG antibodies against the viral envelope neutralize virus, while those against the nucleocapsid do not. Experimentally pregnant mares with antibody to EHV-1 may abort when challenged with EHV-1. The lesions from which virus cannot be isolated suggest an antigen-antibody complex pathogenesis.

Laboratory Diagnosis

In case of abortions, diagnosis is based on characteristic lesions with intranuclear inclusions present in the fetal liver, spleen, lung, and thymus. The same tissues provide a good source of virus, which can be demonstrated by immunofluorescence or immunohistochemical staining of tissue sections or by virus isolation. The virus is usually relatively easy to isolate. The mares' sera may, but does not invariably, demonstrate a rise in titer. Diagnosis of EHV-1-induced myeloencephalitis is difficult antemortem because serology may be confusing and EHV-1 is rarely isolated. Histopathologically there is a vasculitis present also suggesting an antigen-antibody complex mechanism. On several occasions, myeloencephalitis has occurred in North American (California) horses exposed to mules. With a specific enzyme-linked immunosorbent assay (ELISA) now available, it is possible to distinguish EHV-1 from EHV-4 serologically, and a polymerase chain reaction (PCR) assay has been described for the diagnosis of EHV-1 abortion.

Treatment and Control

Limiting traffic in and out of brood-mare bands and weanling fields and minimizing stress to pregnant mares have been suggested to help prevent abortion disease. Vaccines, although widely used, have not been completely effective in eliminating abortion loss. A hamster-adapted live viral vaccine that was fully capable of causing disease in young animals and pregnant mares is no longer used. A modified live viral vaccine of cell culture origin, although capable of evoking antibody responses, has not proven effective. An inactivated cell culture vaccine, given at the fifth, seventh, and ninth months of gestation, was shown to be effective in field trials, but abortions have been seen in mares vaccinated with this product. More recently, combined EHV-1/EHV-4 inactivated vaccines are being used.

EQUINE HERPESVIRUS-2

Disease

Equine herpesvirus-2 (EHV-2) is prevalent in horses worldwide and has been isolated from both clinically healthy and ill horses. It has been isolated from cases of superficial and chronic pharyngeal lymphoid follicular hyperplasia, mild respiratory disease in young animals, and foal pneumonia and from foals with keratoconjunctivitis. There is considerable skepticism by some concerning its role in disease.

Host-Virus Relationship

Distribution, Reservoir, and Transmission

EHV-2 has been isolated from horses worldwide. Both "healthy" and clinically ill horses act as a reservoir for the virus. In ponies experimentally inoculated with EHV-2, the virus was recovered up to 118 days postinoculation. EHV-2 has been associated with signs of upper respiratory tract disease, with the virus persisting for 418 days.

Pathogenesis and Pathology

Little is known about the pathogenesis of EHV-2. Ninety-seven percent of horses less than 1 year old have antibodies to EHV-2, and the virus could be isolated from the leukocytes of 88.7% of normal horses. Similarly, virus was isolated from 68 of 69 foals sampled once between 1 and 8 months of age. It is suggested that infection is initiated in tonsils, with replication in other sites based on an observed viremia and its cell-associated nature.

Laboratory Diagnosis

There are no specific diagnostic features associated with EHV-2 infection. The virus can be isolated from nasal and pharyngeal swabs and from blood buffy coats and identified by PCR assay.

Treatment and Control

Control methods have not been established, and a vaccine is not available for EHV-2.

EQUINE HERPESVIRUS-3 (EQUINE COITAL EXANTHEMA)

Disease

Equine coital exanthema (ECE) is an acute, sexually transmitted disease characterized by the formation of papules, vesicles, pustules, and ulcers on the penis and prepuce of stallions and on the external genitalia and perineal skin of mares. The lesions usually heal after approximately 14 days, leaving depigmented patches on the vulva and erosions and ulcers on the prepuce and penis of the male. Lesions have occurred, infrequently, around the lips, external nares, nasal mucosa, and conjunctiva.

A unique characteristic of equine herpesvirus-3 (EHV-3)

is its inability to grow in cell cultures other than those of equine origin.

Distribution, Reservoir, and Transmission

EHV-3 was first isolated in 1968 concurrently in North America and Australia. The only known reservoir for the virus is the horse and the usual mode of transmission is venereal, but EHV-3 can be spread without coitus. The vulva and vagina need not be damaged for infection to occur. The infection may also spread via fomites, or insects may act as mechanical carriers. It is suggested that in some infected stallions and mares, EHV-3 becomes latent in the nonbreeding season and is reactivated during the breeding season.

Pathogenesis and Pathology

Little is known about the disease pathogenesis, but virus and an antibody increase can usually be demonstrated during development of the lesions. Perivascular and periglandular lymphocytic accumulations suggest that an immune-mediated reaction may play a role in pathogenesis.

Microscopic examination of vulvar tissue demonstrates shallow erosions along with occasional typical intranuclear inclusions scattered in germinal epithelium or in nuclear remnants in necrotic areas.

Host Responses to Infection

Antibodies usually appear during the acute stage of the disease.

Laboratory Diagnosis

Clinical signs, serologic tests, histopathologic examination, and viral isolation can be used in diagnosing ECE.

Treatment and Control

There is no EHV-3 vaccine available. Treatments include use of topical ointments to reduce pain and sexual rest for at least 3 weeks.

EQUINE HERPESVIRUS-4 (EQUINE RHINOPNEUMONITIS)

Clinical manifestations of equine herpesvirus-4 (EHV-4) are seen principally in foals and younger horses, with a seasonal peak of disease in fall and winter. Signs often include malaise and elevated temperature up to 105°F, which may persist for 2 to 5 days; watery nasal discharge, which becomes mucopurulent in the later stages; congested conjunctiva; and, infrequently, enlarged submandibular nodes.

The agent appears to have worldwide distribution; however, it is infrequently isolated. Both inactivated and modified live vaccines are used but results are not uniformly favorable.

EQUINE HERPESVIRUS-5

In a study of multiple equine herpesvirus-5 (EHV-5) isolates, several were found to differ significantly genomically and in their protein composition. EHV-5 has been proposed for this group of viruses that were isolated from equine respiratory tracts. The pathogenic significance of EHV-5 has not been adequately defined.

RUMINANT HERPES VIRUSES

Herpes viruses, representing alpha- and gammaherpesviruses, are responsible for a wide range of conditions in ruminants, including neurologic, genital, fetal, and respiratory diseases. Infections may range from inapparent to fatal. Several herpes viruses infect cattle (bovine herpes viruses [BHV]): infectious bovine rhinotracheitis virus (BHV-1), bovine mammilitis virus (BHV-2), and bovine encephalitis virus (BHV-5) are alphaherpesviruses. BHV-1 causes both respiratory (infectious bovine rhinotracheitis) and genital disease (infectious pustular vulvovaginitis) in cattle. BHV-4 is a gammaherpesvirus, but its role in causing disease is uncertain. Two gammaherpesviruses that previously were designated as BHV-3 have now been named Alcelaphine herpesvirus (AlHV): AlHV-1 is the cause of African malignant catarrhal fever (MCF) associated with wildebeest and AlHV-2 is the cause of atypical MCF associated with the hartebeest. There are two sheep gammaherpes viruses (ovine herpes viruses [OHV] 1, 2): OHV-1 is associated with pulmonary adenomatosis, and OHV-2 is the cause of the sheep-associated form of MCF. Alphaviruses also have been isolated from goats (CpHV-1) and deer (CerHV-1 and CerHV-2), and the CpHV-1 is the cause of reproductive disease in goats.

BOVINE HERPESVIRUSES

BOVINE HERPESVIRUS-1

Disease

Bovine herpesvirus-1 (BHV-1) infection in cattle may present as ocular, genital, respiratory, and, infrequently, neurologic disease. Respiratory disease typically presents as rhinotracheitis (infectious bovine rhinotracheitis [IBR]), which may lead to severe and often fatal bronchopneumonia. Conjunctivitis is common. Occasionally the cornea is involved and a panophthalmitis may occur. BHV-1 can infect genitalia, resulting in abortion, balanoposthitis, and vulvovaginitis (infectious pustular vulvovaginitis [IPV]). Meningoencephalitis in young calves occurs infrequently with BHV-1, and herpes virus isolates from cattle with neurologic disease are most commonly designated BHV-5. BHV-1 has been isolated from vesicular lesions on the udder and teats of a cow.

Etiologic Agent

Infectivity for Other Species and Culture Systems

Although cattle appear to be the major species affected by BHV-1, the virus has been incriminated in swine vaginitis and balanitis, and has been isolated from stillborn and newborn pigs. Approximately 11% of swine tested in parts of North America (Iowa and Texas) had antibodies to IBR. The virus has been isolated from red deer with ocular disease, and could be activated in Malaysian buffalo by steroid administration. It does not appear that BHV-1 virus is a significant pathogen of goats. Only 3% of 1,146 serum samples of captive ruminants in United States zoos had antibodies to IBR virus.

BHV-1 virus can be grown in a wide variety of cells, including bovine, canine, feline, equine, ovine, rabbit, monkey, and human, where it produces a characteristic cytopathic effect.

Host-Virus Relationship

Distribution, Reservoir, and Transmission

The disease occurs worldwide. During the late 1950s, an apparently identical virus to IBR virus was isolated from infectious pustular vulvovaginitis (IPV).

It has been suggested that wildlife may play a role in disease transmission, but in light of demonstrated viral recrudescence, cattle must be considered the primary reservoir. Virus is transmitted by respiratory, genital, and conjunctival secretions of infected cattle.

Pathogenesis and Pathology

The virus replicates in the upper respiratory tract and spreads via the lacrimal ducts. Virus can be recovered from nasal secretions for almost 2 weeks following infection. Although viremia is difficult to demonstrate, experimental infections have yielded virus from various organs, perhaps as a consequence of a leukocyte-associated viremia.

Genital infections are most likely venereally transmitted. Lesions consisting of pustules and later fibronecrotic plaques are usually limited to the vulva and posterior vagina in the female. Similar lesions are seen on the prepuce of affected bulls. Respiratory disease has been produced with genital isolates, and genital lesions have been produced with respiratory isolates. Viral shedding was observed in cows 14 days after experimental genital infection and in males up to 19 days following infection. Virus was shed following prednisolone treatment in these cattle 2 and 7 months, respectively, following initial infection. These observations suggest that the virus may be maintained by periodic shedding when animals are subjected to stress. Although the frequency is low, occasional bulls are encountered that shed BHV-1 intermittently in semen. Insemination of cattle with such semen may result in endometritis, reduced conception, and shortened estrus periods. Experimentally, semen isolates can induce severe rhinotracheitis and vulvovaginitis in cattle. Natural outbreaks of simultaneous respiratory and genital disease are rare.

Abortion is often seen in pregnant cattle with IBR or occasionally following vaccination with modified live virus vaccine. The incubation period between infection of the dam and fetal death varies from 15 to 60 days. Since fetal death occurs several days before abortion, the fetus is often severely autolyzed. Fetal edema, especially of the fetal membranes, occurs along with extensive hemorrhagic edema in the perirenal tissue. Extensive hemorrhagic necrosis of the renal cortex is seen along with a focal necrosis in the liver and usually in the lymph nodes. Some necrosis may be observed in placentomes, which are usually good sources of virus for isolation attempts. Necrotic lesions occur in ovaries of cattle experimentally infected by nongenital routes.

Conjunctivitis is common in BHV-1 infection. Typically it presents with profuse lacrimation and occasionally extends into the cornea, resulting in a keratitis. In some cattle, a multifocal lymphoid hyperplasia may be seen in the palpebral conjunctiva.

Meningoencephalitis has been recorded in natural and experimental disease. Histopathologic lesions include those of a nonsuppurative meningoencephalitis, neuronal necrosis, focal malacia, and often intranuclear inclusion in astrocytes and neurones associated with lesions.

Latent infections have been demonstrated in the trigeminal ganglia of clinically normal cattle. Recrudescent shedding of virus has been observed naturally and in response to corticosteroid administration.

Host Response to Infection

The immune response to BHV-1 involves many factors in addition to the stimulation of neutralizing antibodies, most of which are directed toward surface glycoproteins. IgG and IgM antibodies appear 7 days following exposure. The IgG response during this primary phase is restricted primarily to the IgG1 subclass. Secondary responses seen mainly in the IgG class are due to increase in IgG2 antibody. Secondary intranasal exposure did not produce an increase in IgM antibody, whereas an increase in IgM levels was seen following abortion. The neutralization of extracellular virus prevents extracellular spread of virus stressing the importance of antibody at mucosal surfaces. Antibody can also play a role in the complement-mediated lysis of infected cells and in antibody dependent-cell cytotoxicity. The induction of cytokines can activate effector cells that destroy infected cells directly or through antibody interaction. These actions occur in concert with each other, making it difficult to ascribe a level of importance to each. For vaccine development, it is important that consideration be given to a product's ability to both induce antibody and cell-mediated immunity.

Laboratory Diagnosis

The fibrinonecrotic plaques commonly present in the external nares and on the nasal septum of cattle with infectious bovine rhinotracheitis are good sources of material for viral isolation. The conjunctival form can be tentatively diagnosed by the observation of multifocal white lesions in the palpebral conjunctiva. In their absence, viral isolation is needed. The virus can be readily isolated from the conjunctival swabs. Abortion may be difficult to diagnose as the fetus is often presented in an autolysed condition. If placenta is available and relatively fresh, isolation attempts can be made from the placentomes. While immunofluorescent staining techniques have been used on fetal tissue with varying degrees of success, immunoperoxidase staining that has been positive in IFA negative tissues has improved abortion diagnosis associated with BHV-1. Diagnosis based on serology may be difficult because animals often have high titers at the time of abortion, regardless of cause, making it difficult to demonstrate rising titers. Detection of BHV-1 in semen is difficult by conventional methods. A PCR-based technique has been used to detect BHV-1 in semen.

Treatment and Control

A modified vaccine used intramuscularly was associated with reduction in disease but could cause abortion in pregnant cattle. An intranasal vaccine was shown to be safe for use in cattle. This vaccine containing a temperature-sensitive mutant virus that will replicate only at the lower temperature found only in the upper airways of cattle is promoted as safe and effective for use in pregnant animals. Corticosteroid treatment of animals vaccinated with modified live vaccines has resulted in recrudesence of virus. Despite these uncertainties, modified live BHV-1 vaccines are widely used because of the potentially heavy economic loss resulting from infection.

Inactivated vaccines have not been consistently efficacious. Subunit vaccines have been suggested as an alternative to modified live vaccines, as have gene-deletion mutants.

Eradication

Countries with relatively small cattle populations have used serology to guide eradication efforts; however, common practices in larger countries prevent this approach. Appropriate serology used with genetically engineered vaccines may hold promise.

BOVINE HERPESVIRUS-2 (BOVINE MAMMILLITIS)

Bovine herpesvirus-2 (BHV-2) has been isolated from cattle with generalized skin disease (pseudolumpy skin disease), mammillitis, and stomatitis.

BHV-2 will replicate in a wide range of cells, but bovine kidney cell culture is most widely used. Cattle appear to be primarily infected, with mild experimental disease produced in sheep, goats, and pigs.

BHV-2 has been isolated from cattle skin and mucosal infection in the United States, Africa, Europe, and Australia. Originally virus was isolated from South African cattle with generalized skin disease, subsequently termed *pseudolumpy skin disease*. Mammillitis due to BHV-2 was described in Africa and England, and subsequently in the United States. Stomatitis in bovine and buffalo calves has been described in association with calves nursing cows with mammillitis. Suggested modes of infection include transmission at milking, by insects, or activation of latent virus.

Intravenous exposure produces generalized skin lesions, which are characterized by a severe intercellular edema in the epidermis along with syncytia with intranuclear inclusions. An epidermal mononuclear cell and neutrophil infiltrate is present along with mononuclear and lymphocytic dermal perivascular infiltration.

The diagnosis of pseudolumpy skin disease and mammillitis can be based on clinical signs and viral isolation in cell culture. Serology on paired samples will demonstrate an increase in antibody.

BOVINE HERPESVIRUS-4

Bovine herpesvirus-4 (BHV-4) consists of a group of viruses that have been isolated from different clinical syndromes and normal cattle. Their importance as pathogens is unclear. Only strain DN-599 has been reported to produce conjunctivitis and respiratory disease. Viruses related to this group have been repeatedly isolated from cases of metritis in some North American (California) cattle and are suspected of causing vaginitis in heifers. The North American and European strains appear to be closely related. Latency has been suggested for this group as there appears to be reactivation in response to other inflammatory processes.

BOVINE HERPESVIRUS-5

Nonsuppurative meningoencephalitis has been associated with bovine herpesvirus-5 (BHV-5) infection of cattle. Isolates have been obtained in Argentina, Australia, Hungary, Japan, and the United States from cattle with sporadic cases of encephalitis. BHV-5 strongly cross-reacts with BHV-1 and currently the two cannot be distinguished serologically but can be differentiated by their restriction endonuclease patterns. It appears that BHV-5 has been circulating in cattle for at least 20 years, with only sporadic disease occurrences. Mortality is usually reported to be 100%. Lesions vary as to severity but usually consist of perivascular infiltrates throughout the brain, with neuronal necrosis, disruption of the neuropil, and gliosis. Experimental infections produce similar signs and lesions as those naturally occurring and BHV-5 can be reisolated from the brain.

ALCEPHALINE HERPESVIRUS-1 AND -2 (MALIGNANT CATARRHAL FEVER)

Malignant catarrhal fever (MCF), an often fatal infection of many species of bovidae and cervidae, occurs as two epidemiologically distinct entities: wildebeest-associated and sheep-associated MCF. Alcephaline herpesvirus-1 (AlHV-1) is responsible for wildebeest-derived (or African) MCF, which occurs when cattle and wildebeest graze together. A virus isolated from clinical MCF in cattle in North America (Minnesota) is closely related to AlHV-1. An etiologic agent for sheep-associated (or European and North American) MCF has not been isolated; however, evidence based on competitive-inhibition ELISA and a PCR assay strongly implicate ovine herpesvirus-2 (OHV-2) as the cause of sheep-associated MCF. AlHV-2, which is associated with the hartebeest, has not been incriminated in naturally occurring MCF disease of domestic cattle.

AlHV-1 is a typical gammaherpesvirus. Infectivity is lost by freeze-thawing and sonication of infected cells. The virion is reported to range from 98 nm to 240 nm. Virus has been propagated in bovine thyroid and testicle cell culture.

The clinical disease is limited to cattle, buffalo, and several species of wild exotic ungulates (Pere David deer, banteng, gaurs). Disease is associated with mixing wildebeest and cattle during periods when the wildebeest are calving. Newborn wildebeest calves shed virus in nasal and ocular secretions up to 3 months of age. Viral shedding also occurs in adult wildebeest given corticosteroid. There is no evidence for congenital infection of sheep with OHV-2; rather, lambs appear to become infected during the first year of life. While sheep-associated MCF in cattle has been associated with lambing, it appears that the newborn lamb does not play the same role as the newborn wildebeest. It also appears that all domestic United States sheep carry OHV-2.

Diagnosis of MCF is made based on histopathology and a recently developed PCR test. Affected animals present with mucopurulent nasal and ocular discharge and corneal opacity. Oral lesions may be present, consisting of multiple erosions preceded by a diffuse hyperemia and profuse salivation. Central nervous disturbances are frequent and diarrhea is common.

Histologic lesions are those of a lymphoproliferative disorder characterized by perivascular mononuclear infiltration, necrotizing vasculitis, and tissue lymphoid infiltration. Deposition of immunoglobulin and complement has been described in the glomeruli of affected cattle, suggesting an immune-mediated disease. Viral antigen was rarely detected, however, and virus-specific antibodies were not detected.

CAPRINE HERPESVIRUS-1

A herpesvirus (previously designated BHV-6) was isolated from young goats (1 week) dying in North America (California) with enteric signs and necrosis and ulceration in the rumen, cecum, and colon. Signs of conjunctivitis and rhinitis were observed in Swiss goat kids. Although infection in adults usually is apparent, genital diseases may occur as vulvitis or balanoposthitis. A herpes virus that was isolated from a California sheep fetus was determined by DNA analysis to be caprine herpesvirus (CpHV-1). The California isolate of CpHV-1 replicates in canine, rabbit, feline, equine, bovine, and lamb cells.

Virus was isolated from vaginal secretions of does exposed intranasally, intramuscularly, and intravenously with CpHV-1. Pregnant does abort, but no virus was isolated from the fetuses. Infections were severe in kids, with signs of conjunctivitis, rhinitis, and diarrhea. Fibronecrotic lesions on the nasal septum were remarkably similar to those of cattle with IBR.

Gross lesions are limited to the gastrointestinal tract with necrosis and ulceration in rumen, cecum, and colon. Intranuclear inclusions are present in epithelial cells near the necrotic areas.

The disease can be diagnosed by viral isolation from nasal secretions and fecal material. It appears to be uncommon, and no vaccine is available.

OVINE HERPESVIRUSES

OVINE HERPESVIRUS-1

Ovine herpesvirus-1 (OVH-1) was isolated from the lungs of sheep with pulmonary adenomatosis (jaagsiekte). Although the virus causes experimental pneumonia in lambs, pulmonary adenomatosis is caused by a retrovirus and the pathogenic role of OVH-1 is uncertain.

OVINE HERPESVIRUS-2

Ovine herpesvirus-2 (OHV-2) is proposed to cause the sheep-associated form of malignant catarrhal fever in cattle. The virus has never been isolated; however, OHV-2 DNA has been detected by PCR in cattle with MCF. It shares a close genomic relationship with AlHV-1.

PSEUDORABIES (AUJESZKY'S DISEASE) VIRUS

Disease

Pseudorabies in swine is most severe in younger animals. The virus commonly affects the nervous system and the mortality rate varies from 5% to 100%. Infection of sows during mid- to late pregnancy can result in abortion, fetal death, mummification, or stillbirths. In adult pigs, severe nervous disorders are rare, and pseudorabies usually presents as a rather vague illness of transient pyrexia, dullness, inappetence, incoordination, and ataxia. Respiratory disease can also be seen in pigs of various ages but is most common in grower and finishing pigs. Inapparent or mild disease may be missed or misdiagnosed in older swine. Pseudorabies also occurs in a number of other species, including cattle, sheep, dogs, cats, and raccoons, in which the clinical signs are usually neurologic and manifested by an intense pruritis.

Etiologic Agent

Physical, Chemical, and Antigenic Properties

The pseudorabies virus (PRV) is an alphaherpesvirus that is designated Suid herpesvirus 1 (SuHV-1). Only one serotype has been identified; however, strain variability has been shown by restriction endonuclease digestion of viruses from different geographic areas. Attenuated strains have been demonstrated to have a deletion in their genome, suggesting that specific regions are associated with virulence.

Sensitivity to Physical and Chemical Agents

The PRV is fairly sensitive to high temperatures and is stable in cell culture fluid between a pH of 6 to 8 at cooler temperatures. Virus has been observed to survive in unchlorinated water for 7 days and for 2 days in an anaerobic lagoon. Chemicals that cleave chlorine appear to be the most effective disinfectants.

Infectivity for Other Species and Culture Systems

The disease occurs naturally in cattle, sheep, dogs, cats, and rats. In all but adult swine, the disease is almost always fatal; hence, other animals are essentially "dead-end" hosts. Although one report exists of human infection, PRV is not readily transmitted to humans.

The virus replicates readily in cell cultures from many species and tissues, including cat, dog, cattle, badger, coyote, deer, buzzard, chicken, and goose.

Host-Virus Relationship

Distribution, Reservoir, and Transmission

Pseudorabies is recognized as a severe, highly fatal disease of newborn pigs in Europe and the United States, and has been reported in other parts of the world. The principal reservoir of PRV appears to be the pig and transmission is frequently pig to pig. The virus is transmitted by ingestion and inhalation, and during coitus the virus can be transmitted from boar to sow or vice versa. Transmission can occur in a contaminated environment under crowded conditions.

Feral swine can transmit the virus to domestic swine and among wild animals, the raccoon has been the most studied. Infected raccoons may transmit by close contact with swine and swine may be exposed by consuming infected raccoon carcasses. The pig is the primary source of viral spread to other species. Cases in dogs have been linked to consumption of feral swine tissues. The cat appears to be more sensitive, and infection in cats was observed in 51% of PRV-infected farms where cats were present.

Pathogenesis and Pathology

The virus replicates primarily in the upper respiratory epithelium including the tonsillar tissue. Virus can be isolated from the brain 24 hours following infection, which suggests that the route of infection is via the axoplasm. Viremia is difficult to demonstrate; however, viral shedding may persist in nasal secretions for up to 14 days. Lower airway infection often results, and cardiac and splanchnic ganglia become involved.

The virus produces a nonsuppurative meningoencephalomyelitis with extensive damage to neurons, widespread perivascular cuffing, and gliosis. The brain stem is particularly affected, but lesions also occur throughout the cerebral cortex and cerebellum. There may be intranuclear inclusion bodies in all types of cells. In the respiratory form of the disease, a necrotizing tracheitis and pneumonia occur that result in loss of epithelium in airways and necrosis of alveolar cells.

Microscopic lesions in aborted fetuses include necrosis of many organs, but primarily liver, spleen, visceral lymph nodes, and adrenal glands. Intranuclear inclusion bodies are often present in degenerating hepatocytes, cells of the adrenal cortex, and occasionally mononuclear phagocytic cells of the spleen and lymph nodes. Placental lesions are characterized by degeneration and necrosis of the trophoblasts and mesenchymal cells of the chorion.

Host Response to Infection

IgM antibodies are first detectable about the fifth day after infection followed by measurable IgG antibodies about the seventh day, reaching maximum levels by the twelfth to fourteenth day.

Laboratory Diagnosis

Because signs of the disease in swine vary widely with the age of the animal, the dose of virus received, the strain of virus, and the route of exposure, clinical diagnosis is often difficult.

In the laboratory, a definitive diagnosis of pseudorabies can be made by viral isolation. Immunofluorescent staining of frozen tonsil or brain tissue can provide a rapid diagnosis. Serologic tests for pseudorabies antibodies include solid-phase radioimmunoassay, immunodiffusion tests, enzyme-linked immunosorbent assay (ELISA), complement-fixation test, serum virus-neutralizing test (SVN), counterneuronal immunoelectrophoresis, and indirect hemagglutination. ELISA tests are used to differentiate antibody response to gene-deleted vaccines and field infection. In an acute outbreak, serology may not be helpful because of the time needed for antibodies to develop. In the United States, the most commonly used tests are latex agglutination (LAT), ELISA, and SVN. In eradication efforts, the sensitive LAT, which is quick and easy to perform, is commonly used as a screening assay. For confirmation, the SVN and ELISA are used with specific ELISA tests, which are especially useful in detecting animals vaccinated with gene-deleted vaccines.

Prevention and Control

In an effort to avoid the disease in a breeding herd, a producer should 1) purchase animals from sources free of PRV,

2) require testing prior to purchase, 3) isolate new arrivals and test for antibodies a minimum of 12 days after receipt and isolation, 4) restrict human traffic among the swine and practice hygienic measures, and 5) make efforts to restrict contact of the swine with other animals. Feed is a potential source of virus and appropriate measures should be used.

In infected herds, quarantine is the most urgent obligation and it is recommended that the movement of swine be limited for slaughter only. Porcine origin antiserum with titers of at least 1:256 has proven effective in reducing death losses if administered to neonatal pigs. However, none is commercially available.

Attenuated live vaccines are available and have been successful in reducing death losses in endemic areas. These vaccines do not prevent reinfection with virulent field virus or the shedding of virulent virus for variable periods. Latently infected and vaccinated animals may shed the virus for indeterminate periods while asymptomatic.

Inactivated vaccines are commercially available. Their principal use has been in susceptible sows in endemic areas to provide antibodies to colostrum for protection of newborn pigs during the first few weeks of life. Genetically engineered (gene-deletion) vaccines are currently used in designated states in the United States since control programs utilize differential serology as part of a federal eradication program.

CANINE HERPESVIRUS

Disease

Canine herpesvirus (CHV) causes neonatal deaths, abortions, and mummification as well as fatal systemic infection in newborn pups and relatively mild infections in older dogs. The virus induces a generalized, often lethal infection within the first 2 weeks of life. Pups are either stillborn or die after a short illness.

CHV has been isolated from dogs with respiratory diseases, and, with other viruses and bacteria, may be involved in the "kennel cough" syndrome.

CHV can induce genital lesions in male and female dogs. Affected animals appear healthy but often present a history of infertility.

Etiologic Agent

Physical, Chemical, and Antigenic Properties

Canine herpesvirus is a typical alphaherpesvirus. There is no cross-neutralization between CHV and the viruses of herpes simplex, pseudorabies virus, or infectious bovine rhinotracheitis. However, CHV appears to be antigenically related to herpes simplex virus.

Infectivity for Other Species and Culture Systems

A coyote herpesvirus, shown to be antigenically related to CHV, was found in coyote pups believed to be infected by indirect contact with dogs. No other animals have been reported to show susceptibility to CHV. Limited growth occurs in human lung cells and calf, monkey, pig, rabbit, and hamster kidney cells.

Host-Virus Relationship

Distribution, Reservoir, and Transmission

Canine herpesvirus has been isolated in Europe, Japan, Australia, New Zealand, and the United States. The only known reservoir of CHV in all geographic areas is the dog, with the possible exception of coyotes in the United States.

Modes of transmission of CHV may include transplacental, congenital, oral, and airborne transmission. There is also some evidence of transmission by indirect contact via an animal handler.

Pathogenesis and Pathology

Canine herpesvirus has been associated with respiratory disease in adult dogs, but the severe acute necrotizing and hemorrhagic disease occurs only in puppies infected at less than approximately 2 weeks of age. The virus can be isolated from the nose and pharynx of young dogs exposed intranasally. It can multiply in the respiratory and female genital tracts of older dogs and can be isolated for up to 7 days from the vagina of bitches inoculated intravaginally. It has also been isolated from pharyngeal mucosa. The virus is disseminated hematogenously, resulting in a necrotizing vasculitis in many organs. Grossly, the kidneys may appear mottled and there may be pulmonary congestion and edema, splenomegaly, lymphadenitis, and non-suppurative meningoencephalitis.

Widespread foci of necrosis and hemorrhages characterize the histologic lesions in affected organs such as kidney, liver, and lung. Intranuclear inclusions may be present in areas adjacent to necrotic lesions.

Host Response to Infection

Neutralizing antibodies develop in dogs inoculated with CHV, but the duration of immunity is not known. CHV induces serum-neutralizing antibodies in infected puppies. Reactivation of CHV in experimentally infected pups and dogs has been demonstrated with administration of corticosteroids.

Laboratory Diagnosis

Clinical signs and histopathology can be useful in diagnosis. Definitive diagnosis is by viral isolation and more rapidly by immunofluorescent staining of affected tissues.

Prevention and Control

Commercial CHV vaccines are not available. Hyperimmune globulin may be useful but difficult to obtain because the virus is poorly immunogenic. Removal or separation of infected animals should be considered.

FELINE HERPESVIRUS-1 (FELINE VIRAL RHINOTRACHEITIS)

Disease

Feline herpesvirus-1 (FHV-1) is the cause of feline viral rhinotracheitis (FVR). Along with upper respiratory disease, the virus is also associated with conjunctivitis, ulcerative keratitis, ulcerative stomatitis, abortions, and pneumonia.

Etiologic Agent

Physical, Chemical, and Antigenic Properties

Feline herpesvirus is a typical alphaherpesvirus. Serologic comparisons suggest that FHV from around the world are similar; however, differences in the clinical manifestations caused by various isolates have been observed.

Sensitivity to Physical and Chemical Agents

The infectivity is reduced or eliminated by ether, chloroform and sodium hypochlorite. Virus in cell culture fluid loses 90% of its viability within 6 hours at 37°C, 6 days at 25°C, and 1 month at 4°C. The virus is most stable at pH 6, and complete activity is lost in 3 hours at pH 3 and pH 9. FHV can be recovered for up to 18 hours in a moist environment at 15°C, but for less than 12 hours in a dry room.

Infectivity for Other Species and Culture Systems

Natural infections with FHV have been observed only in the cat family. FHV-1 in vitro growth is limited mainly to cells of feline origin. The virus propagates to high titers with demonstrated cytopathic effect in primary cell cultures of feline testicle, lung, and renal cells.

Host-Virus Relationships

Distribution, Reservoir, and Transmission

Natural cases of the disease have been reported throughout the United States, Canada, Europe, Australia, and New Zealand. Cats serve as reservoirs. Healthy cats that are latently infected with FHV may shed virus when stressed, for example, by corticosteroid administration, and viral transcripts have been detected in trigeminal ganglia of latently infected cats.

The major avenue for spread of FHV-1 is by direct cat-to-cat contact through infectious discharges and aerosolized microdroplets. Indirect or fomite transmission via a contaminated environment, personnel, or feeding and cleaning utensils appears important only in catteries.

Pathogenesis and Pathology

The pathogenesis of the infection differs with the route of inoculation. As FHV-1 infection is often manifested in the upper respiratory tract, experimental studies have been done by nasal and ocular routes. When introduced intranasally, the virus produces rapid, cytolytic infection of epithelial cells of the nasal passages. The virus generally persists in the upper respiratory tract for 2 weeks. Although many cats develop conjunctivitis during the primary disease, very few develop corneal disease. Experimentally, suppression of local immune responses permitted viral access to the cornea. The resulting keratitis appears to be due to the immune response to the virus.

In the respiratory tract, changes occur in both stratified squamous and pseudostratified columnar epithelial cells. Lung changes consist of interstitial pneumonitis with focal necrotic lesions in the bronchi, bronchioles, and alveolar septa with alveolar accumulations of inflammatory cells and fibrinous exudate.

Intranuclear inclusion bodies are numerous in the stratified squamous epithelium of the conjunctiva with conjunctival and corneal lesions. Histologically, corneal ulcers reveal disorientation and degeneration of the epithelial cells, some of which contain nuclear inclusions.

Host Response to Infection

The primary immune response of cats to intranasal infection as measured by serum neutralizing antibodies is not impressive. Antibodies usually persist for 1 to 3 months, although titers have been observed to fluctuate in a cat between 1:48 and 1:256 over a 12-month period. Correlation between presence of antibodies and resistance to infection is not absolute.

Laboratory Diagnosis

Immunofluorescent staining can demonstrate viral antigens in the tissues of experimentally infected cats. Early in the course of FVR, the conjunctival and nasal mucosa contain sufficient numbers of infected cells for antigen detection.

Feline herpesvirus is isolated from tissue samples and from swabs of the ocular, nasal, or oropharyngeal mucosa. The virus can be cultured from nasal or pharyngeal swabbings for 14 to 21 days after infection, but most consistently during the first week.

Virus-neutralizing antibodies can be detected in the serum of convalescent cats. Paired samples, the first collected during acute illness, the other collected 2 or 3 weeks later, can be used for the serologic diagnosis of FVR.

Prevention and Control

Care should be taken to avoid introducing cats with developing, subclinical, or latent infections to a colony. A modified live feline viral rhinotracheitis vaccine is available. Protective immunity appears to be relatively short, and revaccination every 6 to 12 months is recommended. An intranasal vaccine is also available. A recombinant vaccine is reported experimentally to result in a reduced latency load.

SIMIAN HERPESVIRUS B (CERCOPITHECINE HERPESVIRUS-1)

Herpesvirus B causes a natural infection in Old World monkeys (rhesus and cynomolgus species). The infection in monkeys is characterized by oral vesicles similar to the cold sores in humans caused by herpes simplex virus. The disease in monkeys is not fatal and the virus may remain latent in infected animals. Direct contact is the most common means of viral spread in monkeys, since virus can be recovered from saliva and from the central nervous tissues of clinically asymptomatic, persistently infected animals.

The virus can cause fatal central nervous infection in humans and laboratory animals such as rabbits and unweaned mice. Most human infections are caused by a bite from a monkey secreting infectious virus, although handling virus-infected primary monkey kidney cell cultures can also lead to infection. The incubation period in humans is 10 to 20 days. Usually there is local inflammation at the bite site followed by vesicle formation and necrosis of the area. Virus reaches the central nervous system by peripheral nerves, and death may occur due to acute encephalitis or encephalomyelitis.

Herpesvirus B is morphologically similar to other alphaherpesviruses. It is readily inactivated by detergents. The virus can be cultivated on the chorioallantoic membrane of embryonated chick eggs and in rabbit, monkey, and human cell cultures that produce intranuclear inclusion bodies and syncytia formation. Strong cross-reactivity exists between human herpes simplex viruses and herpesvirus B.

Herpes simiae virus infection can be diagnosed by isolating virus from the central nervous tissues of fatal human cases. A PCR-based assay has been developed for viral identification; however, diagnostic detection of herpes B specific antibodies is difficult. There is no treatment for herpesvirus B infection in humans, nor has an effective vaccine been developed. Human gamma globulin that contains virus-specific antibodies should be used immediately after exposure to monkey bites. Caution and wearing of protective gear for handling monkeys remain the best way to avoid infection.

MAREK'S DISEASE

Disease

Marek's disease (MD) is a lymphoproliferative disease of chickens that may involve numerous tissues. Most frequently peripheral nerves are affected. Prior to vaccine development, MD was responsible for heavy losses, and increased losses to MD in vaccinated flocks have suggested an evolution toward greater virulence. There are two species of Marek's disease virus (MDV): gallid herpesvirus-2 (GaHV-2), which is synonymous with MDV type 1, includes isolates that cause mild to severe signs of disease; gallid herpesvirus 3 (GaHV-3), which is synonymous with MDV type 2, includes strains that are nononcogenic. A third species is meleagrid herpesvirus-1 (MeHV-1), which includes viruses from turkeys.

Progressive paralysis of one or more extremities, incoordination, drooping wings, and lowered head position are the most common signs of MD. Mortality varies from 10% with mild MD to over 50% in unvaccinated birds.

Etiologic Agent

Physical, Chemical, and Antigenic Properties

GaHV 1 and 2 and MeHV-1 are alphaherpesviruses.

Resistance to Physical and Chemical Agents

Cell-free virus is readily inactivated at temperatures greater than 37°C and is only relatively stable at 25°C (4 days) and 4°C (2 weeks). MDV can be maintained for long periods at 27°C. Virus is inactivated by pH 3 and pH 11. Infectivity of dried MDV-infected feathers is destroyed by chlorine, organic iodine, a quaternary ammonium compound, cresylic acid, synthetic phenol, and sodium hydroxide.

Infectivity for Other Species and Culture Systems

The chicken is the primary natural host for the MDV, and disease is rare in other species except for quail. Marek's disease virus has not been shown to affect any nonavian animals. No etiologic link has been demonstrated between MDV and human cancer. The virus is most often cultivated on chicken or duck embryo fibroblast cells. Chicken kidney cells have also been used.

Host-Virus Relationships

Distribution, Reservoir, and Transmission

Marek's disease is a major disease of domestic chicken flocks worldwide. The virus can persist in excreta, litter, and poultry house dust, and horizontal infection via aerosols of chickens appears to be the main method of transmission. Egg transmission is doubtful. Marek's disease virus matures to its enveloped infectious form only in the feather follicles and can then be spread to the environment via desquamated cells. Whole live cells from blood or tumor material, or infected whole cell cultures, are infectious experimentally. Cell-free fluid does not appear to be infectious. Certain chicken lines are genetically resistant to MDV, and resistance in most birds is associated with the development of serum-neutralizing antibody.

Pathogenesis and Pathology

The incidence of MD is variable, depending on the strain of the virus and the strain and age of the chicken. It usually occurs in chickens between 2 and 5 months old and is commonly felt not to be seen in birds older than 22 weeks;

however, disease has been observed in birds as young as 3 to 4 weeks and in 60-week-old laying hens. The virus primarily affects the nervous system although visceral organs and other tissues may also be involved. Lesions are present in the nervous system and involve peripheral nerves and spinal roots. The principal nerve trunk involved shows gross lesions consisting of a grayish-white swelling, which histologically are characterized by extensive lymphocytic infiltrations. Edema may be present and myelin degeneration of nerve sheaths may be apparent.

Ocular lymphomatosis is another possible outcome of MDV infection, with blindness resulting due to iris involvement. Histologically, a similar infiltration of lymphocytes is present, which can also occur in the optic nerve.

In the visceral form, lymphoid tumors of varying degrees of severity infiltrate the gonads, liver, lung, and skin. Affected chickens have enlarged visceral organs with white nodular or miliary foci. Oclusive atherosclerosis has been observed experimentally.

Host Response to Infection

The immune response to MDV is complex, in that both humoral and cell-mediated immunity (CMI) develop in normal birds. MDV infection can be immunosuppressive. In addition, the immune response may be involved in tumor formation. Bursectomized birds survive experimental infection, suggesting that CMI is important. In chicks, passively acquired antibody is thought to limit the extent of infection rather than prevent it or clear the virus. Viral-specific antibodies appear within 1 to 3 weeks following infection and neutralizing antibodies persist for the life of the bird. Following infection, transient CMI suppression is common; it may persist in birds that develop neoplasms. Both B and T lymphocytes have been identified in tumors, and thymectomy has been shown to reduce the level of lymphomas in affected birds. It has been suggested that MD might have an autoimmune component based on antibody responses to myelin and peripheral nerves.

Laboratory Diagnosis

On necropsy, gross lesions are common in peripheral nerves, root ganglia, and the spinal roots. Lymphomatous lesions are characteristically composed of small lymphocytes, lymphoblasts, and reticulum cells. Arterial lesions of atherosclerosis are often present. Confirmatory diagnosis is made by viral isolation or by antigen detection using fluorescent antibody, immunoperoxidase, or ELISA on feather follicle cells. Antibodies can be detected by agar gel immunodiffusion, indirect immunofluorescence, and viral neutralization and ELISA assays.

Prevention and Control

Experimentally, MDV-free flocks can be maintained by strict isolation, constant surveillance, and frequent monitoring for virus and antibody, but these techniques have been of limited commercial use. Commercial vaccines are available and have been effective in reducing the inci-

dence of MD. The three live virus serotypes have been used for vaccines resulting in more vaccines becoming available. HVT vaccine (serotype 3) is the most economical to produce and is most effective when exposure is not heavy. Vaccination does not prevent infection or shedding of virulent MDV, but it does prevent tumor formation. Bivalent and polyvalent vaccines have been used successfully where monovalent vaccines have been ineffective. Embryo vaccination is currently used in at least 55% of broiler embryos. Genetically resistant lines of chickens have been maintained experimentally.

Infectious Laryngotracheitis Virus (Gallid Herpesvirus-1)

Disease

Infectious laryngotracheitis virus (ILTV) usually occurs as an acute disease in chickens and represents a serious problem in areas of intense poultry husbandry. The virus produces signs of respiratory distress and coughing that often produce a bloody discharge. Mild enzootic forms of ILTV infection may result in reduced egg production, conjunctivitis, and persistent nasal discharge.

Etiologic Agent

Physical, Chemical, and Antigenic Properties

ILTV is a typical alphaherpesvirus that is also designated as gallid herpesvirus 1 (GaHV-1).

Sensitivity to Physical and Chemical Agents

ILTV is inactivated by 3% cresol, 1% sodium hydroxide, and 1% lye, 24 hours' exposure to ether, and 10 to 15 minutes at 55°C. The virus can be stored for lengthy periods by lyophilization and freezing.

Infectivity for Other Species and Culture Systems

ILTV is primarily a disease of chickens, but the disease has also been reported in pheasants and peafowl. Young turkeys have been infected experimentally, and the virus replicates in embryonated turkey eggs. Starlings, sparrows, crows, doves, ducks, pigeons, and guinea fowl have been found to be resistant to ILTV.

Chicken kidney monolayer cell cultures, embryonated chicken eggs, and chicken embryo (kidney, liver, and lung) cell cultures have been used to culture ILTV.

Host-Virus Relationship

Distribution, Reservoir, and Transmission

ILTV has been identified in almost every country in the world; it occurs primarily in areas with high concentrations of chickens and occasionally occurs in pheasants.

Chickens are assumed to be the primary reservoir and mode of transmission, which occurs by direct contact through droplet infection of the ocular and respiratory secretions. Mechanical transmission can occur via contaminated equipment and litter. Egg transmission of ILTV has not been demonstrated. A carrier state can develop in birds with sublethal disease, and ILTV has been isolated from chickens 2 years after infection. Unvaccinated birds are susceptible to infection from vaccinated birds, and vaccinated birds may become carriers. Acutely infected birds represent a greater source of virus than clinically recovered carrier birds.

Pathogenesis and Pathology

ILTV in natural conditions enters through the upper respiratory tract and ocular tract. In the natural disease, the greatest concentration of ILTV is found in the trachea, since the virus replicates only in the nasal cavity, trachea, and lower respiratory tract. Latent virus has been demonstrated in the trigeminal ganglion. Viremia has not been reported.

In lethal infections of ILTV, thickening of tracheal mucosa, hemorrhage, congestive heart failure, and severe congestion of all internal organs have been found. Histopathology demonstrates fibrinous tracheobronchitis, with detachment of the tracheal epithelium and large intranuclear inclusion bodies in detached cells that are the basis for a strong presumptive diagnosis.

Host Response to Infection

The first signs of ILTV infection usually appear 6 to 12 days following natural exposure. Resistance to disease following the infection or vaccination usually persists for approximately 1 year. Infected birds develop precipitating and serum-neutralizing antibodies; however, the cell-mediated response appears to be important in resistance. Full immunity can be demonstrated in bursectomized chickens in the absence of a humoral response.

Laboratory Diagnosis

Virus can be isolated from tracheal and lung tissue in embryonated chicken eggs, cell culture, and ILTV DNA can be demonstrated by PCR. Immunofluorescent staining of trachea can demonstrate presence of viral antigen up to 14 days postinfection. ELISA-based serology is widely used.

Prevention and Control

Use of live ILTV vaccine results in carriers, which can shed to nonvaccinated susceptible birds. Since the virus can survive for 10 days at temperatures of 13°C to 23°C, the cleaning of infected premises is very important. Complete depopulation and disinfection of premises has been used to control the disease.

Vaccination has been successful via the cloaca, infraorbital sinuses, intranasal instillation, feather follicles, and drinking water. Birds younger than 2 weeks of age do not respond as well as older birds. Water administration of ILTV vaccine does not give as complete or long-lasting immunity as other methods. For water vaccine to be effective, the virus has to penetrate into the nasal cavity or trachea. Cloacal administration of the vaccine leads to rapid absorption of the virus into the bursa of Fabricius and results in an immune response. This route is undesirable, however, since ILTV damages the bursa of young birds. Adequate ILTV vaccination occurs via aerosol procedures. Modified live ILTV vaccines have been associated with disease and chicken embryo origin vaccines have been demonstrated to increase in virulence after in vivo passage. The development of genetically engineered vaccines holds promise for improved control strategies.

55 *Poxviridae*

N. James MacLachlan   Jeffrey L. Stott

Poxviruses infect many vertebrate and invertebrate species. Diseases caused by poxviruses often affect the skin, although some cause systemic infections in which clinical signs of disease may or may not be apparent. Poxvirus infections often cause proliferative epithelial lesions in birds, whereas papular and/or pustular epithelial lesions are characteristic of poxvirus-infected mammals and only in some infections do these become proliferative.

Poxviruses are large and complex and replicate in the cell cytoplasm. Of the two subfamilies of poxviruses, members of the *Chordopoxvirinae* infect vertebrates, whereas viruses within the *Entomopoxvirinae* infect insects. There are eight distinct genera in the *Chordopoxvirinae* (Table 55.1), and there is considerable antigenic cross-reactivity between viruses in the various genera. *Chordopoxvirinae* have pleomorphic, roughly brick-shaped virions (approximately 220–450 nm long x 140–260 nm wide) that include a lipoprotein surface membrane and a biconcave or cylindrical core. The genome is enclosed in the core and consists of a single, very large (up to 130 kilobases) molecule of double-stranded DNA (dsDNA). The viral genome encodes some 150–300 proteins, and approximately 100 of these are contained within virions. Included are many enzymes that are involved in virus replication.

ORTHOPOXVIRUS

Disease

Orthopoxvirus infections cause a variety of papular diseases of humans and animals. Papules are raised epithelial proliferations that often ulcerate rapidly. Lesion development may be confined to specific areas of the skin or the infection may be generalized. Skin lesions often appear first as a rash or papule followed by pustule formation that rapidly is followed by crusting and scab formation.

Etiologic Agent

Orthopoxviruses include vaccinia (and related buffalopox and rabbitpox), cowpox (Fig 55.1), camelpox, monkeypox, ectromelia, and variola (human smallpox). They are morphologically indistinguishable, and there is considerable serological cross-reactivity between the viruses within this genus. Orthopoxviruses contain a hemagglutinin. The various orthopoxviruses can be distinguished on the basis of their genomic DNA sequence, and by pock formation on chick embryo chorioallantoic membranes (pock appearance and the highest temperature at which they develop). The animal host-species of origin is sometimes predictive of the type of orthopoxvirus, but not invariably so.

Host-Virus Relationship

Transmission of orthopoxviruses occurs by contact, aerosol, arthropod bites, or exposure to fomites. The poxviruses tend to be very stable in the environment.

Both cellular and humoral responses are critical to immunity against poxviruses. Cellular immunity facilitates destruction of virus-infected cells and is important in confining the virus to a localized area. Defects in cellular immunity permit widespread distribution of virus, resulting in generalized disease. Neutralizing antibodies are important in recovery from infection. Immunity appears to be of long duration.

Laboratory Diagnosis

Diagnosis of *Orthopoxvirus* infection can be made by electron microscopy of virus extracted from lesions or by viral isolation. Isolation may be achieved by inoculation (scarification) of laboratory animals (especially rabbits), of cell cultures, or of the chorioallantoic membrane of embryonated chicken eggs. The latter procedure has been widely used and may differentiate viral types.

Vaccinia

Vaccinia virus is the genus prototype and was used to vaccinate humans against smallpox (variola), which was a devastating disease prior to its eradication from the world in the second half of the 20th century. Vaccination of humans with vaccinia was responsible for the global elimination of smallpox, using the principle developed by Edward Jenner prior to 1800. Vaccinia was originally believed to be a cowpox, but its origin is uncertain since it is quite distinct from its purported ancestor. Buffalopox and rabbit pox (an infection of laboratory rabbits) are caused by viruses that are closely related or identical to vaccina.

Table 55.1. Genera (Subfamily: *Chordopoxvirinae*) of Significance in Veterinary Medicine

Genus	Members
Orthopoxvirus	Vaccinia (and highly related buffalopox and rabbitpox viruses)
	Cowpox (rodents, cats, cattle, and humans)
	Camelpox
	Mouse pox (ectromelia)
	Monkeypox
	Racoonpox
Parapoxvirus	Bovine papular stomatitis
	Contagious ecthyma of sheep (Orf)
	Pseudocowpox virus of cattle (Milker's nodule of humans)
	Squirrel parapoxvirus
	Sealpox virus
Avipoxvirus	Fowlpox
	Turkeypox
	Junopox (peacocks)
	Quailpox
	Sparrowpox
	Starlingpox
	Canarypox
	Pigeonpox
Capripoxvirus	Sheeppox
	Goatpox
	Lumpy skin disease (Neethling virus)
Suipoxvirus	Swinepox
Leporipoxvirus	Myxoma, rabbit, and squirrel fibroma
Molluscipoxvirus	Molluscum contagiosum
	Unnamed viruses of horses and donkeys
Yatapoxvirus	Yaba monkey tumor virus

Vaccinia may infect cattle via handling (milking) by infected personnel; infected cattle can also infect personnel. Vaccinia infection of cattle can produce lesions that are indistinguishable from those caused by cowpox virus; these occur on the teats and udder and appear as small papules that progress to pustules and, finally, exudative scabs. Buffalopox is a disease of milking water buffalo in Egypt, India, and Southeast Asia that also resembles cowpox. Like vaccinia, buffalopox virus can infect humans.

COWPOX

Cowpox virus is closely related to vaccinia, but antigenically distinct. Cowpox in cattle is characterized by papular, pustular, and crusty exudative lesions on the udder and adjacent areas of skin. Rodents serve as reservoir hosts of the virus, which also is contagious to humans, cats (domestic and large wild cats), and a variety of other animal species. Cowpox appears to be a disease that is confined to Europe including the British Isles.

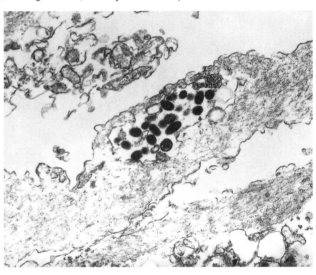

FIGURE 55.1. *Cowpox virus in skin lesions under thin sectioning. 8000X. (Courtesy of A. Castro.)*

CAMELPOX

Camelpox is a severe, generalized pustular disease of the skin of affected camels. It is of economic importance in countries with an indigenous camel population, including those of the Middle East, Africa, and parts of Asia. Disease occurs principally in younger animals and is characterized by fever, generalized rash, and sequential development of papular, pustular, and scabbing lesions on the limbs, neck, and head.

MOUSEPOX (ECTROMELIA)

Mousepox occurs in laboratory mice, although the virus readily is excluded from appropriately managed facilities. Mousepox is a severe, rapidly fatal disease characterized by extensive necrosis of the liver of affected mice. A more chronic form also occurs, characterized by necrosis of the distal extremities (feet, tail, and snout) of affected mice.

PARAPOXVIRUS

Parapoxviruses infect a wide variety of animals, principally ungulates and domestic livestock, although several are also contagious to humans (zoonoses). Parapoxviruses typically produce localized papular and proliferative cutaneous lesions; examples include bovine papular stomatitis virus, orf virus (contagious ecthyma), and pseudocowpox virus (milker's nodule).

Parapoxviruses are morphologically unique in that an organized tubular, threadlike structure forms a crisscross pattern on the virion surface. The viruses are all antigenically related, but the envelope contains antigenically distinct epitopes. The viruses are stable for long periods of time at ambient temperatures.

BOVINE PAPULAR STOMATITIS

Disease

Bovine papular stomatitis is characterized by the presence of papules, which are raised epithelial proliferations, on the muzzle, nares, lips, buccal cavity, dental pad, palate, and tongue. Hyperemic papules, with central necrosis and concentric colored rings, are highly characteristic. The disease is generally of minor importance, although it occasionally can mimic important vesicular diseases of cattle like foot-and-mouth disease and vesicular stomatitis.

Host-Virus Relationship

Bovine papular stomatitis virus infection of cattle occurs worldwide; humans sometimes are infected with the virus. It is believed to persist in a latent state in cattle. Virus is present in oral and nasal secretions and transmission may occur by direct contact.

Laboratory Diagnosis and Control

Bovine papular stomatitis must be differentiated from important vesicular diseases. Virus may be isolated on cell cultures or directly visualized in skin scrapings or biopsy material by electron microscopy. Vaccines have not been developed.

CONTAGIOUS ECTHYMA

Disease

Contagious ecthyma virus (Fig 55.2) is the etiologic agent of contagious ecthyma of sheep and goats (synonyms include scabby mouth, contagious pustular dermatitis of sheep, soremouth, infectious labial dermatitis, and orf). Orf is the term used to describe the disease in humans. Contagious ecthyma of sheep and goats initially is characterized by the appearance of papules and vesicles on the lips, mouth, interdigital skin, genitalia, and udder. Papules and vesicles rapidly progress to pustules, followed by scab formation. Lesions on the lips interfere with suckling or grazing, and thus to loss of condition of affected animals. Young animals are most likely to be affected, and the virus rapidly spreads among susceptible animals.

A related *Parapoxvirus* causes ulcerative dermatosis of sheep, a disease characterized by the presence of ulcerated papules on the lips, face, legs, feet, and external genitalia. Genital infections are transmitted by sexual contact.

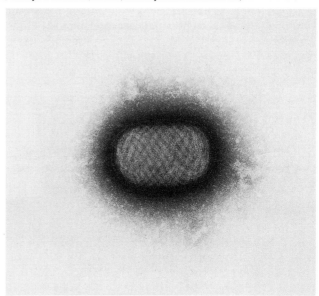

FIGURE 55.2. *Negatively stained preparation of contagious ecthyma virus. 40,000X. (Courtesy of R. Nordhausen.)*

Host-Virus Relationship

In addition to sheep and goats, contagious ecthyma virus may also infect humans (zoonoses), deer, and perhaps other species. Related viruses infect chamois and seals. The virus is distributed worldwide and is maintained in nature by persistent infections of sheep, as well as survival of the virus for prolonged periods in dried scabs. The virus is readily transmitted on rough feed that causes erosions and ulcers in the oral cavity of affected sheep.

Laboratory Diagnosis and Control

Presumptive diagnosis is based upon clinical observations and pathology (e.g., epithelial proliferation with intracellular edema leading to cytoplasmic vacuolation often with the presence of cytoplasmic inclusion bodies). Virus can be identified by electron microscopy and isolated in embryonic sheep skin or testicular cells.

Vaccination is used to control the disease in endemic areas, and immunity is considered to be long term in duration. Virulent virus is used in vaccination by scarification of the skin in areas not affected by the disease; a potential adverse impact of this approach is that it does ensure perpetuation of the virus in nature.

PSEUDOCOWPOX

Pseudocowpox is a mild disease of cattle that particularly affects lactating animals. Teat lesions develop as papules with an ulcerated center that becomes encrusted. This results in a pathognomonic scab with a ring or horseshoe appearance. The causative *Parapoxvirus* is closely related to bovine papular stomatitis virus, and can infect humans via direct contact, producing so-called milker's nodules.

Pseudocowpox occurs in most countries but has little economic significance because most infections are either asymptomatic or very mild. Immunity is of short duration and recurrent infections are common. Cattle occasionally develop chronic infections.

AVIPOXVIRUS

Avipoxviruses infect many avian species (see Table 55.1). Fowlpox virus is the genus prototype.

Disease

Pox is a common disease of commercial chickens and turkeys, and of many different species of pet and wild birds. Fowlpox causes decreased egg production and increased mortality on affected commercial premises. The lesions in affected birds are designated as either cutaneous or diphtheritic. Cutaneous lesions are characterized by nodular, wart-like proliferations of hyperplastic epithelium that involve the skin of the head (comb, wattles, corners of the mouth, nostrils, and eyes). The diphtheritic form is characterized by proliferative lesions on the mucous membranes and may extend into the sinuses; involvement of the larynx and trachea results in dyspnea and rales. The lesions are characterized by inflammation, epidermal hyperplasia, and development of eosinophilic intracytoplasmic inclusion bodies.

Mortality in affected commercial chickens and turkeys, pigeons, and psittacines is typically low, whereas infection in canaries is almost always fatal.

Etiologic Agent

The avipoxviruses are antigenically related but are differentiated by host range, serologic tests, plaque formation in cell cultures, and pock formation on the chorioallantoic membrane of embryonated chicken eggs. The viruses are also distinguished by analysis of their genomic DNA. Like other poxviruses, avipoxviruses are highly resistant to desiccation.

Host-Virus Relationship

Avipoxviruses have a worldwide distribution. Viral transmission can occur by direct contact or mechanical transmission. Virus can survive for long periods in scabs, leading to cutaneous or respiratory infection. The viruses also can be transmitted by biting insects, especially mosquitoes and mites. Chronic infections of individuals may contribute to viral persistence on a given premise.

Humoral and cellular immune responses develop fol-

lowing infection and apparently confer long-term immunity. Maternal antibody does not confer protection to hatched chicks.

Laboratory Diagnosis

Diagnosis of avian poxvirus infections is based on clinical signs and histopathology and electron microscopy. Virus can be isolated by inoculating susceptible birds, the chorioallantoic membrane of embryonated chicken eggs, and cell cultures (chicken and duck embryo fibroblasts).

Treatment and Control

Control of avian poxvirus infections can be aided by providing adequate nutrition, housing, and insect control among birds. Live virus vaccines are used to immunize birds against pox; these vaccines induce a mild disease that leads to protective immunization. Recombinant vaccines recently have been developed and provide a vector for the incorporation of heterologous genes for protective immunization.

CAPRIPOXVIRUS

The genus *Capripoxvirus* includes sheeppox, goatpox, and lumpy skin disease (Neethling) viruses; sheeppox virus is the genus prototype. The viruses are more elongated than other poxviruses and measure about 115 nm x 194 nm; hemagglutinin is absent. The viruses are closely related but differ antigenically. Infection with any virus produces cross-protection to heterologous virus, with the exception of certain strains of goatpox virus. The viruses are predominantly host-specific, though some strains produce lesions in sheep, goats, and/or humans.

SHEEPPOX AND GOATPOX

Disease

Sheeppox and goatpox are important poxvirus diseases of livestock, although infection with these viruses can produce clinical signs that range in severity from inapparent to a severe generalized condition. Animals of all ages are susceptible but disease is more severe in younger animals, especially in endemic areas. Breed and immune status also affect disease severity. Both sheeppox and goatpox viruses cause systemic infections of susceptible hosts, and viremia occurs soon after infection. Virus is disseminated to the skin, lymph nodes, and multiple organs, including the spleen, kidneys, and lungs. The first clinical signs of disease include pyrexia, rhinitis, and conjunctivitis, followed by varying degrees of lesion development on external nares, lips, tongue, gums, and skin (especially where wool or hair is minimal). Skin lesions are initially papules and vesicles that rapidly become pustular and necrotic with scab formation. Infected epithelial cells may contain eosinophilic cytoplasmic inclusion bodies. Lesions may also develop in the respiratory and alimentary tracts, liver, kidneys, and other organs. A nodular form of the disease has been referred to as *stone pox*. Increased mortality rates are associated with secondary bacterial infections and disseminated internal lesions.

Host-Virus Relationship

Infections occur predominantly in Africa, the Middle East, and the Indian subcontinent. Viral transmission is by aerosol, direct contact, and possibly arthropod vectors. Viral persistence is probably due to the survival of virus in scabs and its transmission to susceptible animals within an endemic area.

Antibodies, including those with viral-neutralizing activity, develop within 1 week of lesion development. Immunity is considered to be lifelong.

Laboratory Diagnosis

Histopathology, fluorescent antibody staining, electron microscopy, and serology can help confirm clinical diagnosis. Virus can be isolated in cell cultures of ovine, bovine, and caprine origin. The virus grows relatively poorly in embryonated chicken eggs as compared to orthopoxviruses and parapoxviruses.

Treatment and Control

Preventative measures such as import restrictions are practiced by countries free of the virus. Attenuated and inactivated viral vaccines are used in endemic areas.

LUMPY SKIN DISEASE

Disease

Lumpy skin disease of cattle (and buffalo) is caused by a virus (Neethling virus) closely related to sheeppox and goatpox viruses. Infection is followed by viremia and fever, with the subsequent formation of nodular lesions on the skin (predominantly on the neck, face, muzzle, brisket, flank, legs, perineum, and scrotum) and internally in the respiratory, digestive, and reproductive tracts. The cutaneous lesions are firm, raised and circumscribed, and they often undergo central necrosis and ulceration. Similar lesions occur within the epithelium lining the upper respiratory and alimentary tracts. The virus causes a disseminated infection that results in vasculitis, lymphangitis, and lymphadenopathy.

Host-Virus Relationship

Neethling virus is confined to Africa and Madagascar. Viral transmission probably occurs by direct contact, aerosol and insect vectors. Persistence of virus in nature is probably similar to that described for sheeppox and goatpox, but it is proposed that buffalo may serve as viral reservoirs in some areas.

Laboratory Diagnosis

Definitive diagnosis requires fluorescent antibody staining or electron microscopy of tissues, viral isolation in cell cultures (lamb and calf kidney) or embryonated chicken eggs (development of pocks on the chorioallantoic membrane), or serology.

Treatment and Control

Treatment is confined to supportive therapy. Vaccination results in long-term immunity. Countries free of lumpy skin disease have imposed import restrictions on stock from infected countries.

SUIPOXVIRUS

Swinepox virus is the only member of the genus *Suipoxvirus*. It is the cause of swinepox, a disease characterized by disseminated cutaneous pox lesions.

Disease

Swinepox occurs in pigs of all ages, although younger animals are more commonly affected. The disease usually is very mild, with virtually no mortality. Lesions typically develop on the abdomen and inner thighs and sometimes on other areas of the skin. Lesion development progresses from papular through pustular and scabbing stages. Microscopic lesions are similar to other poxvirus lesion and include hyperplasia of epidermal cells with hydropic degeneration and the formation of eosinophilic intracytoplasmic inclusion bodies. Inflammatory cells are found in the dermis. Vaccinia can cause an identical disease in pigs.

Host-Virus Relationship

Swinepox has a worldwide distribution. Virus may be spread by direct contact or mechanically by lice. Transplacental transmission may also occur. The virus persists for long periods in dried scabs.

Swine develop immunity in the absence of detectable neutralizing antibody, suggesting that local humoral immunity or cell-mediated immunity is important in viral clearance and protection against reinfection.

Laboratory Diagnosis

The skin lesions of swinepox are highly characteristic, and often are associated with lice infestation. Laboratory confirmation may be required to rule out other important vesicular diseases. Definitive diagnosis can be obtained by fluorescent antibody staining, electron microscopic evaluation of lesions for the presence of poxviruses, or virus isolation in porcine cell cultures.

Control

Control of swinepox is best realized by elimination of external parasites. Vaccination is not commonly used.

56 *Picornaviridae*

N. James MacLachlan   Yuan Chung Zee

Jeffrey L. Stott

Picornaviruses comprise a large family of small RNA viruses. The family *Picornaviridae* recently was proposed to include nine genera: *Aphthovirus, Enterovirus, Cardiovirus, Rhinovirus, Hepatovirus, Parechovirus, Erbovirus, Kobusvirus,* and *Teschovirus,* most of which contain members that are important in veterinary medicine (Table 56.1). A variety of avian picornaviruses including duck hepatitis viruses 1 and 3 and turkey hepatitis virus are not yet classified into specific genera.

GENERAL FAMILY CHARACTERISTICS

The viruses included within the various genera of the family *Picornaviridae* have similar general properties. The viruses lack an envelope and exhibit a cubic symmetry with diameters of approximately 30 nm and densities in cesium chloride of 1.33 to 1.45 g/cm^3. The capsid, which is icosahedral, is composed of 60 subunits, each consisting of three surface proteins (VP1, VP2, and VP3 or, respectively, 1D, 1B, and 1C) and (generally) an internal protein (VP4 or 1A) that is closely associated with the genomic RNA. Each of these proteins is derived by systematic cleavage of a single precursor protein, from which 11 or 12 viral proteins eventually are produced by post-translational cleavage.

The viral genome consists of a single piece of single-stranded RNA of 7–8.5 kilobases. The genome is positive-sense RNA, thus it serves as messenger RNA and it also is infectious. A small viral-specified protein, VPg, is linked to the 5' terminus of the genome and may play a role in initiating RNA synthesis and in viral maturation (RNA packaging).

APTHOVIRUS

The genus *Aphthovirus* includes foot-and-mouth disease and equine rhinitis A viruses. These are typical picornaviruses with the notable exception that they are labile below pH 7 (acid-labile) and they have a leader protein that is encoded immediately prior to the capsid proteins. Foot-and-mouth disease virus is the type species. The VP1 protein of aphthoviruses is responsible both for cellular attachment and for viral neutralization.

FOOT-AND-MOUTH DISEASE

Although foot-and-mouth disease (FMD) is not as widely distributed as it once was, particularly in industrialized countries, it remains an enormously important disease of food animals. The economic impact of FMD reflects not only direct losses associated with disease in affected animals, but also interference with international and regional movement of animals. The virus infects all wild and domestic cloven-hoofed animals, but the disease typically is most dramatic in cattle and swine; sheep and goats are usually not as severely affected. Economic losses due to FMD can be vast; the 2001 United Kingdom outbreak, for example, is estimated to have cost producers several billion dollars in lost revenue, and the loss of revenue from reduced tourism that resulted from quarantine measures imposed during the outbreak was estimated to have cost a similar amount.

Disease

FMD in cattle and swine is characterized by fever, depression, excessive salivation, lameness, and formation of vesicles on the mucous membranes of the oral cavity (tongue, dental pad, and gums) and muzzle, epidermis of the coronary band and interdigital spaces, udder, and teats. Vesicles may also develop in the epithelium of the pharynx, larynx, trachea, esophagus, and rumen. Necrosis of the heart muscle occurs in some young animals. The vesicles rapidly erode to leave ulcers that result in reduced food consumption, weight loss, and emaciation. Secondary bacterial infections also occur in the ulcers of some affected animals. While mortality is generally less than 3%, morbidity is very high and economic losses reflect decreased productivity and protracted convalescence of affected animals. Mortality is notably increased in young pigs and sometimes calves.

Etiologic Agent

Physical, Chemical, and Antigenic Properties

FMD viruses are typical picornaviruses (Fig 56.1). There are seven distinct serotypes, designated as O, A, C, SAT1, SAT2,

Table 56.1.   Picornaviridae of Veterinary Significance

Genus	Member	Disease
Aphthovirus	Foot and mouth disease virus	Foot and mouth disease of cloven-hoofed animals
	Equine rhinitis A	Systemic infection with respiratory signs
Enterovirus	Porcine enteroviruses A and B (formerly enteroviruses 8–10)	Reproductive (SMEDI) and dermatitis (skin)
	Swine vesicular disease virus	Vesicular disease
	Bovine enteroviruses 1 & 2	Uncertain
	Simian enteroviruses	Uncertain
Cardiovirus	Encephalomyocarditis virus	Myocarditis
	Theilovirus	Polioencephalomyelitis —Theilers murine encephalomyelitis —Rat encephalomyelitis
Rhinovirus	Bovine rhinoviruses 1, 2, & 3	Upper respiratory (mild)
Hepatovirus	Avian encephalomyelitis-like virus	Neurologic disease
Erbovirus	Equine rhinitis B virus	Respiratory
Teschovirus	Porcine teschoviruses 1–7, 11–13 (formerly porcine enteroviruses 1–7, 11–13)	Neurologic disease (polioencephalomyelitis)
Unassigned	Duck hepatitis virus	Hepatic necrosis
	Turkey hepatitis virus	Hepatic necrosis

FIGURE 56.1.   *Negatively stained preparation of foot-and-mouth disease virus (A12). 108,000X. (Courtesy of B. Baxt.)*

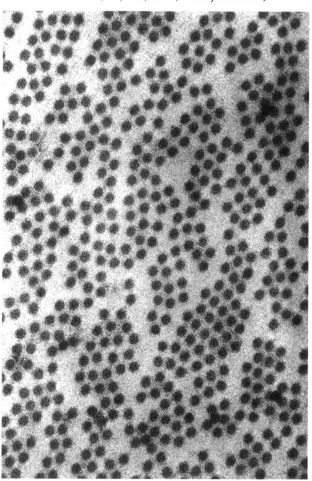

SAT3, and Asia 1. There also is extensive genetic heterogeneity within individual serotypes, with many distinct virus subtypes occurring within each serotype.

The VP1 protein (1D) is responsible for virus neutralization and contains a conserved RGD integrin-binding motif that is responsible for the binding of virus to integrin cellular receptors.

Resistance to Physical and Chemical Agents

FMD virus can survive for extended periods in animal secretions and products. The virus is inactivated by heating above 50°C and is sensitive to both acid (pH less than 6.5) and alkaline (pH greater than 11.0) treatments. FMD virus resists inactivation by lipid solvents. Sodium hydroxide (1%) is recommended for disinfecting premises following outbreaks.

Infectivity for Other Species and Culture Systems

A wide variety of animals are susceptible to infection and disease caused by FMD virus, including cattle, domestic and wild pigs, sheep, goats, certain wild ruminants, buffalo, camels, South American camelids, and humans (rare). Among domestic livestock, cattle and swine are usually most severely affected. Experimental infections of dogs, cats, rabbits, and chinchillas have been reported.

Susceptible laboratory animals include guinea pigs, suckling mice, rats, rabbits, and hamsters. Some viral strains have been propagated in chick embryos, day-old chicks, and several other avian species. FMD virus replicates in a variety of cell cultures of bovine and ovine origin, baby hamster kidney (BHK) cells, and rabbit and mouse cells.

Host-Virus Relationship

Distribution, Reservoir, and Transmission

The worldwide distribution of FMD virus largely mirrors that of the global economic situation, thus the disease occurs principally in developing countries; most industrialized countries are free. FMD is endemic in Africa, South America, and parts of Europe and Asia. North and Central America, the United Kingdom and Ireland, Japan, Australia, New Zealand, Scandinavia, and the Caribbean region are currently free of FMD, although many of these countries have previously suffered outbreaks, some very recently.

The epizootiology of FMD differs somewhat depending upon whether or not FMD virus is endemic in a country/region. Outbreaks of FMD in previously free regions spread very rapidly, as a consequence of the highly infectious nature of the virus and its short incubation period, the large quantities of virus excreted from the respiratory tract of affected animals, and the relative stability of the virus in the environment. Virus may be transmitted by direct contact, aerosol, and fomites and possibly arthropod vectors. Virus may be recovered from all body secretions/discharges (tears, nasal, saliva, urine, feces, milk, vaginal, semen, and the placenta of aborted fetuses). The survival of virus in such excretions depends upon temperature, pH, and humidity. FMD can be transported over long distances via infected animals or their products and is viable for up to 3 months in frozen meat and up to 2 months in ham, bacon, and certain sausages. When discarded as garbage, contaminated pork products constitute a source of FMD virus infection for swine in particular. Animal hides can serve as a source of virus for extended periods of time. Humans may disseminate virus mechanically (fomites) or biologically by becoming infected. Long-distance airborne spread of virus has also been implicated as the source of some outbreaks. It is to be stressed that epidemics of FMD can occur in endemic areas when new serotypes or strains of the virus are introduced and that the severity of any outbreak reflects the inherent biological properties of the infecting virus strain.

Pathogenesis and Pathology

The predominant route of FMD virus infection is respiratory, although ingestion of contaminated food or direct inoculation also are both highly effective in transmitting infection. Viremia precedes development of lesions and overt disease, and virus can be isolated from body fluids and secretions at this time. Virus rapidly moves from the blood during viremia to infect the epithelium of the oral cavity and feet, where lesions develop. The virus can persist in the oral cavity of infected animals for long periods after the acute infection.

The characteristic epithelial lesion of FMD is the vesicle, which forms as a consequence of both intracellular (spongiosis) and intercellular edema. These vesicles rapidly rupture to leave erosions and ulcers in the affected epithelium. In young animals, FMD virus can infect the heart musculature, causing degeneration and necrosis; the characteristic yellow-white streaks of myocardial necrosis are referred to as *tiger heart*.

Host Response to Infection

Serum IgG develops about 2 weeks postinfection and is type-specific. Colostral antibody in newborn calves has been reported to interfere with vaccination. The relative importance of local secretory, systemic, and cell-mediated immunity is not well defined. Duration of immunity is longer in cattle than in swine but apparently persists for only about a year. Serum-neutralizing antibody, actively or passively acquired, appears to correlate with protection in pigs.

Laboratory Diagnosis

Due to the economic and political significance of FMD and its similarity to other vesicular diseases—vesicular stomatitis (VS), swine vesicular disease (SVD), and vesicular exanthema of swine (VES)—a rapid definitive diagnosis is essential. Polymerase chain reaction (PCR) techniques are increasingly used for rapid identification of FMD virus, and sequence analysis of any PCR-positive material then can be used to type the infecting strain of FMD virus and to undertake molecular epidemiologic studies. FMD virus can also be isolated from clinical samples (vesicular fluid and others) by propagation in cell cultures or laboratory animals followed by physicochemical characterization and serology using viral neutralization, enzyme-linked immunosorbent assay (ELISA), fluorescent antibody (FA), or agar gel immunodiffusion (AGID). Electron microscopy (EM) and immuno-EM microscopy also can be used for rapid diagnosis.

Serologic diagnosis of FMD virus infection can be made by ELISA, AGID, and viral neutralization (either in cell cultures or suckling mice). The AGID test can be used to identify antibody to group-reactive antigen (viral infection-associated antigen); such antibody is typically found only in animals that have experienced an active infection and not in animals vaccinated with inactivated virus. Recombinant FMD virus nonstructural proteins (2C and 3AB1) can also be used in serology to distinguish vaccinated from naturally infected animals as vaccinates do not make antibody to these proteins.

Treatment and Control

No specific treatment exists for FMD. However, proper animal husbandry practices and treatment of secondary bacterial infections reduce losses.

Control of FMD is difficult due to its highly contagious nature, multiple hosts, viral stability, multiple antigenic types and subtypes, and transient immunity. Countries free of FMD impose strict import regulations on animals, animal products, and potentially contaminated materials from FMD countries. Previously unaffected countries have often resorted to massive slaughter and quarantine programs to control outbreaks; for instance, more than 4 million ruminants were killed in order to control the recent outbreak of FMD in the United Kingdom.

Quarantine and vaccination programs are also used to control outbreaks and to prevent spread of the disease. Countries with endemic FMD rely heavily on vaccines to control the disease; however, steps still need to be taken to avoid importing additional viral strains since cross-protective immunity between strains is not complete. Inactivated vaccines of tissue culture origin that are administered in adjuvant are most commonly used in FMD-endemic countries. The safety of live attenuated vaccines is questionable, so their use is not widespread. Vaccination is conducted one to three times a year since immunity is short-term. Vaccines must be of the appropriate type/subtype. Current research is directed at developing subunit, synthetic peptide, and recombinant-type vaccines. The latter two approaches have been directed at VP1 with encouraging results.

EQUINE RHINITIS A VIRUS

The equine rhinitis A virus is an economically important pathogen of horses that is closely related to FMD virus. Equine rhinitis A virus produces a systemic infection with respiratory signs in affected horses, and outbreaks of disease have been described. Distinct strains of equine rhinitis A virus have been identified by sequence analysis. Serological surveys indicate widespread infection of horses, although the true impact of equine rhinitis A virus remains uncertain. The virus is difficult to isolate in cell culture, thus it is best detected using polymerase chain reaction (PCR). The virus can be detected in the feces of infected horses, as well as in their respiratory secretions.

ENTEROVIRUS AND *TESCHOVIRUS*

The genus *Enterovirus* encompasses a large number of different viruses that typically are species-specific in their host range, including viruses that infect humans (polio, coxsackie, entero, and echoviruses), cattle (bovine enteroviruses 1 and 2), pigs (porcine enteroviruses A and B [formerly porcine enteroviruses 8, 9, and 10] and swine vesicular disease virus), and monkeys (simian enteroviruses). The porcine *Enterovirus* serotypes 1–7 and 11–13 now are included in a proposed genus *Teschovirus*. Enteroviruses are thermolabile (infectivity destroyed quickly at 50°C), insensitive to detergent treatment, and stable at low pH (can survive pH of 3).

PORCINE ENTEROVIRUSES AND TESCHOVIRUSES

Disease

A variety of enteroviruses and teschoviruses have been described in swine, including swine vesicular disease virus (closely related to human coxsackie B virus), ten serotypes of porcine teschoviruses and two of porcine enteroviruses (A and B). These viruses are the cause of several important diseases of swine. Teschoviruses (especially serotype 1) are the cause of encephalomyelitis in pigs, so-called Teschen and Talfan disease. Infections with porcine enteroviruses are generally asymptomatic, but they also have been associated with infertility (so-called SMEDI, reflecting stillbirth, mummification, embryonic death, and infertility), dermatitis, and pneumonia. Swine vesicular disease virus, which is caused by a distinct porcine *Enterovirus* that is closely related to human coxsackie B virus, is the cause of swine vesicular disease, which must be distinguished from foot-and-mouth disease. The various disease entities caused by these viruses in swine are discussed separately below.

Host-Virus Relationship

Porcine enteroviruses occur in most swine-raising areas. These viruses generally cause asymptomatic enteric infections of swine. Viral persistence is probably facilitated by the continued introduction of susceptible pigs and the presence of carrier animals. Transmission occurs by direct contact and exposure to viral-contaminated feces.

Porcine enteroviruses typically infect the host via ingestion, inhalation, or both. Soon after infection, virus can be isolated from the respiratory system, blood, and intestinal contents. The virus has a tropism for the intestinal tract and may also be isolated from mesenteric lymph nodes, liver, spleen, kidney, tonsils, turbinates, lung, diaphragm, and sometimes the central nervous system (brain and cord) and/or fetuses of pregnant animals. The properties of individual virus strains are clearly variable.

SMEDI infections result in fetal mummification, stillbirths, and reduced litter size, although porcine reproductive and respiratory syndrome virus and porcine parvovirus are more important causes of this syndrome. The consequences (infertility or fetal death/mummification) reflect the stage of gestation when susceptible sows are infected. Sows generally are infected with porcine enteroviruses prior to sexual maturity, thus they are typically immune before they become pregnant, although immunity is serotype-specific.

Laboratory Diagnosis

Definitive diagnosis requires fluorescent antibody staining of the tissues of affected pigs (or fetuses), viral isolation, or PCR. Viral isolation can be attempted on primary pig kidney cell cultures. Serologic diagnosis can be done using paired serum samples to demonstrate seroconversion or an increase in antibody titer.

Control

Control of porcine *Enterovirus* infection is difficult due to the multiplicity of serotypes and their ubiquitous nature in swine operations.

TESCHEN AND TALFAN DISEASES

Disease

Teschen and Talfan are the names given, respectively, to severe and mild forms of polioencephalomyelitis in pigs caused by infection with teschoviruses. The diseases are named after towns in Europe where they first were described in detail. The mild disease (Talfan) also is referred to as *benign enzootic paresis* or *poliomyelitis suum*. Suckling or weaner pigs are most susceptible. Acute disease is characterized by fever, anorexia, weakness, and variable degrees of central nervous system dysfunction. As the disease progresses, animals may have trouble standing or walking and experience tremors, convulsions, and nystagmus with eventual development of paralysis and death.

Host-Virus Relationship

Teschen disease, first described in the Teschen region of Czechoslovakia, still occurs in Central Europe. Milder forms of *Enterovirus*-induced poliomyelitis in young swine (analogous to Talfan disease) have been described throughout the world. There are no characteristic gross lesions in pigs with polioencephalomyelitis. Microscopically, poliomyelitis is most evident in the spinal cord and cerebellum. Lesions are characterized by neuronal degeneration, gliosis, and lymphocytic inflammation. The pathogenesis of polioencephalomyelitis in pigs is analogous to that of human polio (also caused by an *Enterovirus*), with initial virus replication in the intestine and then disseminated to the central nervous system in immunologically naive animals.

Laboratory Diagnosis

The clinical signs described and the histopathologic observation of neuronal necrosis and lymphocytic polioencephalomyelitis cellular aggregations are suggestive, but definitive diagnosis requires demonstration of virus in tissues by immunohistochemical staining, viral isolation, or PCR.

Treatment and Control

Treatment of *Enterovirus*-induced polioencephalomyelitis is usually futile, since most affected pigs die. Inactivated vaccines have been used in Europe with variable success but have not been used elsewhere. Strict quarantine is often used to prevent introduction of the most highly pathogenic forms of the virus to regions free of such viruses.

SWINE VESICULAR DISEASE

Disease

Swine vesicular disease (SVD) resembles foot-and-mouth disease (FMD), vesicular stomatitis (VS), and vesicular exanthema of swine (VES). Affected swine exhibit signs similar to those of FMD, with fever, lameness, and vesicles in and around their feet (coronary bands, soles, and interdigital areas) and, less commonly, the oral cavity and nares.

Host-Virus Relationship

SVD was first described in Italy and still occurs sporadically in Europe and Asia. The causative virus is closely related to human coxsackie virus B5, and SVD is a zoonoses. The virus is highly contagious to swine and is spread by direct contact and by ingestion of contaminated foods. The virus is very stable in pork products such as sausage. Following oral infection, the virus first replicates in the intestinal tract and then is disseminated throughout the body and can be isolated from a variety of tissues and from feces. Encephalitis occurs in some infected pigs. Mortality usually is low in uncomplicated infections.

Laboratory Diagnosis

Rapid diagnosis of SVD is critical because it must be distinguished from FMD and other vesicular diseases like VS and VES. The diagnosis is best done by PCR, and sequence analysis can be used to distinguish SVD virus from other enteroviruses. The virus or viral antigens also can be identified with vesicles by immunohistochemical staining or electron microscopy, or by virus isolation on primary porcine cell cultures or in suckling mice. Serological diagnosis can be accomplished in convalescent animals by ELISA or viral neutralization.

Treatment and Control

No specific treatment for SVD is available, and only experimental vaccines have been described. The real economic importance of SVD is that it readily can be confused with FMD, so control requires strict quarantine and import restrictions in countries free of disease. Strict quarantine and animal depopulation are also used to control incursions of the virus into previously unaffected regions.

BOVINE *ENTEROVIRUS*

Two serotypes of bovine enteroviruses (1 and 2) have been described. These viruses are of uncertain significance because they have been isolated from both healthy and diseased cattle.

HEPATOVIRUS

The genus *Hepatovirus* includes human hepatitis A virus as well as avian encephalomyocarditis-like virus.

AVIAN ENCEPHALOMYELITIS

Disease

Avian encephalomyelitis virus (AEV) causes neurologic disease and high mortality in young chickens (1 to 2 weeks of age). Mortality can be 25% or higher in susceptible young birds, depending on the virulence of the infecting virus strain and flock immunity. Infection of adult birds is usually subclinical.

Etiologic Agent

Although AEV is a typical picornavirus in terms of its virion structure, its nucleotide sequence is dissimilar to those of other picornaviruses. The virus is stable and resistant to acid pH.

Besides chickens and turkeys, Japanese quail and pheasants are susceptible to AEV infection. Ducks, pigeons, and guinea fowl can be experimentally infected. Chick embryos can be infected (the yolk sac route is the most common), but rapid passage of field isolates is required before clinical signs (muscular dystrophy) are observed in the embryo. Cell culture systems for viral propagation include chicken neuroglial cells, embryo fibroblasts, brain cells, and pancreatic cells.

Host-Virus Relationship

Avian encephalomyelitis occurs wherever poultry are raised commercially. The virus replicates in the intestine and then spreads to the central nervous system in susceptible young birds. The virus is transmitted via the feco-oral route, although vertical transmission hen-to-egg also occurs.

Microscopic lesions occur in the brain and spinal cord of affected birds and are those of viral encephalomyelitis, characterized by neuronal degeneration, perivascular cuffing, and gliosis. Visceral lesions, characterized by hyperplasia of lymphoid follicles, occur in the proventriculus, pancreas, and myocardium.

The humoral immune response to AEV results in viral clearance and protection. Neutralizing antibodies develop within 2 weeks of infection. Immunity is apparently of long duration as exposed flocks rarely have recurrent outbreaks. Maternal antibody protects young chicks for several weeks, thus mortality is minimized in immune flocks.

Laboratory Diagnosis

Avian encephalomyelitis must be distinguished from other neurologic diseases, especially other viral diseases like Newcastle disease. Histopathology provides a presumptive diagnosis, which then can be confirmed by virus isolation or by immunohistochemical staining of the tissues of affected birds.

Treatment and Control

No treatment is available for affected birds. Attenuated and inactivated vaccines have been successfully used to control the disease. Birds in high AEV incidence areas may be vaccinated prior to reaching breeding age with live viral vaccine strains. Only part of the flock need be vaccinated since the virus will spread throughout the flock. Inactivated vaccines should be used if breeding flocks are to be immunized. Chickens born to immune hens are resistant to AEV-induced disease.

CARDIOVIRUS

ENCEPHALOMYOCARDITIS VIRUS

Disease

Encephalomyocarditis (EMC) virus naturally infects rodents. The virus is transmitted from rats to humans and domestic animals, in which it can cause myocarditis. In domestic animals, the disease most commonly occurs in young pigs. The disease in swine is typically manifested by sudden death with few, if any, preceding clinical signs. Mortality can be high, especially in young pigs.

Etiologic Agent

There are a number of strains of EMC virus, including mengovirus, Maus Elberfeld virus, and Columbia SK virus.

Host-Virus Relationship

Encephalomyocarditis virus principally infects rodents, but it also can infect nonhuman primates, humans, elephants, squirrels, calves, horses, and pigs. Lack of pig-to-pig transmission following experimental infections suggests that infection usually derives from rodents.

Foci of myocardial necrosis in affected pigs manifest as white tracts of coagulation necrosis with associated lymphocytic inflammation and calcification.

Laboratory Diagnosis

Viral isolation is advised since immune responses require about 5 days and may not develop prior to death. PCR techniques have also been successfully used for diagnosis of infection.

MURINE AND RAT ENCEPHALOMYELITIS

A variety of related strains of cardioviruses cause enteric infections in rodents. Like human polioviruses and porcine teschoviruses, these viruses can spread to the central nervous system to cause polioencephalomyelitis in immunologically naive animals. These viruses can be detected by serological screening, and control is by quarantine, testing, and sanitation.

RHINOVIRUS AND *ERBOVIRUS*

Rhinoviruses are characterized by acid sensitivity (pH of less than 5 to 6). The genus *Rhinovirus* includes human and bovine viruses, whereas equine rhinoviruses 2 and 3 are now tentatively classified together as equine rhinitis B virus in the genus *Erbovirus*. All of these viruses share a tropism for the upper respiratory tract, best exemplified by human rhinoviruses that cause the majority of common colds.

Bovine Rhinovirus

Bovine rhinoviruses infect the upper respiratory tract of susceptible cattle. The majority of infections are asymptomatic or very mild, resulting in minimal serous nasal discharge, mild fever, and coughing. Morbidity is very high, as determined by serologic studies, but the significance of *Rhinovirus* as a pathogen of cattle is uncertain. Rhinoviruses have been implicated in the pathogenesis of the bovine shipping fever complex.

Transmission of the virus is probably by direct contact, aerosol, and contaminated materials.

Protective immunity is best correlated to neutralizing antibody in serum and nasal secretions. Titers of serum antibody to *Rhinovirus* tend to increase with age in cattle, probably due to reinfection with homologous and heterologous viral strains.

Diagnosis of clinical *Rhinovirus* infection is difficult due to the multiplicity of viruses associated with respiratory disease. Viral isolation is often difficult and requires specific bovine cell cultures; a sandwich ELISA has been described for confirmation of bovine *Rhinovirus* identity. Demonstration of a rising neutralizing titer on paired serum samples is sometimes useful.

Equine Rhinoviruses and Erboviruses

Equine rhinitis A virus is an *Aphthovirus* that causes a systemic infection in horses that is sometimes characterized by respiratory disease, whereas equine rhinitis B virus causes inapparent or mild upper respiratory tract infection of susceptible horses. Although rhinitis B virus has been isolated from horses with acute respiratory disease, its true pathogenic significance is poorly defined. Diagnosis is best accomplished using PCR assay, because virus isolation rarely is successful.

UNASSIGNED PICORNAVIRUSES

Duck and Turkey Hepatitis

Disease

Duck hepatitis is a contagious and highly fatal disease of young ducklings. Affected ducklings are depressed and death follows quickly. Morbidity is often high and mortality may approach 90%. A similar disease caused by a related virus occurs in young turkeys.

Etiologic Agent

At least 2 serotypes of duck hepatitis virus (DHV) currently are listed as unassigned members of the family *Picornaviridae,* along with turkey hepatitis virus. These viruses apparently can infect other avian species, and experimental infection of young chickens, pigeons, geese, pheasants, and guinea fowl has been reported, sometimes with high mortality.

The viruses can be propagated by allantoic inoculation of embryonated chicken eggs (ECEs). Infected chick embryos die 5 to 6 days postinoculation and appear stunted and edematous. Various chick, duck, and goose embryonic cell lines support viral replication. Development of cytopathic effect is variable.

Host-Virus Relationship

Duck hepatitis virus appears to have a worldwide distribution. Transmission of virus occurs by direct and indirect contact with contaminated feces. The virus apparently replicates in the intestinal tract of infected birds. The characteristic gross lesion is an enlarged and hemorrhagic liver. Additional lesions may include an enlarged and mottled spleen and congested, swollen kidneys. Microscopic lesions include hepatocellular necrosis, bile duct hyperplasia, and inflammatory responses in various organs.

Immunity develops following infection, and maternal transfer of antibody protects ducklings for several weeks.

Laboratory Diagnosis

Diagnosis is suggested by the rapid spread and peracute nature of the disease. Hemorrhagic lesions in the liver of affected birds are very characteristic, but must be distinguished from other causes of hepatic necrosis. Definitive diagnosis may be made by demonstration of viral antigen in the affected tissues by immunohistochemical staining or by virus isolation in ECE or cell cultures.

Treatment and Control

There is no effective treatment for clinically affected birds. Attenuated and inactivated DHV vaccines are available, and immunization of breeding birds facilitates maternal transfer of antibody. Ducklings may also be immunized directly but successful vaccination of ducklings requires that they be free of maternal antibody.

57 Caliciviridae

Yuan Chung Zee   N. James MacLachlan

Caliciviruses are small (27–40 nm in diameter), nonenveloped, icosahedral viruses with a genome of single-stranded, positive-sense RNA (Fig 57.1). The viral RNA serves as mRNA and is infectious. The name *calicivirus* is derived from the chalice-shaped spheres on the surface of negatively stained viral particles. There are four distinct groups in the family: *Lagovirus*, Norwalk-like viruses, Sapporo-like viruses, and *Vesivirus*. Several members—specifically vesicular exanthema of swine virus, San Miguel sea lion virus, feline calicivirus, European brown hare syndrome, and rabbit hemorrhagic disease viruses—are important animal pathogens.

GENERAL PROPERTIES

The genome of caliciviruses has only two or three open reading frames. Virions are comprised of a single major capsid protein. The nonstructural proteins of caliciviruses share features with those of picornaviruses. Replication of caliciviruses occurs in the cytoplasm, although both cytoplasmic and intranuclear inclusions occur in infected cells.

VESIVIRUSES

Vesicular exanthema and feline calicivirus are classified together in the genus *Vesivirus*. Viruses within this genus are readily propagated in cell culture, in distinct contrast to caliciviruses in the other genera.

VESICULAR EXANTHEMA OF SWINE

Disease

Vesicular exanthema of swine (VES) is an acute viral disease characterized by the formation of vesicles in the oral cavity, interdigital spaces, and coronary band of the foot. VES clinically is indistinguishable from foot-and-mouth disease (FMD), swine vesicular disease, and vesicular stomatitis. The incubation period of the disease is approximately 24 to 72 hours and the course is about 1 to 2 weeks. The disease has a high morbidity but a low mortality. It is of some economic importance as a disease in pigs; however, its main impact is that it mimics FMD, from which it must be distinguished. The last occurrence of this disease occurred in the United States in 1956. Subsequently, the U.S. Department of Agriculture in 1959 declared VES an exotic disease; however, viruses capable of causing VES are endemic in marine mammals, where they also cause vesicular diseases and reproductive failure. A wide variety of seals, sea lions, walrus, and dolphins are infected with these viruses. Outbreaks of VES occur when these marine mammal caliciviruses spread to swine, likely as a result of feeding of dead marine mammals to swine.

Etiologic Agent

Physical, Chemical, and Antigenic Properties

VES virus (VESV) is a typical calicivirus and viral particles are associated with cytoplasmic cisternae in infected swine cells (Fig 57.2) and in crystalline arrays in the cytoplasm (Fig 57.3). VESV is stable at low pH (pH 5). A large number of antigenically distinct types of VESV have been identified (at least 13), and a number of antigenically distinct viruses that originally were isolated from species other than swine are capable of causing VES and so are classified as VES viruses, including bovine calicivirus, Cetacean calicivirus, primate calicivirus, and a number of so-called San Miguel sea lion viruses (17 types). Similar viruses have been isolated from fish, birds, reptiles, and other mammals, including skunks. These viruses are distinguished by serological tests, usually serum neutralization, and the virulence of these viruses to pigs varies significantly.

Resistance to Physical and Chemical Agents

VES virus can persist in the environment and in contaminated meat products for very long time periods. The virus is completely inactivated by 2% sodium hydroxide or 0.1% sodium hypochlorite.

Infectivity for Other Species or Culture Systems

Naturally occurring VES disease is confined only to swine of all ages and breeds. Experimentally, VESV causes vesicles at inoculated sites in seals. Vesicles are also produced at the sites of inoculation in horses and hamsters. Virus is isolated in low titers from some sites of inoculation and draining lymph nodes. VES virus can be propagated in cell lines of swine kidney or Vero monkey kidney.

FIGURE 57.1.

FIGURE 57.1. *Negatively stained preparation of feline calicivirus. 240,000X. (Courtesy of A. Castro.)*

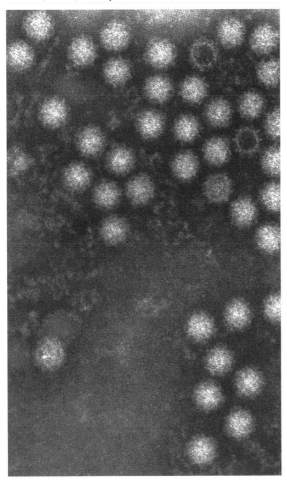

Host-Virus Relationship

Distribution, Reservoir, and Transmission

VES was first described in North America (California) in 1932, and outbreaks were reported every year in California between 1932 and 1951 (with the exception of 1937–1938). The disease first appeared outside of California in 1951, and from 1952 to 1953 it spread to a total of 42 states in the United States. The disease had never been reported elsewhere in the world except Iceland and Hawaii, and these two incidents resulted from shipping contaminated pork products from California.

Marine mammals serve as reservoirs for VESV infection. A calicivirus was first isolated in 1972 from sea lions on San Miguel Island off the coast of southern California. This calicivirus was named *San Miguel sea lion virus (SMSV),* which was indistinguishable from VESV by morphologic, biophysical, and biochemical criteria. Experimental SMSV infection of swine produces a disease indistinguishable from VES. SMSV also has been isolated from asymptomatic domestic swine. Serum-neutralizing antibodies to several serotypes of SMSV and VESV have been demonstrated in marine mammals and both wild and domestic swine in California. Earlier epidemiologic studies during the outbreaks of VES confirmed the relationship between feeding of raw garbage and outbreaks of the disease, and dead sea lions are known to have been utilized as a food source for swine.

Although outbreaks of VES likely originated from feeding SMSV-infected marine animal parts to swine, the infection subsequently spread rapidly within affected herds by direct contact.

Pathogenesis and Pathology

VES is characterized by the appearance of fluid-filled vesicles on the snout, coronary band, and tongue of infected

FIGURE 57.2. *Parallel rows of VESV particles in cytoplasmic cisternae. 72,000X. (Reproduced with permission from Zee YC, Hackett AJ, Talens LT. Electron microscopic studies on the vesicular exanthema of swine virus. II. Morphogenesis of VESV Type H54 in pig kidney cells. Virology 1968;34:596.)*

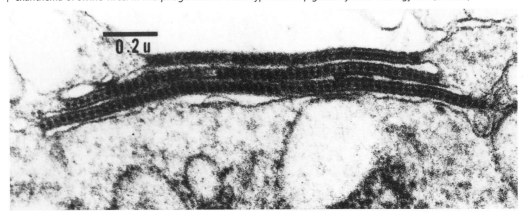

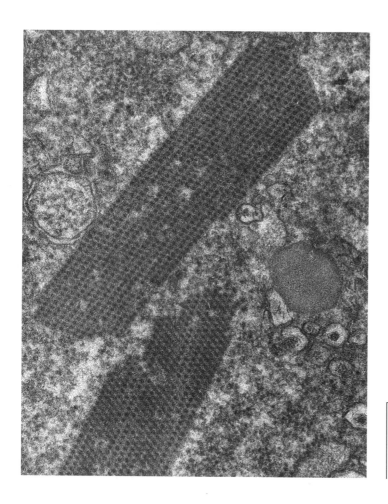

FIGURE 57.3. *Section of a viral crystal in VESV-infected cells. 64,000X. (Reproduced with permission from Zee YC, Hackett AJ, Talens LT. Electron microscopic studies on the vesicular exanthema of swine virus. II. Morphogenesis of VESV Type H54 in pig kidney cells. Virology 1968;34:596.)*

swine. These same lesions develop in swine that are inoculated intradermally with either VESV or SMSV. Infected animals are febrile, and virus is present in blood and nasal-oral secretions for several days after infection. Vesicles appear on the coronary band and interdigital space of the feet at 3 to 4 days after infection. The vesicles rapidly rupture and healing takes place unless complicated by secondary bacterial infection. High titers of virus are present within the fluid in vesicles, which may also contaminate the environment. Mild encephalitis occurs in some swine infected with VESV, and virus also may be recovered from brain tissue of swine infected with SMSV.

Host Response to Infection

Neutralizing antibodies to VESV and SMSV appear in the sera of animals infected with viruses soon after inoculation and titers peak within 7 to 10 days after infection.

Laboratory Diagnosis

VES must rapidly be differentiated from other vesicular diseases of swine, such as FMD, swine vesicular disease, and vesicular stomatitis. Laboratory diagnosis is accomplished by virus isolation in cell cultures, direct electron microscopic examination of vesicle fluid, or polymerase

chain reaction. Although the vesicular diseases all produce similar signs in swine, there are major differences: whereas VES and swine vesicular disease are almost exclusively diseases of swine, vesicular stomatitis frequently affects horses as well as ruminants, and FMD also affects ruminants (Table 57.1).

Table 57.1. Susceptibility of Domestic Animals to Four Viruses That Cause Vesicles in Swine

Animal Species	SVD	VES	FMD	VSV
Cattle	−	−	++	++
Swine	++	++	++	+
Sheep	−	−	+	−*
Horse	−	−*	−	++
Guinea pig	−	−*	+	+
Suckling mice	+	−	+	+
Humans	+	−	−*	+

* Occasional lesions produced by specific virus strains
SVD = Swine vesicular disease
VES = Vesicular exanthema of swine
FMD = Foot-and-mouth disease
VS = Vesicular stomatitis

Treatment and Control

There is no treatment for VES and there are no vaccines for control of the disease. It now is considered to be eradicated in the United States. Enforcement of laws requiring cooking of garbage before feeding it to swine was the most important factor in eliminating the disease.

FELINE CALICIVIRUS

Disease

Feline calicivirus (FCV) infects the oral cavity and upper respiratory tracts of cats to produce fever, sneezing, and nasal and ocular discharges. Clinical signs include rhinitis, conjunctivitis, oral ulcerations, and, in severe cases, pneumonia. Joint or muscle soreness, hyperesthesia, and chronic oral ulceration also have been attributed to FCV infection, and a disseminated highly virulent and fatal systemic disease associated with specific strains of FCV recently has been described. The incubation period of the disease is 2 to 3 days and infected cats usually recover in 7 to 10 days in the absence of secondary bacterial infections. Virulent systemic FCV infection is characterized by alopecia, cutaneous ulcers, subcutaneous edema, and high mortality.

Etiologic Agent

Physical, Chemical, and Antigenic Properties

There are multiple strains of FCV, and the virulence of individual strains varies substantially.

Resistance to Physical and Chemical Agents

Feline calicivirus is resistant to many common disinfectants. It is readily inactivated by a 0.175% sodium hypochlorite solution (Clorox), which is the disinfectant of choice. The virus is stable at a pH of 4 to 5 and is inactivated at 50°C within 30 minutes.

Infectivity for Other Species and Culture Systems

FCV is a ubiquitous pathogen that has been isolated from cats all over the world. There is no evidence that FCV produces disease in laboratory animals. The virus can readily be propagated in feline cell lines. Some strains have been grown in Vero monkey kidney and dolphin kidney cells.

Host-Virus Relationship

Distribution, Reservoir, and Transmission

The disease occurs worldwide, and all species of cats likely are susceptible. Infection and disease are most common in young cats, and older cats usually are immune. Infected cats recovered from the disease may carry virus in their oropharynx for long periods of time and serve as reservoirs of infection. The virus is transmitted by horizontal aerosol infection and by contaminated fomites.

Pathogenesis and Pathology

Cats acquire FCV infection via the respiratory route, either by aerosol or from fomites. The primary sites of viral replication are epithelial cells of the oral cavity and respiratory tract and in the tonsils. Viremia occurs during acute infection.

The characteristic lesions in typical cases of FCV infection in susceptible kittens and young cats are vesicles within the oral cavity (tongue, hard palate) and on the nares. The vesicles rapidly rupture, leaving erosions and ulcers. Highly virulent strains can cause pneumonia in kittens. Regeneration of the oral mucosa occurs rapidly in uncomplicated cases.

Virulent systemic strains of FCV cause epidemics of fatal disease in susceptible cats. Affected animals may exhibit severe oral ulceration, extensive subcutaneous edema, and variable ulceration of the pinnae, paw pads, nares and skin. Some affected cats also have pneumonia as well as liver and splenic necrosis, and FCV antigen is detected by immunohistochemical staining in both epithelial and endothelial cells.

Host Response to Infection

Cats infected with FCV or vaccinated with inactivated or live modified FCV vaccines develop serum-neutralizing antibodies. Kittens born to cats that are immune to FCV acquire maternal serum-neutralizing antibody to FCV via colostrum.

Laboratory Diagnosis

Laboratory tests are required to distinguish FCV infection from other agents that produce similar respiratory signs in cats, particularly feline viral rhinotracheitis (herpesvirus). These include the isolation of FCV in feline cell cultures from nasal secretions, throat swabs, or conjunctival scrapings and the identification of FCV antigen in conjunctival scrapings of tonsillar biopsies by immunohistochemical staining. The characteristic appearance of the virus by electron microscopy can also be used for rapid diagnosis.

Treatment and Control

Treatment for FCV infection in cats is mainly supportive and symptomatic. Broad-spectrum antibiotics help prevent secondary bacterial infections, and fluid therapy is useful in the event of dehydration. All strains of FCV are considered variants of a single serotype because there is considerable serologic cross-reactivity among viruses. Furthermore, cats immunized with one variant of FCV are protected against other strains. Both inactivated and modified live FCV vaccines are commercially available and afford reasonable protection against FCV infection. The FCV vaccines are usually combined with feline rhinotracheitis (a herpesvirus) and feline panleukopenia (a parvovirus) and administered either intranasally or intramuscularly.

FCV infection is controlled primarily by isolating cats that show respiratory signs and disinfecting cages and premises with Clorox before susceptible animals are introduced.

LAGOVIRUSES

RABBIT HEMORRHAGIC DISEASE AND EUROPEAN BROWN HARE SYNDROME

Disease

Rabbit hemorrhagic disease (RHD) and European Brown Hare Syndrome (EBHS) are similar diseases that are caused by related but antigenically distinct caliciviruses. RHD is an acute infectious disease of the European rabbit, *Oryctolagus cunniculus*, and frequently has a very high mortality rate in susceptible rabbit populations. A novel feature of RHD is that the disease is only fatal to rabbits over 2 months of age. The disease is characterized by a short incubation period, followed by fever, disseminated hemorrhage in all body tissues, and rapid death. The disease was first described in China in 1984 and it then rapidly spread throughout much of the rest of the world. EBHS occurs in the European hare, *Lepus europaeus*.

Etiologic Agent

Physical, Chemical and Antigenic Properties

Various strains of RHD and EBHS viruses are recognized and distinguished serologically.

Infectivity for Other Species and Culture Systems

Neither RHD nor EBHS viruses are readily propagated in cell culture, which means that the viruses have been largely characterized using homogenates of the livers of affected animals. The viruses appear to be highly species-specific.

Host-Virus Relationship

Distribution, Reservoir, and Transmission

Although RHD was first reported in China, EBHS had been recognized earlier in Europe. It is possible that a mutation of the EBHS calicivirus led to the emergence of RHDV, causing the lethal pandemic of rabbits. The disease is transmitted by the oral-fecal route.

Pathogenesis and Pathology

Rabbits with RHD have an enlarged spleen, swollen liver, and disseminated hemorrhages. Extensive liver necrosis is highly characteristic and potentially explains the disseminated intravascular coagulation (DIC) that occurs in affected animals. The DIC induced by RHDV is not characteristic of other calicivirus infections, but does occur in such flavivirus-induced diseases as yellow fever and dengue in humans.

Laboratory Diagnosis

Immunofluorescence and ELISA tests have been developed for the rapid diagnosis of RHD. The genome of RHDV has been completely sequenced, so polymerase chain reaction (PCR) readily can be developed and used for rapid diagnosis of the infection.

Treatment and Control

There is no treatment for the acute disease. A formalin-inactivated vaccine that incorporates infected rabbit tissue provides effective immunization against the disease. Control also can be achieved through strict quarantine and isolation to prevent transportation of RHDV-contaminated materials into commercial rabbitries. It is interesting to note that, although most countries have focused on the control and prevention of RHD, RHDV has been used as a biologic weapon to control rabbit numbers in other countries.

UNASSIGNED CALICIVIRUSES

Enteric caliciviruses have been described in cattle, dogs, chickens, and pigs, among others. At least some of these appear to cause clinical signs of intestinal disease analogous to that caused by the Norwalk-like viruses in humans.

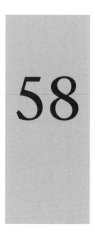

58

Togaviridae and *Flaviviridae*

N. James MacLachlan   Jeffrey L. Stott

TOGAVIRIDAE

The family *Togaviridae* derives its name from "toga," the Latin word for gown or cloak, which refers to the envelope possessed by all members of the family. The family includes two genera, *Alphavirus* and *Rubivirus* (the cause of human rubella). Viruses in the *Alphavirus* genus are arboviruses that are transmitted by mosquitoes; thus they have the capacity to replicate sequentially in insects and vertebrates.

ALPHAVIRUS

Sindbis virus is the prototype of the genus *Alphavirus*. Alphaviruses of veterinary significance include eastern equine encephalitis (EEE), western equine encephalitis (WEE), and Venezuelan equine encephalitis (VEE, including subtype II Everglades) viruses, along with several other viruses (Getah, Highlands J, and Semliki Forest). The three equine encephalitis viruses are also zoonoses, and they are described in detail below.

Disease

EEE, WEE, and VEE all cause encephalitis in horses, but the signs can vary from inapparent to fatal disease. Mild and/or inapparent infections are more common with WEE, whereas EEE and VEE are typically more virulent. Death from VEE may occur in the absence of neurologic signs. Central nervous system (CNS) involvement of horses following encephalitis virus infection is characterized by aimless walking, followed by severe depression and behavioral changes (dummy), central blindness, paralysis, and death soon after the onset of clinical signs. Mortality can be very high (up to 90%), especially with VEE and EEE. Young horses are more susceptible to severe disease.

EEE and WEE may also cause significant disease in domestic birds; EEE is more common and mortality can be very high. Clinical disease is especially common in pheasants and ratites (emus, etc.). EEE also occurs in swine and cattle. Equine encephalitis virus disease in birds is characterized by encephalitis with leg paralysis, torticollis, and tremors. Wild birds may also be infected but rarely experience disease, and they serve as vertebrate reservoirs of virus.

Etiologic Agent

Physical, Chemical, and Antigenic Properties

Alphavirus virions are spherical, enveloped, and approximately 70 nm in diameter. The envelope is derived from the plasma membranes of host cells through which virions bud as they mature. The envelope encloses an icosahedral nucleocapsid that is approximately 40 nm in diameter and consists of a single capsid protein as well as the genome of linear single-stranded positive-sense RNA. The envelope contains a heterodimer of 2 viral glycoproteins (E1 and E2), and some alphaviruses (Semliki Forest virus) have a third glycoprotein (E3). At least four different nonstructural viral proteins are produced in infected cells. The alphaviruses all are antigenically related as determined by serological assays, and are grouped into distinct antigenic complexes with numerous subtypes or strains within each. The extensive genetic and antigenic variation that occurs within the various subtypes and variants of each antigenic complex is reflected by differences in their virulence, biochemical characteristics such as electrophoretic mobility of protein and RNA digests, physicochemical characteristics, host range, geographic distribution, and vector/host tropism.

Resistance to Physical and Chemical Agents

Alphaviruses are sensitive to lipid solvents, chlorine, phenol, acid pH, and heating to 60°C for 30 minutes.

Infectivity for Other Species and Culture Systems

The equine encephalitis viruses can infect a wide host range, including humans, horses, rodents, reptiles, amphibians, monkeys, dogs, cats, foxes, skunks, cattle, pigs, birds, and mosquitoes. Alphaviruses can be propagated in a variety of cell cultures, including chick and duck fibroblasts, Vero, L cells, and mosquito cells; cytopathology is often absent in the latter. A variety of laboratory animals can be experimentally infected, with suckling mice being the most common. Embryonated chicken eggs and young chicks may also be susceptible to infection.

Host-Virus Relationship

Distribution, Reservoir, and Transmission

The equine encephalitis viruses occur in the Western Hemisphere, although related viruses occur elsewhere in the world. EEE occurs in eastern North America (predominantly east of the Mississippi River and the Atlantic Seaboard region in particular), the Caribbean Basin, and Central and South America. WEE occurs throughout much of North America, particularly in areas west of the Mississippi River, and South America. VEE is confined to South and Central America, although incursions into North America have occurred periodically. The United States considers VEE to be a foreign animal disease; however, an avirulent VEE virus (Type II, Everglades) is endemic in portions of Florida.

The equine encephalitis viruses are transmitted by mosquitoes and, despite their names, horses and humans are dead-end hosts that are unimportant to the natural cycle of EEE and WEE virus infections. The viruses all persist in similar but distinct natural cycles of infection that include mosquitoes and birds or rodents that function as the vertebrate reservoirs of each virus. Except in tropical areas where infection occurs year-round, the peak incidence of these diseases typically is in late summer and declines when climatic conditions are less favorable for the mosquito vectors. Mosquitoes are biological vectors of these viruses, which requires that the mosquito actually become infected with the virus rather than simply transmitting it mechanically. For a biological vector to become infected it must obtain a blood meal from a viremic vertebrate host. The level of viremia required to infect the vector is dictated by viral strain, species of mosquito vector, or both. Upon ingestion, the virus infects the insect gut and then spreads to the salivary glands, where replication provides a ready source of virus to infect additional vertebrate hosts during insect feeding. The time required for this process is the extrinsic incubation period. Once infected, the vector remains infected for life.

EEE virus infection causes clinical disease in humans, horses, and birds, especially ring-necked pheasants, ratites, and some commercial poultry (Pekin ducks, etc.). EEE also has been described in cattle and pigs, sometimes with high mortality. EEE virus exists in two distinct ecosystems; North American (eastern United States and Canada) and Caribbean strains of the virus are transmitted by *Culiseta melanura* mosquitoes. The virus is maintained in an enzootic cycle of infection that includes these ornithophilic mosquitoes and the passerine and wading birds that serve as vertebrate virus reservoirs in coastal and inland swamp environments. Periodic spillover of the virus occurs in adjacent horses, humans, birds, and other animals. A variety of mosquito species can transmit the virus during epidemics, and direct horizontal spread occurs among birds when they peck viremic birds. Another mosquito (*Culex melanoconion*) is responsible for transmis-

sion of EEE in Central and South America, where small mammals and birds serve as the vertebrate reservoirs of the virus.

The host-virus relationship of WEE is similar to that of EEE, with the virus being maintained in a transmission cycle between mosquitoes (*Culex tarsalis*) and domestic and passerine birds, with periodic spillover into humans, horses, and domestic birds. Other species of mosquitoes can transmit the virus during outbreaks.

The lifecycle of VEE is more complex. There are several distinct clusters of VEE viruses (Types I-VI), most of which do not cause disease in horses (Type 1, varieties D through F, Types II-VI). These viruses are endemic throughout tropical and subtropical regions of the Americas (including Florida, where VEE Type II [Everglades] occurs). These endemic VEE viruses are maintained in a natural cycle of infection between *Culex* mosquitoes and small rodents in tropical swamps. Only VEE Types 1AB and 1C are virulent to horses, and these are only isolated during the epidemics of VEE that regularly occur in northern South America. It is believed that these epidemic strains emerge after mutation of the E2 envelope glycoprotein of endemic Type 1D strains of VEE that constantly are circulating in endemic areas but are not pathogenic to horses. Once strains of VEE emerge that are virulent to horses and humans, infected horses are a major source of virus because, unlike EEE and WEE, VEE replicates to high titers in horses. Thus, the endemic and epidemic (epizootic) VEE viruses have very different cycles of infection.

Pathogenesis and Pathology

Alphavirus infections can range from inapparent to severe, fatal disease. Infection follows the bite of an infected mosquito. Primary viral replication occurs in regional lymph nodes adjacent to the site of the bite and is followed by generalized infection and viremia in which the virus replicates in the lymphoid tissues throughout the body, bone marrow, and certain other tissues. The encephalitis viruses likely gain entry into the CNS after replication in the endothelial cells lining blood vessels in the brain, and passage of virus to the brain occurs after the acute phase of infection and viremia. Lesions occur throughout the gray matter of the brain and include perivascular cuffing with inflammatory cells, infiltration of neutrophils into the gray matter with neuronal and parenchymal necrosis, and vasculitis, thrombosis, and hemorrhage. Neutrophils are especially characteristic of the early cerebral lesions of EEE and VEE.

Host Response to Infection

The development of neutralizing antibody to encephalitis viruses appears to be important in limiting viral replication and spread and is clearly important in preventing reinfection. Antibodies develop to all viral proteins, and peak titers of neutralizing antibody typically develop within 2 weeks of infection in animals that survive. This antibody may be effective in neutralizing virus, enhancing viral clearance, and lysing infected cells via complement or Natural Killer cells. Cell-mediated immunity also appears to contribute to viral clearance and protective immunity. Cytotoxic T lymphocytes can be identified as early as 3 to 4 days postinfection.

Laboratory Diagnosis

Alphavirus infection may be suspected based on the occurrence of neurologic disease among susceptible animal species in endemic areas, thus prior history and seasonal occurrence can be important. Definitive diagnosis requires laboratory confirmation, which usually is done by serology with an IgM-capture enzyme-linked immunosorbent assay (ELISA) to detect virus-specific antibodies in the serum of acutely affected animals. The diagnosis is unequivocally confirmed by virus isolation from blood or CNS tissue, the latter being preferable due to the variable occurrence of viremia by the time signs of encephalitis are manifest in infected animals. Virus may be isolated in a variety of systems, including cell cultures, chick embryos, and suckling mice.

Treatment and Control

There is no treatment for clinically ill animals. Control of *Alphavirus* infections can be achieved through vaccination and pest management programs. Vector control can be approached through eliminating mosquito breeding sites by water control or spraying programs. In the case of domestic bird farms, the use of tightly screened (insect-proof)

rearing pens and locating such pens away from freshwater swamps is also a possibility. Attenuated (VEE) and inactivated vaccines have been developed for the equine encephalitis viruses. Regular vaccination of susceptible animals is required to maintain immunity if inactivated vaccines are used.

Other Togaviruses

A number of other togaviruses can infect animals, including Sindbis, Semliki Forest, Highlands J, and Getah viruses. Highlands J virus has a similar distribution in North America as EEE virus, but only rarely causes encephalitis in horses. It is, however, an important pathogen of turkeys, pheasants, chukar partridges, ducks, emus, and whooping cranes. Getah virus infects horses and swine in Asia and Southeast Asia. Infection in horses is sometimes characterized by fever, rash, and limb edema (but not encephalitis), and Getah virus also can cause abortion in pregnant swine. Getah virus is included within the Semliki Forest virus complex of alphaviruses, and Semliki Forest virus also can cause a febrile disease of horses in Africa.

FLAVIVIRIDAE

The family *Flaviviridae* contains a large number of viruses within three antigenically distinct genera (Table 58.1): *Flavivirus*, *Pestivirus*, and *Hepacivirus* (human hepatitis C virus). Although not discussed here, the family *Flaviviridae*

Table 58.1. Flaviviruses of Veterinary Importance

Genus	Serogroup/Agent	Vector	Affected species	Distribution
Flavivirus				
	Tick-borne encephalitis group	Ticks	Humans	Europe, Asia
	Louping Ill	Ticks	Sheep	
	Powassan	Ticks	Horses	North America
	Japanese encephalitis group	Mosquitoes		
	Japanese encephalitis virus		Swine, humans, birds	Asia
	Murray Valley encephalitis virus		Humans, birds	Australia
	West Nile virus (Kunjin)		Humans, horses, birds	Americas, Europe, Asia, Australia, Africa
	St. Louis encephalitis virus		Humans, birds	Americas
	Yellow Fever group	Mosquitoes		
	Wesselsbron virus		Sheep	Africa
Pestivirus		None		
	Border disease virus		Sheep	Worldwide
	Bovine virus diarrhea virus 1 and 2		Cattle	Worldwide
	Classical swine fever virus		Swine	Worldwide*

* Eradicated in a substantial number of countries

includes a substantial number of very important human pathogens.

FLAVIVIRUS

Members of the genus *Flavivirus* include arboviruses that are transmitted by either ticks or mosquitoes. The tick-borne flaviviruses include tick-borne encephalitis (European, Far Eastern, and Siberian), Powassan, and Louping-ill viruses. Those that are mosquito-transmitted include the Dengue virus group (the cause of human Dengue hemorrhagic fever), Japanese encephalitis virus group (including Japanese encephalitis, Murray Valley encephalitis, St. Louis encephalitis, and West Nile and Kunjin viruses), and Yellow Fever virus group (including Yellow Fever and Wesselsbron viruses). These viruses cause either encephalitis or systemic hemorrhagic-septicemia in animals and/or humans.

Etiologic Agent

Physical, Chemical, and Antigenic Properties

The name *Flavivirus* is derived from the Latin word *flavus,* which means yellow, since Yellow Fever virus is the family prototype. Members of the genus consist of spherical (50 nm in diameter) enveloped particles with small surface projection (peplomers). A single nucleocapsid protein encapsidates the genome, and the envelope contains two viral membrane proteins (E and M). Several nonstructural viral proteins are also produced in virus-infected cells (NS1-5). The viral genome is a single linear strand of positive-sense RNA. The genomic RNA is infectious and encodes a single large polyprotein that is co- and post-translationally cleaved into the various viral structural and nonstructural proteins.

The flaviviruses are all serologically related as determined by group-specific assays such as ELISA and hemagglutination inhibition. They are distinguished by neutralization assays, although there is considerable cross-reactivity among viruses within the same serogroup (serocomplex). The envelope E protein contains the major determinants of virus neutralization.

Resistance to Physical and Chemical Agents

Virions are stable at a pH of 7 to 9, but are inactivated by acid pH, temperatures above 40°C, lipid solvents, ultraviolet light, ionic and nonionic detergents, and trypsin.

Host-Virus Relationship

Distribution, Reservoir, and Transmission

The flaviviruses of veterinary importance are arboviruses that are transmitted by either ticks or mosquitoes; thus they share the ability for sequential replication in vertebrate and invertebrate hosts. They infect a range of vertebrate species, including mammals and birds.

Pathogenesis and Pathology

Flavivirus infection can produce inapparent to fatal disease. Encephalitis and hemorrhagic fever are characteristic of *Flavivirus*-induced diseases, depending on the specific virus.

Host Response to Infection

Both humoral and cell-mediated immune responses develop in animals following *Flavivirus* infection. Antibodies (HI and viral-neutralizing) develop within a few days after infection. Neutralizing antibodies largely are directed at the E envelope protein, whereas cytotoxic T lymphocyte responses are directed at the nonstructural viral proteins. Humoral responses appear to play an important role in both recovery and long-term protection against reinfection. Cell-mediated immune responses (cytotoxic T lymphocytes) likely contribute to viral clearance. Immunity is probably lifelong after natural infection, but only to the homologous virus.

DISEASES

JAPANESE ENCEPHALITIS

Japanese encephalitis virus (JEV) is the prototype of the JE antigenic complex within the *Flavivirus* genus. The JE complex includes St. Louis encephalitis virus, Murray Valley encephalitis virus, and West Nile virus (and related Kunjin virus), in addition to JEV itself. These are all human pathogens, but JEV and West Nile virus are important veterinary pathogens as well.

JEV infection is typically inapparent but can cause clinical disease in humans, horses, and swine. Infection of dogs and domestic poultry also occurs. The major adverse impact of JEV infection of swine is the occurrence of abortions and neonatal deaths after infection of nonimmune pregnant swine, whereas infected horses can develop severe neurologic disease that resembles eastern equine encephalitis (EEE), although mortality is lower. JEV infection currently is confined to temperate and tropical areas of Asia, where serological surveys indicate that infection of horses, cattle, and swine is widespread. The virus occurs throughout much of Asia, from the Indian Subcontinent to the west to the Pacific Islands in the east. Most infections are inapparent or mild. Horses and humans are unimportant to the epidemiology of JEV infection because viremias are very low-titered in these species, insufficient to serve as a virus reservoir for susceptible mosquito vectors. In contrast, infected swine and birds serve as amplifying hosts for the virus because they have high-titered viremias. *Culex* mosquitoes are the principal vectors of JEV. In swine, virus may also be transmitted from the infected dam to the fetus and from boar to sow via insemination of viral-contaminated semen. The virus is maintained in tropical regions probably by continual transmission between mosquitoes, birds, and swine.

Diagnosis of JEV is accomplished by isolating virus

from the tissues or blood of affected animals using cell cultures (vertebrate or insect) or suckling mice. Viral antigen may also be demonstrated directly in brain tissue sections by immunohistochemical staining. A variety of serological assays also are available, but demonstration of virus-specific IgM (indicative of recent infection) is generally required as IgG assays often detect antibodies to related flaviviruses, which complicates interpretation.

Vaccination is used for control of JEV infection in endemic areas, and both attenuated and killed vaccines are available. Vector control measures are another possible approach.

West Nile and Kunjin Viruses

West Nile virus (WNV), a member of the JEV antigenic complex, occurs throughout Africa as well as portions of Europe, the Middle East, Asia, and Australia (where it is called Kunjin virus). The virus recently emerged in the Western Hemisphere, precipitating a massive epidemic of disease in humans, horses, birds, and an enormous variety of other animals (alligators, squirrels, mountain goats, etc.). The virus is maintained in a mosquito-bird cycle of infection, and humans and horses are "dead-end" hosts because viremia is not sufficient to infect susceptible mosquitoes that feed on infected individuals. There are two distinct genetic lineages of WNV, so-called "lineage 1" and "lineage 2." Lineage 2 viruses are endemic south of the equator in Africa, where they cause little if any disease in horses. In distinct contrast, lineage 1 strains of WNV have been associated with outbreaks of disease in Mediterranean and eastern Europe, North Africa, Asia, and North America.

Whereas many bird species undergo subclinical or asymptomatic infection and have viremias of sufficient magnitude to serve as amplifying reservoir hosts of the virus, other species of birds suffer high mortality similar to horses. The neurological disease that occurs in some WNV-infected horses is characterized by ataxia, weakness, recumbency, muscle fasiculations, and high fatality rates. Among birds, raptors and corvids have been especially hard hit by the WNV epidemic in North America.

Specific species of mosquitoes transmit WNV in endemic areas, whereas a wide variety of mosquito species have been incriminated in the transmission of WNV infection in North America.

Diagnosis of WNV is best done by polymerase chain reaction (PCR), which is rapid and very sensitive. Virus isolation in appropriate cell cultures also is possible. WNV-specific IgM capture ELISA is very useful for the serological identification of animals that are acutely infected with WNV. An inactivated vaccine currently is available for protective immunization of horses.

Wesselsbron

Wesselsbron virus is a member of the Yellow Fever virus antigenic group and causes disease of sheep in sub-Saharan Africa. Subclinical infection of cattle, horses, and swine also occur, and the virus is a zoonotic pathogen. The virus causes extensive liver necrosis, jaundice, subcutaneous edema, gastrointestinal hemorrhage, and fever in infected sheep; mortality in lambs can be high, and abortion is common in pregnant ewes. Wesselsbron virus is transmitted by *Aedes* mosquitoes.

Diagnosis may be based upon viral isolation using a variety of cell cultures (BHK and lamb kidney), chick embryos, or suckling mice. Vaccination and/or prior exposure to other flaviviruses complicate the interpretation of serological assays. Attenuated vaccines are used to prevent the disease in endemic areas.

Louping-Ill

Louping-ill virus is a tick-transmitted flavivirus that naturally infects many animal species, including humans, sheep, horses, deer, and birds. The virus causes encephalomyelitis in sheep, and high mortality may result when susceptible sheep are introduced into an endemic area. Louping-ill is characterized by neurologic signs such as hyperexcitability, cerebellar ataxia, and progressive paralysis. The disease derives its name from the leaping gait sometimes observed in ataxic animals. Louping-ill is a zoonoses, and disease also sometimes occurs in cattle, horses and goats.

Louping-ill is confined to the British Isles and portions of continental Europe. *Ixodes rincinus* ticks are the principal vector. Diagnosis of louping-ill is done by viral isolation, immunohistochemical staining of CNS tissue sections from affected animals, or serology. Virus can be isolated using vertebrate or insect cell cultures and intracerebral inoculation of suckling mice. Propagated virus can be definitively identified by viral neutralization.

Louping-ill can be controlled through tick control by dipping and spraying of sheep. A formalin-inactivated cell culture-origin vaccine is available and effective. Lambs born to immune dams are protected by colostral antibody for approximately 4 months.

Powassan and Related Tick-Borne Encephalitides

Powassan virus is the cause of a tick-transmitted encephalitis of humans and horses in North America. The virus infects a wide variety of animal species, both wild and domestic, as well as several species of ticks. It causes encephalomyelitis in horses that mimics that caused by other flaviviruses like WNV, from which it must be distinguished by either PCR assay or by virus isolation. Similar tick-borne encephalidities of humans are caused by related viruses in Europe and Asia, including Omsk hemorrhagic fever virus, Tick-borne encephalitis viruses (European, Far Eastern, and Siberian), and Kyasanur Forest disease virus. These viruses are maintained in a cycle of infection that includes ticks (which vertically transmit the viruses) and vertebrates (livestock and dogs) that serve as amplifying hosts of the virus. Encephalitis occurs sporadically among animals in areas where these viruses are endemic.

PESTIVIRUS

The genus *Pestivirus* includes the etiologic agents of bovine viral diarrhea (BVDV; Types 1 and 2), border disease (BDV), and hog cholera (also referred to as classical swine fever [CSFV]), all of which are important pathogens of livestock. In contrast to the genus *Flavivirus*, members of the genus *Pestivirus* are not arthropod-borne. They are readily inactivated by low pH, heat, organic solvents, and detergents. Virions are spherical to pleomorphic (40–60 nm in diameter) and enveloped with small surface projections (spikes) emanating from the viral envelope. The virions consist of an envelope and nucleocapsid and include four structural proteins—a nucleocapsid protein (C) and three envelope glycoproteins (E^{rns}, E1, and E2). Some seven or eight viral nonstructural proteins also are produced in infected cells. The genome is a single molecule of positive-sense, single-stranded RNA that contains a single, large open reading frame that encodes a large polyprotein that is co- and post-translationally cleaved into the various structural and nonstructural viral proteins.

The pestiviruses are all antigenically related and include cross-reactive epitopes. Several other pestiviruses have been isolated that are genetically distinct from BVDV (Types 1 and 2), BDV, and CSFV, and it is proposed that pestiviruses isolated from a giraffe and from reindeer, for example, be identified as new species. Neutralizing antibodies are directed against the E^{rns} and E2 envelope glycoproteins. Infected animals also mount a strong immune response against the NS3 protein, whereas the antibody response to other viral proteins is generally weak.

All three viruses are important food-animal pathogens and will be described sequentially. They are very closely related and can only be distinguished by application of monoclonal antibodies and/or molecular biology techniques; however, they tend to be host-specific.

BOVINE VIRUS DIARRHEA VIRUS

Disease

Bovine virus diarrhea virus (BVDV) is responsible for *bovine virus diarrhea-mucosal disease (BVD-MD)*. This disease complex actually includes three distinct disease syndromes:

1. *Type I viral diarrhea* is a usually mild disease of young calves characterized by leukopenia, fever, and erosions and ulcers of the upper gastrointestinal tract, often with accompanying diarrhea. The infection is typically characterized by high morbidity and low mortality.
2. *Type II viral diarrhea* is the consequence of infection of calves with genetically distinct strains of BVDV (so-called *Type II BVDV*). These viruses initially

caused severe, fatal mucosal disease-like signs (see below) in calves when they first emerged, often accompanied by widespread hemorrhages as a consequence of thrombocytopenia. However, Type II strains of BVDV are now increasingly associated with mild disease in calves, similar to that produced by most Type I strains.
3. *Mucosal disease* is characterized by low morbidity but high mortality in cattle of several months to several years of age. It is characterized by severe, fatal disease with extensive ulceration of the upper gastrointestinal tract, diarrhea, and lymphopenia. Mucosal disease occurs only in persistently infected animals that were originally infected with BVDV in utero, thus it has a highly distinctive pathogenesis.

BVDV also causes reproductive losses in cattle from abortion and fetal teratogenesis.

Etiologic Agent

Physical, Chemical, and Antigenic Properties

BVDV is the type species of the *Pestivirus* genus (Fig 58.1); thus it is serologically related to hog cholera and border

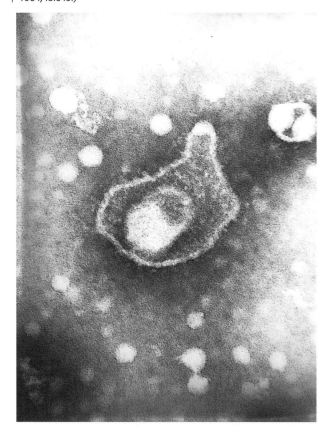

FIGURE 58.1.   *Negatively stained preparation of bovine virus diarrhea virus. 250,000X. (Reproduced with permission from Chu HJ, Zee YC. Morphology of bovine viral diarrhea virus. Am J Vet Res 1984;45:845.)*

disease viruses. The two types of BVDV (Types I and II) are distinguished by genetic and antigenic methods (using monoclonal antibodies in particular). It also is clear that there is enormous genetic variation among field strains of BVDV of both types, which likely influences their biologic properties.

There also are two distinct biotypes of BVDV; one is cytopathogenic for cell cultures and the other is not. The cytopathic strains apparently arise by mutational or recombinational events in noncytopathic strains (deletion or reduplication of the viral genome or insertion of host cell sequences into the genome of the noncytopathogenic virus).

Resistance to Physical and Chemical Agents

BVDV is sensitive to lipid solvents such as ether and chloroform and is inactivated by treatment with trypsin. The virus is most stable in the pH range from 5.7 to 9.3, with maximum stability at pH 7.4. The virus is readily maintained in a lyophilized or frozen state for many years.

Infectivity for Other Species and Culture Systems

Pestiviruses infect cattle, sheep, goats, pigs, and wild ruminants, but BVDV principally is an infectious pathogen of cattle and sometimes sheep. Isolates of BVDV, whether cytopathogenic or noncytopathogenic, can be grown in cell culture systems, including various bovine embryonic cell cultures. Immunofluorescence or other immunohistochemical staining methods are used to detect noncytopathogenic strains of BVDV, which contaminate many commonly used cell lines. Cytopathogenic strains produce plaques and can be used for accurate viral titrations.

Host-Virus Relationship

Distribution, Reservoir, and Transmission

BVDV has a worldwide distribution, and infection of cattle is very common, as determined by serologic surveys. Transmission is by contact and horizontal transfer of virus, particularly from persistently infected carriers of the virus that shed high titers of virus in all of their body secretions and excretions, and transmit the virus vertically to their progeny.

Pathogenesis and Pathology

The consequences of infection of cattle with BVDV vary from an inapparent infection to severe fatal disease. The pathogenesis and consequences of BVDV infection of cattle are dependent on the age and immune status of cattle at infection, as well as the biological properties of the infecting virus strain. Type I and II BVDV infection in calves results in systemic infection of variable severity. Lesions in affected calves range from mild erosion and ulceration of the upper gastrointestinal tract to severe ulceration throughout the gastrointestinal tract and disseminated hemorrhages (characteristic of Type II BVDV).

Highly virulent strains of BVDV can produce severe lesions in susceptible calves that mimic mucosal disease (see below).

Fetal infections are important to both the epidemiology of BVDV infection of cattle and to the pathogenesis of mucosal disease. BVDV infection of bovine fetuses with a noncytopathogenic strain of BVD virus prior to mid-gestation often leads to the birth of calves that are persistently infected with BVDV (if they survive infection). These animals subsequently serve as a reservoir of virus in the herd, which they transmit both horizontally and vertically (to their own progeny); furthermore, they develop weak or no obvious humoral immune response to the virus with which they are persistently infected. Mucosal disease manifests when a cytopathogenic strain of BVD virus emerges in the animal. Interestingly, the noncytopathic and cytopathic strains of BVD virus isolated from cases of mucosal disease are extremely similar genetically. Recent evidence clearly indicates that the cytopathic virus arises from changes (genome deletion or reduplication or insertion of cellular gene sequences into the viral genome) in the original persistent noncytopathic strain. Mucosal disease is characterized by the presence of erosions and ulcers on the muzzle, throughout the oral cavity, esophagus, and small intestine (ulcers over Peyers patches are characteristic). There also is widespread necrosis of lymphocytes. The mechanism of tissue destruction in this fulminant disease currently is uncharacterized but might involve apoptosis of cells.

BVDV is capable of crossing the placenta of immunologically naive pregnant cattle, and BVDV infection of the developing fetus can result in fetal death, developmental abnormalities, or persistent infection in fetuses prior to mid-gestation. Ocular lesions (retinal degeneration and hypoplasia, optic neuritis) and cerebellar atrophy/hypoplasia are characteristic of fetal BVDV infection.

Host Responses to Infection

BVDV infection of cattle usually results in the production of high titers of neutralizing antibodies in serum, and cattle that recover from infection have long-lasting immunity. BVDV infection of animals in utero can result in persistent post-natal infection, and these animals have no or very low titers of virus-specific antibodies.

Laboratory Diagnosis

Clinical diagnosis may be difficult. Mucosal disease must be differentiated from other diseases that cause ulceration of the gastrointestinal tract, including malignant catarrhal fever and rinderpest. Rapid diagnosis is best accomplished by immmunohistochemical staining of the tissues of affected animals with BVDV-specific antibodies, or by polymerase chain reaction to detect viral nucleic acid. Virus isolation also can be used, as can serology; however, the widespread use of vaccines complicates serological diagnosis of BVDV infection, as does the fact that persistently infected cattle have little or no obvious titers to BVDV.

Treatment and Control

Control of BVDV infection of cattle is generally achieved by vaccination with either attenuated (live) or killed BVDV vaccines, and by the identification and removal of persistently infected carriers of the virus. Concerns have been raised about the use of live attenuated BVDV vaccines, including their potential reversion to virulence, dissemination in cattle populations, and potential to cause immunosuppression as well as fetal infections. In the past, inadvertent contamination of bovine cell cultures used for vaccine production with virulent but noncytopathogenic BVDV strains has also occurred. Vaccination of persistently infected cattle with attenuated vaccines can sometimes produce mucosal disease.

Since colostral antibodies may persist for 6 months or more in calves, vaccination prior to this time may not be effective and repeated revaccination may be necessary.

BORDER DISEASE VIRUS

Disease

Border disease (BD) is a congenital *Pestivirus* disease of sheep characterized by the birth of lambs with abnormal ("hairy") wool and tremors that reflect abnormal myelination in the central nervous system (so-called "hairy-shaker" lambs). Expression of disease varies depending on gestational age of the lamb at infection as well as the infecting viral strain. Infection of the developing fetus may result in fetal death, mummification, abortion, stillbirth, or birth of abnormal lambs, whereas infection of adult sheep is subclinical.

Etiologic Agent

Physical, Chemical, and Antigenic Properties

Border disease virus (BDV) is a *Pestivirus* that is genetically and antigenically distinct from bovine virus diarrhea (BVDV) and hog cholera viruses. Multiple strains of BDV have been isolated, most of which are noncytopathic in cell cultures. Some viruses isolated during outbreaks of BD are in fact BVDV.

Resistance to Physical and Chemical Agents

Border disease virus exhibits physicochemical properties similar to BVDV. The virus is inactivated by chloroform, ether, trypsin, and heating to 56°C for 20 minutes.

Infectivity for Host Species and Culture Systems

While BDV is classically associated with infection of sheep, it also can infect cattle and goats, and pregnant sows that were experimentally infected with BDV gave birth to piglets with cerebellar hypoplasia. The virus can be propagated in primary and secondary cell cultures of bovine and ovine origin and in established cell lines, including pig kidney, fetal lamb muscle, and bovine turbinate.

Host-Virus Relationship

Distribution, Reservoir, and Transmission

BDV was initially described in the late 1940s as a congenital disease of sheep in England and Wales. The disease has since been recognized in many European countries, Australia, New Zealand, Canada, and the United States. The virus persists in sheep, likely in a manner similar to that of BVDV in cattle, and extensive outbreaks of BDV can occur when the virus is introduced into immunologically naive flocks. Transmission of BDV is probably most common by the oral and intranasal routes, from infected animals or infected fetuses.

Pathogenesis and Pathology

BDV infection of immunologically naive sheep results in viremia, with subsequent spread of the virus to the fetus in pregnant animals. Generalized infection of the fetus can lead to fetal death, with or without expulsion, or teratogenesis. The consequences of fetal infection are inversely related to fetal age, thus infection during the first trimester is relatively more severe than infection later in gestation. Infection after 80 days' gestation often results in viral clearance without disease. The teratogenic effect of BDV infection also is dependent on fetal age. Infection of the developing central nervous system leads to reduced or altered myelination and demyelinization, resulting in the characteristic congenital tremors of the affected newborn lambs. Necrosis of the developing brain can cause more serious developmental injury, resulting in hydranencephaly, porencephaly, and/or cerebellar dysplasia.

Host Response to Infection

BDV infection of adult sheep usually results in a prompt humoral immune response characterized by the appearance of long-lived neutralizing antibody in serum. The fetal immune response reflects its gestational age at the time of infection. Infection during the first half of gestation usually leads to persistent post-natal infection and a minimal, inadequate immune response. Such animals may remain persistently infected and seronegative to BDV for the remainder of their lives. Infection during the second half of gestation, at a time when the fetus is gaining immunologic competence, usually results in immune responses that resolve the infection.

Laboratory Diagnosis

The clinical signs of BDV in affected lambs are variable, but detailed necropsy and histologic evaluation is often diagnostic, especially when immunohistochemical staining is used to identify viral antigens in the tissues of affected lambs.

Treatment and Control

Control of BDV is difficult. Losses can be high during initial infection of naive animals, whereas losses are relatively minimal when the virus is endemic on a farm. BVDV vaccines are sometimes used.

HOG CHOLERA VIRUS

Disease

Hog cholera (HC, also known as *classical swine fever*) is an important disease of swine worldwide; although it has been eliminated in many intensive swine-producing countries but often reemerges to cause serious, economically devastating outbreaks. HC is characterized by fever (104°F or higher), leukopenia, and loss of appetite. Affected animals may appear dull and drowsy and crowd together as if chilled. Vomiting and diarrhea are common, as is conjunctivitis, erythema of the skin, and neurologic signs such as paralysis and locomotory disturbances. Infection of pregnant sows can result in small litters, fetal death, premature births, stillbirths, and the birth of piglets with cerebellar ataxia or congenital tremors. Morbidity and mortality are both high during epidemics caused by virulent strains of the virus in fully susceptible swine, whereas disease is less apparent when the virus is endemic, making detection and eradication more difficult.

Etiologic Agent

Physical, Chemical, and Antigenic Properties

Hog cholera virus (HCV) is a member of the genus *Pestivirus*, and there is considerable genetic and antigenic variation among strains of the virus.

Resistance to Physical and Chemical Agents

HCV is chloroform- and ether-labile and relatively pH stable. Virions are quickly inactivated by drying but can persist for long periods in uncooked pork or garbage. The virus is completely inactivated in canned hams when an internal temperature of 65°C is maintained for 90 minutes. The virus survives for 3 days at 50°C in defibrinated blood.

Infectivity for Other Species and Culture Systems

Domestic swine and wild hogs are the only naturally susceptible species.

HCV replicates in cultures of porcine cells such as spleen, kidney, testicle, and peripheral blood leukocytes. Most strains of the virus are noncytopathogenic and may persist in culture for many cell passages. The presence of HCV in infected cell cultures is readily demonstrated by immunofluorescent or immunohistochemical staining techniques. Some cytopathogenic strains have been reported.

Host-Virus Relationship

Distribution, Reservoir, and Transmission

HCV occurs worldwide, but it has been eradicated from North America, Great Britain and Ireland, Scandinavia, Australia and New Zealand, and portions of Europe. It is endemic in extensive areas of Asia, Africa, Europe, and South and Central America.

Domestic swine and wild hogs serve as reservoir hosts, often as inapparent carriers. Pigs infected *in utero* may become persistently infected carriers of the virus, analogous to the reservoirs of other pestiviruses like BVDV and BDV. Transmission is by droplet, fomites, and ingestion of infected materials, particularly uncooked garbage.

Pathogenesis and Pathology

Hog cholera is an acute, highly contagious disease that is characterized by disseminated intravascular coagulation leading to hemorrhage and infarction in many tissues. The incubation period is short (3 to 8 days), and the virus first replicates in the lymphoid tissues of the upper respiratory tract or tonsils. The virus then spreads widely and replicates in endothelial cells and mononuclear inflammatory cells throughout the body. The characteristic lesions are petechial hemorrhages on all serous surfaces, lymph nodes (hemorrhagic lymphadenitis), and kidney, and the presence of infarcts in the spleen.

More chronic forms of HC occur in some endemic areas. Affected pigs may exhibit growth retardation (stunting), chronic diarrhea, and secondary bacterial pneumonia.

Host Response to Infection

Animals that recover from hog cholera have a long-lasting immunity. Neutralizing antibody titers correlate with resistance to HCV infection. Suckling pigs acquire colostral antibodies from the immune dam. The half-life of this colostral antibody is 13 days. Pigs that have maternal antibody titers of 1:1000 or above still have some antibody at 4 months.

Pigs infected *in utero* with the virus are often persistently infected carriers, whether or not they are healthy at birth.

Laboratory Diagnosis

Diagnosis of hog cholera can be suspected in free areas by explosive outbreaks of severe disease in pigs, but the diagnosis always requires laboratory confirmation to distinguish it from other septicemias. The virus is identified in the tissues of affected pigs by immunohistochemical staining or by virus isolation from the spleen, tonsils, lymph nodes, and blood. Since many strains are noncytopathogenic in cell culture, the fluorescent antibody method is required for the detection of HCV. Polymerase chain reaction detection now also is available.

The diagnosis of chronic forms of HC is more difficult and requires careful laboratory investigation.

Treatment and Control

Control of HC depends on whether the virus is endemic in a particular country or region. In free areas, exclusion of the virus is accomplished by regulating the movement (importation) of swine from endemic areas and by prohibiting the feeding of garbage and/or food scraps containing pork products to swine. In endemic areas, vaccination and/or eradication are used. Vaccines for HCV are attenuated and, although effective in preventing disease, they complicate efforts to eradicate HCV from a region or country.

59 *Orthomyxoviridae* and *Bunyaviridae*

ALEX A. ARDANS   N. JAMES MACLACHLAN

ORTHOMYXOVIRIDAE

Influenza viruses are included in the family *Orthomyxoviridae,* and are divided into three types (A, B, and C) based on the antigenic differences between their nucleo-protein (NP) and matrix (M) proteins. Type A influenza viruses naturally occur in humans, horses, swine, and birds. Types B and C infect humans, and Type C also infects pigs. Influenza A viruses are further divided into subtypes. The nomenclature system includes the host of origin, geographic origin, strain number, and year of isolation. A description of the two major surface antigens, the hemagglutinin and the neuraminidase, is given in parentheses—for example, A/swine/New Jersey/8/76 (H1 N1). By convention, the host of origin for human strains is now omitted.

Morphology

Influenza virus particles are irregularly shaped spherical particles 80–120 nm in diameter (Figs 59.1, 59.2). The virion envelope is derived from the membranes of host cells. There are two distinct types of surface spikes (peplomers); one is rod-shaped and corresponds to the hemagglutinin (HA), and the other is mushroom-shaped and possesses neuraminidase (NA) activity. Both the HA and the NA are viral glycoproteins that attach to the viral envelope by short sequences of hydrophobic amino acids. The viral envelope surrounds a matrix protein (M) shell, which in turn surrounds the genome of eight (seven in Type C influenza viruses) individual molecules of single-stranded RNA, along with the nucleoprotein (NP) and three large proteins (PB$_1$, PB$_2$, and PA) that are responsible for RNA replication and transcription. Each of the eight genomic RNA species encodes for one, or sometimes two, polypeptides. This independent nature of the individual viral gene segments results in the phenomena of high frequency recombination (reassortment of gene segments from two parental viruses to generate progeny with new genotypes) during mixed infections, and explains the origin of some new pandemic strains of influenza virus.

Viral Proteins

Hemagglutinin

All strains of influenza are capable of agglutinating erythrocytes from humans, guinea pigs, and chickens as well as many other species. Antibodies to the HA prevent infection of host cells. The HA and NA are the two major strain-specific surface antigens and are important to host immunity. In fact, it is the variation of these molecules that is primarily responsible for emergence of new strains of the virus leading to new outbreaks of influenza, and the failure to control them by vaccination. The HA functions in initial virus attachment to its cellular reception, and subsequent HA cleavage allows fusion of the viral envelope with an intercellular membrane allowing transfer of the nucleocapsid into the cell cytoplasm. There are now 15 recognized influenza HA proteins.

Neuraminidase

The NA is responsible for the cleavage of the sialic acid-containing receptor and the elution of the viral particle from the host cell. This phenomenon prevents self-aggregation and promotes release of the virus from the infected cell. Antibody against the NA does not protect against infection but does confer protection against disease and reduces transmissibility. There are nine recognized NA subtypes.

Nucleoprotein

The nucleoprotein (NP) was originally designated the soluble, or S, antigen and is the innermost component of the influenza virion. It is coiled into a double helix 50 nm to 60 nm in diameter and is intimately associated with each RNA segment and the three different polymerases.

The NP is one of the type-specific antigens used to distinguish genera of influenza virus, and can be identified by enzyme-linked immunosorbent assay (ELISA), double immunodiffusion, complement fixation, single radial diffusion, agar-gel precipitation, and the hemagglutination inhibition tests.

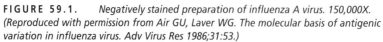

FIGURE 59.1.   *Negatively stained preparation of influenza A virus. 150,000X. (Reproduced with permission from Air GU, Laver WG. The molecular basis of antigenic variation in influenza virus. Adv Virus Res 1986;31:53.)*

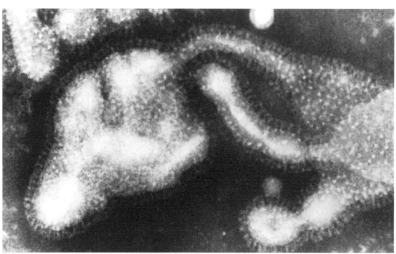

FIGURE 59.2.   *Diagram of influenza virus. The diagram illustrates the main structural features of the virion. The surface of the particle contains three kinds of spike proteins—the hemagglutinin (HA), the neuraminidase (NA), and matrix (M2) protein— embedded in a lipid bilayer derived from the host cell and covers the matrix (M1) protein that surrounds the viral core. The ribonucleoprotein complex making up the core consists of at least one of each of the eight single-stranded RNA segments associated with the nucleoprotein (NP) and the three polymerase proteins (PB2, PB1, PA). RNA segments have base pairing between their 3' and 5' ends forming a panhandle. Their organization and the role of NS2 in the virion remain unresolved. (Reproduced with permission from Murphy B, Weneter RG. Orthomyxoviruses. In: Fields B, Knipe DM, Howley PM, et al., eds. Fields virology. 3rd ed. New York: Lippincott-Raven, 1996:1401.)*

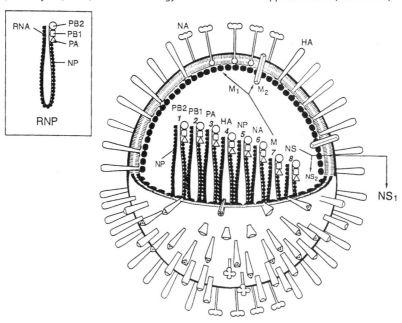

Matrix Protein

The nonglycosylated matrix protein is also a type-specific antigen of influenza viruses. However, antibodies against M provide little, if any, protection against infection. This structural protein surrounds the nucleoprotein to form the inner part of the viral envelope.

Nonstructural Proteins

There are at least two nonstructural proteins, NS1 and NS2. Their function is at this time unknown.

Polymerase Proteins

The polymerase proteins (PB_1, PB_2, PA) localize with the NP and viral RNA. They are the largest of the viral proteins and are responsible for RNA polymerization of the viral genome. PB_1 and PB_2 are necessary for complementary RNA synthesis, while PA and NP are required for viral RNA synthesis.

Viral Genome

The influenza A genome contains at least 10 different open reading frames (genes) in its 8 segments of negative-sense RNA. The segmented genome of influenza viruses facilitates reassortment, resulting in the production of new strains. Influenza viral variation is frequent and occurs in two ways, drift and shift. Antigenic drift is due to point mutations resulting in amino acid substitutions mainly in the HA protein. Antigenic shift occurs with reassortment of individual RNA segments when a cell is infected with two different influenza viruses, generating new viruses that cause pandemics of human influenza.

EQUINE INFLUENZA

Disease

Influenza is an acute respiratory disease of horses. While horses of all ages are affected, those between 2 and 6 months of age are at greatest risk. The mortality rate of equine influenza is low whereas the morbidity rate can approach 100%. The incubation period lasts from 1 to 3 days. Disease is manifested by a high fever, up to 106°F, which lasts about 3 days. Other clinical signs include a frequent, strong, dry cough lasting 1 to 3 weeks, a nasal discharge that is initially serous in character but that later becomes mucoid, anorexia, depression, photophobia, lacrimation with a mucopurulent ocular discharge, and corneal opacity (sometimes with loss of sight). Limb edema and muscle soreness can occur and, in some severe outbreaks, acute deaths due to fulminant pneumonia have occurred. Enteritis was described in a 1989 outbreak in northern China due to a new equine influenza virus, A/equine/2/Jilin; this virus is considered to have emerged from birds into horses.

Equine influenza viruses are Type A viruses. They have been divided into two subtypes, A/equine/1 (H7N7) and A/equine/2 (H3N8), based on antigenic differences in their HA. A/equine/1 has one prototype, A/equine/1/Prague. Antigenic drift has occurred among A/equine/1 viruses with the subsequent designation of two subgroups that do not appear to differ significantly in terms of their immunity after vaccination. Significant drift has occurred among A/equine/2 viruses from the original prototype A/equine/2/Miami/63 first isolated from a severe 1963 outbreak in Florida horses. Additional prototypes A/equine/2/Fountainbleu, A/equine/2/Kentucky, along with other variants including the 1989 Chinese virus, have shown that considerable drift occurs in the A/equine/2 viruses, which may have implications for efficacious vaccination. Influenza occurs in horses worldwide, with the notable exceptions of countries such as New Zealand and Australia, and is a common and troublesome problem when horses are congregated at shows, sales, stables, and racetracks.

Etiologic Agent

Resistance to Physical and Chemical Agents

Equine influenza virus is usually inactivated at 56°C in 30 minutes. Like Type A influenza viruses, the virus is inactivated by phenol, lipid solvents, detergent, formalin, and oxidizing agents such as ozone.

Infectivity for Other Species and Culture Systems

Equine influenza virus infects horses, asses, and mules. It can be experimentally adapted to infect mice when introduced intranasally. All orthomyxoviruses, including equine influenza virus, can be propagated in the amniotic cavity of embryonated chicken eggs. Equine influenza virus can also be grown in chick embryo kidney, bovine kidney, rhesus monkey kidney, and human embryo kidney cells.

Host-Virus Relationship

Pathogenesis and Pathology

Equine influenza virus infects both the upper and lower respiratory tracts. There is an early lymphopenia with accompanying enlargement of the lymph nodes of the head. Initially there may only be a slight serous nasal discharge, which later becomes mucoid. Fatal pneumonia can occur in foals and on occasion in older animals. Occasionally there is ventral edema of the trunk and lower limbs. A/equine/2 has been known to cause a postinfection encephalopathy in foals. Catarrhal and even hemorrhagic enteritis may occur. Necrotizing bronchiolitis in which the bronchioles are progressively obstructed is characteristic of equine influenza. Severe necrotizing myositis with elevated serum enzyme levels has been observed with A2 infections. Most animals recover within 2 to 3 weeks; those that do not may develop chronic obstructive pulmonary disease (COPD). Prolonged recovery and severity of disease appear to be related to the level of stress an affected horse undergoes, thus adequate rest is important for recovery.

Equine influenza virus is most commonly transmitted via aerosol and can spread extremely rapidly due to the frequent, violent cough of infected horses. Infected animals continue to shed virus for about 5 days after the first signs appear. The virus also can be spread by fomites.

Laboratory Diagnosis

A tentative clinical diagnosis of equine influenza can be made from the characteristic rapid spread of the disease, especially among stabled horses, and the frequent dry cough of affected horses. A definitive diagnosis requires isolation of the virus, demonstration of viral antigen, or demonstration of rising antibody titers between acute and convalescent sera by complement fixation (CF) and hemagglutination inhibition (HI) tests. During outbreaks it is important for the success of future vaccination programs to isolate and type the causative strains of influenza virus.

Treatment and Control

Vaccination is somewhat effective in preventing influenza in horses. Protection, however, is dependent on the manner of vaccination and the quality of the vaccine, with particular emphasis placed on proper selection of vaccine strains. Available vaccines contain inactivated virus of both A/equine/1 and A/equine/2 subtypes. Classically, A/equine/Prague/56 (H7N7) and A/equine/Miami/63 (H3N8) have been used as the prototype A/equine/1 and A/equine/2 strains, respectively. There is increasing evidence of antigenic diversity among contemporary equine influenzas that circulate in nature, suggesting that the effectiveness of the conventional vaccine strains in providing protection will become limited with time. For this reason, current vaccines include some of the newer variant A/equine/2 viruses. The various inactivated vaccines available are incorporated with adjuvants that have proved to significantly augment their immunogenic potential. Initial immunization requires two doses of vaccine 2 to 4 weeks apart. These should be followed by a single booster when the horse is 1 year of age and then repeated every 6 months until the horse is about 3 years of age, at which time the booster interval may be increased to not more than 1 year.

In horses, a relationship has been shown between titers of nasal antibody to influenza virus and resistance to infection. The presence of prechallenge serum antibody has also been shown to shorten the duration of viral excretion and febrile response.

In addition to vaccination, isolation and quarantine measures are advised during outbreaks to reduce the spread of disease, and disinfection of affected premises, equipment and clothing is essential to prevent mechanical transmission of the virus.

SWINE INFLUENZA

Disease

Swine influenza is an acute upper respiratory disease of pigs. The natural disease commonly affects large numbers of animals in the herd almost simultaneously. Swine influenza occurs more frequently during colder months. Disease caused by swine influenza alone is usually mild; however, disease may be severe when secondary infections occur.

The incubation period is short, requiring at most several days. Disease symptoms include fever, anorexia, leukopenia, extreme weakness, and prostration. Respiratory signs also occur, including hyperpnea, dyspnea, sneezing, painful coughing, and a nasal discharge. Some animals develop conjunctivitis, pulmonary edema, or bronchopneumonia. Most animals recover uneventfully in 2 to 6 days but with considerable weight loss.

Swine influenza was first recognized during the massive human influenza pandemic in 1918, and subsequent studies confirm that a similar H1N1 virus caused disease in both humans and swine. Swine influenza virus can spread from pigs to humans causing illness, and there is concern that swine may serve as a reservoir from which influenza virus can emerge to precipitate human epidemics.

Swine influenza occurs in many parts of the world, including Europe, Asia, and North America. The H1N1 virus is most commonly responsible for disease outbreaks in swine worldwide, although H3N2 viruses also circulate in some regions.

Antigenic differences among strains of swine influenza virus have not been great enough to justify the designation of subtypes.

Host-Virus Relationship

Pathogenesis and Pathology

On postmortem examination of swine with influenza, the mucosa of the upper respiratory tract is congested and the cervical and mediastinal lymph nodes are edematous. Affected lung lobes may be atelectatic and emphysematous. There may be pneumonia with consolidation. The spleen is often moderately enlarged, and the gastric mucosa is often hyperemic.

Transmission of the disease is by droplet infection. Viral maintenance and swine exposure were previously thought to depend on earthworms containing viral-infected larvae of the pig lungworm (*Metastrongylus* spp.). Pigs fed such earthworms and simultaneously exposed to *Haemophilus (para) suis* often developed typical swine influenza. A less elaborate explanation assumed that recovered animals acted as viral carriers. Previous evidence of transplacental infection has been disputed by recent studies. Transmission of influenza viruses between pigs and birds has been suggested by the isolation of an influenza from sick turkeys of an H1N1 virus strain antigenically and genetically identical to viruses isolated from pigs.

Laboratory Diagnosis

Swine influenza is suspected whenever there is an "explosive" appearance of upper respiratory disease involving many pigs, particularly during the fall or winter months. A definitive diagnosis requires either viral isolation from nasal secretions or the lung or demonstration of a rising titer between acute and convalescent sera. Swine influenza virus can be cultivated in 10- to 12-day-old embryonated chicken eggs and various tissue culture monolayer systems involving primary or stable cell cultures.

Treatment and Control

Swine that have recovered from influenza develop H1, serum neutralizing (SN), complement fixing (CF), precipitating, and neuraminidase-inhibiting antibodies. There is a controversy as to whether recovered animals are immune. Some researchers believe they are and that subsequent respiratory outbreaks in a herd in a given season must be caused by another agent. Others have demonstrated that pigs with neutralizing antibody may still succumb to challenge with swine influenza virus and *H. (para) suis* combined. Pigs born to immune sows are protected for as long as 13 to 18 weeks by passive transfer of maternal antibodies.

Immunization using various viral preparations has been attempted with little success. In the United States, there are no commercial vaccines for swine influenza.

Treatment entails supportive measures including a draft-free environment with clean, dry, dust-free bedding; fresh clean water; and a good source of feed. Antibiotics given on a herd basis may help prevent secondary bacterial infection. Recovery often occurs as suddenly as the onset of disease.

AVIAN INFLUENZA

Disease

Avian influenza affects the respiratory, enteric, or nervous systems of many species of birds. Viruses of relatively low virulence may cause few signs whereas others cause high mortality. Most outbreaks produce respiratory signs such as sneezing, coughing, rales, sinusitis, and lacrimation. Other signs include depression, diarrhea, and a decline in egg production or fertility. The disease caused by a highly pathogenic virus was once called *fowl plague*. Viruses that cause virulent disease should be classified as highly pathogenic avian influenza (HPAI) viruses. Domestic turkeys, in particular, have often been infected by influenza, which has caused substantial losses over the years. There is marked genetic diversity among avian viruses and at least 15 HA and 9 NA proteins have been identified among avian influenza viruses. Thus, a large number of subtypes of avian influenza viruses are possible, and birds serve as the natural reservoir of influenza. Evidence exists that all HA subtypes are maintained in aquatic bird populations, including ducks, gulls, and shorebirds. Most infections in aquatic birds produce no clinical signs. In wild ducks, influenza virus replicates in intestinal mucosal cells and is excreted in high concentrations. Virus has been isolated from lake and pond water, and surveys have demonstrated that as many as 60% of juvenile birds may be infected as they congregate prior to migration.

Host-Virus Relationship

Geographic Distribution, Reservoir, and Mode of Transmission

Highly virulent avian influenza is a major threat to the world's poultry industry. To date, it has been found in Asia and South and North America, and historically has been associated with HA subtypes H5 and H7. In both the Pennsylvania outbreak of 1983–1984 and the recent outbreak in Mexico involving H5N2 virus, early isolations yielded virus of low pathogenicity. It appears that the HA gene is important in pathogenicity in that highly pathogenic viruses possess HAs that are readily cleaved. Early Pennsylvania isolates had a glycosylation site in the cleavage region that may have blocked cleavage. It appears that a single mutation removed that glycosylation site, which resulted in a highly pathogenic virus. Similarly, in the Mexican outbreaks differences were observed in low- and high-pathogenicity H5N2 viruses involving the cleavage site. As a result, it is recommended that the HA cleavage site sequence also be determined in evaluating pathogenicity of isolates.

The disease is transmitted through poultry flocks mainly through ingestion of virus, but it may also be transmitted by inhalation and by mechanical means involving movement of personnel throughout flocks or between premises. Furthermore, some believe that for waterfowl, a fecal-water-cloacal route of transmission may be important in addition to the fecal-water-oral route. Outbreaks of highly virulent avian influenza may be self-limiting because few birds survive the disease to serve as carriers.

Waterfowl have been implicated as the major natural reservoir for influenza. Infected ducks can shed virus for prolonged periods without showing clinical signs or producing a detectable antibody response. There is evidence that influenza can persist in some birds for several months after infection. In the past, although avian influenza has frequently been isolated from imported exotic birds, prompting strict quarantine measures on newly imported birds, there is no evidence for spread in this manner as has been demonstrated with Newcastle disease virus. Furthermore, avian influenza may be transmitted on such objects as shoes, clothing, and crates that come in contact with infected birds or premises. While the possibility of vertical transmission of avian influenza through infected eggs exists, no evidence exists for its spread by this means.

Avian influenza viruses have been found to be capable of infecting a wide range of mammalian species in addition to birds. In fact, avian strains have been implicated in the deaths of mink during an epidemic in Sweden and in the disease of seals as well as the emergence of new strains in northern China affecting horses. Avian influenza virus can be propagated in cell cultures of human, bovine, canine, chicken, and rabbit origin.

Pathogenesis and Pathology

The pathogenesis of avian influenza varies widely depending on strain of virus, age and species infected, concurrent infections, and husbandry. At necropsy, lesions include foci of necrosis of various sites including the skin, comb, wattles, spleen, liver, lung, kidney, intestine, and pancreas. There may be fibrinous exudates in the air sacs, oviduct, pericardial sac, or peritoneum. Other lesions include petechiation of the heart muscle, abdominal fat, and the mucosa of the proventriculus, a nonsuppurative encephalitis, and a serofibrinous pericarditis.

Laboratory Diagnosis

A definitive diagnosis requires viral isolation and identification or the demonstration of rising antibody titer by HI, viral neutralization tests, soluble antigen fluorescent antibody test, agar gel precipitation, or ELISA technique. Avian influenza can be cultivated in chick embryos; duckling, calf, and monkey kidney cell cultures; and from samples of trachea, lung, air sac, sinus exudate, or cloacal swabs. Antigen capture ELISA tests have been used for rapid viral detection.

Treatment and Control

Recovered birds remain immune to subsequent challenge by a homologous strain for at least several months. Birds immunized parenterally with inactivated vaccines are completely protected against challenge by a heterologous strain with the same HA and are partially protected against heterologous strains possessing the same neuraminidase. Following immunization, chickens remain immune for at least 84 days, approximately twice as long as turkeys remain immune. It has been demonstrated that anti-HA antibody is important for protection against infection while antineuraminidase antibody protects against disease and reduces virus shedding but does not prevent infection.

In practice, however, appropriate vaccines are rarely available to the poultry industry owing to great genetic and antigenic diversity among avian viruses. In several states in North America (such as Minnesota and California), the rapid isolation of virus during outbreaks has permitted the development of inactivated vaccines felt to be effective in limiting the severity of an outbreak. There is hope that a polyvalent vaccine with a broader protective range may be developed.

For the most part, control of avian influenza is through the prevention of exposure. Careful husbandry to prevent the introduction of the virus into the flock is important. New birds should not be introduced into a started flock, and careful precautions should be taken to prevent either direct or indirect contact with wild, migratory, or exotic birds. Since turkeys have been found also to be susceptible to a strain of influenza typically associated with pigs, it is a good management practice not to have pigs on the same farm as turkeys. Eggs for hatching should come from flocks demonstrated to be free of the virus. Virus has been demonstrated to persist for 105 days in liquid manure following depopulation. Strict measures should be employed to eliminate movement of personnel and equipment, potentially contaminated by manure, between flocks and premises. During an outbreak, isolation of a flock along with orderly marketing of the flock should be considered.

Drugs such as amantadine, used for human influenza prevention, have not been cleared for use in birds for consumption and to date there is no satisfactory treatment for avian influenza. Treatment of infected flocks with broad-spectrum antibiotics is useful in controlling secondary bacterial infections, and proper nutrition and husbandry may help reduce mortality.

Zoonotic Significance of Animal Influenzas

A growing body of evidence suggests that pandemic strains of human influenza arise as a result of recombination between human and animal strains of influenza virus. Waterfowl appear to be of particular significance in the origin of new human isolates. Ducks appear to act as a "melting pot" where various strains of influenza can come together and undergo genetic reassortment, resulting in the generation of new strains of influenza. Swine have also been implicated as intermediate hosts of "avian-like" and "human-like" influenza viruses. Since the internal genes are critical for host range, and the HA and NA are important to host immunity, recombination events can result in the formation of new virus strains that contain the same or similar internal genes but possess very different HA and NA proteins. The novel viruses generated in this manner might still be infective to humans but possess surface antigens that are very different than those to which the human population previously was exposed (and immune). The result could be a substantial influenza pandemic as the new strain rapidly spreads through a susceptible population.

In the past, major antigenic shifts have taken place among human influenza viruses leading to pandemics in the human population. Each of the last three shifts had its origin traced to China. The role of China in the emergence of these pandemic strains has not been completely resolved; however, China is known to contain a large reservoir of different influenza A viruses among wild and domestic species, particularly ducks. Furthermore, the mass production of ducks and the proximity of human habitations to the farms, also in close association with swine, have been implicated by some as an ideal situation for establishing new antigenic strains and introducing these viruses to the human population.

BUNYAVIRIDAE

The family *Bunyaviridae* includes the genera *Bunyavirus, Hantavirus, Nairovirus, Phlebovirus,* and *Tospovirus.* There are several hundred bunyaviruses, and viruses of veterinary significance are classified within the genera *Bunyavirus*—California encephalitis serogroup viruses and Akabane virus (as well as Aino and Cache Valley viruses); *Phlebovirus*—Rift Valley fever virus; and *Nairovirus*—Nairobi sheep disease virus. Many of the bunyaviruses are arboviruses that are transmitted by arthropods such as mosquitoes, ticks, biting flies, etc., and thus have the capacity to alternately replicate in vertebrate animals and insects.

Several bunyaviruses are important zoonotic pathogens, including hantaviruses (the cause of *Hantavirus* pulmonary syndrome and hemorrhagic fever with renal syndrome in people), which are carried by rodents and infection of humans occurs by inhalation of virus-contaminated rodent excreta and detritus; Rift Valley fever virus; Crimean-Congo hemorrhagic fever virus; and Nairobi sheep disease virus.

General Family Properties

Bunyaviruses are enveloped, pleomorphic viruses, 80–120 nm in diameter, with surface projections (spikes) emanating from the envelope surface of mature virions. The virions consist of four structural proteins, including two external glycoproteins in the envelope, a nucleocapsid protein that encapsidates the genome, and a transcriptase protein (L). The envelope glycoproteins are responsible for neutralization and hemagglutination. A variety of nonstructural proteins also are encoded by the viral genome.

The nucleic acid is helical and included in three distinct segments (large [L], medium [M], and small [S]), each comprised of single-stranded, negative-sense RNA.

There is considerable genetic diversity and serologically cross-reactivity among viruses within the various genera of the *Bunyaviridae*.

GENUS *BUNYAVIRUS*—AKABANE, AINO, AND CACHE VALLEY VIRUSES

Akabane virus is the cause of periodic outbreaks of fetal malformation in ruminants, especially cattle, in Asia, Australia, the Middle East, and Africa. The virus is transmitted by mosquitoes and *Culicoides* midges and causes distinctive teratogenic defects of the musculoskeletal and nervous systems (arthrogryposis-hydranencephaly) in fetuses that are born to dams that become infected during pregnancy. The gestational age of the fetus at infection determines the type of lesions that will be present at birth; fetuses infected prior to mid-gestation are typically born with their limbs held in rigid flexion (arthrogryposis), with variable deviation of their vertebral columns. The brains of affected fetuses may lack cerebral hemispheres, or

these may be represented only as fluid-filled sacs as a consequence of virus-mediated destruction of the developing cerebrum during gestation (hydranencephaly). An inactivated vaccine is used to protectively immunize ruminants prior to conception.

Aino virus causes a similar disease as Akabane virus and has much the same global distribution. Cache Valley virus has been documented as the cause of outbreaks of arthrogryposis-hydranencephaly of sheep in the western and southwestern United States.

CALIFORNIA ENCEPHALITIS SEROGROUP VIRUSES

California encephalitis serogroup viruses are related (serologically cross-reactive) mosquito-transmitted viruses of the genus *Bunyavirus* and include La Crosse, snowshoe hare, and Jamestown Canyon viruses. These viruses occur in endemic cycles of infection in different regions of North America and, although infection occurs in a variety of mammalian species, encephalitis is rarely documented even in humans.

Other members of the genus *Bunyavirus* have been sporadically incriminated as the cause of encephalitis in animals—Main Drain virus in horses, for example.

GENUS *PHLEBOVIRUS*—RIFT VALLEY FEVER

Rift Valley fever virus (RVFV) is a zoonotic, mosquito-transmitted virus that causes epidemics of severe, frequently fatal systemic disease of ruminants, especially sheep and goats. Mortality is highest in young animals, and pregnant ruminants often abort following infection. RVFV causes extensive liver necrosis in affected sheep and goats, and widespread hemorrhages are common. Encephalitis with neuronal necrosis also occurs in some affected animals.

Rift Valley fever (RVF) is endemic in sub-Saharan Africa and periodically incurs into adjacent northern regions such as Egypt. Climatic conditions influence the occurrence of epidemics, particularly high rainfall that results in rapid expansion of the populations of *Aedes* mosquitoes that harbor the virus. RVF is a zoonoses, and human mortality can be very high during epidemics.

RVFV is widely feared because of its virulence to humans and animals, as well as its capacity for rapid spread by a variety of species of mosquito during epidemics. Thus, rapid diagnosis is imperative, usually by virus isolation or serology. An inactivated vaccine is available, and unvaccinated veterinarians and laboratory staff working with RVFV-infected material are at risk of infection.

GENUS *NAIROVIRUS*—NAIROBI SHEEP DISEASE

Nairobi sheep disease (NSD) and related viruses cause severe disease of ruminants, principally sheep and goats, in

Africa and Asia. The virus is transmitted by the brown ear tick. NSD is characterized by high fever, intestinal hemorrhage, and death of susceptible ruminants. Pregnant animals typically abort. NSD is a highly virulent zoonotic pathogen.

Other members of the genus *Nairovirus* that are of potential veterinary significance include Crimean-Congo hemorrhagic fever, a zoonotic disease that occurs throughout Africa, eastern Europe, the Middle East and Asia. The virus is transmitted by ticks, and both wild and domestic animals can serve as reservoirs of the virus, although disease apparently is rare in species other than humans.

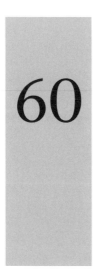

60

Paramyxoviridae, Filoviridae, and *Bornaviridae*

Yuan Chung Zee   N. James MacLachlan

The order *Mononegavirales* includes viruses within the families *Paramyxoviridae, Filovirdae, Bornaviridae,* and *Rhabdoviridae* (Chapter 61). These viruses are ancestrally related as reflected by their common features, including genome of a single-strand of negative-sense RNA, similar replication strategy and gene order, and virion morphology that includes an envelope.

PARAMYXOVIRIDAE

The *Paramyxoviridae* family is subdivided into two subfamilies, the *Paramyxovirinae* and the *Pneumovirinae* that are further subdivided into three (*Respirovirus, Rubulavirus, Morbillivirus*) and two genera (*Pneumovirus, Metapneumovirus*), respectively (Table 60.1). Viruses in this family cause a number of serious respiratory and/or systemic diseases of humans, animals, and birds.

Paramyxoviruses are characterized by virions that are enveloped, pleomorphic (filamentous or spherical; approximately 150 nm or more in diameter), and contain a genome of linear, negative-sense, single-stranded RNA. The viral nucleocapsid has helical symmetry and is approximately 13–18 nm in diameter (Fig 60.1). At least three proteins are associated with the nucleocapsid, including an RNA-binding protein (N or NP), a phosphoprotein (P), and the viral polymerase (L). The nucleocapsid is enclosed by a lipoprotein envelope derived from the host cell plasma membrane, and contains two or three transmembrane viral glycoproteins that form spikes (8–12 nm) that project from the surface. The spikes are formed by the attachment protein (hemagglutinin [H] or hemagglutinin-neuraminidase [HN] in the *Paramyxovirinae;* G protein in the *Pneumovirinae*) and the fusion protein (F) that is essential for virus infectivity and for cell-to-cell spread. Another protein, the matrix (M) protein, lines the inner surface of the envelope. Various nonstructural viral proteins are also formed in infected cells.

PARAMYXOVIRINAE

MORBILLIVIRUSES

Although the various morbilliviruses are all closely related as evidenced by extensive serological cross-reactivity between them, they are distinguished on the basis of their individual host range, genome sequences, and antigenic differences. These viruses all have a hemagglutin (H) surface protein, but only rinderpest virus has a neuraminidase(HN).

CANINE DISTEMPER

Disease

Canine distemper (CD) is an important viral disease of dogs. Acute CD is characterized by any combination of diphasic fever, ocular and nasal discharges, anorexia, depression, vomiting, diarrhea, dehydration, leukopenia, pneumonia, and neurologic signs. The severity of clinical signs exhibited by individual animals can vary markedly. The disease has an incubation period of 3 to 5 days. The mortality rate depends largely on the immune status of the infected dog, and is highest among puppies. Animals that survive the acute disease may develop other signs, including hyperkeratosis of the footpads (hard pad disease) and neurologic disease that is characterized by any combination of convulsions, tremor, myoclonus, locomotory disturbances, paralysis, and blindness. The onset of neurologic signs frequently is delayed until several weeks after the systemic signs of acute CD are manifest. Old dog encephalitis is a rare form of chronic neurologic disease caused by defective CD virus.

Etiologic Agent

Physical, Chemical, and Antigenic Properties

Canine distemper virus (CDV) exhibits the properties described above for paramyxoviruses. The surface H protein

Table 60.1.   Major Subgroups of the Family *Paramyxoviridae*

Subfamily	Genus	Vernacular Name	Natural Host
Paramyxovirinae			
	Respirovirus	Bovine parainfluenza virus 3	Cattle
	Human parainfluenza virus 1,3	Humans	
	Sendai virus	Mice	
	Rubulavirus	Avain paramyxovirus 2–9	Birds
	Human parainfluenza virus 2, 4	Humans	
	Mumps virus	Humans	
	Newcastle disease virus	Birds	
	Porcine *Rubulavirus*	Pigs	
	Simian virus 5 (similar to canine parainfluenza virus 2)		
	Morbillivirus	Measles virus	Humans
	Canine distemper	Canines	
	Phocine distemper virus		
	Cetacean *Morbillivirus*		
	Rinderpest virus	Ruminants	
	Peste des petits ruminants virus	Goats and sheep	
	Equine (Hendra) *Morbillivirus*	Fruit bats	
Pneumovirinae			
	Pneumovirus	Bovine respiratory syncytial virus	Cattle
	Human respiratory syncitical virus	Humans	
	Murine pneumonia virus	Mice	
	Metapneumovirus	Turkey rhinotracheitis virus	Birds

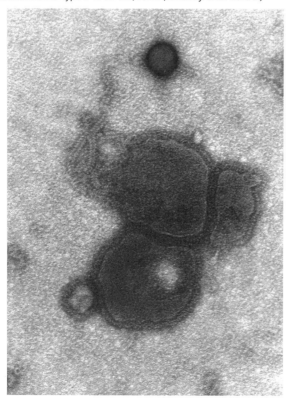

FIGURE 60.1.   *Negatively stained preparations of bovine parainfluenza Type 3 virus. 120,000X. (Courtesy of A. Castro.)*

lacks neuraminidase activity, and is responsible for attachment of CDV to cells. There is only one antigenic type of CDV, although distinct strains of the virus with different biologic properties clearly occur.

Resistance to Physical and Chemical Agents

Canine distemper virus is labile to environmental factors such as extremes of temperature, pH, and to several disinfectants. It is inactivated by visible and ultraviolet light, and heating at 60°C for 30 minutes. The virus can survive in tissues for 48 hours at 25°C and for 14 days at 5°C. Viral infectivity is lost above pH 10.4 or below pH 4.4, and the virus is most stable at pH 7. Canine distemper virus is readily inactivated by disinfectants, quaternary ammonium compounds (such as 0.2% Roccal), and 0.75% phenol solution. Labile viruses like CDV persist longer in cool, shady environments or in serum or tissue debris.

Infectivity for Other Species and Culture Systems

Canine distemper virus infects a wide range of animals. In addition to dogs, other members of the Canidae (e.g., fox, coyote, wolf, wild dogs), Ailuridae (red panda), Hyaenidae (hyena), Mustelidae (e.g., ferret, mink, skunk, badger), Tyassuidae (javelinas [collared peccaries]), Ursidae (bears), Viverridae (civet, mongoose), and Procyonidae (e.g., raccoon, panda) are all susceptible. Some members of the Felidae (lion, tiger, and leopard) also are susceptible, and devastating outbreaks of distemper recently have occurred among lions in Africa.

Canine distemper virus can be isolated and propagated in primary canine and ferret kidney cell cultures.

The virus has been successfully adapted to embryonated chicken eggs and various cell cultures including bovine kidney, Vero monkey kidney, and human amnion or fibroblast continuous cultures. The virus can also be adapted to newborn Swiss mice and weanling hamsters.

Host-Virus Relationship

Distribution, Reservoir, Transmission

Canine distemper occurs worldwide, and remains endemic in many areas despite the widespread use of vaccines that are highly effective in preventing the disease. Dogs are the principal reservoir of CDV. Infected dogs secrete virus in their nasal and ocular secretions, and CDV is present in the urine of experimentally infected dogs 6 to 22 days after infection. Feces of infected dogs may also contain CDV. Infection usually is transmitted by aerosol or by direct contact, leading to respiratory infection of susceptible animals.

Pathogenesis and Pathology

The CDV is pantropic and has an especially strong tropism for epithelium and lymphoid tissues. The lungs are also central to the pathogenesis of CDV infection. Initial replication of CDV occurs in macrophages in the bronchial lymph nodes and tonsils immediately following respiratory infection. The virus then is spread to other lymphoid tissues (lymph nodes, spleen, thymus, and bone marrow) where further replication occurs prior to viremia that disseminates CDV to virtually all organs of the body, including the central nervous system (CNS) and eyes. This generalized dissemination of CDV to the epithelium of the alimentary, respiratory, and urogenital tracts; the skin and mucous membranes; and endocrine glands and the CNS occurs at approximately 8 or 9 days after infection and only in dogs that fail to develop sufficient titers of neutralizing antibodies to CDV by that time.

The lesions of CD occur in the organs in which the virus replicates, and the respiratory and alimentary tracts are especially affected. The lungs of dogs with acute CD have diffuse interstitial pneumonia characterized by necrotizing bronchiolitis and alveolitis with thickening of the alveolar septae. Secondary bacterial pneumonias are common in dogs with primary CDV-induced interstitial pneumonia. Characteristic eosinophilic intranuclear and intracytoplasmic inclusion bodies are often present within respiratory epithelium and in the epithelium lining the stomach, urinary bladder, and renal pelvis. Extensive necrosis of lymphocytes is characteristic of acute CD, leading to lymphoid depletion and immune suppression. Immune suppression predisposes affected dogs to secondary bacterial pneumonia and may assist the virus in gaining access to the nervous system.

Dogs that survive acute CD may subsequently develop neurologic signs that result from virus-induced demyelination. The lesions within the central nervous system of these dogs begin as focal areas of demyelination that increasingly are accompanied by lymphocytic inflammation and accumulation of macrophages. Lesions occur within the cerebellum, brain stem, and cerebrum, and CDV inclusion bodies may occur in astrocytes, ependymal cells, and neurons. Although CDV predominately replicates in astrocytes and microglial cells within the brains of infected dogs, direct virus-mediated injury to oligodendrocytes is proposed to be responsible for much of the initial virus-induced demyelination that occurs in demyelinating forms of CD.

Old dog encephalitis is a rare disease of mature dogs that results from very long-term persistent CDV infection of the central nervous system, leading to dementia. The disease is characterized by severe lymphocytic encephalitis with neuronal degeneration and, often, the presence of CDV inclusion bodies. Demyelination is less prominent than in typical neurologic CD. It is proposed that a replication defective form of CDV is responsible for old dog encephalitis, analogous to the role of defective measles virus in subacute sclerosing panenecephalitis (Dawson's disease) of humans.

Host Response to Infection

Canine distemper virus infection induces long-lasting immunity in dogs that recover from natural infection. Neutralizing antibodies first appear in serum of infected dogs 8 to 9 days after infection and persist for years thereafter. Cell-mediated immune responses are also generated by dogs infected with CDV and are likely important to recovery from the disease. Virus-induced immune suppression contributes to the pathogenesis of CDV infection by predisposing affected dogs to secondary bacterial infections and by facilitating spread of the virus to the CNS.

Laboratory Diagnosis

Since the clinical signs of CD are variable and sometimes nonspecific, definitive diagnosis requires identification of CDV by virus isolation or the staining of CDV antigen in the cells or tissues of affected dogs using CDV-specific antibodies and the immunofluorescent or immunoperoxidase techniques. Alternatively, serological diagnosis can be done by demonstration of rising IgG titers in paired sera by enzyme-linked immunosorbent assay (ELISA).

Treatment and Control

Treatment for CD is supportive, such as the use of antibiotics to prevent secondary bacterial infections and electrolyte solutions to restore fluids and electrolytes. Vaccination against CD is the best means of preventing the disease. Both modified live and inactivated CD viral vaccines are available, and vaccination has greatly reduced the incidence of this disease in dogs. New generation recombinant distemper vaccines are increasingly being developed, including canary pox virus-based vectors.

Maternally derived antibody to CDV can interfere with the successful vaccination of puppies against CDV. Puppies should be vaccinated for CD at an age when maternally derived antibody has declined to a level that does not interfere with immunization. Although both inactivated and modified live virus CDV vaccines safely have been used to immunize a variety of wild animal species, including foxes, ferrets, mink, bush dogs, and maned wolves, there have been reports of vaccine-induced CD in a variety of species, including mink, kinkajous, and lesser pandas after immunization with modified live CDV vaccine. Similarly, instances of vaccine-induced CD have been described in dogs.

PHOCINE DISTEMPER

Phocine distemper is an infectious disease of seals that resembles canine distemper (CD). The disease first was recognized in the late 1980s when massive die-offs of seals occurred in the Baltic and North seas. The lesions and clinical signs in affected seals were remarkably similar to those of CD, and the disease of seals subsequently was shown to be caused by phocine distemper virus (PDV), a *Morbillivirus* that is closely related to CD virus. A similar disease caused by dolphin distemper virus caused extensive mortality among dolphins on the Atlantic coast of North America in the early 1990s. The dolphin and phocine distemper viruses are closely related, and other genetically distinct morbilliviruses have been shown to cause similar diseases in other pinnipeds and cetaceans. Like CD, pneumonia dominates the clinical and pathological manifestations of morbillivirus-induced distemper in marine mammals.

EQUINE *MORBILLIVIRUS* (HENDRA) DISEASE

Equine *Morbillivirus* disease is unique to Australia, where it was first recognized in 1994 during an outbreak of severe respiratory disease that killed a number of horses and their trainer. The disease also is known as Hendra (and the causative agent Hendra virus) after the town in which the disease was first described. Affected horses develop severe interstitial pneumonia and pulmonary edema that rapidly is fatal. The disease is caused by a unique paramyxovirus that tentatively is classified as a *Morbillivirus*. The virus is harbored asymptomatically by several species of fruit bat (flying foxes). Although fruit bats are the reservoir of equine *Morbillivirus,* the virus is contagious between horses and to humans by direct contact with nasal secretions or fomites that contain the virus. A similar virus (Nipah) is endemic in fruit bats in Malaysia and adjacent regions of Southeast Asia, and periodically emerges to cause fatal disease in humans and swine.

RINDERPEST

Disease

Rinderpest (also known as cattle plague) has long been recognized as a devastating pandemic viral disease of domestic cattle, buffalo, and some wild ruminant species. Rinderpest is characterized by fever, lymphopenia, nasal and lacrimal discharges, diarrhea, and erosions and ulcers throughout the oral cavity (ulcerative stomatitis). The disease has an incubation period of 3 to 8 days and the virus is extremely contagious, so morbidity rates are very high. The mortality rate also can be high (up to 100%) in cattle that have no immunity, but varies depending on the virulence of the infecting virus strain. The disease has been eradicated from many parts of the world, but it persists in parts of Asia, the Middle East, and Africa and thus continues to pose a serious threat to cattle production worldwide. The international community has embarked on an ambitious program to completely eradicate rinderpest by 2010.

Etiologic Agent

Physical, Chemical, and Antigenic Properties

There is only one antigenic type of rinderpest virus, but at least three distinct genetic lineages of the virus currently exist. One lineage is present in Asia and two different lineages occur in eastern Africa. Strains of rinderpest vary in their virulence to cattle.

Resistance to Physical and Chemical Agents

Rinderpest virus is inactivated by sunlight within 2 hours and is rapidly inactivated by ultraviolet light. The virus is inactivated by heat exponentially, but small amounts of virus may survive heating at 56°C for 50 to 60 minutes or at 60°C for 30 minutes. Rinderpest virus is relatively stable between pH 4.0 to 10.2. It is inactivated by lipid solvents or disinfectants, such as phenol or strong alkaline compounds.

Infectivity for Other Species and Culture Systems

Rinderpest virus infects all species of the order *Artiodactyla*, which includes cattle, water buffalo, pigs, warthogs, sheep, and many species of African antelope. The virus can be adapted to grow in laboratory animals, such as rabbits, mice, and guinea pigs, and in embryonated chicken eggs. Rinderpest virus can be cultivated in primary or continuous cell cultures of bovine, ovine, and porcine origin.

Host-Virus Relationship

Distribution, Reservoir, and Transmission

Rinderpest historically occurred throughout Europe, Africa, and Asia but never became established in either the Americas or in Australasia. The virus currently is enzootic only in certain regions of Asia, the Middle East, and Africa.

Domestic and wild animals infected with rinderpest virus serve as reservoirs for the disease, especially those species that have a high innate resistance to the disease. These species, including certain breeds of indigenous cattle, Thompson's gazelle, and others, do not show clinical signs of the disease but can shed virus for long periods of time. Similarly, swine, goats and sheep can serve as important reservoir hosts that disseminate virus to susceptible cattle. Rinderpest virus is present in high titers in the nasal discharges, saliva, ocular secretions, and excretions of infected animals, and transmission requires direct contact of susceptible animals with secretions and excretions of infected animals.

Pathogenesis and Pathology

Rinderpest virus infection normally occurs through the upper respiratory tract, although cattle can be experimentally infected by any parenteral route of inoculation. The virus first replicates in the tonsils and regional lymph nodes, and a predominantly lymphocyte-associated viremia then disseminates the virus throughout the body. The virus replicates in lymphoid tissues (spleen, bone marrow, lymph nodes), and the mucosa of the alimentary and upper respiratory tracts. Nasal and ocular secretions contain high titers of virus at this time. Fever (up to 107°F) and leukopenia occur prior to the appearance of oral ulcers and onset of diarrhea that may contain blood (dysentery). Titers of virus in the tissues and secretions of infected cattle decline after the appearance of neutralizing antibodies in serum. The convalescent phase begins with the healing of mouth lesions, and complete recovery from the disease may take 4 to 5 weeks.

Lesions of rinderpest occur in the tissues in which the virus replicates. Oral ulcers are characteristic of severe cases of rinderpest in cattle, and these begin as areas of necrosis with the basal cell layer of the epithelium. Necrosis also occurs in the mucosa of the abomasum and small intestine. The presence of syncitial cells within the affected epithelium is highly characteristic of rinderpest, but not other ulcerative diseases like malignant catarrhal fever or bovine viral diarrhea. There also is extensive necrosis of gut-associated lymphoid tissues as a result of virus-mediated destruction of lymphocytes, and similar lympholysis occurs in other lymphoid tissues (lymph nodes, spleen, bone marrow).

Host Response to Infection

Cattle recovered from rinderpest develop a long-lasting immunity that is likely mediated by the presence of neutralizing antibody in their serum. In cattle vaccinated with modified live rinderpest viral vaccine, both IgM and IgG_2 serum antibodies appear 2 weeks after vaccination.

Laboratory Diagnosis

Initial diagnosis of rinderpest is based on the clinical signs and "explosive" nature of the disease in naive cattle, characteristic lesions, and herd history of recent introduction of animals from a rinderpest-infected area. Given current efforts to eradicate the virus and the very serious consequences of incursion of rinderpest into free areas of the world, laboratory diagnosis is required to confirm the diagnosis and to differentiate rinderpest from other infectious diseases such as bovine viral diarrhea, infectious bovine rhinotracheitis, malignant catarrhal fever, and foot-and-mouth disease. The rinderpest virus can be isolated in appropriate cell cultures. The presence of viral antigens or viral nucleic acid in tissues or ocular secretions of infected animals can rapidly be confirmed using agar gel immunodiffusion or PCR assay, respectively. The competitive ELISA and virus neutralization tests are used for serological diagnosis of rinderpest virus infection.

Treatment and Control

There is no effective treatment for rinderpest. Control is accomplished by vaccination in endemic areas and rigorous quarantine of ruminants from infected areas as outbreaks of rinderpest in areas free of disease are always associated with the introduction of infected animals. Inactivated rinderpest virus vaccine was previously used to immunize cattle, but it has been replaced by modified live vaccines that induce a longer-lasting immunity. Recombinant rinderpest vaccines also have been developed that induce strong protective immunity.

PESTE DES PETITS RUMINANTS

Peste des petits ruminants (PPR) virus is a *Morbillivirus* that produces a rinderpest-like disease in goats and sheep. The virus is closely related to rinderpest virus, thus distinction between the two is very important given the current effort to eradicate rinderpest from the world. Of particular importance is the fact that PPR virus infections of small ruminants frequently are subclinical, thus small ruminants are the major reservoir of this virus.

RUBULAVIRUSES

The rubulaviruses are included in the subfamily *Paramyxovirinae*, family *Paramyxoviridae*. All viruses within this genus have both hemagglutinin and neuraminidase (HN) proteins. Included in the rubulaviruses are nine different species of avian paramyxoviruses (avian paramyxoviruses 1–9) that are distinguished on the basis of their lack of significant cross-neutralization and cross-protection. Avian paramyxovirus 1 is the cause of Newcastle disease (ND).

NEWCASTLE DISEASE

Disease

Newcastle disease (ND) is a highly contagious disease of chickens that is characterized by respiratory distress, diarrhea, and neurological signs. The severity of the disease is dependent upon the age and immune status of the birds, and on the virulence of the strain of ND virus that is responsible for the infection. The most virulent strains are designated as *velogenic* and produce mortality rates in affected birds as high as 90% or more. The disease caused by *mesogenic* strains is less severe and the mortality rate is often less than 25%. The *lentogenic* strains are relatively avirulent and are often used as vaccines.

Etiologic Agent

Physical, Chemical, and Antigenic Properties

The properties of ND virus are similar to those of other members of genus and subfamily.

Resistance to Physical and Chemical Agents

Newcastle disease virus (NDV) can be inactivated by heat, ultraviolet light, pH, oxidation, and chemicals (lysol, phenol, detergents, and butylated hydroxytoluene). The rate of viral inactivation varies with the strain of NDV, quantity of virus initially exposed, time of exposure, and presence of organic matter in the environment. Infectious virus has been recovered from contaminated areas and eggshells several weeks following an outbreak of ND, and can survive for long periods in eggs and in frozen carcasses.

Infectivity for Other Species and Culture Systems

Newcastle disease virus infects chickens, guinea fowls, turkeys, and a large number of species of domestic and wild birds. Sea birds are less susceptible but may act as carriers. Humans accidentally infected with NDV when exposed to infected birds or live viral vaccines may develop a self-limiting conjunctivitis.

Newcastle disease virus can be propagated in the chorioallantoic cavities of 10- to 12-day-old embryonated chicken eggs. The most commonly used cell cultures for the cultivation of NDV are primary chick embryo kidney, primary chick fibroblast, and baby hamster kidney (BHK) cells.

Host-Virus Relationship

Distribution, Reservoir, and Transmission

Newcastle disease occurs worldwide and domestic birds are the major reservoir for NDV. Although NDV has been isolated from a large number of wild birds such as sparrows, crows, ducks, and geese, they appear to play a minimal role in transmitting this disease. The epizootic outbreak of the exotic velogenic strain of NDV in North America (California) in 1971 has been attributed to the introduction of caged birds.

Aerosol respiratory infection is the most common route for transmission of NDV. Infected birds begin to shed virus 2 to 3 days after exposure from their respiratory tracts and continue to shed virus for several weeks. The virus also is readily spread by fomites because of its stability.

Pathogenesis and Pathology

Initial replication of NDV occurs in the mucosa of the upper respiratory tract following aerosol infection. Viremia then disseminates the virus throughout the body, and widespread multiplication of virus in cells of parenchymal organs leads to a secondary viremia, which in some instances leads to the infection of the cells of the CNS. Disease takes several different forms in chickens, depending on the virulence of the strain involved. The very virulent velogenic strains cause very rapidly fatal infections involving the visceral organs or the CNS. Mesogenic strains of NDV cause respiratory and, occasionally, neurologic disease in infected chickens with low mortality, while lentogenic strains produce a mild or often inapparent disease. Differences in the virulence of individual strains of NDV are correlated with differences in the cleavage and activation of their HN protein, and thus these strains rapidly can be differentiated by sequence analysis of the gene encoding HN.

Lesions in ND vary greatly. Inapparent infections cause few, if any, lesions whereas hemorrhagic necrosis that affects the intestinal tract, respiratory tract, and visceral organs is characteristic of more severe forms. In chickens with CNS involvement, necrosis of the glial cells, neuronal degeneration, perivascular cuffing, and hypertrophy of endothelial cells are often present.

Host Response to Infection

Chickens infected with NDV produce antibodies 6 to 10 days after infection. Antibodies to the envelope glycoprotein, HN, exhibit viral neutralizing and hemagglutination inhibition activities and are responsible for host immunity to the disease. Humoral antibodies (IgM and IgG), secretory antibody (IgA), and cell-mediated immunity all appear to play a role in immunity to ND.

Laboratory Diagnosis

As the clinical signs and pathologic lesions of ND are variable and nonspecific, definitive diagnosis of the disease must depend on laboratory methods to identify NDV. This now is best accomplished using PCR, and sequence and/or nucleic acid hybridization analysis to distinguish whether the virus is a velogenic field strain or a live vaccine strain. Alternatively, NDV can be isolated by inoculating embryonated eggs or cell cultures with respiratory exudate or tissue suspensions (spleen, lung, or brain), and NDV antigen in affected tissues or cell cultures can be identified by immunofluorescence or immunohistochemical staining. Serological diagnosis requires demonstration of rising NDV antibody titers by the hemagglutination inhibition, neutralization, or ELISA methods.

Treatment and Control

Sanitary management to prevent exposure of susceptible chickens to NDV is an important aspect of control against the disease. Since there is only one serotype of NDV, vaccination with either inactivated or live virus vaccines is also used to prevent ND. The majority of live vaccines incorporate lentogenic strains of NDV administered in drinking water or applied as aerosols.

RESPIROVIRUSES

The respiroviruses are included in the subfamily *Paramyxovirinae,* family *Paramyxoviridae.* All viruses within this genus have both hemagglutinin and neuraminidase (HN) proteins. Included in the respiroviruses are parainfluenza viruses from cattle, primates, and mice (Sendai virus). The parainfluenza viruses are distinguished by their host range and serological reactivity. They are frequently associated with upper respiratory infections in humans and animals.

CANINE PARAINFLUENZA TYPE 2

Canine parainfluenza virus 2 has been implicated as a cause of infectious tracheobronchitis (kennel cough) in dogs, along with canine adenovirus and *Bordetella bronchiseptica.* The disease is characterized by sudden onset, mild fever, slight to copious nasal discharge, and a harsh, nonproductive cough. Parainfluenza Type 2 virus is antigenically related to the SV-5 virus of monkeys, and it appears that the same or very similar viruses infect a wide variety of animal species. Live modified parainfluenza Type 2 viral vaccines are available, usually combined with other canine viral vaccines such as canine distemper and canine hepatitis or with a *Bordetella bronchiseptica* vaccine.

BOVINE PARAINFLUENZA 3

Parainfluenza Type 3 virus (PI-3) has been implicated in so-called "shipping fever" of cattle, a clinical disease syndrome in the bovine respiratory disease complex. The disease is characterized by high fever (107°F or above), conjunctivitis, respiratory distress, mucopurulent rhinitis, and pneumonia, and occurs after cattle are congregated on feedlots. The disease is widespread in the United States and remains one of the major causes of economic losses in the cattle industry. A number of viruses including PI-3 and bacteria, especially *Mannheimia haemolytica,* have been implicated in the pathogenesis of "shipping fever," but the precise role of PI-3 virus in the disease, if any, is poorly defined. Similar viruses have been isolated from upper respiratory infections of humans, sheep, horses, and water buffaloes.

Inactivated and modified live PI-3 viral vaccines are available, usually combined with other viral vaccines or with bacterins.

PNEUMOVIRINAE

PNEUMOVIRUSES

The genus *Pneumovirus* is included in the subfamily *Pneumovirinae* in the family *Paramyxoviridae* (see Table 60.1). Viruses within the genus include respiratory syncitial viruses that infect humans, cattle, and mice, as well as those that infect sheep and goats, which are closely related to bovine respiratory syncitial virus. The viruses within this genus are distinguished on the basis of their host range and lack of cross neutralization. The members of this group lack neuraminidase and the nucleocapsid has a diameter of 13–14 nm, which is smaller than the nucleocapsid of the paramyxoviruses (18 nm). All members of the genus *Pneumovirus* are antigenically related but are antigenically distinct from other paramyxoviruses. Their hemagglutin protein is designated as G, as compared to H or HN in members of the subfamily *Paramyxovirinae.*

BOVINE RESPIRATORY SYNCYTIAL VIRUS

Bovine respiratory syncytial virus (BRSV) causes an acute pneumonia in calves, which show such clinical signs as coughing, fever, anorexia, nasal discharge, and respiratory distress. The pneumonia is characterized by bronchitis and alveolitis with multinucleated syncytia and alveolar epithelial hyperplasia. The disease has been reported in North America, Japan, Europe, and Australia. Not all cattle infected with BRSV show clinical signs of the disease. Infected animals serve as the reservoir of the disease and the virus is shed in the nasal secretions of infected animals. BRSV infection can be diagnosed by direct staining of nasopharyngeal smears with immunofluorescent antibody to BRSV.

Cattle infected with BRSV develop serum-neutralizing antibody 3 days after viral exposure, reaching a peak after 3 to 4 weeks. There is also evidence of a cell-mediated immune response in cattle to BRSV. An attenuated live bovine respiratory syncytial viral vaccine is available.

METAMOVIRUSES

Metapneumoviruses are distinguished from pneumoviruses on the basis of their gene order and virion protein composition. Turkey rhinotracheitis virus (avian pneumovirus) is assigned to this group. This virus causes upper respiratory tract disease in young turkeys and chickens.

FILOVIRIDAE

Viruses within this family are characterized by enveloped, pleomorphic (filamentous) virions and a genome of single-stranded molecule of negative-sense RNA. There are two major groups of filoviruses: Ebola and related viruses, and Marburg and related viruses. Viruses within these groups cause severe, fatal diseases of humans that are characterized as "hemorrhagic fevers" because of the spectacular diseases they cause in affected humans. These viruses infect primates and can be adapted to laboratory animals.

BORNAVIRIDAE

Viruses within this family are characterized by enveloped spherical virions of approximately 90 nm in diameter, and a genome of single-stranded, negative-sense RNA. Borna disease virus (BDV) is the prototype virus of this family. Sheep and horses are considered to be the natural reservoir host of BDV, but infection occurs in a variety of other animal species including humans, cattle, rabbits, goats, dogs, cats, and selected species of birds. The BDV is neurotropic and it has been incriminated as a cause of a variety of behavioral disorders in humans and encephalitis in animals. Borna disease is described as severe neurologic disorder of horses that largely is confined to regions of central Europe, whereas apparently asymptomatic BDV infection of humans and horses apparently occurs worldwide. The precise significance of BDV as a veterinary pathogen remains to be adequately defined.

61 *Rhabdoviridae*

Yuan Chung Zee   N. James MacLachlan

Rhabdoviruses (the Greek word *rhabdo* means rod) are bullet-shaped, enveloped, single-stranded RNA viruses that have a broad host range. Members of the family *Rhabdoviridae* are included in four genera (*Lyssavirus, Vesiculovirus, Ephermerovirus, Novirhabdovirus*) and infect vertebrates, invertebrates (arthropods), and plants. Rhabdoviruses cause a variety of important diseases: rabies (and rabies-related virus diseases), vesicular stomatitis, bovine ephemeral fever, and diseases of fish that include spring viremia of carp, infectious hematopoetic necrosis, and viral hemorrhagic septicemia of salmon (Table 61.1). Rhabdoviruses share a common morphology, require a viral RNA-dependent polymerase for replication, and have mature virions that bud from plasma membrane or into intracytoplasmic vacuoles (Figs 61.1, 61.2).

RABIES

Disease

Rabies virus infects all warm-blooded animals, including humans, causing a severe and invariably fatal disease of the central nervous system (CNS). The incubation period is prolonged, varying from 2 weeks to 6 months and even longer in exceptional circumstances. Clinical signs involve the CNS but vary depending on the species of animal that is affected. The early signs and symptoms of human rabies are headache, extreme thirst, vomiting, and anorexia. More advanced signs and symptoms include painful spasms of the pharyngeal muscles when drinking (hydrophobia), excitement to sensory stimuli, and generalized paralysis. Death is the inevitable outcome once clinical signs develop. The course of rabies in dogs usually lasts only 3 to 8 days. Behavioral changes are common during the early phases of disease, and fever, dilation of the pupils, and photophobia are sometimes present. The furious form of rabies occurs later, when the affected dog becomes nervous and progressively irritable. Affected dogs may bite without provocation. Clinical signs include profuse salivation and frothing at the mouth, difficulty in swallowing and drinking, convulsions, and muscular incoordination. Some affected dogs exhibit only a paralytic or "dumb" stage without going through a furious phase. Characteristic clinical signs of this form of rabies are paralysis of the muscles of the pharynx and lower jaw, and incoordination that progresses to coma and death. The clin-

ical signs of rabies in cats are similar to those in dogs, but rabid cats have an even greater tendency to hide in secluded places and are often more vicious than affected dogs. Clinical signs of rabies in horses often include progressive ataxia and eventual paralysis, and difficulty in swallowing. Cattle affected with rabies are usually excitable and restless. Typical signs include salivation, choking, absence of rumination, rectal straining, and paralysis of the hindquarters.

Several viruses that are closely related to rabies virus can also cause a rabies-like disease in infected animals and humans (see Table 61.1). Bats are an important reservoir host of several of these viruses.

Etiologic Agent

Physical, Chemical, and Antigenic Properties

The virion of rabies virus is shaped like a cone or a bullet, approximately 180 nm in length and 80 nm in width, and contains an envelope with short spikes (peplomers 6 nm to 7 nm in length). A central cylindrical core of ribonucleoprotein runs throughout the longitudinal axis. The virus has a buoyant density of $1.20 g/cm^3$ in cesium chloride. The viral RNA is single-stranded, negative-sense, and encodes five subgenomic mRNAs that are translated into five major proteins designated as L (the RNA-dependent RNA polymerase), G (the glycoprotein that forms the envelope spikes, N (the nucleoprotein), P (a part of the viral polymerase) and M (or M_2 for rabies virus). The major surface glycoprotein G contains the neutralizing epitopes of the virus. The nucleocapsid consists of viral RNA and the N, NS, and L proteins, and the M protein links the nucleocapsid to the lipid envelop that contains the G glycoprotein.

Strains of rabies virus isolated from naturally occurring cases are referred to as "street virus," and attenuated laboratory strains are referred to as "fixed virus." These strains differ in their biologic properties in laboratory animals—for example, virulence, length of the incubation period, and distribution and nature of histologic lesions in target tissues. The antigenic variation between street and fixed strains of rabies virus can be distinguished by their reaction with monoclonal antibodies. It has been shown that vaccinated mice were protected against challenge with the field strain that was more closely related to the vaccine strain than more antigenically distant strains. Thus, the selection of appropriate strains of the virus for vaccine production can be critical.

Table 61.1.   Major Genera of Rhabdoviruses

Genus	Virus	Natural Host	Disease
Vesiculovirus			
	Vesicular stomatitis	Horses, cattle, swine	Vesicules and ulcers
	Alagoas virus		
	Indiana virus		
	New Jersey virus		
	Spring viremia of carp	Carp	Abdominal distention
Lyssavirus			
	Rabies	All warm-blooded animals	Rabies
	Australian bat lyssavirus	Bat	Rabies-like
	European lyssavirus (1 & 2)	Bat	Rabies-like
	Lagos bat	Bat	Rabies-like
	Mokola	Shrews	Rabies-like
Ephemerovirus			
	Bovine ephemeral fever	Cattle	Systemic infection; fever
Novirhabdovirus			
	Infectious hematopoietic necrosis	Salmonids	Systemic; nervous system
Ungrouped			
	Viral hemorrhagic septicemia	Salmonids	Tissue necrosis and hemorrhage

FIGURE 61.1.   *Vesicular stomatitis virus budding from plasma membrane of an infected L cell. 40,000X. (Reproduced with permission from Zee YC, Hackett AJ, Talen L. Vesicular stomatitis virus maturation sites in six different host cells. J Gen Virol 1970;7:95.)*

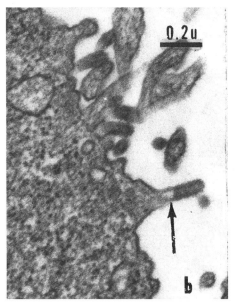

Rabies virus is included in the genus *Lyssavirus,* along with rabies-related viruses like Australian bat lyssavirus, European bat lyssaviruses 1 and 2, Lagos bat virus, and Mokola virus, all of which can induce a rabies-like disease in humans (see Table 61.1).

Resistance to Physical and Chemical Agents

Rabies virus is inactivated by heating at 56°C for 30 minutes and by chemical agents such as formalin (1%), cresol (3%), and beta-propiolactone (0.1%). The virus may persist in infected brain tissue for up to 10 days at room temperature and for several weeks at 4°C, but is relatively susceptible to disinfection.

Infectivity for Other Species or Culture Systems

Rabies virus infects and replicates in all warm-blooded animals. The virus can be readily propagated in chicken embryo or duck embryo as well as in a number of cell cultures, especially in baby hamster kidney cells (BHK21) and human diploid cells (WI-26).

Host-Virus Relationship

Distribution, Reservoir, and Transmission

Rabies is distributed throughout the world, with the notable exception of Australia (although Australian bat *Lyssavirus* is closely related to rabies virus and causes an identical disease in humans), the United Kingdom and Ireland, Cyprus, Japan, New Zealand, and Scandinavia. The disease is endemic in many countries in Africa, Asia, North and South America, and Western Europe. Extensive epizootics of rabies have occurred in Asia and Africa in particular. Rabies recently has been eradicated from extensive portions of Europe by vaccination of wildlife reservoir hosts of the virus, especially foxes.

Of the many animals that are susceptible to rabies, dogs, foxes, skunks, wolves, raccoons, mongooses, coyotes,

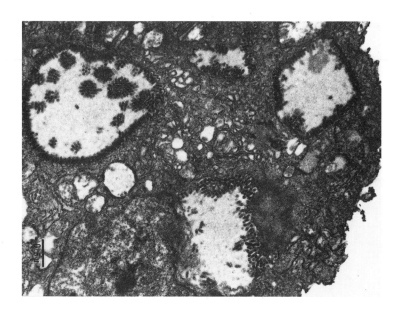

FIGURE 61.2.   *Vesicular stomatitis virus budding into the lumen of cytoplasmic vacuole in an infected chick fibroblast. 17,000X.*

skunks, and bats all can serve as reservoirs of rabies virus. The significance of individual reservoir host species differs between geographic regions. For example, foxes are an important reservoir host of rabies virus in Western Europe. Similarly, foxes are the most important reservoir hosts of rabies virus in portions of Canada, Alaska, and the desert southwestern regions of the United States, whereas skunks and raccoons are the critical reservoir of rabies virus in other regions of North America. The mongoose is an important reservoir of rabies virus in Africa and Asia. The domestic dog, however, remains the most important source of rabies for humans, especially in the developing countries of Africa, Asia, and Latin America.

Most rabies cases stem from the bite of a rabid animal—the saliva of most infected animals contains infectious virus. However, transmission from bats is an increasing problem, and rabies virus may be transmitted from bats to humans without any history of a bite. Rabies may be acquired by inhaling aerosol containing rabies virus in infected bat caves or by virus passing through intact mucous membranes.

Pathogenesis and Pathology

The primary route of infection in rabies is through the bite of a rabid animal that contains infectious virus in its saliva. Several factors, including the virulence of the infecting virus strain, the quantity of infectious virus in the saliva, and the susceptibility of the species, are important in determining whether or not infection is established in the recipient animal. Foxes, cattle, hamsters, and coyotes are particularly susceptible to rabies, and dogs and cats are more susceptible than either humans or rodents. The length of the incubation period after viral exposure varies greatly and depends on the anatomic distance between the bite site and the CNS, the severity of the bite, and the amount of infectious virus in the saliva.

Following viral exposure, the rabies virus persists in the local muscle tissues for hours or days, and viral replication takes place in striated muscle cells near the inoculation site. There is no evidence that a viremia is necessary for dissemination of rabies virus to the CNS; rather, rabies virus is taken up at motor and sensory nerve endings and the virus then ascends within the axons of nerve cells to the ventral horn cells of the spinal cord at a rate of 12 mm to 24 mm per day. Antibodies do not inhibit viral transport once virus is present within the axon. Viral replication occurs in the spinal cord cells and subsequently spreads to the brain. The virus then disseminates within the brain leading to the clinical signs and symptoms of rabies. It should be pointed out, however, that the virus can persist in the brain of infected skunks, rats, raccoons, bats, and foxes for many months without producing overt clinical signs. It has been shown experimentally in rodents that rabies virus after peripheral inoculation can be found in the spinal cord 24 to 72 hours after inoculation and in the brain 96 to 192 hours after inoculation. Rabies virus ultimately spreads from the CNS to other organs, such as salivary glands, cornea, and tonsils, via the peripheral nerves. Viral replication in salivary glands occurs rapidly, and infected saliva is the major source of infection.

Lymphocytic polioencephalomyelitis with perivascular cuffing is the most prominent histologic lesion in the brains of animals with rabies, although the severity of this change is highly variable. The presence of acidophilic intracytoplasmic inclusion bodies (Negri bodies) in the infected neurons of the hippocampus or cerebellum is characteristic of rabies.

Host Response to Infection

Animals and humans vaccinated with rabies virus vaccine develop circulating neutralizing antibodies to the virus within 2 to 3 weeks of vaccination. High titers of neutralizing antibody may occur in animals with rabies; thus it is likely that antibodies must be present at the time of exposure to rabies virus if they are to be protective. Both cellular and humoral immune responses are important in preventing rabies in vaccinated animals, although neither mechanism is effective in preventing disease in naive animals.

Laboratory Diagnosis

The diagnosis of human rabies centers on a history of an animal bite and, logically, every effort should be taken to locate and quarantine the suspected animal. Clinical diagnosis of rabies in animals requires differentiation from other infectious or noninfectious diseases of the CNS. Rabies should be suspected in endemic or epizootic areas when an animal exhibits abnormal behavior and/or paralysis. The definitive laboratory diagnosis is typically done by direct immunofluorescent antibody staining of sections of brain, which is a very rapid and accurate diagnostic test. Direct immunofluorescent staining of the skin can be used as an antemortem diagnostic test also. Highly sensitive PCR assays have been developed for laboratory confirmation. The diagnosis can be confirmed by intracerebral inoculation of young mice with brain suspension from suspected animals. Inoculated mice usually develop clinical signs within 17 days of inoculation, and Negri bodies are usually present in their neurons at the time of death. Monoclonal antibodies directed against the glycoprotein of rabies virus can be used to distinguish rabies virus from rabies-related viruses, and to confirm cases of vaccine-induced rabies in dogs, cats, and foxes.

Treatment and Control

Rabies in animals can be controlled by eliminating or immunizing wild animal reservoir hosts, and by vaccinating susceptible domestic animals. Strict quarantine of imported wild and domestic animals for up to 6 months from rabies-endemic regions has kept island nations such as New Zealand, Australia, the United Kingdom and Hawaii, free of rabies. The elimination of wild animal reservoir hosts is difficult and increasingly unacceptable in many countries, thus vaccination of these hosts is a more acceptable and successful strategy.

Various types of inactivated and live attenuated rabies vaccines are commercially available for vaccinating dogs and cats, including new generation recombinant vaccines that do not include infectious rabies virus. New generation vaccines do not suffer from the instances of vaccine-induced rabies that sporadically occurred with the original live-attenuated low-egg passage vaccine. Caution should be exercised when live vaccines are used, especially in a different species.

There is no effective treatment for rabies in animals.

VESICULAR STOMATITIS

Disease

Vesicular stomatitis (VS) virus causes an acute febrile disease of horses, cattle, and swine in the western hemisphere.

The disease in cattle is characterized by the formation of vesicles in the mucosal lining of the mouth and tongue. Lesions range from mild punctate erosions on the dental pad to severe ulcers on the tongue. Formation of vesicles is also observed on the teats, on the skin of the coronary band, and in the interdigital spaces of the foot. The lesions of VS in cattle and pigs mimic those of foot-and-mouth disease, and in swine they also mimic those of swine vesicular disease and vesicular exanthema; thus the major impact of VS is the restrictions imposed on animal movement that adversely impact trade and commerce. The important distinction, however, is that only VS occurs in horses, and horses frequently are the sentinel species affected during outbreaks of VS. Indeed, spectacular epidemics of VS occurred in the past when horses were congregated in the United States during times of military conflict.

Vesicular stomatitis is a relatively benign and self-limiting disease, and infected animals usually recover uneventfully. However, milk production can be markedly impacted in dairy cattle, and affected animals and the oral lesions can be painful so that affected animals cease eating and lose condition. The VS virus produces an acute, influenza-like illness in humans, and severe conjunctivitis when virus directly is introduced to the eye. Experimental infection of mice with VSV can produce fatal encephalitis, and the susceptibility of VSV in mice is age-dependent.

Etiologic Agent

Physical, Chemical, and Antigenic Properties

The VS virus generally resembles rabies virus in its morphology, genome, and protein structure. Three different species of VS virus occur in the Americas; New Jersey, Indiana, and Alagoas viruses.

Resistance to Physical and Chemical Agents

Vesicular stomatitis virus is inactivated by high temperatures (50°C to 60°C for 30 minutes) and by light, ultraviolet light, and lipid solvents. It is also sensitive to common disinfectants such as sodium hypochlorite and quaternary ammonium compounds (Clorox, Roccal, respectively), phenol, and formalin. The virus is more resistant to lye (NaOH); 2% to 3% lye fails to inactivate VS virus after an exposure of 2 hours. The virus can be preserved for years at −70°C and by freeze-drying under vacuum.

Infectivity for Other Species or Culture Systems

Vesicular stomatitis virus infects and causes diseases in horses, mules, cattle, swine, deer, and humans. Most mammalian species can be infected with VSV, and the virus can be propagated in laboratory animals such as mice and guinea pigs and in embryonated chick eggs. Vesicular stomatitis virus readily is propagated in a wide variety of cell cultures and produces a cytopathic effect and visible plaques. The virus can also replicate in mosquitoes and certain other insects.

Host-Virus Relationship

Distribution, Reservoir, and Transmission

Vesicular stomatitis is a disease of North, Central, and South America. Vesicular stomatitis virus is endemic in regions closest to the equator, and epidemic incursions of the virus into adjacent temperate regions (such as the United States) occur at regular intervals (3–10 years or so). Both New Jersey and Indiana viruses cause epizootics of VS in North America, although New Jersey now is more common. Molecular epidemiologic studies indicate that each VS epidemic in North America is caused by a single genetic variant of VS virus, suggesting that the virus emerges from an endemic focus further to the south. Multiple genetic lineages of VS viruses occur in tropical regions of the Americas.

The definitive reservoir host of VS virus is uncertain, and insects have been implicated as biological vectors. Direct contact is an important mode of transmission of VSV as large quantities of virus are present in the vesicles in the mouth, thus contamination with infected saliva can transmit the infection to healthy animals. Cattle can also be experimentally infected by the aerosol route. Several insects (stable fly, tabanids, mosquitoes) have been demonstrated to be mechanical carriers of VSV and presumably can transmit the disease. Sandflies perpetuate the virus in tropical and subtropical regions of the Americas, including Ossabaw Island off the coast of Georgia in the United States. Epizootics of VS typically end after the first killing frost in temperate regions of North America, and the seasonal occurrence of outbreaks of VS in the warmer months further implicates insects in the dissemination of the virus.

Pathogenesis and Pathology

Vesicular stomatitis has a short incubation period in animals infected through an abrasion, after which the virus rapidly disseminates to a wide variety of tissues. Cattle with VS are febrile (103°F to 104°F) and develop oral lesions that begin as papules that progress to vesicles which rapidly ulcerate, leaving punctate erosions on the dental pad and ulcers that can be extensive on the tongue and oral mucosa. In severe cases, sloughing of the mucous membrane on the surface of the tongue causes extensive salivation and anorexia. Ulcerated vesicles can be extensive in the mouths of affected horses. High titers of virus are present in the vesicle fluid and saliva but not in the blood. These lesions usually heal rapidly, although recurrent and/or chronic ulcers can develop. Similar vesicular lesions that rapidly ulcerate occur on the feet and teats of affected cattle and swine, and these can become secondarily infected with bacteria.

Histologic changes in affected areas of oral mucosa and skin adjacent to the hoof include epithelial hyperplasia with marked intracellular and intercellular edema. Neutrophils infiltrate affected regions, which rapidly undergo necrosis leading to epithelial ulceration.

Host Response to Infection

Infected or vaccinated animals develop high neutralizing antibody titers (>32,000; 80% plaque reduction assay) 10 days after exposure. Serologic response can also be measured by the complement fixation test and enzyme-linked immunosorbent assay (ELISA). Immunity, however is transient, and animals with high titers of neutralizing antibody can be susceptible to reinfection with the homologous virus. There is little cross-protection between the Indiana and New Jersey viruses.

Laboratory Diagnosis

Diagnosis of VSV is important because its lesions resemble those caused by foot-and-mouth disease; horses are not affected by foot-and-mouth disease, whereas they are commonly affected in outbreaks of VS. Laboratory diagnosis is required for the definitive identification of VSV infection. The animal inoculation test was once the only one available for the differential diagnosis of vesicular diseases, but now the following laboratory tests are used to detect VSV: 1) electron microscopy or immunoelectron microscopy on vesicle fluid, 2) immunofluorescence antibody staining of vesicle tissues, 3) isolation of VSV using susceptible cell cultures, and 4) demonstration of a rise in antibody titer by the ELISA method.

Treatment and Control

A variety of VSV vaccines are available to prevent economic losses from interruption of milk production in dairy cattle. There is no effective treatment for the disease other than providing good nursing care. Sick animals should be separated from clinically healthy ones.

BOVINE EPHEMERAL FEVER

Bovine ephemeral fever (BEF), also known as *3-day sickness,* is a noncontagious disease of cattle and water buffalo that is characterized by fever, lameness, and nasal discharge. The morbidity of the disease is high but the mortality is very low. Economic loss is associated with loss of milk production in infected cows. Bovine ephemeral fever virus (BEFV) can infect other species of ruminants. The virus can be propagated in suckling mice, mammalian cell cultures such as BHK-21, Vero cells, and insect cell cultures such as *Aedes albopictus* cells.

Like rabies and VS viruses, BEF viruses are bullet-shaped or cone-shaped particles with a length of 140 nm to 200 nm and a diameter of 60 nm to 80 nm. The genome and virion organization also are similar. The virus is inactivated by heat (10 minutes at 56°C) and by high pH (12.0) or low pH (2.5).

Bovine ephemeral fever is enzootic in tropical and subtropical regions of Africa, Australia, the Middle East, and Asia. It has never been reported in the Americas. The disease is not transmitted by direct contact, and BEFV has been isolated from mosquitoes and biting midges (*Culicoides*) that serve as vectors.

Lesions described in fatal cases of BEF include serofibrinous polyserositis with accumulation of fluid in the joints and pericardial, peritoneal, and pleural cavities, and congestion of lymph nodes. Histologic lesions include necrosis of muscle, generalized hyperemia and edema, and vasculitis that apparently is mediated by neutrophils.

Diagnosis is accomplished by the demonstration of BEFV by isolation in cell culture or intracerebral inoculation of suckling mice with blood of infected animals, or by the detection of a rise in neutralizing antibody titer in paired serum samples. Animals infected with BEFV are immune for several years. Experimental attenuated live, recombinant, and inactivated vaccines have been developed.

DISEASES OF FISH CAUSED BY RHABDOVIRUSES

Infectious hematopoietic necrosis, Spring viremia of carp, and viral hemorrhagic septicemia of salmonids are diseases of fish that are all caused by rhabdoviruses, and there are several others. Infectious hematopoietic necrosis is a disease of salmon and trout that cause substantial losses in hatcheries in North America, Asia, and Europe. Disease is characterized by anemia and hemorrhage. Viral hemorrhagic septicemia is the cause of a similar disease of salmonids. Spring viremia of carp virus causes a fatal disease of carp that also is characterized by hemorrhages and edema of abdominal viscera leading to abdominal distention.

62

Coronaviridae and *Arteriviridae*

UDENI B. R. BALASURIYA   JEFFREY L. STOTT

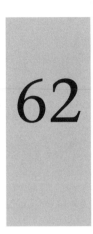

The virus families *Coronaviridae* and *Arteriviridae* are included in the order *Nidovirales* (Table 62.1), along with the newly identified family *Roniviridae*. All members of the order *Nidovirales* are enveloped viruses with linear, positive-sense, single-stranded RNA (ssRNA) genomes. They share a strikingly similar genome organization and replication strategy, but differ considerably in their genetic complexity and virion architecture. "Nido" derives from the Latin word *nidus* for *nest,* which refers to the 3' co-terminal nested subgenomic viral mRNA that is produced during replication of these viruses.

The family *Coronaviridae* is further divided into two genera, *Coronavirus* and *Torovirus.* The *Coronavirus* genus contains numerous pathogens of veterinary significance, and coronaviruses commonly are associated with respiratory and enteric infections of a variety of animal species. The toroviruses infect humans and animals (horses, cattle, and pigs) and are predominantly associated with enteric disease. The family *Arteriviridae* (genus *Arterivirus*) contains four species—specific viruses that infect horses and donkeys (equine arteritis virus), pigs (porcine reproductive and respiratory syndrome virus), monkeys (simian hemorrhagic fever virus), and mice (lactate dehydrogenase elevating virus). The outcome of *Arterivirus* infections is highly variable and includes persistent asymptomatic infections, respiratory disease, reproductive failure (abortion), and lethal hemorrhagic fever. The family *Roniviridae* (genus *Ronivirus*) contains a number of closely related viruses that infect farmed prawns in Australia and Asia, but will not be further discussed here because these viruses are not yet well characterized.

CORONAVIRUS

Coronaviruses have a unique morphologic appearance. They are spherical, enveloped virions with large club-shaped surface projections (peplomers) extending from the viral envelope. The envelope encloses an icosahedral internal core structure within which is a helical nucleocapsid (Fig 62.1). Virion size ranges from 80 nm to 220 nm in diameter. *Coronavirus* genomic ssRNA (linear, positive-sense) is the largest viral RNA genome and ranges in size from 27.6 to 31 kb.

Two viral-specified structural glycoproteins (spike [S] and M) are present in the envelope. Glycoprotein S is largely external to the membrane perimeter and forms the club-shaped projections (approximately 20 nm in length) from the virion membrane. Neutralizing antibodies and cell-mediated cytotoxicity are directed against epitopes in the S glycoprotein, which also is responsible for binding of virions to host cell membranes. Glycoprotein M is a transmembrane protein that is more deeply embedded in the envelope. Antibodies directed against M may neutralize the virus in the presence of complement. The small envelope protein (E), together with the M protein, plays an essential role in *Coronavirus* particle assembly. Some of the coronaviruses contain a hemagglutinin-esterase (HE) protein that forms short surface projections. The nucleocapsid protein (N) is a basic phosphoprotein that forms a long, flexible, helical nucleocapsid enclosing the genomic RNA. The M and N proteins form an internal core structure in at least two coronaviruses (transmissible gastroenteritis virus and mouse hepatitis virus).

Coronaviruses infect a wide range of mammals (including humans) and birds. They exhibit a marked tropism for epithelial cells of the respiratory and enteric tracts, as well as macrophages for some viruses. Coronaviruses cause a remarkably diverse spectrum of different diseases in different hosts (see Table 62.1). They typically have a restricted host range, infecting only their natural host and closely related animal species. Based on their serological cross-reactivity, coronaviruses are divided into three antigenic groups, including two groups of mammalian coronaviruses and a single group of avian coronaviruses.

TRANSMISSIBLE GASTROENTERITIS VIRUS AND PORCINE RESPIRATORY CORONAVIRUS

Disease

Transmissible gastroenteritis (TGE) is a highly contagious enteric disease of swine caused by TGE virus (TGEV). The disease is characterized by severe diarrhea, vomiting, dehydration, and high mortality in young piglets (less than 2

Table 62.1. Important Animal Viruses in the Order *Nidovirales*, Which Includes Three Virus Families: *Coronaviridae* (Genera *Coronavirus* and *Torovirus*), *Arteriviridae* (Genus *Arterivirus*), and *Roniviridae* (Genus *Ronivirus*)

Family	Genus	Species	Primary host	Disease/Tissue affected
Coronaviridae	Coronavirus	Transmissible gastroenteritis virus (TGEV)[a]	Swine	Enteric infection
		Porcine respiratory coronavirus (PRCoV)[a]	Swine	Respiratory infection
		Feline coronavirus (FECoV)[a]	Feline	Enteric infection
		Feline infectious peritonitis virus (FIPV)[a]		Peritonitis, respiratory, enteric, and neurological infection
		Canine coronavirus (CCoV)[a]	Canine	Enteric infection
		Rabbit coronavirus (RbCoV)[a]	Rabbit	Enteric infection
		Human coronavirus (HCoV 229E)[a]	Human	Respiratory infection
		Porcine epidemic diarrhea virus (PEDV)[a]	Swine	Enteric infection
		Porcine hemagglutinating encephalomyelitis (HEV)[b]	Swine	Enteric, respiratory, and neurological infection
		Canine respiratory coronavirus (CRCoV)[b]	Canine	Respiratory infection
		Bovine coronavirus (BCoV)[b]	Bovine	Enteric and respiratory infection
		Enteric bovine coronavirus (EBCoV)		
		Respiratory bovine coronavirus (RBCoV)		
		Mouse hepatitis virus (MHV)[b]	Mouse	Hepatitis, enteric, and neurological infection
		Rat coronavirus—syn. Sialodacryadenitis virus (SADV)[b]	Rat	Sialodacryadenitis
		Human coronavirus (HcoV-OC43)[b]	Human	Respiratory infection
		Sever acute respiratory syndrome coronavirus (SARS-CoV)[b]	Human	Respiratory infection
		Equine coronavirus (ECoV)[b]	Equine	Enteric infection
		Infectious bronchitis virus (IBV)[c]	Avian (chicken)	Respiratory, reproductive, and kidney infection
		Turkey coronavirus (TCoV)[c]	Avian (turkey)	Respiratory and enteric infection
	Torovirus	Equine torovirus (ETV)	Equine	Enteric infection
		Bovine torovirus (BoTV)	Bovine	Enteric infection
		Porcine torovirus (PoTV)	Porcine	Enteric infection
		Human torovirus (HuTV)	Human	Enteric infection
Arteriviridae	Arterivirus	Equine arteritis virus (EAV)	Equine	Respiratory and reproductive infection
		Porcine reproductive and respiratory syndrome virus (PRRSV)	Porcine	Respiratory and reproductive infection
		Simian hemorrhagic fever virus (SHFV)	Simian	Hemorrhagic fever
		Lactate dehydrogenase elevating virus (LDV)	Murine	Neurological infection
Roniviridae	Ronivirus	Gill-associated virus (GAV)	Prawns	Lymphoid organ
		Lymphoid organ virus (LOV)	Prawns	Lymphoid organ
		Yellow head virus (YHV)	Prawns	Lymphoid organ

[a] Antigenic group I
[b] Antigenic group II
[c] Antigenic group III

weeks of age). Mortality in older pigs (greater than 5 weeks) is usually low.

Porcine respiratory coronavirus (PRCoV) is a deletion mutant of TGEV (deletion of nucleotides 621 to 681 in the S gene) and has a tropism for respiratory epithelium and alveolar macrophages. PRCoV is nonenteropathogenic and can infect pigs of all ages by aerosol or direct contact transmission. PRCoV infections are generally subclinical, but strains of the virus differ in the severity of the clinical signs they induce. Clinical signs include moderate to severe respiratory disease with interstitial pneumonia. In addition, PRCoV infection can be concurrently associated with other respiratory virus infections, such as with porcine reproductive and respiratory syndrome virus, which can alter the severity of disease and associated clinical signs.

Etiologic Agent

Physical, Chemical, and Antigenic Properties

TGEV is antigenically related to coronaviruses of humans, dogs, and cats. Only one serotype of TGEV is recognized, and TGEV and PRCoV antigenically cross-react, although some antigenic sites of TGEV are absent from PRCoV because of the deletion in the amino terminus of the S protein in PRCoV.

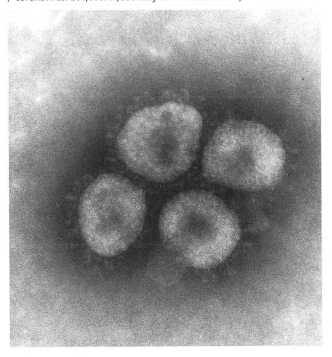

Resistance to Physical and Chemical Agents

TGEV and PRCoV are inactivated by lipid solvents (ether and chloroform), sodium hypochlorite, quaternary ammonium compound, iodines, heating at 56°C for 45 minutes, and exposure to sunlight. Both viruses are stable when frozen but somewhat labile at room temperature. TGEV resists inactivation by trypsin and acidic pH (pH of 3) and is relatively stable in pig bile.

Infectivity for Other Species and Culture Systems

TGE has only been described in swine; however, TGEV has been isolated from the feces of experimentally infected cats, dogs, foxes, and starlings (*Sturnus vulgaris*) for up to 20 days. Serologic studies have also suggested natural infection of skunks, opossums, muskrats, and humans. Virus has also been demonstrated in house flies (*Musca domestica Linneaus*) following experimental and natural infection.

TGEV has been propagated in various cell culture systems, including pig kidney, testis, salivary gland, and thyroid; organ cultures of esophagus, intestine, and nasal epithelium; canine kidney cell cultures; and embryonated chicken eggs (amniotic cavity). Pig kidney and swine testicle (ST) cell lines have been the choice of cells for virus isolation from the feces or gut contents of infected pigs. Development of cytopathic effect may require multiple passages in cell culture.

PRCoV replicates in pig kidney and ST cells, as well as a cat fetus cell line.

Host-Virus Relationship

Distribution, Reservoir, and Transmission

TGEV infection of swine occurs worldwide and has been documented in North, Central, and South America; Europe; and Asia. Epizootics of TGE are often seasonal in the United States, occurring in the winter months. The primary mode of TGEV transmission appears to be ingestion of feed contaminated with infected feces (fecal-oral).

Persistence of TGEV in nature is likely via the fecal carrier/shedding state in recovered swine; thus the virus is maintained in endemically infected herds through ongoing fecal-oral infection of susceptible pigs. Infection of swine in endemically infected herds is often subclinical or mild, whereas the virus spreads rapidly in nonimmune herds and can cause devastating outbreaks of disease. In addition to movement by infected swine, TGEV is potentially transmitted between herds by fomites and other animals.

PRCoV virus has been isolated in North America and Europe. The virus is not shed in the feces, and therefore there is no evidence for the fecal-oral transmission. Infected pigs shed virus in their respiratory secretions, and PRCoV may persist in herds by continuous infection of newly weaned pigs.

Pathogenesis and Pathology

TGEV survives in the gastrointestinal tract after ingestion because of its resistance to low pH and trypsin, thus it passes through the stomach without inactivation. Six to twelve hours following intragastric inoculation, viral replication occurs in villus epithelial cells of the small intestine with highest titers of virus in the jejunum. TGEV infects and destroys the columnar epithelial cells lining the intestinal villi, resulting in atrophy of the villi. Villous blunting and increased crypt depth (as a consequence of replication of the progenitor cells in the crypts in an effort to repopulate the denuded villi) occurs 24 to 40 hours postinfection and coincides with the occurrence of severe diarrhea. The loss of enterocytes lining the villi results in malabsorption and maldigestion, which in turn results in diarrhea and dehydration. Undigested lactose in the intestinal contents passes to the large bowel, where it exerts an osmotic effect that further exacerbates the diarrhea.

Affected piglets are dehydrated with fecal staining around the perineum. The typical lesions include thinning of the interstitial wall, villous atrophy, and gastrointestinal distension with yellow fluid containing curds of undigested milk.

The characteristic microscopic lesion of PRCoV infection is diffuse intestinal pneumonia, whereas the intestine does not exhibit atrophy of the villi.

Host Response to Infection

Neutralizing antibodies develop within approximately 7 days of TGEV infection of swine. The presence of secretory

IgA plays a major role in protective immunity and viral clearance. Intramuscular immunization of pigs with TGEV results in development of a humoral IgG response but not protective immunity. Conversely, pigs immunized orally with TGEV develop protective virus-specific IgA in their intestinal mucosal secretions. Infection of sows with TGEV results in the secretion of protective IgA in colostrum (so-called lactogenic immunity), which is protective in suckling pigs. Cell-mediated immunity also is likely important in the immune response to TGEV infection, as passive transfer of mononuclear leukocytes from immune donor pigs to susceptible histocompatible piglets results in reduced disease expression. High levels of Type I interferon are produced by infected intestinal cells, which also may play a role in controlling viral replication.

Pigs infected with PRCoV develop neutralizing antibodies to the virus. Antibodies against PRCoV provide partial protection against TGEV, and therefore the incidence and severity of TGE may decline in swine herds with endemic PRCoV infection.

Laboratory Diagnosis

TGEV infection of young pigs is usually diagnosed through the demonstration of viral antigen in mucosal scrapings or frozen sections of jejunum and ileum by immunohistochemical or immunofluorescent staining with virus-specific antibodies. Definitive diagnosis can be done by viral isolation through inoculation of animals (pigs 2 to 7 days old) or cell cultures (pig kidney, testis, or thyroid). Electron microscopy (EM) or immuno-EM can also be used on fecal contents or intestine.

Serologic diagnosis is appropriate when acute and convalescent sera are available. However, serologic diagnosis is complicated by the finding that both PRCoV and TGEV induce neutralizing antibodies that cross-neutralize each other. Therefore, TGEV strains are not distinguished from its nonenteropathogenic variant PRCoV by the virus neutralization test but can be distinguished by a blocking ELISA test.

Treatment and Control

Treatment of TGEV-infected pigs is usually unrewarding. Replacement of fluids and antibacterial drugs to reduce complications associated with enteropathogenic *Escherichia coli* may be of benefit.

Inactivated and modified live attenuated virus vaccines are available for vaccination of pigs to prevent TGE. These can be used for vaccination of newborn piglets or immunization of sows, or both. Vaccination of pregnant sows provides lactogenic immunity that is passively transferred to piglets via colostrum. Vaccines have been variably successful in preventing TGE. Oral immunization provides optimal stimulation of local immunity (secretory IgA) in the intestine. The practice of infecting sows with virulent TGEV at least 3 weeks prior to farrowing to induce an immune response by providing colostral immunity to piglets is complicated by the fact that this practice contaminates the environment with virulent TGEV that subsequently can spread to susceptible pigs.

HEMAGGLUTINATING ENCEPHALOMYELITIS VIRUS

Disease

Hemagglutinating encephalomyelitis virus (HEV) is the cause of vomiting and wasting disease (VWD) of young swine, a disease that is characterized by encephalomyelitis, vomiting, and wasting. VWD occurs in pigs less than 3 weeks of age, although older swine may exhibit milder signs of the disease. VWD in young piglets is characterized by anorexia, lethargy, vomiting, constipation, and signs of central nervous system disturbance (hyperesthesia, muscle tremors, paddling of the legs). Mortality is high, up to 100%; pigs also may develop chronic infections and eventually die from starvation or secondary infections.

Etiologic Agent

Physical, Chemical, and Antigenic Properties

HEV is antigenically related to bovine coronavirus. The virus hemagglutinates chicken, rat, mouse, hamster, and turkey erythrocytes.

Resistance to Physical and Chemical Agents

HEV is sensitive to lipid solvents, including sodium deoxycholate; it is also heat labile and relatively stable when frozen.

Infectivity for Other Species and Culture Systems

HEV grows in primary pig kidney (PK) or pig thyroid (PT) cells with formation of characteristic syncytia.

Host-Virus Relationship

Distribution, Reservoir, and Transmission

HEV was first isolated and associated with VWD in Canadian swine in 1958. Subsequently, the virus has been identified in swine in many areas of the world. Pigs are the only known host of HEV, and subclinical or inapparent carrier states likely exist. Nasal secretions contain virus and horizontal aerosol and direct animal contact are mechanisms of transmission.

Pathogenesis and Pathology

The pathogenesis of HEV infection has been characterized by experimental inoculation of colostrum-deprived day-old pigs. Following oronasal inoculation, primary viral replication occurs in the epithelial cells of the nasal mucosa, tonsils, lungs, and small intestine. Virus subsequently spreads along peripheral nerves to the central nervous system (CNS). Prior to disease expression, viral antigen is present in the trigeminal, inferior vagal, and superior cervical ganglia, solar and dorsal root ganglia of the lower thoracic region, and the intestinal nerve plexuses. Infection in the brain stem is initiated in the trigeminal and vagal sensory nuclei and subsequently spreads to other nuclei and the rostral portion of the brain stem. Later stages of the infection may be characterized by viral replication in the cerebrum, cerebellum, and spinal cord; virus is typically found in nervous plexuses of the stomach late in infection.

There are few characteristic gross lesions in natural HEV infections; a mild catarrhal rhinitis is sometimes evident in encephalomyelitis cases, and gastroenteritis is sometimes observed in VWD.

Lesions in the CNS are of a nonsuppurative encephalomyelitis characterized by perivascular cuffs of mononuclear cells, formation of glial nodes, neuronal degeneration, and meningitis. Respiratory tract lesions consist of focal or diffuse interstitial peribronchiolar pneumonia with cellular infiltrates composed of monocytes, lymphocytes, and neutrophils.

Host Response to Infection

Humoral immune responses may be quantitated by viral neutralization, hemagglutination inhibition (HI), and agar gel immunodiffusion (AGID). The clinical disease is self-limiting in pig populations and is due to the rapid development of maternal antibodies and their transfer by colostrum.

Laboratory Diagnosis

Diagnosis of HEV encephalomyelitis or VWD in piglets requires immunohistochemical staining of viral antigens in the tissues of affected pigs, virus isolation on primary PK or PT cells, or demonstration of a rising antibody titer by neutralization or hemagglutination inhibition assays.

Treatment and Control

No effective treatment has been described for HEV-induced encephalomyelitis or VWD. Clinical outbreaks are self-limiting. No vaccines are available and good animal husbandry practices are essential for the prevention and control of the disease.

Porcine Epidemic Diarrhea Virus

Coronavirus-like viruses have been isolated from swine with diarrhea, thus their designation as porcine epidemic diarrhea viruses (PEDV). These viruses are antigenically distinct from TGEV and HEV, and cause diarrhea, vomiting, and dehydration in inoculated swine. Pathogenesis studies indicate that PEDV replicates in both the small and large intestines, but lesions are confined to small intes-

tines. Affected pigs have small intestines that are distended with yellow fluid; the lesions are similar to those of TGE.

PEDV particles can be demonstrated in the feces of infected pigs by direct EM, and the virus can be propagated in some African green monkey (Vero) cell lines and not in others. Viral growth depends on the presence of trypsin in the cell culture medium. Generally, field strains of PEDV need to be adapted to grow in cell culture before they can be used as a routine diagnostic assay. A direct IF test and immunohistochemical technique applied on a section of small intestine are the most sensitive, rapid, and reliable methods of diagnosis of PEDV. A serologic diagnosis can be made by demonstration of PEDV antibodies by IF and ELISA.

Currently there is no vaccine for prevention of PEDV infection in pigs, thus control is dependent on management and husbandry practices.

Bovine Coronavirus

Disease

Bovine coronavirus (BCoV) is an enteric pathogen that is responsible for both neonatal diarrhea in newborn calves (1 to 3 weeks) and winter dysentery in adult cattle. The clinical disease in newborn calves is characterized by anorexia and a liquid, yellow diarrhea that persists for 4 to 5 days. Winter dysentery is a sporadic acute disease in adult cattle that is characterized by explosive bloody diarrhea accompanied by decreased milk production, depression, and anorexia. The BCoV strains that are isolated from diarrhea fluid or intestinal fluid are now identified as enteropathogenic bovine coronaviruses (EBCoV).

Other strains of bovine coronavirus more recently have been identified as respiratory pathogens in cattle; these strains of coronavirus have been isolated from the nasal secretions and lungs of cattle with severe shipping fever pneumonia, and are designated as respiratory bovine coronaviruses (RBCoV). Respiratory disease caused by RBCoV typically occurs in calves aged 6 to 9 months, and is characterized by fever, nasal discharge, and respiratory distress.

Etiologic Agent

Physical, Chemical, and Antigenic Properties

BCoV particles hemagglutinate erythrocytes from hamsters, mice, and rats. BCoV is antigenically related to coronaviruses of other species. Although there are significant phenotypic, antigenic and genetic differences between EBCoV and RBCoV strains, the precise relationship between enteric and respiratory strains of BCoV is uncertain.

Resistance to Physical and Chemical Agents

BCoV is acid stable (pH of 3.0), but is inactivated by lipid solvents, detergents, and high temperatures.

Infectivity for Other Species and Culture Systems

Infection with BCoV is limited to cattle (bovids), but the virus has been propagated in suckling mice, and following such passage, will infect suckling rats and hamsters by both intracerebral and subcutaneous routes. EBCoV has been propagated in Madin-Darby bovine kidney (MDBK), African green monkey kidney (Vero), bovine fetal thyroid (BFTy) cells, and bovine fetal brain (BFB) cells. Trypsin treatment of the latter two fetal cell cultures enhances plaque formation and cell fusion. Certain isolates are difficult to propagate in vitro and may require passage in the natural host. In contrast, only a human rectal tumor cell line (HRT-18) is permissive for initial isolation of RBCoV.

Host-Virus Relationship

Distribution, Reservoir, and Transmission

The distribution of BCoV is worldwide, and transmission of EBCoV is likely fecal-oral by ingestion of virus from contaminated feed, teats, and fomites. RBCoV is shed in respiratory tract secretions of infected animals, and thus is spread horizontally by aerosol.

Pathogenesis and Pathology

Diarrhea develops within 24 to 30 hours following oral infection of calves with EBCoV. Four hours after onset of diarrhea, viral antigen is detectable in the epithelium of the small intestine and colonic crypts. Initiation of infection is facilitated by proteolytic enzymes in the intestinal tract since trypsin treatment of coronaviruses in cell culture results in enhanced viral growth. The virus also infects the adjacent mesenteric lymph nodes. Destruction of the mature enterocytes that line the intestinal villi leads to atrophy and fusion of affected villi, with subsequent intestinal maldigestion and malabsorption, rapid loss of fluids and electrolytes, and, in severe cases, dehydration, acidosis, shock, and death.

RBCoV infection in calves causes interstitial pneumonia with congestion, hemorrhage, and edema of the interlobular septa of the lung. Histologically there is interstitial pneumonia with infiltration of mononuclear inflammatory cells and thickenings of alveolar septa.

Host Response to Infection

Both EBCoV and RBCoV infections in calves result in a humoral immune response that readily can be quantitated by viral neutralization, hemagglutination inhibition (HI), hemadsorption inhibition (HAI), and ELISA tests. Local immune responses play an important role because circulating antibodies do not protect calves from infection. Neonatal ingestion of colostral IgA protects the intestinal lumen against EBCoV infection for a limited period of time.

Laboratory Diagnosis

Diagnosis of EBCoV-induced neonatal diarrhea requires identification of the virus in fecal samples or intestinal sec-

tions. This can be achieved by viral isolation, electron microscopy, fluorescent antibody or immunohistochemical staining. Nasal swabs collected during the acute stage of upper respiratory tract disease are the specimens of choice for the diagnosis of RBCoV. Respiratory epithelial cells present in the nasal swabs are spotted onto slides for examination by direct fluorescent antibody test.

Treatment and Control

Treatment is dictated by the severity and type of disease. Electrolyte solutions can be administered for dehydration in calves with diarrhea caused by EBCoV infections, and antibiotic therapy may be used to control secondary infections. All BCoV infections are best controlled by good management practices to minimize exposure to these viruses, such as by avoiding introducing new (infected) animals into an intensive calving operation. It is difficult to control enteric disease by vaccination because very young calves are most affected, before they have the opportunity to respond to vaccination. The alternative is to immunize the dam to increase antibody levels in colostrum.

CANINE CORONAVIRUS

Disease

Canine coronavirus (CCoV) infection of dogs is highly contagious and generally causes inapparent or mild gastroenteritis. The virus occasionally is associated with more severe enteric disease, and puppies are most susceptible to CCoV-induced enteritis. Signs include anorexia, lethargy, vomiting, and diarrhea. More recently, CCoV also has been proposed to be an important cause of tracheobronchitis ("Kennel-cough") in dogs as well.

Etiologic Agent

Physical, Chemical, and Antigenic Properties

Canine coronavirus (CCoV) is antigenically related to other coronaviruses, including transmissible gastroenteritis virus, feline enteric coronavirus, and feline infectious peritonitis virus. Multiple antigenically and genetically distinct strains of CCoV have been recognized, including a novel respiratory coronavirus.

Resistance to Physical and Chemical Agents

Canine coronaviruses are inactivated by lipid solvents and are heat-labile. The viruses are acid-stable (pH of 3.0) and retain infectivity under cool conditions.

Infectivity for Other Species and Culture Systems

Canine coronavirus infects domestic and wild canine species; several primary and continuous canine cell cultures, including primary kidney and thymus; and continuous lines of thymus, embryo, synovium, and kidney (line A-72). The virus also infects feline kidney and embryo fibroblast cell lines.

Host-Virus Relationship

Distribution, Reservoir, and Transmission

Canine coronavirus was first isolated in 1971 from an epidemic of diarrhea in dogs in Germany. The virus since has been recognized virtually worldwide, including North America, Europe, Australia, and Asia.

Infected dogs excrete virus in their feces for 2 weeks or longer, and fecal contamination of the environment is the primary source for its transmission via fecal-oral infection.

Pathogenesis and Pathology

Following an incubation period of 1 to 4 days, the virus causes infection of intestinal epithelial cells that progressively passes through the gastrointestinal tract. Diarrhea occurs 1 to 7 days postinfection, virus being present in feces within 1 to 2 days following the appearance of clinical signs. Viral replication in the intestinal epithelium results in desquamation and shortening of the villi. The diarrhea associated with CCoV infection occurs as a consequence of intestinal maldigestion and malabsorption.

While CCoV infection is widespread, mortality is typically very low. Thus, necropsy of CCoV-infected dogs is unusual.

Host Response to Infection

Mucosal immunity appears to be protective because dogs orally infected with CCoV become immune and those immunized parenterally do not.

Laboratory Diagnosis

Virus or viral antigens can be visualized by electron microscopy (EM) or fluorescent antibody (FA) staining of feces or necropsy tissues. Antiserum, specific for CCoV, is commonly used to aggregate virus prior to negative staining for EM. Virus can be isolated from feces or intestinal tissue on cell culture. A reverse-transcriptase-polymerase chain reaction (RT-PCR) assay has been developed to detect CCoV in feces. Serum virus neutralization and ELISA tests for detection of CCoV antibodies have been developed.

Treatment and Control

Treatment of CCoV-associated gastroenteritis is limited to relief of dehydration and electrolyte loss in severe cases.

Inactivated and modified live virus vaccines are available for parental administration for protection against CCoV infection. However, their use is questionable due to the apparent importance of local immunity at the level of the intestinal mucosa.

FELINE INFECTIOUS PERITONITIS AND FELINE ENTERIC CORONAVIRUS

Disease

Feline infectious peritonitis (FIP) is a contagious, progressive and highly fatal disease of domestic and some wild feline species. The signs are highly variable and reflect the tissues affected by the disease, but persistent fever, weight loss, lethargy, dyspnea, and abdominal distension all are common clinical signs. The disease can occur in cats of all ages but is especially common in young and very old cats.

Two distinct forms of FIP are recognized: 1) an effusive (wet) and 2) a noneffusive (dry) form. The effusive form, which is two to three times as common as the dry form, is characterized by accumulation of protein-rich fluid (exudate) in the peritoneal cavity. The noneffusive form is characterized by formation of granulomas in internal organs, CNS, and eyes. Mortality rates are high.

FIP has an unusual and highly complex pathogenesis that involves the mutation of relatively nonpathogenic feline enteric coronavirus (FECoV) into FIP virus (FIPV) that replicates in macrophages to produce an immune-mediated disease in affected cats.

Etiologic Agent

Physical, Chemical, and Antigenic Properties

FIPV is antigenically related to other coronaviruses and is very closely related to feline enteric coronaviruses (FECoV) that do not produce FIP; it now is evident that FIPV arises by mutation of FECoV. The virulence to cats of strains of FIPV is directly correlated to their ability to grow in cultured feline macrophages. The virus is resistant to acid and trypsin but is readily inactivated by most disinfectants, including lipid solvents.

Infectivity for Other Species and Culture Systems

In addition to infecting domestic cats, FIPV has been associated with disease in wild *Felidae* such as lions, mountain lions, leopards, jaguar, lynx, caracal, sand cats, and pallas's cats. Young pigs can be experimentally infected with FIPV, resulting in development of lesions similar to those induced by TGEV. Suckling mice are susceptible to infection, with virus replicating in the brain. FIPV primarily replicates in macrophages, but virus can be propagated in vitro in feline organ cultures, cell lines, and mononuclear phagocytes.

Host-Virus Relationship

Distribution, Reservoir, and Transmission

FECoV and FIPV occur worldwide. Persistently infected cats serve as the virus reservoir, and the virus is readily spread horizontally between cats.

Pathogenesis and Pathology

The pathogenesis of FIP is complex, and much remains to be resolved. Initial FECoV infection rarely is characterized by obvious disease, but results in persistent, low-level infection of macrophages in many tissues. The development of clinical FIP is associated with increased viral replication, usually secondary to some immunosuppressive event that suppresses cellular immunity. Increased virus replication results in the emergence of viral variants (FIPV) that replicate with increasing efficiency in macrophages where they persist, safe from immune clearance. Antibody exacerbates the disease, which suggests that FIP is at least in part an immune-mediated disease. Virus-specific antibody actually facilitates uptake of FIPV by phagocytes in which pathogenic strains of the virus replicate.

Both "wet" and "dry" forms of FIP are characterized by the appearance of granulomas (or pyogranulomas) around blood vessels. It is proposed that deposition of complexes of FIPV and specific antibody (immune complexes) in the walls of blood vessels is responsible for the characteristic perivascular location of these lesions. These perivascular granulomas can occur in the bowel, kidneys, liver, lungs, CNS, eyes, and lymph nodes of affected cats, and are especially common on the serosa of the abdominal viscera in cats with the wet form of FIP.

Host Response to Infection

The basis of immunity to FIPV is poorly understood. Cats develop humoral and cellular immune responses soon after FECoV infection, and these responses hold the infection in check until some stress or concurrent infection causes immune suppression. Antibodies to FECoV cross react with FIPV, and these cause disease expression rather than protection; this antibody facilitates viral uptake by phagocytic cells where the virus effectively replicates, and viral antigens complexed with specific antibodies (and complement) contribute to immune-mediated vasculitis.

Laboratory Diagnosis

FIP is a common disease of cats that often can be diagnosed based upon the characteristic clinical signs coupled with serology and hematology. Fluid accumulation in the peritoneal or pleural cavity, as determined by paracentesis, in association with a positive serum or fluid antibody titer is indicative of effusive FIP. Noneffusive FIP is more difficult to diagnose and must be differentiated from other infectious, granulomatous, and neoplastic conditions. Histologic examination for pyogranulomatous or fibronecrotic inflammatory lesions and vasculitis, in association with serology, facilitates diagnosis. Reverse transcription-polymerase chain reaction (RT-PCR) techniques have been developed for identification of FIPV sequences in clinical material, as has immunohistochemical staining for FIPV.

Serologic diagnosis may be determined by viral neutralization, ELISA, or indirect fluorescent antibody techniques. A serum titer of greater than 1:3200 supports the diagnosis of FIP although cats with FIP can have low titers of virus-specific antibody and, conversely, unaffected cats may have high titers of antibody to the virus.

Treatment and Control

No treatment for FIP has been described that consistently reverses the disease process.

A temperature-sensitive mutant FIPV is available for vaccination of cats. Its use is not recommended in seropositive cats. Control of FIP is best realized by decontaminating (with quaternary ammonium compounds) infected premises, isolating serologically positive cats from those with no titer, and screening newly acquired cats for serum antibody.

MOUSE HEPATITIS VIRUS

Mouse hepatitis virus (MHV) is highly contagious and causes "explosive" outbreaks of disease in mouse colonies throughout the world. The severity of the clinical disease depends on several factors. These factors can be broadly distinguished into viral (strain, dose, and route of infection) and host factors (strain of mice, age, and immune status). There are many different strains of MHV, each with characteristic tissue tropism and associated clinical manifestations. Infection of mice with different virus strains can cause enteritis, hepatitis, nephritis, and demyelinating encephalomyelitis. For example, the A59 strain of MHV induces moderate to severe hepatitis, whereas the MHV-4 strain does not.

The enteropathogenic strains of MHV cause severe diarrhea in suckling mice, with nearly 100% mortality. The intestines are distended and filled with yellowish fluid. Older mice develop jaundice, lose weight, and cease breeding. Characteristic histological lesions include blunted (club-shaped) intestinal villi with extensive syncytium formation. All mice develop acute hepatitis with focal hepatocellular necrosis and inflammatory cell infiltration. Other strains of MHV are the cause of respiratory and central nervous system (CNS) disease in mouse colonies. CNS infection with neurotropic strains of MHV causes paralysis due to demyelination (used as a model of chronic demyelinating diseases of humans, such as multiple sclerosis).

MHV infection in mouse colonies is diagnosed with the detection of characteristic gross and histological lesions in the intestines and liver, although some strains of MHV are highly attenuated and cause little pathology or disease. The diagnosis is confirmed by immunohistochemistry and serology using an enzyme immunoassay. Virus can be isolated using any of several mouse cell lines.

The virus persists following epidemics in persistently infected mice that continually infect susceptible mice that are introduced into the colony. Control is achieved by breaking this cycle of transmission through the use of strict quarantine measures.

Sialodacryadenitis Virus (Rat Coronavirus)

Sialodacryadenitis virus is the etiologic agent of sialodacryadenitis in laboratory rats. It is a severe, self-limiting inflammatory disease of the salivary and nasolacrimal glands of rats. The virus is highly contagious and causes high morbidity and low mortality in infected colonies. Clinical signs of infection include swelling of the face and neck, excessive lacrimation and blinking, squinting, and exophthalmia. Lesions in the lacrimal duct may lead to corneal drying. Lesions typically resolve within 2 weeks. The virus is transmitted by aerosol, direct contact, and by fomites.

Equine Coronavirus

Coronavirus-like virions have been isolated from both mature horses and foals experiencing enteritis. The viruses found in horses were antigenically distinct from group 1 (e.g., TGEV and HCV 229E) and group 3 (e.g., IBV and TCoV) coronaviruses, but had a close antigenic and/or genetic relationship with group 2 coronaviruses (e.g., BCoV). However, the pathogenicity of these equine coronaviruses, as well as their role in enteric disease has not been examined in detail.

Avian Infectious Bronchitis Virus

Disease

Avian infectious bronchitis virus (IBV) causes respiratory disease in chicks 10 days to 4 weeks of age; however, all ages, sexes, and breeds are susceptible to infection, although mortality is low in birds greater than 6 weeks of age. The virus also causes disease of the reproductive tract and kidneys. The respiratory disease is characterized by respiratory distress, rales, coughing, nasal discharge, and depression. The clinical course lasts 6 to 18 days. Morbidity is 100% and mortality may exceed 25%. Chicks with no maternal antibody may experience permanent oviduct damage and fail to lay eggs when mature. Infection of laying flocks results in a drop of egg production and hatchability. Pullets in good condition return to normal production within a few weeks.

IBV-associated renal disease is dependent upon viral strain. Many viral strains with an affinity for the kidneys cause only mild or inapparent respiratory signs, but can cause substantial mortality in susceptible birds.

Etiologic Agent

Physical, Chemical, and Antigenic Properties

IBV is antigenically distinct from other coronaviruses, and multiple distinct virus strains have been identified and grouped by serologic techniques, polypeptide patterns in polyacrylamide gel electrophoresis (PAGE), oligonucleotide fingerprinting, and nucleotide sequencing. Strain-specific epitopes for viral neutralization and hemagglutination have been identified on the S1 protein with monoclonal antibodies.

Resistance to Physical and Chemical Agents

Most strains of IBV are inactivated within 15 minutes at 56°C. The virus is quite stable at cold temperatures. Stability at acidic pH is strain-variable; with some strains surviving at pH 3 for 3 hours at 4°C. Lipid solvents inactivate the virus.

Infectivity for Other Species and Culture Systems

The chicken is the only known natural host of IBV. However, quail and gulls have been experimentally infected. Suckling mice can be infected by intracerebral inoculation. The virus can be cultivated in developing avian embryos, cell cultures, and organ cultures. Turkey embryos have also been successfully infected with IBV, but less efficiently.

IBV can be grown in chick embryo cells (kidney, lung, and liver), embryonic turkey kidney cells, and monkey kidney (Vero) cells. Organ cultures have been used to propagate IBV including tracheal and oviduct cultures.

Host-Virus Relationship

Distribution, Reservoir, and Transmission

IBV has a worldwide distribution. The virus likely persists in persistently infected birds and/or continuous cycles of transmission. Virus has been recovered for up to 49 days from infected chickens held in isolation and for even longer periods in those held under natural conditions.

Viral transmission occurs by inhalation, the respiratory tract being the primary site of infection. Virus is shed in respiratory and fecal materials, with subsequent spread by contaminated fomites and aerosol.

Pathogenesis and Pathology

The incubation period of IBV infection is 18 to 36 hours. Virus gains entry via the respiratory tract and the respiratory form of IBV results in tracheitis and bronchitis. Mortality may be as high as 25% in young chicks. Strains exhibiting an affinity for the kidneys damage the renal tubules, resulting in renal failure.

Infection produces primarily a serous, catarrhal, or caseous exudate in the trachea, nasal passages, and sinuses. The air sacs may contain a caseous exudate, and small foci of bronchopneumonia may be apparent. Young chicks may experience a more severe infection, with lesions developing in the oviduct. Chickens infected with nephrotropic viral strains develop renal tubular necrosis characterized by swollen and pale kidneys with accumulation of uric acid crystals causing distension of the tubules and ureters.

Microscopic lesions of the respiratory tract include cellular infiltration, mucosal edema, vascular congestion, and hemorrhage.

Host Response to Infection

IBV elicits humoral and cellular immune responses. Humoral responses can be measured by viral neutralization and hemagglutination inhibition (HI) tests. Titers of passively transferred maternal antibody decrease to negligible levels within 4 weeks of hatching.

Chickens recovered from natural infection are resistant to homologous viral challenge. The duration of immunity is variable and difficult to determine due to the multiplicity of IBV strains. Passive transfer of maternal antibody does not confer total protection to the chick but reduces disease severity and mortality.

Local tracheal immunity appears to play a major role in resistance to IBV. The relative importance of humoral versus cellular immunity is unclear. The observation that chickens may be protected in the absence of demonstrable antibody would suggest an important role for cell-mediated immunity.

Laboratory Diagnosis

Diagnosis of infectious bronchitis may be based upon direct visualization of viral antigen in tracheal smears using immunohistochemical or fluorescent antibody staining, viral isolation, or serology. Infectious bronchitis must be differentiated from other acute respiratory diseases of birds, such as Newcastle disease, laryngotracheitis, and infectious coryza.

Viral isolation is conducted by inoculation of tracheal or respiratory exudates into the chorioallantoic sac of 10- to 11-day-old embryonated chicken eggs (ECE). Serial passage in ECEs may be required before embryo dwarfing or mortality occurs.

Serologic diagnosis of IBV infection requires paired serum samples and the use of IBV-specific viral neutralization, hemagglutination inhibition (HI), agar gel immunodiffusion (AGID), or ELISA assays.

Treatment and Control

No specific treatment for infectious bronchitis is available. Proper husbandry practices that reduce environmental stress are logical. Control of infectious bronchitis may be approached through management procedures and vaccination. Spread of the virus may be reduced by strict isolation of an affected flock, and restocking with day-old chicks reared in isolation. Attenuated and inactivated vaccines have been developed for the control of IB. Inactivated vaccines induce neutralizing antibodies, but their efficacy has been questioned. Live viral vaccines attenuated by serial passage in embryonated chicken eggs have reduced pathogenicity but also decreased immunogenicity. Vaccines may be administered via aerosol or in drinking water. High passage vaccine viruses apparently

have a reduced invasiveness and generally require aerosol administration.

The multiplicity of IBV strains and serotypes has made it difficult to develop efficacious vaccines. No single strain has been identified as capable of inducing more than limited protection to heterologous viruses. Multivalent vaccines are available, but in certain instances prolonged reactions to vaccination and some interference between vaccine strains have been reported.

TURKEY CORONAVIRUS

Disease

Turkey coronavirus (TCoV) is the causative agent of coronavirus enteritis (CE) of turkeys. It is an acute and highly contagious disease of turkeys of all ages. Synonyms of the disease include bluecomb disease, mud fever, transmissible enteritis, and infectious enteritis. It is of major economic importance to the turkey industry and affects turkeys of all ages. The disease affects primarily the alimentary tract and is characterized by depression, subnormal body temperature, anorexia, inappetence, loss of body weight, and wet droppings. Darkening of the head and skin and tucking of the skin over the crop are characteristics of infected growing turkeys. A rapid drop in egg production with formation of chalky eggshells occurs in producing breeder hens. Morbidity is essentially 100%, and mortality varies with age and environmental conditions.

Etiologic Agent

Physical, Chemical, and Antigenic Properties

TCoV is inactivated by lipid solvents and detergents, but is resistant to acidic pH (pH of 3 at 20°C for 30 minutes). The virus is resistant to 50°C for 1 hr. TCoV is apparently unrelated antigenically to other coronaviruses. TCoV agglutinates rabbit and guinea pig erythrocytes, but not those from cattle, horse, sheep, mouse, goose, monkey, or chickens.

Infectivity for Other Species and Culture Systems

TCoV infection is confined to turkeys. Laboratory propagation of the virus has been limited to turkey and chicken embryos, and attempts to grow TCoV in cell cultures have been unsuccessful.

Host-Virus Relationship

Distribution, Reservoir, and Transmission

CE has been described in North America and Australia. The virus persists in turkeys for life following recovery from the disease. It is stable in frozen feces and survives throughout the winter months in infected droppings, thus transmission of TCoV principally is fecal-oral from the infected feces of carrier birds. Introduction of virus onto a premise may occur via carrier turkeys, feces-contaminated fomites such as personnel and equipment, and possibly mechanical transmission by free-flying birds.

Pathogenesis and Pathology

The incubation period of CE varies from 1 to 5 days. Gross lesions are largely confined to the intestinal tract, with petechial hemorrhages sometimes apparent on the serosal surface. Lesions are most distinct in the jejunum but may also occur in the duodenum, ileum, and cecum. Gas and fluid typically distend the small intestine and ceca. The breast muscles are typically dehydrated and the carcass generally appears emaciated.

Microscopic lesions include destruction of enterocytes lining the intestinal villi, leading to their shortening, loss of microvilli, and mononuclear cell infiltration of the lamina propria of the affected bowel.

Host Response to Infection

Turkeys respond to TCoV infection with humoral and cellular immune responses. Serum antibodies (IgM, IgA, and IgG) develop following infection but by 21 days only IgG is present. Local IgA antibody appears in intestinal secretions and bile for at least 6 months. Passive transfer of maternal immunity has not been observed and administration of antiserum to young poults does not afford protection.

Laboratory Diagnosis

Definitive diagnosis of CE requires identification of viral antigen in intestinal tissue sections by immunohistochemical staining, viral isolation, or demonstration of serum antibody. Virus may be isolated by inoculation of embryonated turkey eggs or young poults and its presence confirmed by fluorescent antibody staining of infected tissues. Serologic diagnosis can be conducted on paired serum samples by viral neutralization or indirect FA tests.

Treatment and Control

No specific treatment is effective in reducing morbidity of CE, although various treatments may be used to prevent other intestinal infections. TCoV vaccines are not available, but prevention of infection is possible. The disease has been eliminated in some areas by depopulation and decontamination of affected premises. An alternative to viral elimination is exposing poults (5 to 6 weeks of age) to recovered carrier birds under ideal environmental conditions for the purpose of inducing protective immunity. Such a program is recommended only on farms with continued problems and when all other methods of control have failed.

TOROVIRUS

Toroviruses resemble coronaviruses in their genome organization and replication strategy but differ in virion morphology. Toroviruses are pleomorphic and measure 120–140 nm in diameter. Spherical, oval elongated, and kidney-shaped particles have all been observed. Toroviruses are enveloped with a tubular nucleocapsid of helical symmetry. The nucleocapsid forms a doughnut-shaped structure, and the envelope contains a large number of spikes that resemble the peplomeres of coronaviruses. *Torovirus* particles consist of at least four structural proteins: nucleocapsid protein (N), unglycosylated membrane protein (M), spike glycoprotein (S), and hemeagglutinin-esterase protein (HE). The *Torovirus* genome consists of a polyadenylated, positive-sense, linear molecule of ssRNA, which is estimated to be 20 to 30 kb in length. The members of this genus *Torovirus* include equine torovirus (ETV; formally named Beren virus), bovine torovirus (BoTV; originally named Breda virus), porcine torovirus (PoTV) and human torovirus (HuTV). Toroviruses have also been detected by electron microscopy in the feces of dogs and cats.

Toroviruses infect the epithelial cells of the small and large intestine extending from mid-jejunum to colon. ETV was originally isolated from the rectal swab of a horse with diarrhea. BoTV has been identified as a pathogen causing gastroenteritis and diarrhea in calves and possibly pneumonia in older cattle. Antibodies to BoTV have been demonstrated in several countries around the world. PoTV was originally isolated from the feces of piglets that did not show any signs of enteritis or diarrhea, but it since has been isolated from pigs with diarrhea at the time of weaning. Much remains to be determined regarding the pathogenic importance of *Torovirus* infections of animals.

ARTERIVIRUS

The members of family *Arteriviridae*, genus *Arterivirus*, include equine arteritis virus (EAV), porcine reproductive and respiratory syndrome virus (PRRSV), lactate dehydrogenase-elevating virus (LDV), and simian hemorrhagic fever virus (SHFV). Three of these viruses were first discovered and characterized long ago (EAV-1953, LDV-1960, and SHFV-1964), whereas PRRSV was first isolated in North America in 1987 and in Europe in 1990. The arteriviruses are each antigenically distinct, but LDV and PRRSV are most closely related to each other. There are two genetically distinct subspecies of PRRSV (European, Type I; American, Type II). The arteriviruses are highly species-specific, but share many biological and molecular properties, including their virion morphologies, unique properties of their structural proteins, and the ability to establish persistent infection. EAV and PRRSV are of veterinary significance and will be discussed in detail.

Etiologic Agent (EAV, PRRSV, LDV, and SHFV)

Physical, Chemical, and Antigenic Properties

Arterivirus virions are spherical, 45 to 60 nm in diameter and consist of an isometric (probably icosahedral) nucleocapsid of 25 to 35 nm in diameter, surrounded by a lipid envelope. The envelope includes 12–15 nm diameter ring-like structures. The large spikes that are typical of coronaviruses are absent from the *Arterivirus* envelope. The *Arterivirus* genome is a linear, positive-sense, ssRNA molecule of 12.7 to 15.7 kb. The buoyant density of arteriviruses ranges from 1.13–1.17 g/cm³ in sucrose, whereas the sedimentation coefficient is 214S to 230S.

Arterivirus particles consist of a nucleocapsid protein (N) and six envelope proteins (E, GP2, GP3, GP4, GP5, M). However, three additional envelope proteins (GP2, GP4b, and GP7) have been reported for SHFV. The GP5 (glycosylated) and M (unglycosylated) are the major envelope proteins of the arteriviruses and they form a disulfide-linked heterodimer in the mature virus particles. In addition, the *Arterivirus* envelope contains a heterotrimer of three minor membrane glycoproteins (GP2, GP3, and GP4) and an unglycosylated envelope protein (E). The GP5 protein contains the known neutralization determinants of EAV, PRRSV, and LDV, and monoclonal antibodies (MAbs) specific to the GP4 of PRRSV also neutralize the virus indicating that some of the neutralization epitopes are also localized in this protein.

Resistance to Physical and Chemical Agents

Both EAV and PRRSV are readily inactivated by lipid solvents (ether and chloroform) and by common disinfectants and detergents. EAV survives 75 days at 4°C, between 2–3 days at 37°C, and 20 to 30 minutes at 56°C. Tissue culture fluid or organ samples containing EAV can be stored at −70°C for years without significant loss of the infectivity. PRRSV infectivity is lost within 1 week at 4°C, but is stable for a long time (months to years) when frozen −70°C or −20°C. PRRSV is rapidly inactivated by low and high pH (below 6 and above 7.5). LDV is not stable at −20°C and rapidly loses its infectivity.

Infectivity for Other Species and Culture Systems

EAV can infect horses, donkeys, mules, and zebras, and replicates in primary cultures of equine pulmonary artery endothelial, horse kidney, rabbit kidney, and hamster kidney cells. It also replicates in cell lines such as BHK-21, RK-13, African green monkey kidney cells (Vero), rhesus monkey kidney (LLC-MK2), hamster lung (HmLu), SV-40 transformed equine ovary, and canine hepatitis virus-transformed hamster tumor cells (HS and HT-7). PRRSV primarily infects pigs, but recently, chickens and ducks that were exposed to PRRSV in drinking water shed the virus in their feces, suggesting that they are susceptible to infection with the virus. North American PRRSV (Type II) isolates replicate in porcine alveolar macrophages (PAM), CRL-11171, and African green monkey cell line (MA-104), and derivatives thereof (CL2621 or MARC-145). Most, if not all, European PRRSV (Type I) isolates replicate best or exclusively in PAMs. However, European PRRSV isolates have been adapted to grow in CL2621 cell lines. Vaccine strains of PRRSV replicate much more efficiently (100 to 1000 times) in derivatives of monkey kidney cell lines than in PAMs. LDV primarily replicates in primary cultures of mouse macrophages from 1- to 2-week-old mice and other mouse macrophage cell lines, but not other cell lines.

SHFV infects and replicates in primary cultures of peritoneal macrophages from rhesus and patas monkeys and also replicates in the MA-104 cell line.

EQUINE ARTERITIS VIRUS

Disease

EAV is the causative agent of equine viral arteritis (EVA) in horses, a respiratory and reproductive disease that occurs throughout the world. There is only one serotype of EAV; however, field strains differ in their virulence and neutralization phenotype. The clinical signs displayed by EAV-infected horses depend on a variety of factors, including the age and physical condition of the horse(s), challenge dose and route of infection, strain of virus, and environmental conditions. The vast majority of EAV infections are inapparent (or subclinical), but acutely infected animals may develop a wide range of clinical signs, including pyrexia, depression, anorexia, dependent edema of (scrotum, ventral trunk, and limbs), stiffness of gait, conjunctivitis, lacrimation and swelling around the eyes (periorbital and supraorbital edema), respiratory distress, urticaria, and leukopenia. The incubation period of 3 to 14 days (usually 6 to 8 days following venereal exposure) is followed by pyrexia of up to 41°C that may persist for 2 to 9 days. The virus causes abortion in pregnant mares, and abortion rates during natural outbreaks of EVA can vary from 10 to 60% of infected mares. EAV-induced abortions can occur at any time between 3 and 10 months of gestation. EAV infection of neonatal foals can cause a severe fulminating interstitial pneumonia, and of older foals a progressive pneumoenteric syndrome. A high proportion of acutely infected stallions (30 to 60%) become persistently infected and shed the virus in semen; however, there is no evidence of any analogous persistent infection of mares, geldings, or foals. The virus persists in the ampula of the male reproductive tract and the establishment and maintenance of the carrier state in stallions is testosterone-dependent.

Host-Virus Relationship

Distribution, Reservoir, and Transmission

The EAV is distributed throughout the world, although the seroprevalence of EAV infection varies between countries and horses of different breeds and age in the same country. In the United States, some 70 to 90% of adult Standardbred horses are seropositive to EAV, as compared to only 1–3% of the Thoroughbred population. Similarly, a high percentage of European warmblood horses are seropositive to EAV. Seroprevalence to EAV increases with age, indicating that horses may be repeatedly exposed to the virus as they age. Persistently infected carrier stallions function as the natural reservoir of EAV and disseminate the virus to susceptible mares at breeding. The two principal modes of EAV transmission are horizontal transmission by aerosolization of infectious respiratory tract secretions from acutely infected horses and venereal transmission during natural or artificial insemination with infective semen from persistently infected stallions. EAV also can be transmitted through indirect contact with fomites or personnel. Congenital infection results from transplacental transmission (vertical transmission) of virus when pregnant mares are infected late in gestation.

Pathogenesis and Pathology

Most information on the pathogenesis of EAV infection is derived from experimental studies in horses inoculated intranasally with a highly virulent strain of EAV. Initial multiplication of virus takes place in the alveolar macrophages in the lung, and the virus soon appears in the regional lymph nodes, especially the bronchial nodes. Within 3 days the virus is present in virtually all organs and tissues (viremia), where it replicates in macrophages and endothelial cells.

EAV infection of adult horses is almost never fatal. EAV infection of pregnant mares can result in the abortion of fetuses, which are usually partially autolyzed at the time of expulsion. Aborted fetus may exhibit interlobular pulmonary edema, pleural and pericardial effusion, and petechial and ecchymotic hemorrhages on the serosal and mucosal surfaces of the small intestine. Neonatal foals occasionally develop a very severe, acute interstitial pneumonia.

The characteristic histologic feature of EVA is a severe necrotizing panvasculitis of small vessels. Affected muscular arteries show foci of intimal, subintimal, and medial necrosis, with edema and infiltration of lymphocytes and neutrophils. Prominent vascular lesions are also seen in the placenta, brain, liver, and spleen of the aborted fetuses. Lungs of affected neonatal foals have severe interstitial pneumonia.

Host Response to Infection

Animals that recover from EAV infection or those that are vaccinated with either inactivated or attenuated strains of EAV develop neutralizing antibodies and are resistant to subsequent challenge with EAV. Neutralizing antibodies are detected within 1 to 2 weeks following exposure to the virus, reach maximum titers between 2 to 4 months, and persist for 3 years or more. With the exception of persistently infected stallions, EAV is eliminated from the tissues of infected horses by 28 days after the exposure. Foals born to immune mares are protected against clinical EVA by passive transfer of neutralizing antibodies in colostrum. Neutralizing antibodies appear a few hours after colostrum feeding, peak at 1 week of age, and gradually decline to extinction between 2 to 6 months of age.

Laboratory Diagnosis

EVA is uncommon in horses, and other, more important viral respiratory infections clinically resemble EVA. Conformation of a diagnosis of EVA currently is based on virus isolation and/or serological demonstration of raising neutralizing antibody titers (fourfold or greater) in paired serum samples taken at a 21- to 28-day interval. EAV can be isolated from nasal swabs or anticoagulated blood collected from adult horses with signs of EVA, or the tissues (including placenta) of aborted equine fetuses. Carrier stallions are first identified by serology because they always are seropositive, and persistent infection is confirmed by virus isolation from semen in cell culture, by test-breeding using seronegative mares (and monitoring these for seroconversion to EAV after breeding), or by RT-PCR to identify viral nucleic acid in semen. Histopathologic examination coupled with immunohistochemical staining also is useful for diagnosis of abortion in particular, as are RT-PCR assays.

Treatment and Control

There is no specific treatment for horses infected with EAV. Currently there are no means available of eliminating the carrier state in stallions persistently infected with EAV other than castration. Modified live attenuated and killed virus vaccines are available for prevention of EAV infection in horses. Colts should be vaccinated with attenuated vaccines after they lose colostral immunity but before puberty.

Outbreaks of EVA can be prevented by the identification of persistently infected stallions and the institution of management practices to prevent the introduction of EAV-infected horses. Carrier stallions should be kept physically isolated and bred only to mares that are seropositive from previous natural exposure or vaccination. Mares should be kept isolated from other seronegative horses after being bred by carrier stallions.

PORCINE REPRODUCTIVE AND RESPIRATORY SYNDROME VIRUS

Disease

The European (Type I; prototype Leylystad virus [LV]) and American (Type II; prototype VR-2332 virus) isolates of PRRSV represent genetically and antigenically distinct groups of the same virus. Both viruses are associated with outbreaks of similar reproductive and respiratory disease in pigs, despite the fact that there is only 55 to 70% nucleotide identity in the various genes of the two types. Clinical signs of porcine reproductive and respiratory syndrome (PRRS) are extremely variable and influenced by strain of virus, immune status of the herd, and management practices. Low-virulence strains of PRRSV may result in widespread infection of swine with minimal occurrence of disease, whereas highly virulent strains can cause severe clinical disease in susceptible herds. All ages of pigs are susceptible to infection with PRRSV in immunologically naive herds. Acute PRRSV infection of susceptible pigs is characterized by anorexia, fever (39° to 41°C), dyspnea, and lethargy. Affected swine are lymphopenic, and exhibit transient cutaneous hyperemia or cyanosis of extremities that is most visible on the ears, snouts, mammary glands, and vulvas. Transplacental transmission of PRRSV occurs most efficiently in the third trimester of pregnancy (usually after 100 days of gestation), and the abortion rate in affected sows can range from 10 to 50%. Sow mortality is considerably lower. Affected liters contain a variable mixture of normal pigs, weak small pigs, stillborn pigs, and partially or completely mummified fetuses (so-called *SMEDI*: stillbirth, mummification, embryonic death, and infertility). Infected sows also can exhibit nervous signs such as ataxia and circling. PRRSV infected boars may continue to shed virus in their semen for prolonged periods of time.

Host-Virus Relationship

Distribution, Reservoir, and Transmission

Despite its very recent recognition, PRRSV appears to be endemic in virtually all swine-producing countries of the world. The original source of the virus and the circumstances under which it was introduced into the domestic swine population are unknown. Transmission of PRRSV usually occurs by close contact between infected and uninfected animals. Swine are susceptible to PRRSV by a number of routes of exposure, including oral, intranasal, vaginal, intramuscular, and intraperitoneal. PRRSV is shed in respiratory tract secretions, saliva, semen, mammary secretions, urine, and feces of infected animals. Susceptible pigs are naturally infected by inhalation of infectious aerosols or ingestion of PRRSV-contaminated food. Congenital infection results from transplacental transmission (vertical transmission) of virus. Transmission of PRRSV to females has been demonstrated during breeding with semen from persistently infected carrier boars. PRRSV also can be transmitted through indirect contact with fomites or personnel, and some pigs harbor the virus in their tonsils long after the virus is cleared from other tissues.

Pathogenesis and Pathology

PRRSV replicates in macrophages and dendritic cells, especially those in the lungs and lymphoid tissues. Viremia occurs soon after infection, and can last for 1 to 2 weeks in mature animals and 8 weeks in young pigs. Gross lesions are usually observed in only a few organ systems (e.g., respiratory and lymphoid). Microscopic lesions of PRRS include diffuse interstitial pneumonia, myocarditis, vasculitis, and encephalitis. Lymphoid tissues exhibit lymphoid hyperplasia and follicular necrosis with mixed inflammatory cell infiltration. Clinical outbreaks of PRRSV can be complicated by bacterial pneumonia, septicemia, or enteritis.

Host Response to Infection

Pigs infected with PRRSV mount an immune response and virus-specific antibodies have been identified using a variety of assays. The antibody response is detected by the appearance of virus-specific IgM by 7 days and specific IgG by 14 days after infection. Antibody titers peak by 5 to 6 weeks postinfection and persist for the life of commercial feeder pigs. However, neutralizing antibodies appear slowly, usually between 4–5 weeks postinfection, and peak at about 10 weeks postinfection. Piglets born to immune sows acquire anti-PRRSV antibodies by ingestion of colostrum. The cell-mediated immune response to PRRSV has not been well characterized; however, T lymphocyte proliferation responses in pigs infected with PRRSV have been demonstrated between 4 and 12 weeks after infection.

Laboratory Diagnosis

Diagnosis of PRRSV may be complicated by the fact that many infections are inapparent, but PRRS should be considered when there are clinical signs of respiratory disease associated with reproductive failure in a herd. PRRSV antibodies are detected by using a variety of serological assays, including ELISA, immunofluorescence assay (IFA), immunoperoxidase monolayer assay (IPMA), and serum virus neutralization assay (SVN). Serological examination of acute and convalescent pig sera may provide evidence of seroconversion. Virus isolation from clinical specimens such as bronchioalveolar lavage fluid, lung, lymph node, buffy coat, and serum can be done in PAMs, MA104 and its derivatives, and CRL-11171 cell lines, although different strains or isolates of PRRSV vary in their ability to replicate in different cell types. Various PCR assays have been developed to detect viral nucleic acid in blood, semen, and other clinical specimens.

Treatment and Control

There is no effective treatment for PRRSV infection in pigs. Both modified live attenuated (MLV) and killed vaccines are available for prevention of PRRSV infection. They can be used to immunize sows or weanling piglets; however, there is considerable variation in the relative safety and efficacy of MLV vaccines. MLV vaccines induce long-lasting protection as compared to killed vaccines, but do not completely prevent reinfection with wild-type virus and subsequent virus transmission. Furthermore, there have been reports of under-attenuation and reversion of MLV vaccine viruses to a more virulent type that can be spread from vaccinated to unvaccinated swine. Control programs have been developed to eradicate the virus from infected herds.

LACTATE DEHYDROGENASE-ELEVATING VIRUS

Lactate dehydrogenase-elevating virus (LDV) can cause a lifelong persistent infection in inbred laboratory strains of mice, although infection of laboratory mice now is very uncommon. The virus has also been isolated from wild house mice (*Mus musculus domesticus*) in several countries, although the worldwide incidence is not known. Attempts to infect *Peromyscus* mice, rats, guinea pigs, and rabbits with LDV have been unsuccessful. LDV replicates in permissive macrophages in the spleen, lymph nodes, thymus, and liver of infected mice. The subpopulation of macrophages that are permissive to LDV infection also are responsible for the normal clearance of the lactate dehydrogenase (LDH) enzyme from circulation. The continuous destruction of these macrophages by LDV leads to elevated levels of LDH in blood, thus the name of the virus. The persistent infection that characterizes LDV infection of mice is maintained by replication of LDV in new permissive macrophages that are continuously regenerated from apparently nonpermissive precursor cells. Other than the elevated LDH level and subtle changes in host immunity, persistent LDV infection of mice generally is asymptomatic. However, infection of mice of certain strains (C58, AKR, PL/J, and C3H/FgBoy) by neurovirulent strains of LDV can lead to fatal age-dependent poliomyelitis.

Anti-LDV antibodies begin to appear 4 to 5 days postinfection and peak at 3 to 4 weeks. Antibodies that neutralize LDV appear in mice only after 4 weeks postinfection, and these antibodies are directed against the GP5 protein of the virus. The replication of LDV in macrophages allows it to avoid host defense mechanisms, although the precise mechanism of immune evasion and persistent infection is still unclear.

LDV transmission between mice is relatively inefficient, despite the lifelong viremia that occurs in infected mice and the secretion of the virus in urine, feces, and saliva. LDV transmission from mother to offspring through the placenta or via breast milk is highly efficient if the mother is immunologically naive. However, transmission via these routes from persistently infected mothers is rare because anti-LDV antibodies block transplacental transmission of the virus and its release into milk. Generally horizontal transmission of LDV between mice is restricted by mucosal barriers, although horizontal transmission of LDV does occur among laboratory mice that fight and bite one another. The sexual transmission of LDV has not been demonstrated.

LDV can only be quantitated by an end-point dilution assay in mice, which is based on the increase in plasma LDH activity that accompanies LDV infection in mice. The presence of LDV in mice or in other materials is readily detected by injecting plasma, tissue homogenates, or other materials (e.g., transplantable mouse tumors) into groups of two to three mice and assaying their plasma LDH activity 4 to 5 days later. Transplantable mouse tumors can be readily freed of LDV by a 3-week in vitro propagation or passage in a host animal other than mice.

Simian Hemorrhagic Fever Virus

Simian hemorrhagic fever (SHF) virus (SHFV) was first isolated from rhesus macaques suffering from hemorrhagic fever, in primate research centers in both the former Soviet Union and the United States. African monkeys of three genera (African green monkey [*Ceropithecus aethiops*],

patas [*Erythrocebus patas*], and baboon [*Papio anuibus*]) are persistently infected in the wild with the SHFV, and they do not exhibit any clinical signs of disease. Accidental transmission of SHFV from African monkeys to any of three species of Asian macaque monkeys (*Macaca mulatta, Macaca arctoides, and Macaca fascicularis*) results in a generally fatal hemorrhagic fever. Clinical signs of SHF in macaques include anorexia, fever, cyanosis, skin petechia, and hemorrhages, nosebleeds, facial edema, bloody diarrhea, dehydration, adipsia, and proteinuria. Death generally occurs 5 to 25 days after the onset of clinical signs, and mortality approaches 100%. The high lethality observed in macaque monkeys may be due to an extreme sensitivity of their macrophages to cytocidal infection by SHFV. Infection of captive patas monkeys with SHFV from persistently infected patas monkeys results in persistent infection without any clinical signs. However, infection of captive patas monkeys with SHFV from diseased macaques results in transient mild disease, indicating selection of more virulent variants during epizootics in macaque monkeys. The humoral immune response against SHFV varies with the species of monkey and the infecting virus strain. SHFV induces neutralizing antibodies in patas monkeys 7 days after experimental infection. However, only low levels of anti-SHFV antibodies are found in many persistently infected patas monkeys.

The prevalence and incidence of SHFV infection among African monkeys in endemic areas of Africa is not known, but the incidence of persistent subclinical infections in wild patas monkeys appears to be high. The method of transmission of SHFV among African monkeys in the wild is unclear. Infection most likely occurs through wounds and biting, but sexual transmission has not been ruled out. SHFV is not transmitted transplacentally from persistently infected mothers to their offspring. Several epizootics of SHF in captive macaque colonies originated from accidental mechanical transmission of SHFV from asymptomatic, persistently infected African monkeys. Once illness becomes apparent in the macaque colony, the SHFV spreads rapidly throughout the colony, most likely by direct contact and aerosols.

Persistently infected monkeys can be identified by the presence of SHFV that replicates in primary cultures of peritoneal macrophages from rhesus and patas monkeys. The most sensitive method for detection of persistent infection is experimental inoculation of macaque monkeys, and currently there are no molecular diagnostic assays for detection of SHFV. Indirect immunofluorescent assay (IFA), ELISA, and neutralization assays are available for serological diagnosis of SHFV infection. However, these assays are not reliable because of the low level of anti-SHFV antibodies found in many persistently infected monkeys. Accidental transmission of SHFV from persistently infected African monkeys to macaque monkeys in primate centers can be minimized by strict adherence to proper sanitary conditions and animal care practices.

63 *Reoviridae*

N. James MacLachlan   Jeffrey L. Stott

Viruses in the *Reoviridae* family infect a wide range of species, including mammals, fish and shellfish, insects, and plants. All of the viruses in this family have a segmented genome of double-stranded RNA (dsRNA), and the number of individual genome segments varies between genera. The family is grouped into nine genera: *Orthoreovirus, Orbivirus, Rotavirus, Aquareovirus, Coltivirus, Oryzavirus, Cypovirus, Phytoreovirus,* and *Fijivirus*. The latter four genera are confined to insects, plants, or both. The *Coltivirus* genus includes Colorado tick fever virus, which is an insect-transmitted human pathogen. Orthoreoviruses (Fig 63.1) and rotaviruses (Fig 63.2) infect a wide variety of vertebrate species. The host range of orbiviruses includes both vertebrates and invertebrates, with bluetongue virus serving as the prototype. The aquareovirus host range includes fish and shellfish, with golden shiner virus serving as the prototype. Table 63.1 includes a list of genera and species that are important in veterinary medicine.

ORTHOREOVIRUSES

MAMMALIAN ORTHOREOVIRUSES

Disease

Reoviruses (genus *Orthoreovirus*) have been isolated from the respiratory and/or gastrointestinal tract of many animal species, including nonhuman primates, rodents, horses, cattle, sheep, swine, cats, and dogs. Reoviruses are usually isolated from healthy animals, thus their designation as "respiratory enteric orphan" viruses because they typically are not associated with any disease. However, reoviruses are sometimes isolated from animals with mild respiratory and/or enteric disease, and reovirus infection of infant (neonatal) mice can cause severe systemic disease. Experimental infection of kittens with reovirus serotype 3 has caused conjunctivitis, photophobia, gingivitis, serous lacrimation, and nasal discharge. All three serotypes of reovirus have been isolated from sheep, and experimental infections with serotype 1 have been reported to cause enteritis and pneumonia.

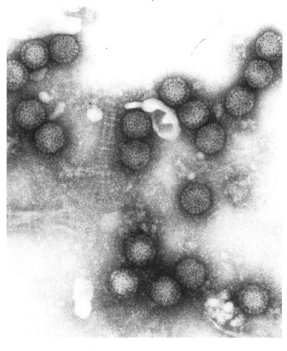

FIGURE 63.1.   *Negatively stained preparations of avian orthoreoviruses. 204,000X. (Courtesy of R. Nordhausen.)*

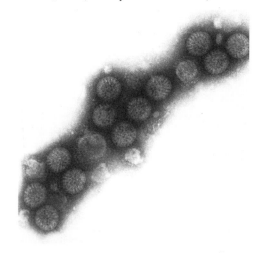

FIGURE 63.2.   *Negatively stained preparations of bovine rotaviruses. 204,000X. (Courtesy of R. Nordhausen.)*

Etiologic Agent

Physical, Chemical, and Antigenic Properties

There are three serotypes (1, 2, and 3) and many strains of mammalian reoviruses. Strains of reovirus that vary in virulence have been identified by sequence analysis of individual viral genes and proteins. Mammalian reoviruses all possess a genome of ten distinct segments of dsRNA. The genome segments are of different sizes (grouped as large, medium, and small). Each encodes a single protein except the S1 gene, which includes two distinct open reading frames. The complete reovirus particle has no envelope and exhibits icosahedral morphology with a diameter of approximately 85 nm. The reovirus particle consists of eight structural proteins arranged into inner and outer protein capsids (coats). The inner protein core contains the viral RNA-dependent RNA polymerase (transcriptase), as well as other enzymes that mediate mRNA synthesis and capping, helicase activity, and other functions that are necessary for virus replication. The predominant outer coat protein sigma 1 is the primary determinant of virus serotype and hemagglutination and also is the cell attachment protein. Enzymatic digestion of the outer capsid protein sigma 3 from intact reovirus particles generates infectious subviral particles, and removal of the outer capsid proteins sigma 1, sigma 3, and mu 1 generates core particles. All three particles are important in the lifecycle of reovirus replication. Genetic diversity of strains of reovirus occurs through accumulation of mutations within individual viral genes (genetic drift) and by the exchange of entire genes (reassortment) between viruses during mixed infections with more than one reovirus strain or serotype.

Resistance to Physical and Chemical Agents

Reoviruses are stable at low temperatures (4°C to room temperature) and are resistant to high temperature (55°C) for short periods of time. Reoviruses are also resistant to detergents and many disinfectants and stable over a wide pH range (pH 2 to 9). They are inactivated by exposure to 95% ethanol and sodium hypochlorite.

Infectivity for Other Species and Culture Systems

Reoviruses infect most mammals and they replicate in a variety of cell cultures.

Host-Virus Relationship

Distribution, Reservoir, and Transmission

Mammalian reoviruses have a wide geographic distribution and are commonly present in river water, untreated sewage, and stagnant water, likely reflecting fecal contamination by infected animals and/or humans. The mode of transmission is apparently by direct contact or exposure to materials contaminated by virus-infected feces (orofecal) and/or respiratory discharge.

Table 63.1.   Genera Within the *Reoviridae* That Include Viruses Relevant to Veterinary Medicine

Genus	Serogroup	Minimum Number of Serotypes
Orthoreovirus	Mammalian	3
	Avian	11
Orbivirus	Bluetongue	24
	Epizootic hemorrhagic disease	8 (possibly 9)
	African horsesickness	9
	Equine encephalosis	7
	Palyam	11
Rotavirus	5 major groups	Uncertain
Aquareovirus	Not designated	Uncertain

Pathogenesis and Pathology

Studies in mice have shown that reoviruses can infect either intestinal or respiratory epithelial cells after, respectively, orofecal enteric or aerosol respiratory infection. Initial virus replication occurs in regional lymphoid tissues after reovirus infection of either the gastrointestinal (Peyers patches) or respiratory (bronchus-associated lymphoid tissues) tracts. The virus sometimes gains entry to the systemic circulation in infected neonatal mice, leading to pancreatitis, myocarditis, myositis, encephalomyletitis, or hepatitis, with the specific disease process and pathogenesis reflecting the properties of the individual infecting strain of reovirus as well as the age and resistance of the infected mouse. Reoviruses can cause encephalitis and hepatitis in primates.

Host Response to Infection

Both respiratory and enteric infection of mice with mammalian reoviruses results in induction of humoral and cellular immune responses, natural killer cells, as well as interferons and other cytokines, all of which are potentially important in terminating infection.

Laboratory Diagnosis

Reovirus infections can be diagnosed by virus isolation or detection, and by serology. Virus can be isolated from tissues and from rectal, nasal, and throat swabs by cell culture techniques, although blind passage may be required before cytopathic effect (CPE) becomes visible. Virus isolates can be serotyped by either hemagglutination inhibition (HI) or virus neutralization (VN) testing with serotype-specific antisera. Reoviruses can be identified in tissues or cell culture by immunofluorescent antibody staining (FA) or immunohistochemistry. Serologic testing is done using paired sera and VN or ELISA.

Treatment and Control

Since reovirus infection in mammals is usually mild, treatment is not required. No vaccines or control measures have been described and are unlikely to be developed in the future unless reoviruses are determined to be of greater importance as animal pathogens.

Avian Orthoreoviruses

Disease

Avian reoviruses (genus *Orthoreovirus*) are of economic significance to the poultry industry. Systemic reovirus infections of poultry can cause a variety of clinical syndromes, including gastroenteritis, hepatitis, myocarditis and pericarditis, pneumonia, and ill-thrift. Acute reovirus infections also lead to increased mortality and carcass condemnations in affected flocks, as well as poor growth and food conversion efficiency (stunting syndrome). Arthritis and tenosynovitis are common in birds that survive acute reovirus infection; reoviruses are a major cause of avian arthritis, and this disease occurs principally in broiler chickens and, less often, in layer birds and turkeys.

Etiologic Agent

Physical, Chemical, and Antigenic Properties

The avian reoviruses largely resemble their mammalian counterparts but differ in that they produce cell fusion in cell cultures (syncitia), lack hemagglutinating activity, and are typically unable to grow in mammalian cell lines. Avian and mammalian reoviruses exhibit varying degrees of antigenic relatedness. At least 11 serotypes of avian reovirus have been described, and strains of avian reoviruses vary significantly in their virulence. All share common antigens as determined by agar gel immunodiffusion (AGID) and complement fixation (CF).

Infectivity for Other Species and Culture Systems

Avian reoviruses replicate in embryonated chicken eggs, primary avian cell cultures, and, once adapted, certain established mammalian cell lines.

Host-Virus Relationship

Distribution, Reservoir, and Transmission

Avian reoviruses are prevalent worldwide in chickens, turkeys, and other avian species. Avian reoviruses persist in nature through environmental contamination and by continued transmission of the virus from infected birds, including those persistently infected with the virus, to susceptible birds. Transmission occurs both horizontally and vertically. Horizontal transmission is predominantly by the orofecal route and occurs through both direct and indirect contact. Vertical transmission has been demonstrated following oral, tracheal, and nasal inoculation of breeder chickens.

Pathogenesis and Pathology

Infection with avian reoviruses is usually inapparent, and the occurrence of disease reflects the age of the bird at infection (young birds are predisposed), the virulence of the infecting virus strain, and the route of exposure. Reovirus-induced arthritis is initially characterized by acute inflammation within affected joints that progresses to pannus formation with erosion of articular cartilage; thus, reovirus-induced arthritis in chickens somewhat mimics human rheumatoid arthritis. Gross lesions in affected chickens often also include extensive swelling of the digital flexor and metatarsal extensor tendons that can lead to chronic hardening and fusion of the tendon sheaths.

Host Response to Infection

Antibody responses to avian reoviruses have been demonstrated by AGID, CF, and VN tests. The mechanism or mechanisms responsible for protective immunity are poorly defined, and variable degrees of cross-strain protection have been reported.

Laboratory Diagnosis

Reovirus-induced avian arthritis must be differentiated from arthritis and synovitis caused by other viruses and bacteria. A definitive diagnosis requires demonstration of reovirus infection by direct FA staining of tissues (tendon sheaths), virus isolation, or serology.

Treatment and Control

There is no treatment for avian viral arthritis, and the infection is best controlled by proper management procedures and vaccination with either attenuated or killed vaccines.

ORBIVIRUSES

Orbiviruses are important pathogens of livestock. Fourteen serogroups have been described and five are of real or potential veterinary significance: 1) bluetongue virus (BTV), 2) epizootic hemorrhagic disease virus (EHDV), 3) Palyam virus, 4) African horsesickness virus (AHSV), and 5) equine encephalosis virus (EEV). Like mammalian reoviruses (orthoreoviruses), orbiviruses have a double capsid structure, possess a segmented dsRNA genome (10 segments), and replicate in the cytoplasm of infected cells. Orbiviruses are distinguished from orthoreoviruses and rotaviruses because they replicate in both insects and mammals, and by the fact that they are not enteric pathogens of vertebrates. Orbiviruses replicate within the digestive tract of the hematophagous (blood sucking) insects that transmit these viruses between susceptible mammalian hosts.

Bluetongue Virus

Disease

Bluetongue (BT) is an arthropod-transmitted virus disease of domestic and wild ruminant species caused by BT virus (BTV). BT occurs most commonly in sheep (soremuzzle, catarrhal fever) and certain species of wildlife, particularly white-tailed deer. BT in sheep and deer is characterized by congestion, hemorrhage, and ulceration of the mucous membranes of the mouth, nose, and upper gastrointestinal tract. Other characteristic lesions include hyperemia of the coronary band and necrosis of both cardiac and skeletal muscles. BTV infection of sheep and deer is sometimes fatal, with terminal occurrence of disseminated intravascular coagulation. Sheep that survive severe bouts of BT are frequently emaciated, weak, and lame, and have a protracted convalescence during which they are susceptible to secondary infections. Breaks may occur in the wool fiber of convalescent sheep. Cattle are commonly infected with BTV in endemic areas, but clinical disease is extremely uncommon. Vaccine strains of BTV and those propagated in cell culture can cross the placenta of pregnant sheep and cattle to infect the developing fetus, leading to fetal death, abortion, stillbirths, or teratogenic defects in progeny.

The major economic impact of BT is that it is included in List A of the Organization Internationale des Epizooties, along with foot-and-mouth disease and some fourteen other diseases that are considered to have major adverse economic and societal ramifications. As a consequence, the international movement of ruminants and their germplasm from BTV-endemic countries is frequently restricted by non-tariff trade barriers pertaining to BT. The validity of these trade barriers is highly conjectural given that distinct strains and serotypes of BTV, along with unique species of insect vectors, occur in different regions of the world, implying that the global spread of BTV was not a recent event and certainly not associated with recent trade in animals or their germplasm.

BTV recently was recognized as a potential pathogen of carnivores. Inadvertent infection of pregnant dogs with a BTV-contaminated vaccine caused abortion and death. Serologic evidence of BTV infection has also been demonstrated in African carnivores.

Etiologic Agent

Physical, Chemical, and Antigenic Properties

The genome of BTV and other orbiviruses includes 10 segments of dsRNA, each of which encodes at least one protein (Table 63.2). The BTV particle is composed of seven structural proteins, two of which form the outer coat and

Table 63.2. Molecular Constituents of Orbiviruses

Gene	Encoded protein	Role
1	VP1	RNA polymerase; minor component of viral core particle
2	VP2	Receptor binding; serotype determination; component of outer capsid
3	VP3	Interacts with genomic RNA; structural component of viral core particle
4	VP4	RNA capping enzymes; minor component viral core particle
5	VP5	Structural interactions with VP2; component of outer capsid
6	NS1	Virus tubules; not a virion component; nonstructural
7	VP7	Group antigen; structural component of viral core particle
8	NS2	Binds RNA; virus inclusion bodies; nonstructural
9	VP6	Helicase; binds RNA; minor component of viral core particle
10	NS3/3A	Virus egress from infected cells; nonstructural

five the inner core. The outer capsid protein, VP2, contains the serotype-specific epitopes recognized by neutralizing and hemagglutination-inhibiting (HI) antibodies. The other outer coat protein, VP5, contributes to the conformation of the neutralizing epitopes on VP2. Four nonstructural (NS) proteins also occur in BTV-infected cells, with NS-1 forming cytoplasmic macrotubular structures that are characteristic of orbivirus-infected cells. The core protein VP7 contains epitopes that are common to all serotypes and strains of BTV, which is the basis of group-specific serological assays such as agar-gel immmunodiffusion (AGID) and competitive enzyme-linked immunosorbent assay (cELISA).

There is considerable heterogeneity within the BTV serogroup, with 24 distinct virus serotypes and many strains, each with potentially distinct biological properties. This genetic diversity has arisen as a consequence of both genetic drift of individual gene segments as well as the reassortment of gene segments during mixed infections of either insect or ruminant hosts with more than one BTV serotype or strain. Interestingly, recent sequence and phylogenetic analyses have shown that prolonged co-evolution of BTV with the different species of vector insects that occur in various regions of the world has resulted in strains of BTV that are unique to each region, so-called virus "topotypes."

Infectivity for Other Species and Culture Systems

BTV commonly infects domestic (sheep, cattle, and goats) and wild (deer, antelope, wild sheep species, etc.) ruminants. The viruses can be adapted to growth in suckling mice, embryonated chick eggs (ECEs), and a variety of mammalian and insect cell cultures. Replication of BTV in ECEs is facilitated by an incubation temperature of 33.5°C.

Host-Virus Relationship

Distribution, Reservoir, and Transmission

Bluetongue virus has been isolated from ruminants in all continents except Antarctica. Infection occurs throughout tropical, subtropical, and temperate regions of the world, coincident with the distribution of susceptible ruminants and competent vector insects (*Culicoides* spp.). The virus is not contagious between ruminants; rather, infection occurs only following the bites of BTV-infected *Culicoides* insects. Subclinical and/or asymptomatic BTV infection of ruminants occurs throughout endemic regions of the world. Outbreaks of BT occur only sporadically, most often at the northern and southern extremities of the virus' range following incursions of BTV into immunologically naive populations of ruminants.

Vector *Culicoides* insects become persistently infected with BTV after feeding on a viremic ruminant. These hematophagous insects are true biologic vectors of BTV because they only transmit virus to other ruminants after an extrinsic incubation period of approximately 10 days. During this time the virus disseminates from the midgut of the infected insect to its salivary glands. Replication of BTV within the insect vector is dependent on ambient temperature; thus increased replication of BTV in vector insects occurs at higher temperatures, but the lifespan of these insects is inversely proportional to temperature. Transmission of BTV can occur year-round in climates that permit insect (*Culicoides*) activity in all seasons, with the virus persisting in a perpetual vector-ruminant cycle of infection. In contrast, transmission of BTV is highly seasonal in regions of the world at the northern and southern extremities of the virus' range (approximately 35 degrees latitude south and 45 degrees latitude north). In these areas BTV transmission typically occurs only in the late summer and fall when vector populations peak and when ambient temperatures are highest (likely reflecting the influence of temperature-dependent virogenesis). The traditional global range of BTV has recently expanded into Mediterranean Europe after the northern spread of competent vectors, perhaps as a consequence of global warming.

Pathogenesis and Pathology

Sheep and some species of deer are most susceptible to BT, whereas cattle are resistant. The pathogenesis of BTV infection appears to be identical in all ruminant species. The virus multiplies initially in the lymph node(s) draining the site of infection, and viremia occurs as early as 3 days later with a subsequent febrile response. Upon systemic distribution, virus replicates in mononuclear phagocytic cells and the endothelium of small blood vessels, resulting in vascular injury, thrombosis, and infarction of the affected tissues; these include the upper gastrointestinal and respiratory tracts, the coronary bands, the heart, and skeletal muscle. Disseminated intravascular coagulation likely contributes to the vascular injury, hemorrhage, and tissue infarction that are characteristic of severe cases of BT in sheep and deer.

Viremia in BTV-infected ruminants is highly cell-associated. Virus initially is associated with all blood cell types, and titers of virus in each cell fraction reflect the proportion of each cell type in blood; thus BTV initially is most associated with platelets and erythrocytes, and less so leukocytes. Late in the course of infection, however, virus appears to be exclusively associated with erythrocytes. It is this association of BTV with erythrocytes that facilitates both prolonged infection of ruminants as well as infection of the hematophagous *Culicoides* insect vectors that feed on them. It is to be stressed that although BTV infection of ruminants can be prolonged (up to approximately 60 days), persistent BTV infection of ruminants does not occur.

The gross lesions of BT include facial edema and hyperemia, with or without hemorrhage (petechial and ecchymotic) of the oral and nasal mucosa, skin, and coronary band. Ulcerations and erosions also may occur in and around the mouth, especially on the hard palate. Hemorrhages at the base of the pulmonary artery are very characteristic of severe cases of BT. Petechial hemorrhages may also occur in the myocardium, pericardium, skeletal musculature, and the tissues of the upper gastrointestinal tract.

Host Response to Infection

BTV-infected ruminants develop both humoral and cellular immune responses. Virus-neutralizing (serotype-specific) and non-neutralizing (group-specific) antibodies develop 7 to 14 days after infection. However, virus can co-exist in blood with high titers of neutralizing antibody for several weeks because of the intimate association of BTV with the cell membrane of infected erythrocytes. Varying degrees of cross-serotype viral neutralization may occur following infection of an animal with a single BTV serotype and subsequent exposures to additional serotypes can generate production of broadly cross-reactive neutralizing antibody, including antibodies that neutralize serotypes of BTV other than those with which the animal was infected.

Laboratory Diagnosis

Initial diagnosis of BT in sheep and deer is based on the characteristic clinical signs of affected animals in known BTV-endemic areas. BT typically occurs in the late summer and fall. Confirmation of the diagnosis requires virologic testing, usually by either polymerase chain reaction (PCR) assay or by virus isolation using inoculation of susceptible sheep, ECEs, suckling mice, or cell cultures. The cell cultures most often used include Vero and BHK; multiple blind passages are often required before cytopathic effect is observed. Upon adaptation to cell culture, virus can be identified by fluorescent antibody staining or virus neutralization assay. BTV is very commonly detected in the blood of healthy ruminants in endemic areas, especially if sensitive nested PCR assays are used because these can detect BTV nucleic acid for up to 200 or more days after infection. Thus, the mere demonstration of BTV or BTV nucleic acid in the blood of ruminants certainly is not proof of disease causality.

Serologic diagnosis can be performed using tests for group-specific (AGID, CF, ELISA, IFA) or type-specific (viral neutralization, HI) antibodies. Paired serum samples are required to demonstrate seroconversion or an increase in titer. A single serological test is often meaningless because a high proportion of ruminants are seropositive in BTV-endemic areas, and the vast majority of these animals never experience obvious clinical disease following BTV infection.

Treatment and Control

There is no specific treatment for BT, although stress appears to exacerbate expression of disease. Furthermore, transmission of BTV to unaffected ruminants can be prevented by moving animals indoors (if feasible) where insect vectors are not present. Vaccination of sheep with attenuated strains of BTV has been practiced for many years in South Africa and North America; the South African vaccine incorporates a large number of different BTV serotypes, and requires vaccination on three different occasions. Potential disadvantages of live attenuated vaccines include reversion to virulence and their ability to be transmitted in nature. Furthermore, live attenuated vaccines potentially can reassort their genome segments with field strains of BTV to create novel variant viruses. Finally, live attenuated vaccine strains of BTV repeatedly have been shown to be able to cross the placenta to cause fetal death or injury, whereas field strains of the virus apparently cannot. Recombinant baculovirus-expressed virus-like particles recently have been used as a BTV vaccine, avoiding the problems inherent to live attenuated vaccines.

EPIZOOTIC HEMORRHAGIC DISEASE AND IBARAKI VIRUSES

Epizootic hemorrhagic disease (EHD) is an arthropod-transmitted virus disease of wild ruminants caused by EHD virus (EHDV). EHDV is an important cause of disease and mortality in white-tailed deer in North America and, to a lesser extent, pronghorn antelope and bighorn sheep. Although EHDV infection of domestic ruminants is common in endemic areas, EHDV is not regarded as a pathogen of domestic livestock, and authentic cases of EHD in domestic livestock are lacking. A notable exception is Ibaraki disease of cattle in Japan and Korea; the causative agent, Ibaraki virus, is closely related to EHDV serotype 2. EHDV shares many features with BTV, and EHD of white-tailed deer closely resembles fulminant bluetongue with hyperemia, hemorrhage and ulceration of the upper gastrointestinal tract, necrosis of cardiac and skeletal muscle, and terminal disseminated intravascular coagulation with widespread bleeding. Additional features of Ibaraki disease in cattle include marked dysphagia as a consequence of necrosis of muscles of the larynx, pharynx, esophagus, and tongue.

Like BTV, EHDV infection occurs throughout tropical and temperate regions of the world, and EHDV infection of ruminants has been described in Africa, Asia, and the Americas. EHDV closely resembles BTV in terms of its epidemiology, including dissemination by *Culicoides* insect vectors, pathogenesis of infection of ruminants, replication strategy, molecular structure, and methods of diagnosis. There currently are eight recognized serotypes of EHDV—nine if Ibaraki virus is classified as EHDV serotype 7, as recently has been proposed. With the exception of Ibaraki virus, vaccines are not widely available for EHDV.

PALYAM VIRUS

Palyam viruses are insect-transmitted orbivruses that cause abortion and teratogenesis among cattle in Africa, Asia, and Australia. Fetuses that survive infection with Palyam viruses prior to mid-gestation may develop brain malformations, including hydranencephaly and/or false porencephaly. Like the other orbiviruses of veterinary importance, Palyam viruses are disseminated by *Culicoides* insect vectors. There are 11 serotypes of Palyam viruses, and the pathogenesis and teratogenic effects of Chuzan (Kasaba) virus infection of fetal cattle have been especially well described.

AFRICAN HORSESICKNESS VIRUS

Disease

African horsesickness (AHS) is an arthropod-transmitted *Orbivirus* disease of equids, including horses, mules, and donkeys. The causative agent, AHS virus (AHSV), is zoonotic, although fatal infection of humans only rarely has been described. Fatal AHSV infection of dogs also has been described. AHS of horses varies greatly in severity, depending on the infecting strain of virus and the susceptibility of the infected horse. Several distinct forms of AHS have been described, including 1) a peripheral form characterized by edema of the head; 2) a central form characterized by pulmonary edema, high fever, severe depression, coughing, discharge of fluid from the nostrils, and rapid death of many affected horses; 3) an intermediate form that is characterized by fever, edema of the head and subcutis (supraorbital edema is highly characteristic), and significant mortality of affected horses; and 4) horse sickness fever, which is a febrile disease with a more benign course.

Etiologic Agent

Physical, Chemical, and Antigenic Properties

The causative agent of AHS belongs to a distinct serogroup within the genus *Orbivirus*. Nine serotypes of AHSV have been identified by cross-neutralization studies in mice. All types share common group-specific antigens.

Infectivity for Other Species and Culture Systems

AHSV infections have been documented in horses, donkeys, mules, zebras, goats, dogs, and large African carnivores such as lions. Disease has been described in horses and dogs. The virus can be propagated in suckling mice and adapted to grow in ECEs and cell cultures (Vero and BHK).

Host-Virus Relationship

Distribution, Reservoir, and Transmission

African horsesickness occurs throughout southern Africa, with periodic epizootics in northern Africa, the Middle East, Asia (the Indian subcontinent), and, on occasion in the past, Mediterranean Europe (the Iberian Peninsula). AHS is not contagious; rather, the virus is transmitted only by *Culicoides* insects that serve as true biologic vectors. Like bluetongue, AHS occurs most commonly in the late summer and fall in endemic areas, and the distribution of AHSV is dependent on the presence of competent insect vectors and ambient temperatures that facilitate temperature-dependent virogenesis within these vectors. Zebras have been implicated as potential mammalian reservoirs of AHSV in southern Africa, because AHSV infection is asymptomatic in zebras and AHSV viremia is more prolonged in zebras than in horses. Dogs may become infected with AHSV by eating infected horse meat, and serological surveys have shown that antibodies to AHSV are common among large wild carnivores in southern Africa.

Pathogenesis and Pathology

The incubation period of AHS is generally less than 7 days following the bite of an AHSV-infected *Culicoides* insect. The incubation period is shortest in horses infected with virulent strains of AHSV, and mortality in susceptible horses infected with highly virulent AHSV can reach 95%. AHSV replicates in mononuclear cells of the lymph nodes, spleen, thymus, and pharyngeal mucosa, and in vascular endothelium. The lesions of AHS result from vascular injury to small blood vessels, although it is uncertain whether the vascular injury that characterizes AHS is a result only of direct virus-mediated endothelial injury or if vasoactive mediators released from AHSV-infected mononuclear phagocytic cells also contribute. The severe central form of AHS is characterized by pulmonary edema, hydrothorax, and hydropericardium, with epicardial and endocardial hemorrhages. Subcutaneous edema can be extensive in horses that suffer a more protracted form of the disease.

Host Response to Infection

All serotypes of AHSV share common group antigens and induce development of antibodies that may be recognized by CF, AGID, and indirect FA. Viral neutralizing antibodies also develop following infection; these are predominantly serotype-specific, but some cross-neutralization activity has been observed.

Laboratory Diagnosis

Field diagnosis of AHS, especially in nonendemic areas, should be supported by viral isolation or serology to distinguish other infections that can produce similar clinical signs. Polymerase chain reaction tests are available, which provide a rapid and accurate result if done properly. The presence of virus also can be rapidly identified in tissue specimens using an AHSV-specific capture ELISA. Virus isolation is a slower but accurate method of virus detection. Intracerebral inoculation of suckling mice with blood or tissue suspension is a very sensitive method of isolating AHSV, although time-consuming serial passage may be required for viral adaptation. Cell cultures are not as efficient in isolating virus as mouse or horse inoculation. Virus can be identified by virus neutralization, HI, or FA.

Serologic diagnosis requires paired serum samples for demonstrating seroconversion or an increase in antibody titer. Assays routinely used for such purposes include competitive ELISA and CF, which are group-specific tests and detect antibodies to AHSV regardless of the infecting virus serotype, and viral neutralization assay, which is very sensitive but serotype-specific.

Treatment and Control

No specific treatment of AHS is available. Hyperimmune horse serum confers transient protection. Stabling of horses in insect-secure facilities is assumed to reduce exposure of animals to the *Culicoides* vector. Annual vaccination of horses with attenuated virus vaccines that include the nine recognized serotypes of AHSV is widely practiced in southern Africa, and to control incursions of AHSV into Europe. There are several potential problems inherent to use of multivalent modified live AHSV vaccines, including lack of protection against all serotypes of the virus, reversion to virulence of vaccine strains of virus, acquisition and dissemination of vaccine viruses by vector insects, and reassortment of gene segments between different virus strains/serotypes during mixed infections.

EQUINE ENCEPHALOSIS VIRUS

Equine encephalosis virus (EEV) has been isolated from horses with hepatic lipidosis and vague neurologic signs, but its importance as a primary pathogen is uncertain. The virus has also been isolated from aborted fetuses. Serologic studies have shown that EEV infection is very widespread and common among horses in southern Africa. The seven recognized serotypes of equine encephalosis virus (EEV) share common group antigens and closely resemble African horse sickness viruses (AHSV). The epidemiology of EEV infection is also like that of AHSV, with transmission by *Culicoides* insects.

ROTAVIRUSES

Disease

Rotaviruses cause enteritis and diarrhea in many mammalian species (including humans) and birds. *Rotavirus* infections are an important cause of diarrhea in young farm animals, including calves, lambs, foals, and piglets. The virus infects mature adsorptive cells at the tips of the intestinal villi with resulting malabsorption, maldigestion, and diarrhea. The clinical severity of the infection depends on factors such as the age and susceptibility of the affected animal, the virulence of the infecting strain of *Rotavirus,* and the presence of other enteropathogenic organisms.

Etiologic Agent

Physical, Chemical, and Antigenic Properties

Rotaviruses represent a distinct genus within the family *Reoviridae*. The viruses are nonenveloped, contain a segmented (11 segments) dsRNA genome, and exhibit a double-shelled capsid morphology with an overall diameter of the mature virion of approximately 100 nm (see Fig 63.2). At least 13 different rotavirus proteins have been identified, with 2 of the 11 gene segments encoding 2 distinct proteins. Of these 13 proteins, 7 are structural virion components (including enzymes) and 6 are nonstructural proteins that are produced in *Rotavirus*-infected cells but that are not incorporated into virions.

The rotaviruses currently are organized into five major groups (A–E), with two possible additional species (F,G). Many distinct strains and/or serotypes of *Rotavirus* occur within each group. Rotaviruses within each group share common antigens, can reassort their genome segments during mixed infections, have considerable sequence homology of conserved viral genes, and tend to infect the same species of animals. Neutralizing antibodies are induced by the outer capsid proteins VP7 and VP4, whereas VP6 expresses determinants common to each rotavirus group and subgroup.

Infectivity for Other Species and Culture Systems

Although rotaviruses obtained from one species can sometimes infect other species, strains of *Rotavirus* are largely species-specific in their tropism. Rotaviruses are difficult to propagate in cell culture. A major advance in the propagation of rotaviruses was the discovery that low concentrations of trypsin are required to initiate virus infection and replication in cell culture. Trypsin cleaves the viral outer coat protein, VP3, to facilitate infection of cell cultures, and once adapted rotaviruses grow well in cell culture. The most common cell lines used are kidney epithelial cells, especially the rhesus monkey kidney cell line, MA104.

Host-Virus Relationship

Distribution, Reservoir, and Transmission

Rotaviruses are considered to be distributed worldwide, and occur in many different animal species. High titers of virus are excreted in the feces of infected animals, and the virus is very stable in the environment if associated with feces. Transmission to other animals occurs by ingestion of virus, following either direct or indirect orofecal transmission.

Pathogenesis and Pathology

The pathogenesis of *Rotavirus* infection is similar regardless of the animal species affected. After oral infection, the virus infects the mature adsorptive epithelial cells that line the apical (lumenal) aspects of the intestinal villi. The infection progresses from the upper to the lower portions of the small intestine, and in some species, to the colon. Destruction of these mature villus enterocytes leads to villus atrophy, and the mature absorptive cells that line the villi are replaced by more immature cells from the intestinal crypts, leading to maldigestion, small intestinal malabsorption, and diarrhea. Interestingly, the NSP4 protein of rotavirus alone can induce intestinal hypersecretion from crypt cells, suggesting that both malabsorption and hypersecretion of fluid and electrolytes contribute to the diarrhea of rotaviral enteritis. The disease is worst in young animals and can rapidly lead to fatal acidosis, dehydration, and hypovolemic shock.

Animals that die of *Rotavirus* enteritis are dehydrated and have very liquid intestinal contents. Diarrhea is fluid and yellow/white (the so-called *white scours*), which frequently stains the perineum of affected animals. Histologic lesions include villus atrophy with loss of mature adsorptive cells covering the villi, and hyperplasia of the immature cells within the intestinal crypts.

Host Response to Infection

Animals infected with *Rotavirus* develop local and systemic humoral immune responses that can be identified by various serologic techniques. Viral-neutralizing antibody is serotype-specific and directed at VP4 and VP7. The *Rotavirus* ELISA detects antibodies to group and subgroup determinants. Local immunity within the bowel is very important in preventing severe rotaviral enteritis in young animals; thus ingestion of colostrum with high titers of *Rotavirus*-neutralizing antibody provides temporary immunity against disease in neonates.

Laboratory Diagnosis

Diagnosis of *Rotavirus*-induced diarrhea requires identification of the virus in feces or in tissues obtained at necropsy. Electron microscopy (EM), immune EM, and fluorescent antibody (IFA) staining of feces and/or intestinal tissue sections all facilitate direct visualization of virus or viral antigens, but *Rotavirus* in feces is most easily detected by antigen-capture ELISA. The ELISA is very sensitive and, depending on the capture antibody used, can distinguish different types. Direct examination of the dsRNA genome of rotaviruses in the feces of animals can be done by polyacrylamide gel electrophoresis, which also identifies the specific group of *Rotavirus* that is present. Polymerase chain reaction assays also are available.

Virus isolation is usually done on MA104 cells in the presence of low concentrations of trypsin. Avian rotaviruses are isolated on primary chicken embryo liver and kidney cells.

Serologic diagnosis can be done by ELISA or virus neutralization assays; however, the utility of data obtained usually is uncertain because of the widespread distribution of *Rotavirus* infection, which means that a high proportion of animals are seropositive regardless of disease status.

Treatment and Control

Treatment of clinically ill animals is guided by disease severity, and treatment of severe cases involves replacement fluid therapy to treat dehydration and acidosis, minimization of environmental stress, and treatment of secondary infections.

Control is often difficult because of the stability of the virus in feces leading to long-term environmental contamination. Although often challenging to implement, stringent sanitation practices can minimize exposure. Vaccine strategies are best directed at the dams of suckling neo-

nates, to ensure that high titers of antibody are present in the colostrum and milk of these animals.

AQUAREOVIRUSES

Aquareoviruses are morphologically and physicochemically similar to orthoreoviruses, but have 11 segments of dsRNA. Seven of the 12 proteins (genome segment 11 encodes two proteins) are structural, with VP7 representing the major capsid protein. Six genotypes (A–F) have been proposed for *Aquareovirus*. Viruses in this genus infect both fish and shellfish, causing necrosis in the parenchymal organs of infected fish and high mortality in fish hatcheries. Aquareoviruses replicate in fish or shellfish cell lines at 16°C and can induce syncytia formation.

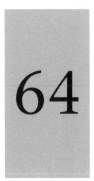

64 *Birnaviridae*

N. James MacLachlan   Jeffrey L. Stott

The family *Birnaviridae* includes three genera: *Avibirnavirus* (infects poultry), *Aquabirnavirus* (infects fish), and *Entomobirnavirus* (infects insects). Infectious bursal disease virus (genus *Avibirnavirus*) is the best studied. Infectious pancreatic necrosis virus (genus *Aquabirnavirus*) is a significant pathogen of salmonid fish.

INFECTIOUS BURSAL DISEASE

Disease

Infectious bursal disease (IBD), also known as *Gumboro disease* after the town in Delaware (North America) where it was first identified, is an economically important virus disease of young chickens. The IBD virus replicates in immature B lymphocytes in the Bursa of Fabricius, leading to reduced immunologic responsiveness. The virus can cause relatively high mortality in chickens 3 to 6 weeks of age, and profound immunosuppression in birds infected earlier in life. The clinical disease in birds over 3 weeks of age is characterized by soiled vent feathers (birds often peck at their own vents), diarrhea, depression, anorexia, trembling, severe prostration, dehydration, and eventual death. In the United States, economic losses are typically due not so much to bird death but rather to reduced weight gain and carcass condemnation due to hemorrhages in skeletal muscle, whereas highly virulent strains of IBD virus that cause high mortality in affected flocks are increasingly important in Europe and other regions of the world. Infection of birds less than 3 weeks of age results in economically devastating inapparent infection. Such birds are extensively immunocompromised and exhibit increased susceptibility to a variety of other infectious diseases. Furthermore, affected birds respond poorly to vaccination.

Etiologic Agent

Physical, Chemical, and Antigenic Properties

Infectious bursal disease virus (IBDV) particles are nonenveloped with icosahedral symmetry (60 nm in diameter; Fig 64.1). The genome includes two segments of double-stranded RNA (dsRNA), designated A and B, that encode five proteins. Segment A has two open reading frames and encodes a nonstructural protein (VP5) as well as a polyprotein that is cleaved into two structural proteins (VP2, VP3) and the viral protease (VP4). Gene segment B encodes the viral RNA-dependent RNA polymerase (VP1). There are two serotypes of IBDV and marked antigenic and genetic variation within each type. Strains of IBDV serotype 1 cause disease in chickens throughout the world.

Resistance to Physical and Chemical Agents

Infectious bursal disease virus is extremely stable and resists inactivation following acid treatment (stable at pH 3), lipid solvents, various disinfectants, and heat (survives 60°C for 30 minutes).

Infectivity for Other Species and Culture Systems

Infectious bursal disease virus principally affects chickens, although turkeys, ducks, and some other species of domestic and wild birds also can be infected with the virus. The virus can be propagated in embryonating chicken eggs, with subsequent embryo mortality, as well as in a variety of avian cell cultures.

Host-Virus Relationship

Distribution, Reservoir, and Transmission

Infectious bursal disease occurs worldwide in intensive poultry-raising areas. The virus persists in nature because of its stability. The virus has reportedly persisted in poultry houses, following depopulation, for over 100 days. There is no evidence of a true carrier state in birds.

Transmission of IBDV occurs by ingestion of virus from feces or feces-contaminated fomites, feed, and water.

Pathogenesis and Pathology

Initial replication of IBDV occurs in the intestinal tract within hours of ingestion of the virus, from where it disseminates to numerous tissues, including the bursa of Fabricius (BF). Other lymphoid organs such as thymus, spleen, and tonsils also may be affected, and disseminated lymphoid atrophy is especially characteristic of birds infected with very virulent strains of IBDV.

The striking age-dependent nature of the response of chickens to IBDV likely reflects the maturation of the BF at the time of infection. Specifically, birds are most susceptible to IBD from 3 to 6 weeks of age, whereas bursectomized birds of the same age do not develop disease. Birds older

FIGURE 64.1. *Negatively stained preparations of infectious bursal disease virus. 250,000X. (Courtesy of R. Nordhausen.)*

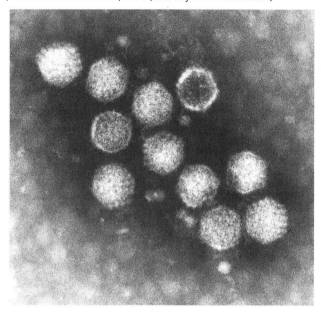

Laboratory Diagnosis

Field diagnosis can usually be made based upon the characteristic clinical signs and high morbidity and rapid recovery of most affected birds. Atrophy of the cloacal bursa is characteristic of inapparent IBDV infection in young chicks. Definitive diagnosis of IBD can be carried out by direct fluorescent antibody (FA) staining of sectioned tissues or viral isolation from the bursa and spleen. Isolation can be made by inoculation of embryonated chicken eggs or cell cultures. Serology is also useful for diagnostic purposes.

Treatment and Control

No treatment has been described for affected birds. Control of the disease may be facilitated by proper sanitation practices. Vaccination programs are widely used to control IBD. Immunization of breeder flocks is done to facilitate passive transfer of immunity to chicks. Vaccination of chicks is also practiced, but to be effective, levels of maternal antibody must be low. Both attenuated and killed virus vaccines are available.

than 6 weeks also do not develop severe disease, nor do those infected prior to 3 weeks of age. The impaired immunologic responsiveness that occurs in chicks infected early in life has been attributed to bursal injury, which results in failure to seed B lymphocytes to peripheral lymphoid organs and diminished humoral immunity. Cellular immunity also is reduced in IBDV-infected young chicks.

Gross lesions may include dehydration, darkened pectoral muscles, and hemorrhages in the pectoral and leg muscles. The appearance of the BF is dependent on the state of disease. The BF initially becomes enlarged due to edema and hyperemia, but this rapidly is followed by progressive atrophy that is marked by approximately 8 days after infection. Bursal necrosis and hemorrhage are characteristic of advanced disease.

Histologically, the epithelial surfaces of the BF have multiple erosions, and there is extensive necrosis of lymphocytes within lymphoid follicles so that these become depleted of lymphocytes. Edema and infiltration of heterophils occurs initially in the affected BF, followed by formation of cystic cavities bound by columnar epithelial cells and lymphoid depletion. Pathology in other lymphoid organs is less severe and recovery more rapid, except in birds infected with very virulent strains of IBDV.

Host Response to Infection

Following infection, birds develop a humoral immune response that is measured by viral neutralization, agar gel immunodiffusion, and enzyme-linked immunosorbent assay (ELISA) tests. Adult birds transfer maternal antibody to developing embryos, and if present in sufficient titer, the antibody lends protection to the hatched chick for variable periods of time.

INFECTIOUS PANCREATIC NECROSIS

Infectious pancreatic necrosis virus (IPNV) is the cause of a highly contagious and fatal disease of salmonid fish (trout and salmon) that is increasingly important to the aquaculture industry worldwide. The disease is especially severe in fish that are less than 6 months old, but also occurs in older fish following stresses such as that associated with relocation from fresh to salt water. Affected fingerlings appear dark in color and swim with a rotating action (whirling). Petechial hemorrhages may be present in the abdominal viscera of affected fish, along with necrosis of the pancreas. The virus also affects commercially raised yellowtails with high mortality and is classically referred to as *viral ascites* due to accumulation of fluid in the abdomen (ascites) and associated abdominal distension. Eels can be infected with resulting clinical disease. Fish that survive infection with IPNV become carriers and serve as a source of infection to other fish, especially under hatchery conditions. The virus is very stable in the environment. The virus can be identified in the tissues of affected or carrier fish by virus isolation in fish cell cultures or reverse-transcriptase-polymerase chain reaction (RT-PCR) techniques. Up to 10 serotypes of IPNV have been described, with the neutralizing epitopes being mapped to VP2. Efforts to develop effective vaccines are complicated by the multiple serotypes of IPNV and the difficulty in immunizing very young fish that are especially susceptible to the virus. Control is based on husbandry efforts that maximize hygiene and sanitation and minimize crowding, stress, and introduction of infected replacement stock and/or eggs. Vigorous identification and culling of carrier fish is advocated as a method of controlling the disease.

65

Retroviridae

RICHARD M. DONOVAN   FREDERICK J. FULLER

Retroviruses (family *Retroviridae*) are enveloped, single-stranded RNA viruses that replicate through a DNA intermediate using an RNA-dependent DNA polymerase (reverse transcriptase). This large and diverse family includes members that are oncogenic, are associated with a variety of immune system disorders, and cause degenerative and neurologic syndromes.

Classification

The family *Retroviridae* is classified into seven genera (Table 65.1). Classification is based on genome structure and nucleic acid sequence, in addition to older classification criteria based on morphology, serology, biochemical features, and the species of animal from which the retrovirus was isolated.

The genus *Lentivirus* (Latin *lenti*, meaning slow) includes the human immunodeficiency viruses (HIV) as well as many important animal retroviruses. Lentiviruses are most often associated with chronic immune dysfunction and neurologic diseases. The genus *Spumavirus* (Latin *spuma*, meaning *foam*) are nononcogenic viruses found in spontaneously degenerating cell cultures, causing the formation of multinucleated vacuolated (foamy) giant cells. No diseases have been associated with spumaviruses in humans or animals. The remaining retrovirus genera are termed the oncoviruses (Greek *onkos*, meaning tumor) or the RNA tumor viruses because of their ability to induce neoplasia, although they are now known to cause other kinds of diseases as well. These genera are the *Alpharetrovirus* (e.g., Avian leukosis virus), *Betaretrovirus* (Mouse mammary tumor virus), *Gammaretrovirus* (e.g., Murine leukemia virus), *Deltaretrovirus* (e.g., Bovine leukemia virus) and *Epsilonretrovirus* (e.g., Walleye dermal sarcoma virus).

Several additional features need to be considered in the classification and description of the *Retroviridae*. Exogenous retroviruses spread horizontally (or vertically but nongenetically) from animal to animal, similar to the mechanism of transmission of other kinds of viruses. In contrast, endogenous retroviruses are transmitted genetically. These retroviruses persist as integrated DNA proviruses that are passed from generation to generation through the DNA in the gametes of the host animal species. Thus, the endogenous proviral genome occurs in each cell of the animal. Many vertebrates possess such endogenous retroviral DNA sequences. These endogenous retroviruses are usually not

pathogenic for their host animals and are often not expressed. When replication of endogenous viruses does occur in the host cell of origin, it is usually restricted. Cells from animal species other than the host species are sometimes unrestricted, however, and can support the replication of the retrovirus in an exogenous manner. The endogenous mode of transmission occurs in many of the oncoviruses, but is not known to occur in the lentiviruses or the spumaviruses.

Some members of the oncoviruses are also classified by their interaction with cells of different species. Ecotropic strains replicate only in cells from animal species of origin and xenotropic strains replicate only in cells of other species. Amphotropic strains replicate in both. Most of the endogenous retroviruses are also xenotropic.

The morphology of retroviruses in transmission electron micrograph is also useful in classification (Fig 65.1). The size range of retrovirus particles is from 80 nm to 130 nm. Type A particles occur only inside cells and consist of a ring-shaped nucleoid surrounded by a membrane. B-type virions have an eccentric core, and C-type virions a central core. D-type virions have a morphology intermediate between B and C virions with an elongated, dense core. The core of lentiviruses has a shape that resembles an ice-cream cone.

GENERAL FEATURES OF RETROVIRUSES

Many of the features of retroviruses are known in great detail because of the extensive work done on the oncoviruses in cancer research and the lentiviruses in acquired immunodeficiency syndrome (AIDS) research. The members of the family *Retroviridae* share many common features in their composition, organization, and life cycle, although the details of individual retroviruses vary.

Components of Retroviruses

A typical retrovirus virion is composed of 2% nucleic acid (RNA), 60% protein, 35% lipid, and 3% (or more) carbohydrate. Its buoyant density is 1.16 to 1.18 g/mL.

Retroviral Lipids

Retroviral lipids are mainly phospholipid and occur in the virion envelope. They form a bilayered structure similar to

Table 65.1.   Genera and Selected Species of *Retroviridae*

Genus	Species
Alpharetrovirus	Avian Leukosis Virus
	Avian Erythroblastosis Virus
	Avian Myeloblastosis Virus
	Avian Myelocytomatosis Virus
	Rous Sarcoma Virus
Betaretrovirus	Mouse Mammary Tumor Virus
	Simian Type D Retrovirus[a]
	Ovine Pulmonary Adenocarcinoma Virus
	Squirrel Monkey Retrovirus
Gammaretrovirus	Murine Leukemia Virus
	Feline Leukemia Virus
	Porcine Type C Oncovirus
	Feline Sarcoma Viruses
	Murine Sarcoma Virus
	Woolly Monkey Sarcoma Virus
	Avian Reticulendotheliosis Virus
Deltaretrovirus	Bovine Leukemia Virus
	Human T-lymphotropic Virus 1
	Human T-lymphotropic Virus 2
	Simian T-lymphotropic Virus
Epsilonretrovirus	Walleye Dermal Sarcoma Virus
Lentivirus	Visna/Maedi Virus[b]
	Caprine Arthritis Encephalitis Virus
	Equine Infectious Anemia Virus
	Bovine Immunodeficiency Virus
	Feline Immunodeficiency Virus
	Primate Lentiviruses (HIV-1, HIV-2, SIV)
Spumavirus	Human Spumavirus
	Simian Foamy Virus
	Bovine Syncytial Virus
	Feline Syncytial Virus

[a]Simian AIDS-related virus (SRV).
[b]Ovine progressive pneumonia virus is synonomous with maedi virus.

the outer cell membrane from which the retrovirus envelope is derived.

Retroviral Nucleic Acid

Retroviral RNA. Retroviral particles contain RNA as their genetic material. This genomic RNA is present in each viral particle as a dimer of two linear, single-stranded, positive-sense copies that are noncovalently joined near their 5′ ends (Fig 65.2A). Hence, the virion is diploid. The genomic RNA has a sedimentation size of 60 to 70S in neutral sucrose gradients. Upon denaturation, each RNA copy has a sedimentation coefficient of 38S. The molecular weight of monomer RNA determined by electrophoresis in polyacrylamide gels is approximately 2 to 5 x 10^6 daltons, or about 7 to 11 x 10^3 bases. Host cell transfer RNA (tRNA) is associated with genomic RNA near the 3′ terminus and serves as a primer for the synthesis of DNA by the reverse polymerase. The type of tRNA packaged in the virion is useful

in the classification of retroviruses. The 3′ terminus of each RNA monomer has a poly (A) tract. The 5′ terminus has a methylated nucleotide cap.

Proviral DNA. Within a cell, the retroviral RNA genome is reverse transcribed into a DNA copy, and it is the proviral DNA form that serves as the intracellular retroviral genome. The retroviral DNA is several hundred bases longer than the retroviral RNA genome due to duplication of repeated and unique terminal sequences present in the RNA genome during the reverse transcription process. These sequences form the long terminal repeats (LTR) that flank the genes in the retroviral DNA (see Fig 65.2B). The proviral DNA is covalently integrated in the DNA of the infected host cell. This integration is facilitated by a viral enzyme, appropriately termed integrase, which is encoded in the polymerase open reading frame.

Retroviral Nucleic Acid Structure and Sequence. The sequence of structural genes of retroviruses, from the 5′ end to the 3′ end of genomic RNA, is Gag-Pol-Env. Some retroviruses, such as the lentiviruses, spumaviruses, and deltaretroviruses have additional genes (*tax* and *rex*) that regulate expression of the retroviral genome and other accessory functions. Highly oncogenic retroviruses often have an oncogene in place of a portion of the Pol and/or Env gene.

Retroviral Proteins

Retroviral Structural Proteins. Retroviral structural proteins are encoded by the Gag gene and the Env gene (Fig 65.3). Gag (group specific antigen) proteins form the core of the virus and consist of three major proteins. The nucleocapsid (NC) is a small protein (about 5 kd to 10 kd) that interacts with retroviral RNA. The capsid (CA) protein (about 25 kd) forms the major structural element of the retroviral core. The matrix (MA) protein (about 15 kd) serves to join the retroviral core with the retroviral envelope. In some retroviruses, there are additional small core proteins.

The Env (envelope) gene is responsible for the synthesis of two glycoproteins that are non-covalently linked. These two glycoproteins form trimeric multimers in some retroviruses. The glycoprotein outside of the retrovirus (SU, surface) is a knob-like glycoprotein (about 100 kd) that is responsible for binding the retrovirus to its cellular receptor during infection. The other glycoprotein (TM, transmembrane) is a spike-like structure (about 50 kd) that attaches the SU protein to the retroviral envelope.

Retroviral Enzymes. The Pol gene encodes several proteins with enzymatic activities that are important for the replication of retroviruses. These enzymatic proteins are found within the retroviral particle, but in a much lower molar concentration than the retroviral structural proteins.

The reverse transcriptase (RT) enzyme is responsible for the production of the retroviral DNA genome from the retroviral RNA genome. To accomplish this, reverse transcriptase possesses several catalytic functions, including an RNA-dependent DNA polymerase and an RNase H activity. RT requires the presence of a divalent cation to function, and the type of divalent cation (magnesium or manganese) that a particular retrovirus requires is useful in retroviral classification. The measurement of reverse tran-

FIGURE 65.1.   *Transmission electron photomicrographs of budding and mature virions of feline immunodeficiency virus (A,B); feline leukemia virus (C,D); feline syncytium-forming virus (E,F); human immunodeficiency virus (G,H); simian immunodeficiency virus (I,J); and visna-maedi virus (K,L). Uranyl acetate and lead citrate stain. (Reproduced with permission from Yamamoto JK, Sparger E, Ho EW, et al. Pathogenesis of experimentally induced feline immunodeficiency virus infection in cats. Am J Vet Res 1988;49:1246.)*

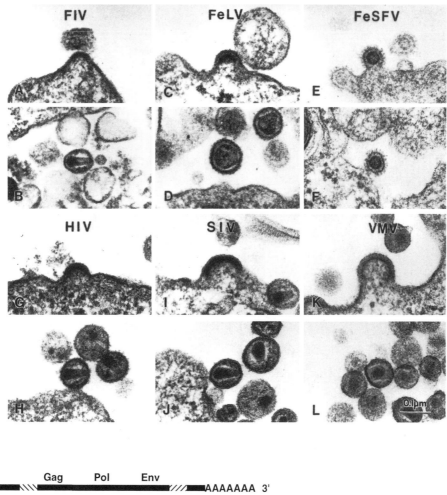

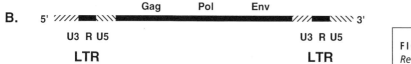

FIGURE 65.2.   *The nucleic acid of a retrovirus. Retroviral RNA (A); retroviral DNA (B).*

scriptase activity is one of the principal laboratory methods for the detection and assay of retroviruses.

The Pol gene also encodes other enzymes. The retroviral protease (PR) mediates cleavage of Gag and Pol polyproteins during retroviral assembly and maturation. The retroviral integrase (IN) functions to covalently link the retroviral DNA into the host cell's DNA as an integrated

provirus. Some retroviruses also encode a deoxyuridine triphosphatase enzyme (dUTP) that is required for virus replication in nondividing cells.

Other Retroviral Proteins. For many members of the *Retroviridae,* only the proteins encoded by the Gag, Pol, and Env genes are present. Other retroviruses contain additional genes whose products serve functions such as controlling

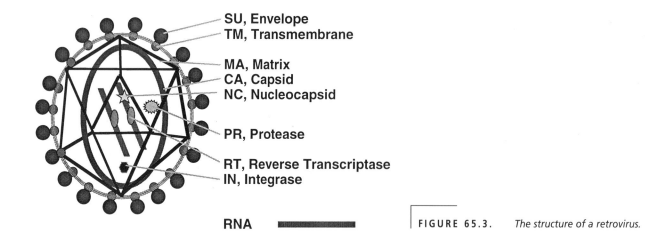

SU, Envelope
TM, Transmembrane

MA, Matrix
CA, Capsid
NC, Nucleocapsid

PR, Protease

RT, Reverse Transcriptase
IN, Integrase

RNA

FIGURE 65.3.   *The structure of a retrovirus.*

FIGURE 65.4.   *The life cycle of a retrovirus.*

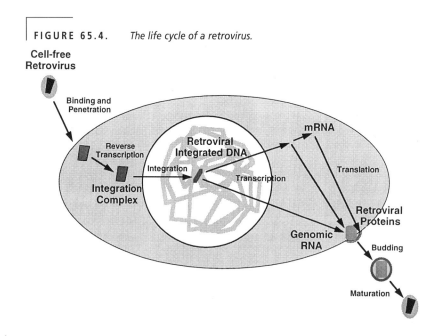

Cell-free
Retrovirus

Binding and
Penetration

Reverse
Transcription

Retroviral
Integrated DNA

mRNA

Integration

Transcription

Translation

Integration
Complex

Retroviral
Proteins

Budding

Genomic
RNA

Maturation

the level of provirus transcription, facilitating transport of retroviral mRNA, and enhancing retroviral replication in specific cell types.

Retroviral Replication

A general scheme of retroviral replication is shown in Figure 65.4. A retroviral particle binds to a specific receptor on the surface of a target cell via the SU protein. The retrovirus penetrates the cell and the retroviral core undergoes specific structural changes. The retroviral RNA within the modified core is reverse transcribed by RT using the associated tRNA primer, first to an RNA/DNA hybrid form, then to a linear double-stranded DNA form with long terminal repeats. The newly made retroviral DNA is still associated with some viral core proteins and enzyme activities in a structure termed the *integration complex*. In some retroviruses, infection must occur within dividing cells so that the integration

complex can access the host DNA, while in other retroviruses the integration complex is actively transported into the nucleus of the cell, allowing such retroviruses to replicate in nondividing or terminally differentiated cells.

The retroviral DNA is integrated into the host cell's DNA by the activity of the IN enzyme. The integration of retroviruses is not at a specific site within the cellular DNA, rather integration can occur at many sites. The integrated DNA provirus behaves very much as a eukaryotic gene. It may be transcribed into mRNA and genomic RNA using host cell enzymes to produce more virus, or it may remain latent for long periods of time and replicate when the cellular DNA is replicated by the cell.

New retroviral particles are produced by budding from cellular membranes. Immature retroviral Gag polyprotein and genomic RNA assemble and acquire envelopes as they exit infected cells by budding through the plasma membranes into which retroviral SU and TM envelope proteins have been inserted.

In the final step, the retroviral protease (PR) cleaves the Gag polyprotein into the mature structural proteins of matrix, capsid, and nucleocapsid.

Immunologic Characteristics of Retroviruses

Retroviral proteins possess various types of antigenic sites. Type-specific antigens that define the serologic subgroups are associated with the envelope glycoproteins. Group-specific antigens are shared by related viruses and, in general, are associated with the virion core proteins. There are also interspecies antigens that are shared by otherwise unrelated viruses derived from different host species. Reverse transcriptase (RT) is also antigenic and contains type-, group-, and interspecies-specific determinants.

Oncogenic Viruses and Oncogenes

Oncogenic viruses can produce inappropriate cell growths in the tissues of susceptible hosts. Cancers are malignant tumors that are characterized by loss of normal cellular controls resulting in unregulated growth and ability to invade adjacent tissues and to metastasize to other parts of the body. Cancers are classified by their tissue of origin: sarcomas are malignant tumors of connective tissue (mesenchyme); carcinomas are malignant tumors of epithelial origin.

The ability of oncogenic viruses to cause cancers under either natural or experimental conditions has been the subject of intense study for almost a century and this work has made significant contributions to the understanding of viruses, neoplasia, and cell biology. The fundamental discovery in the field is that oncogenic viruses cause cancer via genes they carry or activate. These genes are termed *oncogenes.*

Oncogenesis by Retroviruses

There are several mechanisms by which retroviruses are associated with cancer. Highly oncogenic or acutely transforming retroviruses cause cancer rapidly and efficiently, often within days or weeks of infection. Such retroviruses are rare in natural animal populations, but are used extensively in the laboratory for the study of cancer. Rous sarcoma virus (RSV) of chickens, which was discovered in 1910, is the prototype highly oncogenic retrovirus.

In highly oncogenic retroviruses, all or part of an oncogene exists in the viral genome, usually in place of viral genes. This retroviral oncogene is responsible for the ability of a highly oncogenic retrovirus to cause oncogenic transformation of a cell. There are more than 20 different retroviral oncogenes known. Each of these has a corresponding gene that can be found in the genome of normal cells. The normal gene that corresponds to a viral oncogene is termed a *c-oncogene* or *proto-oncogene*, and the viral version is called a *v-oncogene*. In a normal cellular environment, the gene products of proto-oncogenes usually have some function in growth regulatory pathways, such as protein kinases, growth factors or their receptors, GTP binding proteins, or transcriptional activation factors. When they are part of a retroviral genome, these proto-oncogenes are under the control of the retroviral LTR rather than being regulated by normal cellular mechanisms, and are often expressed at high levels. The v-oncogene may also be truncated, contain point mutations, or be fused with another retroviral gene. This aberrant expression of mutant protein can lead to abnormal growth of the infected cell and the beginning of progression to neoplasia.

For example, in RSV the *src* oncogene is responsible for sarcomatous transformation. The v-*src* gene was originally acquired from the normal c-*src* cellular proto-oncogene when illegitimate recombination occurred between retroviral and the cellular genomic sequences for c-*src*. The c-*src* gene product is a 60 kd protein that has protein kinase activity and is located near the inner surface of the plasma membrane. The kinase activity is part of an intricate cellular signal transduction pathway that mediates cell growth. Other examples of v-oncogenes with c-oncogene counterparts in normal cells are found in other acute transforming retroviruses, for example, *myb* (avian myeloblastosis virus), *erb* (avian erythroblastosis virus), *myc* (avian myelocytomatosis virus), and *ras* (mouse sarcoma virus).

Highly oncogenic retroviruses are usually defective. The reason they are defective is that they lack their full complement of Gag-Pol-Env genes because the v-oncogene takes the place of a portion of the retroviral genome. In order to replicate, these defective retroviruses require a replication-competent helper virus to supply the missing gene products. The helper retrovirus is usually a closely related retrovirus that is not defective and contains the usual Gag-Pol-Env complement of genes. Since the defective, highly oncogenic virus is packaged into a virion composed of the envelope proteins of the helper virus, the host range of the highly oncogenic virus is dependent upon the helper virus. The presence of the genome of one retrovirus with the protein components of another virus is termed a *pseudotype.*

Weakly oncogenic (nonacutely transforming) retroviruses cause neoplasia less rapidly and much less efficiently than do highly oncogenic retroviruses. Such viruses exist in domestic animals. Weakly oncogenic retroviruses do not carry a v-oncogene and do not require a helper virus. However, examination of the tumors produced by the weakly oncogenic viruses usually shows a clonal proliferation of cells with a retroviral genome near a cellular oncogene. For example, avian leukosis virus is often integrated near or in the c-*myc* gene. The mechanism by which weakly oncogenic retroviruses cause cancer is known as *insertional or cis-activational oncogenesis.* During retroviral replication, proviral DNA is inserted into many random locations in the host genome. Occasionally the integration of the provirus occurs close to a cellular proto-oncogene. This can sometimes produce inappropriate transcription of the oncogene, either by read-through from the retroviral promoter, or by enhancer activity by the retroviral LTR. Integration of the provirus near a proto-oncogene tends to be a very rare event and therefore occurs much less frequently and at much lower efficiency than when the retrovirus carries its own oncogene. The tumors are clonal in origin because, although many cells are infected, only one rare cell has undergone insertional oncogenesis and progresses to a tumor. In addition, the inappropriate activation of a proto-oncogene is just one event in a multifactorial process that leads to cancer.

A third mechanism of retroviral oncogenesis occurs in the bovine leukemia virus-human T lymphotropic virus genus of *Retroviridae*. These viruses have a regulatory gene called Tax in addition to Gag, Pol, and Env. The protein product of Tax functions as a transactivator to upregulate retroviral transcription by binding to specific DNA sequences in the LTR of the retrovirus. Under some circumstances, the Tax protein can sometimes also bind to transcriptional activator sequences in cellular genes and may disrupt regulatory pathways of the infected cell. Unlike insertional oncogenesis, the integrated provirus is not necessarily adjacent to a proto-oncogene, since it is the Tax protein that produces the oncogene activation (in trans), rather than the retroviral DNA itself. Like insertional oncogenesis, the transactivation of a proto-oncogene is just one event in a multifactorial process that leads to cancer.

Oncogenesis by DNA Viruses

Many of the DNA viruses, including the adenoviruses, papovaviruses (polyoma, papilloma), herpesviruses, hepadnaviruses, and poxviruses, have oncogenic potential. In contrast to highly oncogenic retroviruses, the v-oncogenes of DNA viruses are not cellular derivatives but are true viral genes. The normal function of these viral genes is to activate cellular pathways for DNA replication. This activation is required for DNA viruses to multiply in resting cells that lack the enzymes and materials the virus needs for its own DNA replication. The mechanism of neoplastic transformation by oncogenic DNA virus is that the viral genes that activate cellular DNA replication are functional, but the genes for viral production for some reason are not. This causes the infected cell to get inappropriate activation signals without the subsequent viral production that destroys the cell. The result is inappropriate cell activation and division, and is one of the initial steps that can lead to the development of a cancer. Like the weakly oncogenic retroviruses, insertion and transactivation mechanisms are also known for DNA viruses.

FELINE LEUKEMIA/SARCOMA VIRUS

Disease

Feline leukemia virus (FeLV) causes a variety of important diseases of cats. The most significant consequence of persistent FeLV infection is severe immunosuppression that results in the development of opportunistic secondary infections. Clinical syndromes produced by FeLV infection in cats also include tumors of the hemolymphatic system (lymphoma, leukemia), refractory anemia, ulceration of the oral cavity, a feline panleukopenia-like syndrome, FeLV-

induced neurologic syndrome, and immune-complex glomerulonephritis.

Lymphoma (lymphosarcoma) is the most common neoplasm in cats, although only about 70% of all lymphomas in cats are caused by FeLV infection. Multicentric lymphosarcoma that affects a variety of tissues (including liver, gastrointestinal tract, kidneys, spleen, bone marrow, and central nervous system) is the most common tumor in FeLV-infected cats, whereas thymic and alimentary (gastrointestinal) forms predominate in uninfected cats. Young cats with lymphoma tend to be infected with FeLV, whereas older cats with lymphoma tend not to be. Cats with lymphoma typically present with weight loss, often accompanied by any combination of respiratory difficulty, diarrhea, vomiting, and constipation. FeLV can also cause abnormal proliferation of erythroid and myeloid cells, resulting in a variety of myeloproliferative disorders including leukemias.

Transmissable fibrosarcoma in cats is associated with infection by feline sarcoma virus (FeSV) and typically occurs in young cats. The more common fibrosarcomas that occur in older cats are not associated with FeSV. The FeSV-induced fibrosarcomas tend to be poorly differentiated and more invasive than non–FeSV-induced tumors.

Etiologic Agent

Classification

Three subgroups of exogenous FeLV (A, B, and C) are distinguished by viral interference tests and antibody neutralization tests. These two properties are associated with the envelope glycoprotein.

Feline sarcoma viruses (FeSV) are replication defective, highly oncogenic (acute transforming) viruses that have acquired an oncogene through recombination of the FeLV genome with one of several cellular oncogenes. FeSVs are thought to arise de novo in FeLV-infected cats and not to be naturally transmitted from cat to cat.

Cats also have endogenous feline retroviruses such as RD-114 that are transmitted genetically. Multiple copies of the RD-114 provirus are found in all cat cells. These endogenous viruses are not associated with any known feline disease.

Physical, Chemical, and Antigenic Properties

Morphologically, the feline retroviruses are typical mammalian Type C retroviruses of the *Gammaretrovirus* genus. FeLV is composed of two envelope proteins, gp70 (SU) and p15E (TM), and three Gag proteins, p10 (NC), p15 (MA), and p27 (CA). The Gag proteins are produced in great excess in infected cells and are useful in laboratory diagnosis of FeLV infection of cats.

Resistance to Physical and Chemical Agents

Like most enveloped viruses, FeLV is sensitive to inactivation by lipid solvents and detergents. FeLV is rapidly inactivated at 56°C, but only minimal inactivation occurs at

37°C for up to 48 hours in culture medium. The virus is rapidly inactivated by drying.

Infectivity for Other Species and Culture Systems

FeLV-A replicates exclusively in cat cells, whereas FeLV-B and FeLV-C replicate in a variety of cell types, including human cells. The host range specificity of FeLV is associated with the envelope glycoprotein, gp70. No relationship has been shown between FeLV and human disease, and there is no evidence that FeLV disease is transmissible to humans.

Since the much rarer sarcoma virus, FeSV, is defective, the host range of this virus is dependent upon the helper leukemia virus that supplies the protein for its envelope. Most experimental studies have been conducted with the FeSV (FeLV-B) pseudotype. FeSV can transform fibroblasts from nonfeline species, including dog, mouse, guinea pig, rat, mink, sheep, monkey, rabbit, and human. FeSV has been found to be oncogenic in many of the animal species tested, although inoculation of fetal or newborn animals is generally required to show oncogenesis of FeSV in species other than cats.

Host-Virus Relationship

Distribution, Reservoir, and Transmission

FeLV infection of cats occurs throughout the world, and the cat is the only known reservoir of the virus. About 2% of the cats in the United States are seropositive, indicating either past or current infection, and some 50% of these seropositive cats are positive for FeLV antigens by immunofluorescent antibody test (IFA) of their peripheral blood leukocytes, indicating current infection. FeLV-A occurs in infected cats either alone (50%) or in combination with FeLV-B or FeLV-C.

FeLV is excreted in saliva and tears and possibly the urine. Transmission appears to occur during close contact via biting or licking (grooming). It is possible that infection may occur via contaminated feeding dishes. Prolonged, extensive cat-to-cat contact is required for efficient spread. In environments with multiple cats, the presence of one infected cat greatly increases the risk of infection for other cats. FeLV is also transmitted congenitally, and most kittens exposed in utero or before 8 weeks of age become persistently viremic.

Pathogenesis and Pathology

Upon penetrating the oral, ocular, or nasal membranes, the FeLV replicates in lymphocytes in the local lymph nodes of the head and neck. Acute FeLV disease, manifested by fever, lymphadenopathy, and malaise, develops 2 to 4 weeks after infection; however, these signs are seldom conspicuous. In about one-half of infected cats, the animals recover quickly and become FeLV antibody positive, FeLV antigen negative. Some of these cats have probably cleared the virus and the virus remains latent in others. The long-term significance of latent FeLV infection has

not been determined, and FeLV-viremia may be reactivated under conditions of stress or corticosteroid therapy in some of these cats.

In cats that do not mount an adequate immune response, the FeLV replicates in the rapidly dividing cells of the bone marrow. These cats are persistently infected with FeLV and are positive for FeLV antigen by the IFA test in peripheral blood leukocytes. The cycle of infection is complete after viral replication in epithelial cells of the salivary glands, where infectious FeLV is shed in the saliva.

The time from the onset of viremia to the appearance of the later signs of FeLV infection is termed the *induction period*. This period ranges from months to years, with an average of about 2 years. Most persistently viremic cats die within 3.5 years of infection. Persistently infected cats often develop leukopenia, immune deficiency, and secondary opportunistic infections. FeLV-induced immune deficiency must be distinguished from that induced by feline immunodeficiency virus (FIV), which is a different retrovirus.

Host Response to Infection

About half of FeLV-infected cats produce protective amounts of neutralizing antibodies to the major envelope glycoproteins while FeLV is confined to cells of the local lymph nodes, and the virus is eliminated or remains latent. These cats do not become persistently infected with FeLV, and usually live out a normal life span. The response to FeLV infection depends on the age of the cat, the dose of virus received, and probably other genetic and virologic factors. Kittens tend to respond poorly and, as a result, are predisposed to persistent FeLV infection.

Laboratory Diagnosis

Because some cats are able to clear a FeLV infection, and many cats have been vaccinated against FeLV, tests for antibody to FeLV are of limited utility. The most useful tests for FeLV diagnosis detect FeLV antigens. An enzyme-linked immunosorbent assay (ELISA) is available for FeLV antigens in serum or saliva and is especially useful as a rapid screening method. An immunofluorescence antibody test (IFA) is used to detect FeLV antigens inside of infected cells, which is evidence that the virus is replicating in the bone marrow and that the cat is persistently viremic.

Treatment and Control

Vaccines against FeLV are available, although their efficacy under field conditions is controversial. Current FeLV vaccines either contain the inactivated ("killed") whole virus or a subunit protein preparation of the virus. Kittens should be vaccinated twice starting at 9 to 10 weeks of age, with the second dose of the vaccine given 3 to 4 weeks later, and with annual booster vaccinations. Eight-five percent of cats under 12 weeks of age, if exposed, become persistently infected, but cats over 6 months of age have only a 10%–15% chance of becoming persistently infected if exposed. Use of FeLV vaccines are thus potentially most beneficial in young cats.

FeLV infection in catteries can be controlled by test and removal procedures and can be combined with FeLV vaccination, since vaccination will not interfere with the laboratory detection of FeLV antigen in infected cats.

A diagnosis of FeLV infection does not necessarily dictate euthanasia, since an FeLV-positive healthy cat may live for years. Because the cat is probably shedding virus that could infect other cats, however, precautions to reduce the chance of spreading the virus and contact with opportunistic pathogens should be instituted.

SIMIAN TYPE D RETROVIRUS

Disease

Simian Type D retrovirus, which is a member of the *Betaretrovirus* genus (Simian AIDS-related virus, SRV), produces a fatal immunosuppressive disease in monkeys. Infected animals show an initial generalized lymphadenopathy and splenomegaly accompanied by fever, weight loss, diarrhea, anemia, lymphopenia, granulocytopenia, and thrombocytopenia. Profoundly immunosuppressed animals develop diseases caused by opportunistic pathogens, the most common of which is disseminated cytomegalovirus (CMV) infection.

Etiologic Agent

Classification

Primate retroviruses are represented in four distinct genera: 1) *Betaretrovirus* genus, which includes the simian type D retrovirus (SRV); 2) the *Deltaretrovirus* genus, which includes the simian T-lymphotropic viruses (STLV) and human T-lymphotropic viruses (HTLV); 3) the primate lentiviruses, which include the human immunodeficiency viruses Types 1 and 2 (HIV-1 and HIV-2) and the simian immunodeficiency viruses (SIV); and 4) the simian and human spumaviruses. Although SRV is in a separate genus from the primate lentiviruses (HIV and SIV) that cause acquired immunodeficiency in humans (AIDS) and simians (SAIDS), many aspects of the immunodeficiency and associated opportunistic infections are similar.

The Mason-Pfizer monkey virus (MPMV) was the original SRV to be isolated.

Physical, Chemical, and Antigenic Properties

SRV is a Type D retrovirus (*Betaretrovirus* genus). The Type D viruses are characterized by the formation of cytoplasmic Type A precursor core particles. Mature Type D viruses are pleomorphic in shape, spheroid, enveloped, and 80 nm to 100 nm in diameter. The nucleocapsid is isometric to spherical with an asymmetric, spherical nucleoid.

The RT of SRV has a preference for Mg^{2+} and uses $tRNA^{Lys}$ as a primer for negative-strand DNA reverse transcription.

SRV consists of at least five serotypes based on neutralization properties of the envelope.

Infectivity for Other Species and Culture Systems

SRV infects several species of monkeys. Serologic surveys have shown no conclusive evidence of SRV infection in animal handlers who work with monkeys.

SRV isolates replicate in both T and B lymphocytes as well as in macrophages. Various human and monkey cell lines of T and B lymphocyte, macrophage, and fibroblast origin support the growth of SRV. SRV induces syncytia in Raji cells, which can be used as a method to quantitate the virus.

A human counterpart of SRV—a human Type D retrovirus—has been reported. The distribution and clinical significance of this virus remains to be determined, as does its relationship to SRV.

Host-Virus Relationship

Distribution, Reservoir, and Transmission

SRV is indigenous and widespread in Asian macaques but does not naturally infect African monkey species. In one study, about 25% of captive macaques in United States primate centers were seropositive; however, the prevalence varies widely based on the location and the species studied.

SRV is transmitted primarily in the saliva by biting. Mortality has been estimated to be 30% to 50%, and often occurs at an early age. Inapparent carriers that are viremic but antibody negative may be an important reservoir for SRV.

Pathogenesis and Pathology

SRV infects both T and B lymphocytes in vivo and causes a profound depletion of both of these kinds of lymphocytes leading to fatal immunosuppressive disease. The absolute lymphocyte count decreases but the CD4/CD8 ratio remains relatively stable. In the lymph nodes there is a depletion of lymphocytes and an absence of plasma cells. SRV also infects macrophages, but not granulocytes.

Host Response to Infection

Some infected monkeys die acutely 7 to 20 weeks after experimental inoculation, whereas some remain persistently infected, and some develop neutralizing antibody and become nonviremic and remain healthy.

Laboratory Diagnosis

Serologic screening methods include ELISA and Western immunoblotting. Because infected monkeys may be seronegative, however, it is necessary to include virus isolation as part of the screening process. Techniques based on antigen capture and polymerase chain reaction (PCR) have also been developed.

Treatment and Control

It is important to establish and maintain specific retrovirus-free breeding colonies, both for animal health as well as improving the quality of nonhuman primates used in biomedical research and, potentially in the future, transplantation. A serial test and removal program can eliminate SRV infection in group-housed monkeys.

Vaccines against SRV have demonstrated effectiveness under experimental conditions.

AVIAN LEUKOSIS/SARCOMA COMPLEX

Disease

The avian leukosis/sarcoma complex of viruses (ALSV) induce a wide variety of diseases in chickens. These have been of great economic importance to the poultry industry, as well as being important research tools for the understanding of cancer. These diseases include lymphoid leukosis, erythroblastosis, myeloblastosis, myelocytomatoses, sarcomas, osteopetrosis, hemangiomas, and nephroblastoma. The signs of disease produced by the ALSVs are not specific, and differential diagnosis requires careful histopathologic examination and laboratory testing.

In lymphoid leukosis, the most common and economically important disease caused by ALSVs, the comb may be pale, shriveled, and occasionally cyanotic. Inappetence, emaciation, and weakness occur frequently. Enlargement of the liver, bursa of Fabricius, kidneys, and the nodular nature of the tumors can sometimes be detected on palpation.

ALSV also causes sporadic cases of nonlymphoid tumors, such as erythroblastosis, myeloblastosis, and myelocytomatoses. Clinical signs of these diseases include lethargy, general weakness, and pallor or cyanosis of the comb. In more advanced disease, weakness, emaciation, diarrhea, and occasionally profuse hemorrhage from feather follicles are observed.

Osteopetrosis, in which the long bones of the limbs are commonly affected, is also caused by ALSV. Thickening of the diaphyseal or metaphyseal region can be detected by inspection or palpation. Affected chickens are usually stunted, pale, and walk with a stilted gait or limp.

Reticuloendotheliosis virus (REV) is a retrovirus found in chickens and turkeys that is unrelated to the viruses of the *Alpharetrovirus* genus (leukosis/sarcoma group). REV is actually classified in the genus *Gammaretrovirus* based on nucleic acid homology and biochemical properties. REV causes neoplastic disease and nonneoplastic runting in several species of poultry.

Etiologic Agent

Classification

ALSVs are classified into five subgroups, A to E, on the basis of differences in their viral envelope glycoprotein antigens that determine virus-serum neutralization properties and viral interference patterns with members of the same or different subgroups. Subgroup E viruses include ubiquitous endogenous leukemia viruses of low pathogenicity. Additional subgroups (F, G, H, I) comprise retroviruses from pheasants, quail, and partridges and have antigenic properties and host range distinct from that of the viruses in subgroups A to E.

It is important to note that many of the highly oncogenic avian alpharetroviruses (type C) that are used in research studies are defective and require a helper virus to replicate. These viruses are packaged as pseudotypes using the envelope proteins of a helper virus. They therefore take on the interference and neutralization properties of their helper virus.

Physical, Chemical, and Antigenic Properties

In size, shape, and ultrastructural characteristics, viruses of the avian leukosis/sarcoma complex are alpharetroviruses (Type C) and are indistinguishable from one another. ALSVs within a subgroup cross-neutralize to varying extents. Viruses of different subgroups do not cross-neutralize except for partial cross-neutralization between subgroups B and D.

Resistance to Physical and Chemical Agents

The infectivity of ALSVs is abolished by treatment with lipid solvents such as ether or detergents (sodium dodecyl sulfate). These viruses are rapidly inactivated at higher temperatures, whereas viruses of this group can be preserved for long periods at temperatures below 26°C. The stability of viruses of this group changes little between pH 5 and pH 9. Outside this range, however, inactivation rates are markedly increased.

Infectivity for Other Species and Culture Systems

ALSVs occur in chickens and have also been isolated from pheasants, quail, and partridges. More distantly related retroviruses occur in turkeys. Experimentally, some of the ALSVs have a wide host range, especially RSV. Some strains of RSV induce neoplasms in other species of birds and even mammals, including monkeys, although only very young or immunologically tolerant animals generally are susceptible.

The avian oncoviruses, like many retroviruses, are not cytocidal for the cells in which they replicate. In chicken embryo fibroblast cell culture, RSV and other highly oncogenic members of the ALSV group induce rapid transformation of cells characterized by alterations in cell growth properties and cell morphology. These cells proliferate to produce discrete colonies or foci of transformed cells within a few days. The number of transformed foci is inversely proportional to the viral dilution and can be used as a gauge of viral concentration. Various strains of sarcoma virus can induce transformation in mouse, rat, and hamster embryo fibroblasts, as well as in chickens.

Although members of the weakly oncogenic ALSV group induce neoplastic disease, they produce no obvious cytopathic effects or detectable levels of transformation in chicken fibroblast culture. Their presence is assessed by an immunofluorescence focus assay with type-specific chicken antisera or by their ability to induce resistance to transformation by RSV. This resistance occurs when the glycoproteins (attachment sites) of an identical or related virus block the cell receptors for the super-infecting virus. Stocks of leukosis virus originally detected by interference with RSV are referred to as *resistance-inducing factor* (RIF) strains.

Host-Virus Relationship

Distribution, Reservoir, and Transmission

ALSVs occur naturally in chickens and most flocks of chickens worldwide harbor various strains of ALSV, except for those derived from specific pathogen-free (SPF) birds. Even in infected flocks, the frequency of lymphoid tumors is typically low and mortality is usually 2% or less, although sometimes losses can be much higher. The reservoir host for ALSV is the infected chicken.

Transmission can be either vertical (from hen through egg) or horizontal. Vertically infected chicks are immunologically tolerant to the virus and fail to produce neutralizing antibodies, and remain viremic for life. Horizontal infection is through infected saliva and feces and is characterized by transitory viremia followed by the development of antibodies. Tumors are more frequent in vertical than horizontal infections.

Endogenous leukosis viruses, such as those of subgroup E, are usually transmitted genetically in the germ cells in the form of a DNA provirus. Many of these endogenous ALSVs are defective, but some (RAV-O) are released in an infectious form and can be transmitted horizontally, although most chickens are genetically resistant to infection.

Pathogenesis and Pathology

ALSVs induce a wide variety of neoplasms. The pathogenesis of infection of birds with ALSVs depends on whether the particular ALSV in question carries an oncogene or not. ALSVs containing a v-oncogene are highly oncogenic retroviruses, transform cells in culture, are usually defective, and are most often products of the research laboratory and occur only sporadically in nature, if at all. ALSV strains that contain a particular v-oncogene usually cause a rapid and relatively reproducible type of neoplastic disease in a high percentage of infected chickens.

In contrast, naturally occurring ALSVs are weakly oncogenic, cause disease by insertional oncogenesis, do not transform cells at detectable levels in culture, are usually not defective, and are naturally transmitted. The oncogenic spectrum of non-oncogene-containing strains of ALSVs tends to overlap, so that a given strain of ALSV can induce many kinds of tumors depending on other factors, such as the amount of virus, age, and genotype of chicken, and route of infection. This is consistent with the concept of insertional oncogenesis for these viruses in which the ALSV infects and replicates in a variety of cell types but, in order to produce neoplastic transformation, must integrate near an appropriate cellular proto-oncogene.

Under natural conditions, the most common disease caused by ALSV is lymphoid leukosis. Transformation of lymphocytes occurs in the bursa of Fabricius, usually at a few months after infection. These early ALSV-induced lesions sometimes regress, while others enlarge and eventually spread to other visceral organs. Grossly visible neoplasms are of variable size and organ distribution, almost always involve the liver (a synonym for lymphoid leukosis is *big liver disease*), spleen, and bursa of Fabricius. Individual neoplasms are soft, smooth, and glistening and are usually miliary or diffuse, but may be nodular, or a combination of these forms. These neoplastic masses are composed of large B lymphocytes that express surface immunoglobulin. There are often no consistent or significant hematologic changes in circulating blood, and frank lymphoblastic leukemia is rare. Fully developed lymphoid leukosis occurs in birds at about 4 months of age and older.

Erythroblastosis occurs sporadically in ALSV-infected chicken flocks. The liver and spleen are enlarged by a diffuse infiltration of proliferating erythroblasts, and the bone marrow is effaced by the same cells. Affected chickens become anemic and thrombocytopenic. Blood smears show an erythroblastic leukemia. Induction of erythroblastosis by naturally occurring, slowly transforming ALSV involves activation of the cellular oncogene c-*erb*B by insertional oncogenesis. Highly oncogenic, laboratory strains of ALSV carry the v-form of this oncogene and are termed *avian erythroblastosis virus* (AEV). Some strains of AEV can kill chickens by erythroblastosis within a week after experimental infection.

Myeloblastosis is relatively uncommon under natural conditions and tends to occur in adult chickens. The target organ in this disease is bone marrow, and the first neoplastic alteration is in the form of multiple foci of proliferating myeloblasts, which is followed by leukemia and invasion of other organs, especially liver, kidney, and spleen. Microscopic examination reveals massive intravascular and extravascular accumulations of myeloblasts with variable proportions of promyelocytes. The v-*myb* gene is carried by the highly oncogenic avian myeloblastosis virus (AMV) strains. These laboratory strains produce mortality a few weeks after experimental infection.

Myelocytomatosis is another form of leukosis that occurs sporadically in chickens. In this disease, tumors characteristically occur on the surface of bones in association with the periosteum and near cartilage, and at the costochondral junctions, posterior sternum, and cartilaginous bones of the mandible and nares. They consist of compact masses of uniform myelocytes. Earliest changes occur in bone marrow in which there is crowding of intersinusoidal spaces by myelocytes, destruction of sinusoid walls, and eventual overgrowth of the bone marrow. Tumors may crowd through the bone and extend through the periosteum. The v-*myc* oncogene is carried by the highly oncogenic avian myelocytomatosis virus.

Various benign and malignant connective tissue tumors occur sporadically in ALSV-infected chickens. There are a number of laboratory strains of avian sarcoma virus (ASV), the most famous of which is Rous sarcoma virus (RSV). ASVs induce sarcomas (tumors of connective tissue), including fibrosarcoma and fibroma; myxosarcoma and myxoma; histiocytic sarcoma, osteoma, and osteogenic sarcoma; and chondrosarcoma. These highly oncogenic ASVs carry an oncogene such as *src* (in RSV), *fps, ros,* or *yes.*

Infection with ALSV is important in its own right. As compared with specific pathogen-free chickens, ALSV-infected chickens exhibit poor growth and egg production even in the absence of tumor formation. The pathogenesis of subclinical ALSV infection of birds is poorly understood.

Host Response to Infection

Chickens exposed to ALSV virus fall into four classes: 1) no viremia, no antibodies; 2) no viremia, antibody; 3) viremia, antibody; and 4) viremia, no antibody. Category 1 includes birds that are genetically resistant. Most exposed chickens are included in category 2, and antibody persists throughout the life of these birds and is passed via the yolk to progeny chicks. The passive immunity provided by such antibodies generally lasts for 3 to 4 weeks. In addition to the neutralizing antibodies directed against the envelope proteins, antibodies are produced to the internal group-specific antigens (Gag proteins), which are nonneutralizing and not protective. Although virus-neutralizing antibodies restrict the amount of virus, they have little direct effect on growth of the virus-induced neoplasms. Few chickens occur in the third category, which may represent chickens that are in the process of clearing an acute infection with ALSV. Most chickens in category 4 acquire ALSV vertically when in the egg and are immunologically tolerant to the virus. Hens in category 4 transmit virus to a high proportion of their progeny through the egg.

Since there are multiple subgroups (A to D) that commonly occur in chicken flocks and are not cross-neutralized by antibody, the status of a chicken for one subgroup of ALSV is independent of other viral subgroups.

Laboratory Diagnosis

ALSV can usually be isolated from plasma, serum, tumor tissue, and albumin, or from the embryo of infected eggs. Since ALSV is generally not cytopathogenic, complement fixation, fluorescent antibody, or radioimmunoassay (RIA) tests must be used to detect and identify the viruses in cell culture. An ELISA test is used for direct detection of virus in egg albumen or vaginal swabs. These tests have been used directly on test material (egg albumin) or indirectly on the cell cultures used for viral isolation. All tests require a source of chicken embryos free from endogenous ALSV.

Another means of identifying virus is based on phenotypic mixing of viruses. Chicken fibroblasts that are transformed with envelope-defective strains of RSV are nonpro-

ducers (NP) of infectious RSV. Superinfection of NP cultures by another ALSV acting as a helper virus results in production of infectious RSV, which produces transformed foci on susceptible chicken embryo fibroblasts.

Treatment and Control

Attempts to produce effective vaccines have been largely unsuccessful. Moreover, congenitally infected chicks, which constitute the major source of virus and are most likely to develop neoplasms, are immunologically tolerant to ALSV and cannot be immunized.

It is possible to eradicate ALSV from chickens by establishing breeder flocks that are free of exogenous ALSVs. Hens are selected that are negative for ALSV antigens in their eggs. The fertile eggs laid by the selected hens are hatched and the chicks reared in isolation in small groups. The birds without leukosis virus antigen or antibody are used as the breeders for a leukosis virus-free flock. The flock must then be maintained in isolation from untested chickens.

BOVINE LEUKEMIA VIRUS

Disease

Bovine leukemia virus (BLV) is a cause of lymphoma (lymphosarcoma; lymphoreticular neoplasia) in older cattle—so-called enzootic bovine leukosis (EBL), which occurs very sporadically in BLV-infected cattle. Cattle with EBL are usually older than 3 years, with the peak of tumor incidence between 5 and 8 years. Affected cattle typically are afebrile with nonpainful enlargement of peripheral lymph nodes (lymphadenopathy). Depending on the involvement of different organs, affected cattle can exhibit signs of gastrointestinal dysfunction, paralysis, exopthalmus, and cardiac dysfunction. Neoplastic lymphocytes can invade the blood to cause lymphoid leukemia in some affected cattle. The forms of lymphomas that occur in calves (less than 6 months of age) and juvenile cattle (6–18 months of age) are not associated with BLV infection.

Etiologic Agent

Classification

Because of its genome structure, nucleotide sequence, and size and amino acid sequence of the structural and nonstructural viral proteins, BLV has recently been grouped in a genus (*Deltaretrovirus*) with the human T-lymphotropic viruses (HTLV-I and HTLV-II), and the closely related simian T-lymphotropic viruses (STLV). These viruses can induce diseases with similar pathologies, characterized by low viremia, long latency period, and a lack of preferred proviral integration sites in the tumors (i.e., the provirus is not necessarily found near an oncogene).

Physical, Chemical, and Antigenic Properties

Morphologically, BLV resembles other Type C retroviruses. Antibody to gp51 is neutralizing.

Resistance to Physical and Chemical Agents

The infectivity of BLV is abolished by lipid solvents, periodate, phenol, trypsin, and formaldehyde. Infectivity is rapidly destroyed at 56°C but can be retained for prolonged periods at less than 50°C. Pasteurization destroys the infectivity of this virus, which is of interest because infected lymphocytes are found in the milk of infected dairy cattle.

Infectivity for Other Species and Culture Systems

BLV has been shown to be infectious for several animal species other than cattle, including sheep, goats, and pigs. Under natural conditions, the oncogenic potential of BLV appears to be expressed only in cattle and sheep. Since there are no significant antigenic or genetic differences between bovine and ovine isolates, the agent designated *ovine leukemia virus* is regarded as BLV infecting a heterologous host.

BLV replicates in cell culture from a wide variety of species, including bovine, human, simian, canine, caprine, and equine cells. Although BLV replicates in human cells, humans are not known to be infected. Seroepidemic studies among high-risk humans (veterinarians, farmers, animal keepers, and slaughterhouse personnel) revealed no infections, and BLV has not been associated with human neoplasms.

Host-Virus Relationship

Distribution, Reservoir, and Transmission

The geographic distribution of BLV is worldwide. The reservoir is infected cattle. Disease is directly related to BLV prevalence, which can vary widely but is highest in intensive dairy areas (up to 50% or even higher). In addition to production losses associated with BLV infection of cattle, additional losses result from exportation restrictions by foreign countries that halt export of BLV-positive cattle or semen from infected bulls.

BLV is transmitted horizontally under conditions of close contact, and most commonly occurs when heifers are introduced into the milking herd. The virus is highly cell-associated, and transmission is by blood or tissue containing lymphocytes between animals, by trauma, contaminated veterinary equipment, or other less defined routes. Transmission of BLV can occur through the skin and the reproductive, alimentary and reproductive tracts, and is easily transmitted to susceptible calves or sheep by as few as 2500 lymphocytes from infected animals. Experimental transmission has also been accomplished with milk and colostrum, both of which contain lymphocytes, but this route is likely unimportant. In utero transmission of BLV has been documented, but occurs infrequently. The transmission of BLV by hematophagous flies and ticks has been demonstrated experimentally; how-

ever, field observations do not support a major role for such vectors. BLV-infected cattle with virus-induced persistent lymphocytosis are major reservoirs of the virus and pose the greatest risk for transmission.

Pathogenesis and Pathology

Most BLV infections are asymptomatic. There is a brief viremia soon after infection of susceptible cattle, followed by a long incubation period when the virus remains quiescent as provirus that is randomly integrated into the genome of infected cells. Only a low percentage of BLV-infected animals ever develop lymphoma, suggesting that the incubation period for induction of neoplasia is longer than the lifespan of many infected animals. Some cattle develop only a transient viremia without seroconversion, and after 3 to 4 months virus can no longer be isolated, whereas others develop persistent lymphocytosis within months or years after infection.

Neoplasms in cattle with enzootic bovine leukosis typically involve any combination of internal and superficial lymph nodes, heart, abomasum, intestines, kidneys, uterus, liver, spleen, epidural space of the lumbar spinal cord, and retrobulbar fat (of the eye). Distribution of the tumor is unpredictable, but blood is often not involved. Both T lymphocytes and B lymphocytes can be infected with BLV but the tumors are composed only of proliferating B lymphocytes.

Host Response to Infection

Most BLV-infected cattle develop antibodies to BLV structural proteins. A greater response is usually detected to the glycosylated proteins gp51 and gp30 than to the internal proteins p24, p15, p12, and p10 and to the reverse transcriptase. Whereas most infected cattle develop high titers of virus-specific antibodies, some remain persistently seronegative.

Antibodies to BLV are also detected in the milk and colostrum and are partially protective against infection of calves. Antibodies do not provide protection against tumor development in infected animals, however, and do not prevent the spread of infectious BLV by carriers.

Laboratory Diagnosis

A variety of serologic tests (agar gel immunodiffusion [AGID], immunofluorescence, and ELISA) that detect BLV-specific antibody can be used. The animal usually becomes seropositive 4 to 12 weeks after viral exposure.

Bovine leukemia virus induces syncytia in target cells.

Treatment and Control

Infection, once established, appears to be lifelong in infected cattle. There is no treatment for lymphoma or BLV infection in cattle. BLV can be eliminated from a herd by repeated serologic testing and immediate removal of positive animals.

Visna/Maedi/Progressive Pneumonia Viruses and Caprine Arthritis Encephalitis Virus

Disease

These viruses cause several different diseases that involve the lungs, joints, mammary glands, and central nervous system of affected sheep and goats. Initial signs of visna are subtle and insidious, consisting of a slight aberration of gait, especially of the hindquarters; trembling of the lips, unnatural tilting of the head; and in rare instances, blindness. The signs progress to paresis or even total paralysis. Fever is absent. Unattended animals die of inanition, hence the name *visna*, which means "wasting" in Icelandic. Signs of visna typically occur in sheep over 2 years of age, and the clinical course is protracted.

Maedi and progressive pneumonia viruses cause a similar chronic pneumonia in infected sheep. Early manifestations include progressive loss of condition accompanied by dyspnea. Eventually, breathing requires the use of accessory muscles and is accompanied by rhythmic jerks of the head. There is sometimes a dry cough, but no nasal discharge. The clinical phase is protracted, although affected animals often die from secondary bacterial pneumonia.

Caprine arthritis-encephalitis virus (CAEV) induces several disease syndromes in domestic goats, including chronic progressive arthritis, mastitis, and occasionally interstitial pneumonia in older goats, and an acute paralytic syndrome in kids that is characterized by hind limb ataxia, weakness, and paralysis.

Etiologic Agent

Classification

The agent of visna/maedi/progressive pneumonia and the closely related organism of CAEV are lentiviruses. The name designations are largely historical and refer to the site of virus isolation or the predominant pathology in an individual animal. Ovine progressive pneumonia virus is synonomous with maedi virus.

Physical, Chemical, and Antigenic Properties

The virion is composed of four structural proteins designated gp135, p30, p16, and p14. Minor structural proteins include a reverse transcriptase, integrase, and dUTPase. Neutralization tests have shown that variations in virus strains occur during infection in individual animals. If an animal is inoculated with plaque-purified virus, many months later a virus can be isolated that is not neutralized by antiserum that neutralizes the original inoculum strain. Both the inoculum strain and the variant strains can be isolated simultaneously, indicating that new strains do not replace parental virus. With time, neutralizing antibodies are produced to the new strains.

The RT of these viruses has a preference for Mg^{2+} and uses tRNA^{Lys} as a primer for negative-strand DNA reverse transcription.

Visna/maedi/progressive pneumonia virus and CAEV show extensive cross-reaction by immunodiffusion assays involving the major structural protein.

Resistance to Physical and Chemical Agents

Lentiviruses are relatively resistant to ultraviolet irradiation. Infectivity is abolished by lipid solvents, periodate, phenol, trypsin, ribonuclease, formaldehyde, and low pH (less than 4.2). Infectivity is relatively stable at 0 to 4°C in the presence of serum, but infectivity is rapidly destroyed at 56°C.

Infectivity for Other Species and Culture Systems

Visna and ovine progressive pneumonia have been described only in sheep and goats. Some breeds of sheep appear to be more susceptible, especially Icelandic sheep, which are highly inbred. The visna virus infects cells derived from many vertebrate species but replicates efficiently only in sheep cells. Unadapted virus isolates replicate best in macrophage cultures.

Host-Virus Relationship

Distribution, Reservoir, and Transmission

These viruses cause disease in sheep and goats throughout much of the world. The frequency of infection varies widely based on control programs, but can range to greater than 75% in some flocks in the United States. Infected sheep serve as the reservoir.

Transmission is via respiratory exudates and aerosol. Virus is excreted in the milk, and lambs raised on infected ewes are infected at a young age. Infection rates are increased by practices that pool milk. Intrauterine transmission is infrequent.

Pathogenesis and Pathology

The ovine lentiviruses infect cells of the monocyte-macrophage system. Visna is a chronic and progressive encephalomyelitis characterized by multifocal areas of chronic inflammation with accompanying demyelination. The process begins immediately beneath the ependyma bordering the ventricles, but spreads throughout the brain and spinal cord.

The lungs of sheep with progressive pneumonia are markedly expanded, with as much as a two- or threefold increase in lung weight. The histopathologic changes include thickening of the interalveolar septa as a result of infiltration of lymphocytes, monocytes, and macrophages. The thickening may be so pronounced as to obliterate the alveoli. Lymphoid accumulations with the formation of follicles and germinal centers are scattered throughout the lung parenchyma.

Some adult sheep infected with ovine lentiviruses develop chronic arthritis and/or mastitis.

Caprine arthritis encephalitis virus (CAEV) causes a peculiar motor spinal dysfunction in goat kids at 2–4 months of age. The lesions in affected goats resemble those of visna. Goats that survive infection with CAEV as kids often develop progressive, chronic arthritis, mastitis, and, occasionally, interstitial pneumonia that resembles ovine progressive pneumonia.

Host Response to Infection

Most lentivirus infections of ruminants are subclinical, likely because of the prolonged incubation period of the diseases these viruses induce. Lesions in all of these diseases include chronic, ongoing inflammation; thus the lesions themselves likely result in part from the host's immune response.

In experimental infections, complement-fixing antibodies appear a few weeks after inoculation, rise to a maximum within 2 months, and remain constant throughout the course of disease. Neutralizing antibodies appear later, reach a maximum at about 1 year, and then remain constant. However, the virus persists despite a vigorous humoral immune response, possibly because most infected cells are not producing viral antigens and are therefore undetectable by the immune surveillance mechanisms.

Laboratory Diagnosis

In its early stages, visna is difficult to distinguish from other central nervous system (CNS) diseases; however, the progressive protracted course, the absence of fever, and the pleocytosis in the cerebrospinal fluid (CSF) are all characteristic of visna. Tremor of the head, grinding of teeth, and intense itching are more characteristic of scrapie than visna.

Virus can be isolated from CNS, lung, spleen, peripheral blood leukocytes, and CSF, but because of the limited viral replication that occurs in vivo, tissue explantation and blind passage are often required. Group-specific tests that detect antibodies that appear early and are maintained throughout the disease are preferred over serum neutralization for serologic diagnosis. Neutralization tests are of less value in diagnosis because they become positive much later in disease and are strain-specific. Thus, serologic tests such as agar gel immunodiffusion are now used to identify lentivirus-infected sheep and goats.

Treatment and Control

No effective vaccine currently exists and no useful therapeutic agents are available. Control of these viruses and their diseases is by serologic testing and the elimination of infected animals. Visna and maedi were eliminated from Iceland as the result of an eradication program.

Equine Infectious Anemia Virus

Disease

Equine infectious anemia virus (EIAV) can cause severe anemia in horses, but the clinical presentation of EIA is highly variable. In the acute form, signs develop suddenly 7 to 21 days postinfection. Signs can include fever, anorexia, thrombocytopenia, and severe anemia. There may also be profuse sweating and a serous discharge from the nose. Such attacks often last for 3 to 5 days, after which the animal appears to recover. Horses in the acute stage of the disease are seronegative for EIA.

Subacute disease often follows the acute infection after a convalescence of 2 to 4 weeks. Acute signs are repeated along with weakness, edema, petechiae, lethargy, depression, anemia, and ataxia. The animal again appears to recover and the cycle may then recur.

Chronic EIA is the classical presentation of so-called "swamp fever," which resembles the subacute form but is milder and seldom leads to death. The cycle of fever, weight loss, anorexia, and clinical signs can recur six or more times. Each episode usually lasts 3 to 5 days, and the interval between cycles is irregular (weeks to months). The frequency and severity usually decrease after 6 to 8 episodes, usually within the first year. Most horses are then without clinical signs but carry the virus for the remainder of their lives. EIA can be induced by stress or immunosuppressive drugs.

EIAV infection in horses generally results in clinical signs that are inapparent, subclinical, or mild. These horses remain asymptomatic but have antibody to the virus and are lifelong carriers of the virus. Asymptomatic but chronically viremic animals have been observed for periods in excess of 18 years.

Etiologic Agent

Classification

EIAV is a *Lentivirus,* and was the first animal disease to be identified as caused by a filterable virus (1904).

Physical, Chemical, and Antigenic Properties

EIAV is composed of two envelope-encoded glycoproteins (gp 90 = SU and gp 45 = TM) and four major nonglycosylated proteins (p26 = CA, p15 = MA, p11 = NC, and p9). The p26 is the major core protein and demonstrates group specificity, while the envelope-associated glycoproteins demonstrate hemagglutination activity and are type-specific.

The EIAV genome is highly mutable. When the virus is placed under selective pressure by the host immune system, individual nucleotide substitutions (mutations) produce novel antigenic variants of the gp 45 and gp 90 envelope proteins. It is thought that these antigenic variants cause EIA's characteristic episodic recurrence. In cell culture (where there is no immune selection), antigenic types remain stable and neutralizable by serum antibodies from the horse from which the virus was isolated. When introduced into a new horse, these same strains produce new antigenic viral variants that no longer are neutralized by the original antibodies.

Resistance to Physical and Chemical Agents

EIAV is readily inactivated by common disinfectants that contain detergents. The virus is also inactivated by sodium hydroxide, sodium hypochlorite, most organic solvents, and chlorhexidine. EIAV heated in horse serum at 58°C for 30 minutes shows no infectivity for horses. However, at 25°C, EIAV remains infectious on hypodermic needles for 96 hours.

Infectivity for Other Species and Culture Systems

Horses, ponies, donkeys, and mules are susceptible to infection by EIAV. There is only one report of human infection, and no cases of EIA-like disease have been identified. Attempts to propagate the virus in lambs, mice, hamsters, guinea pigs, and rabbits have failed. Primary isolates of EIAV can be propagated only in equine leukocyte cultures, where it grows in cells of the monocyte/macrophage lineage. Laboratory strains of EIAV can be propagated in a variety of cell lines from several species, including human fetal lung fibroblasts. These laboratory strains display significant sequence differences from primary isolates, particularly in the U3 region of the LTR.

Host-Virus Relationship

Distribution, Reservoir, and Transmission

The distribution of EIAV is worldwide but is most prevalent in warm climates. Infection rates vary widely but the disease is increasingly rare in countries such as the United States. Horses, donkeys, and mules are the only known reservoirs and natural hosts of the virus.

Mechanical inoculation of blood is considered the major mode of EIAV transmission. EIAV is naturally transmitted by hematophagous insects, especially deer and stable flies. EIAV does not replicate in the insect cells, but flies can transmit the virus by simple mechanical transfer of infected blood. The transmission of EIAV via blood can also be through contaminated needles; thus it is important not to share needles or use unsterilized needles in veterinary procedures. Viral transmission to the nursing foal from a carrier mare is well documented. EIAV can also be transmitted in utero but this is probably rare.

Pathogenesis and Pathology

Acute EIA is related to massive viral replication. Anemia reflects reduced life span of red blood cells (RBCs) as a consequence of hemolysis and erythrophagocytosis by activated macrophages. A decrease in complement levels and the presence of complement-coated erythrocytes have been observed in EIAV-infected horses. Decreased erythropoiesis levels and pertubations in iron metabolism also contribute to anemia in chronic cases.

Lesions of EIA reflect the duration and severity of infection and disease, and can include widespread hemorrhage and necrosis of lymphatic tissues, anemia, edema, and emaciation. Microscopic lesions include activation of the mononuclear phagocytic system in all lymphoid tissues, activation of Kupffer cells, and hemosiderin deposition in many organs. Immune complex–mediated glomerulonephritis and hepatic centrolobular necrosis are common,

the latter as a consequence of severe, acute-onset anemia. Granulomatous ependymitis, meningitis, choroiditis, subependymal encephalitis, and hydrocephalus are associated with ataxia.

Host Response to Infection

Horses infected with EIAV develop persisting antibody titers within 45 days. Most animals become ELISA-positive within 12 days and AGID-positive within 24 days of infection.

Laboratory Diagnosis

Laboratory diagnosis depends on the detection of specific antibody using an agar gel immunodiffusion test (the Coggins test). More sensitive ELISA tests are also now available.

Treatment and Control

No specific treatments are available. Supportive therapy is the most important factor in recovery.

Affected animals should be either euthanized because the virus is contagious or physically isolated. Spread of EIAV can be reduced by control of stable flies and mosquitoes. Repeated use of hypodermic needles and transfusions from untested donors must be avoided.

Infected stallions should not be bred to seronegative mares, although the reverse need not be true. Uninfected foals can usually be obtained from positive mares and positive stallions if they are isolated from the infected mare and her milk.

A vaccine against EIAV is used in some countries (Cuba, China) but probably does not provide broad protection against all variants of EIAV.

BOVINE IMMUNODEFICIENCY VIRUS

Disease

Despite its provocative name, the significance of bovine immunodeficiency virus (BIV) as a cause of immune dysregulation and chronic inflammation in cattle is uncertain. Unsubstantiated reports implicate BIV as a cause of lethargy, mastitis, pneumonia, lymphadenopathy, and chronic dermatitis, but these reports are viewed with increasing skepticism.

Etiologic Agent

Classification

BIV is a *Lentivirus* that is not closely related to any other known *Lentivirus*.

Physical, Chemical, and Antigenic Properties

The morphology and physical properties of BIV closely resemble those of other lentiviruses. BIV has an SU glycoprotein of 100 kd and a TM glycoprotein of 45 kd, and Gag proteins, MA, CA, and NC, of 16, 26, and 7 kd, respectively. BIV also produces several nonstructural proteins. The RT of BIV has a preference for Mg^{2+}.

Infectivity for Other Species and Culture Systems

Experimental infection of rabbits and sheep with BIV is possible, but these animals do not develop disease. BIV can be cultured in cells from a variety of species, including bovine, rabbit, and canine, but not primates or humans.

Host-Virus Relationship

Distribution, Reservoir, and Transmission

The distribution of BIV is probably worldwide. In the United States, the prevalence of BIV infection is low but may be much higher in individual herds. Herds infected with BIV are often also infected with BLV.

Pathogenesis and Pathology

Cells of the monocyte/macrophage support replication of BIV in infected cattle.

Host Response to Infection

BIV infection in cattle results in a strong host antibody response. However, like most other lentiviruses, BIV induces a chronic lifelong infection. The vast majority of infections are subclinical.

Laboratory Diagnosis

Infected cattle can be detected by serologic tests for antibodies to BIV. BIV isolation from blood can also be used to detect infected animals.

Treatment and Control

There is no vaccine or treatment for BIV infection. The importance of BIV infection as a pathogen of cattle remains most uncertain.

FELINE IMMUNODEFICIENCY VIRUS

Disease

Feline immunodeficiency virus (FIV) infection of cats produces acute fever and lymphadenopathy, followed by an asymptomatic carrier phase. In some cats, FIV infection causes profound immunodeficiency leading to secondary chronic infections. FIV infection of cats shares common features with AIDS of humans, and FIV infection of cats has become an important animal model for AIDS research.

Etiologic Agent

Classification

FIV is a *Lentivirus* that is not closely related to any other known *Lentivirus*.

Physical, Chemical, and Antigenic Properties

The morphology and physical properties of FIV closely resemble those of other lentiviruses. FIV has an SU glycoprotein of 95kd and a TM glycoprotein of 41 kd, and Gag proteins, MA, CA, and NC, of 16, 27, and 10 kd, respectively. FIV also codes for several nonstructural proteins. The RT of FIV has a preference for Mg^{2+}.

Resistance to Physical and Chemical Agents

FIV is inactivated by appropriate concentrations of disinfectants such as chlorine, quaternary ammonium compounds, phenolic compounds, and alcohol. It survives at 60°C for only a few minutes.

Infectivity for Other Species and Culture Systems

FIV infects domestic cats, although there is serologic evidence that FIV-like viruses infect wild *Felidae* in Africa (lions, cheetahs) and the Americas (puma, bobcats, jaguars). FIV isolates replicate in primary cultures of feline mononuclear cultures stimulated to divide with mitogen and supplemented with interleukin-2 (IL-2; T cell growth factor). Some isolates of FIV are also able to replicate in established feline cell lines. FIV does not replicate in nonfeline cell lines. There is no link between FIV and any human disease, including AIDS.

Host-Virus Relationship

Distribution, Reservoir, and Transmission

FIV is endemic in cats throughout the world, although the virus is not as contagious as FeLV. FIV is shed in saliva, and the most important route of transmission is probably through bites. Free-roaming male cats, which are most likely to fight, are most frequently infected with FIV. The virus is not efficiently spread by casual, nonaggressive contact among cats. Sexual contact probably is also not a primary means of spreading FIV. Transmission from an infected queen to her kittens can occur.

Cats remain infected with FIV for life, although the majority of FIV infections are clinically silent.

Dual infection of FIV and FeLV is not uncommon, and cats infected with both FIV and FeLV appear to have a more severe disease course.

Pathogenesis and Pathology

There are no definitive gross or histologic changes in the tissues of FIV-infected cats, even in more advanced stages of disease. Following initial infection, the virus replicates in regional lymph nodes, then spreads to lymph nodes throughout the body, sometimes resulting in a transient generalized lymphadenopathy. Most infections are asymptomatic, whereas lymphoid depletion and immune suppression occur in some cats that are then susceptible to secondary opportunistic infections. FIV appears to infect both CD4 and CD8 lymphocytes, as well as macrophages in vivo. Many cats manifest an absolute decrease in the number of CD4 lymphocytes with an inversion of the CD4/CD8 ratio.

Host Response to Infection

Infected cats typically respond with vigorous humoral (antibody) and cell-mediated immune responses. These responses appear to be sufficient to limit the initial acute phase of the disease. Like most lentiviruses, however, FIV is never eliminated. It probably produces various degrees of subclinical immune dysfunction in the majority, and clinically significant immunodeficiency and associated secondary infections in a minority, of infected cats.

Laboratory Diagnosis

FIV infection is most easily diagnosed by detecting antibodies in the blood. Antibody to FIV can be detected using ELISA tests, Western immunoblotting, and indirect fluorescent antibody (IFA). ELISA is often used as a first screening test, followed by Western blot as a confirmatory test. FIV infection can also be diagnosed by virus isolation and polymerase chain reaction (PCR) to detect FIV nucleic acid.

Young kittens may be antibody positive (and thus have a positive test result) without actually being infected with FIV due to passive transfer of FIV antibodies from their mother.

Treatment and Control

Treatment of FIV-associated disease is largely supportive. Secondary and opportunistic infections are treated with appropriate antimicrobial therapy. Control of FIV infection is by avoiding contact with stray cats and avoiding cat fights. Experimental vaccines appear promising.

SIMIAN IMMUNODEFICIENCY VIRUS

Disease

The simian immunodeficiency virus (SIV) comprises a number of lentiviruses indigenous in many simian species living in the wild in Africa. In their natural African simian hosts, these viruses apparently cause little or no disease. In contrast, the Asian macaques, which are not infected with SIV in the wild, are susceptible to a fatal immunosuppressive syndrome called *simian AIDS* (*SAIDS*) when infected by some strains of SIV.

SIV-infected Asian macaques often develop a transient skin rash soon after infection. Lymph nodes and spleen may be initially enlarged. The architecture of lymph nodes becomes disrupted and eventually atrophies. The main clinical features of SAIDS in Asian macaques are wasting and persistent diarrhea. Opportunistic infections occur and often persist in the immunocompromised monkey. Virtually all Asian macaques infected with pathogenic SIV strains develop fatal SAIDS within 2 months to 3 years.

The fatal immunodeficiency disease caused by SIV in Asian macaques is the major animal model for AIDS in humans. Further, an awareness of the biology of SIV is important for the occupational health of animal caretakers, technicians, and veterinarians who handle monkeys, as well as use of primates in biomedical research and medicine. Artificially generated Simian/Human Immunodeficiency virus (SHIV) strains of virus have been constructed that contain HIV-derived envelope genes with SIV-derived genomes that have been used extensively in the laboratory for studying immunity and pathogenesis to HIV envelope proteins in a nonhuman primate model system.

Etiologic Agent

Classification

The primate lentiviruses exist as a broad continuum. For example, the prototype SIV isolate from Asian macaques (designated SIVmac) is only about 50% related to HIV-1, but is 75% related to HIV-2 based on nucleic acid sequence. Other SIV isolates from chimpanzees (SIVcpz) are much more closely related to HIV-1 than to HIV-2. Further, some SIV isolates from other African primate species are even closer to HIV-2 than is SIVmac. Many isolates of SIV and HIV have been made and their nucleic acids sequenced and classified in phylogenetic trees of sequence relatedness in an effort to understand the origin of AIDS and the diversity and epidemiologic potentials of the primate lentiviruses.

Physical, Chemical, and Antigenic Properties

The morphology and physical properties of SIV closely resemble those of other lentiviruses. SIV has an SU glycoprotein of 120kd and a TM glycoprotein of 32 kd, and Gag proteins, MA, CA, and NC, of 16, 28, and 8 kd, respectively. SIV also codes for several nonstructural proteins that function in regulation of viral expression and accessory functions.

The RT of SIV has a preference for Mg^{2+} and uses $tRNA^{Lys}$ as a primer for negative-strand DNA reverse transcription.

On the basis of seroepidemiologic data, as many as 30 distinct SIV strains may be harbored in their African monkey hosts. The prototype SIVmac strain is antigenically more closely related to HIV-2 than to HIV-1, in agreement with the sequence homology overall. SIV isolated from chimpanzees, SIVcpz, however, is more closely related to HIV-1 than to other SIV types.

Infectivity for Other Species and Culture Systems

SIV isolates replicate in primate (including human) lymphocyte cultures in stimulated cells that have a CD4 receptor. SIV isolates do not replicate in nonprimate cells. Cross-species transmission of SIV to humans is possible and SIV has infected humans in laboratory accidents. HIV is able to infect chimpanzees, although it is not highly pathogenic.

Host-Virus Relationship

Distribution, Reservoir, and Transmission

SIV is carried as an apparently harmless infection in its natural hosts, species of African nonhuman primates (*Cercopithecus*, including African green monkeys, and *Cercocebus*, including sooty mangabeys). The prevalence of infection in both zoos and in the wild is variable, but can be over 50%. In Asian macaques, in which the SIV is not found in nature, SIV produces a fatal immunodeficiency disease that has many features in common with AIDS.

Transmission of SIV is by biting and also by poor veterinary practices or intentionally by experimental protocol. Mother-to-infant and sexual transmission is thought to occur rather inefficiently in nature.

Pathogenesis and Pathology

Asian macaques in the initial stages of illness tend to have hyperplastic lymphoid tissues, whereas lymphoid depletion characterizes later stages of the disease. The types of lesions vary greatly depending on the presence of secondary infections and the stage of disease. SIV persists in both Asian macaques and its natural hosts despite a strong humoral and cellular immune response; however, fatal immunosuppression soon occurs in infected macaques. Neutralization escape mutants arise and become the dominant phenotype. The kinetics of viral infection and alteration of CD4 lymphocytes parallel those observed in human HIV-1 infection and provide reliable markers for disease progression.

Host Response to Infection

Infected monkeys generally respond with vigorous antibody responses and cell-mediated immune responses. These responses appear to be sufficient to limit the initial acute phase of SIV infection. Like most lentiviruses, however, SIV is never eliminated in either its natural host or in Asian macaques.

Laboratory Diagnosis

SIV infection is most easily diagnosed by detecting antibodies in the blood. Antibody to SIV can be detected using indirect fluorescent antibody, Western blots, and ELISA tests. SIV infection can also be diagnosed by virus isolation, detection of viral antigen, and PCR to detect SIV nucleic acid.

Treatment and Control

Experimental vaccines and therapies are being evaluated as part of the current massive efforts in AIDS research and development.

66 Transmissible Spongiform Encephalopathies

BRADD C. BARR   YUAN CHUNG ZEE

Transmissible spongiform encephalopathy (TSE) is the collective term given to a unique group of progressive, uniformly fatal, degenerative, central nervous system (CNS) diseases of humans and animals that share a similar pattern of clinical disease, neuropathology, and etiology. While some human TSEs are inherited or sporadic, most TSEs are infectious diseases that can be transmitted to susceptible hosts. For many years the identification of the infectious cause remained elusive, but Stanley Prusiner postulated in 1982 that an abnormal host protein called a *prion* (derived from *pro*teinaceous *in*fectious particals; abbreviated as PrP^{Res}) was the infectious agent and that propagation of this protein was a post-translational event, not requiring nucleic acid or genetic material. Prusiner's prion hypothesis incorporated mechanisms to explain both the heritable and infectious disease presentations of the TSEs. Since his initial proposal, a large body of exquisite research work by Prusiner, colleagues, and other researchers (working mostly with scrapie) has been amassed that supports his original hypothesis, and Prusiner received the Nobel Prize for this work in 1997. The concept of the prion as an infectious agent is now widely accepted, and few believe that genetic material still may be found. Counter hypotheses include 1) the virion hypothesis, which suggests the infectious organism has a small central core of nucleic acid protected and/or surrounded by protein; and 2) some sort of unconventional virus. Given the vast amount of research work supporting the prion hypothesis, and the apparent lack of data supporting the other hypotheses, the remainder of this discussion is based on the premise that the prion is the infectious etiology for this group of diseases.

TSEs generally have a limited host range. With one apparent exception, the human TSEs are limited to humans (excluding experimental studies). They include two forms of Creutzfeldt-Jakob disease (CJD), Gerstmann-Straussler-Scheinker syndrome (GSS), fatal insomnia (FI), Kuru, and new variant CJD (vCJD), which is the exception because of its relationship with bovine spongiform encephalopathy (BSE). Some of these human TSEs (familial CJD, GSS, and fatal familial insomnia) are inherited, while sporadic CJD occurs spontaneously in a small percentage of humans. The animal TSEs are all considered to be infectious and, with the notable exception of BSE, they have a narrow host range. The animal TSEs and their respective natural hosts include scrapie in sheep and goats, BSE in cattle and other species (exotic ungulate species, felids where it is known as feline spongiform encephalopathy, and compelling evidence to suggest it is also responsible for vCJD), transmissible mink encephalopathy (TME) in mink, and chronic wasting disease (CWD) in deer and elk. While there are many similarities shared by all TSE diseases, there are also salient differences in the behavior of the various TSEs, most notably related to their tissue distribution and detection within hosts, their means of transmission, and very importantly the zoonotic potential of BSE. Scrapie, the prototypical TSE has been studied most extensively.

SCRAPIE

Disease

Scrapie is a chronic, progressive, and uniformly fatal degenerative CNS disease that occurs naturally in only sheep and goats. There is no evidence to indicate that scrapie is a zoonoses. Scrapie occurs throughout the world, with a few exceptions (e.g., Australia, New Zealand). The disease incidence, based on current detection methodology, is low in endemic countries. Scrapie is caused by an abnormal prion protein designated PrP^{Sc} (*Prion Protein, Scrapie*). Within the world's sheep population, there is a varying degree of susceptibility and resistance to scrapie following exposure to PrP^{Sc}. The reasons for this diversity in disease susceptibility are complex and poorly understood, although sheep breed and genotype, as well as PrP^{Sc} strain diversity, likely all play some role. For scrapie the genotype of individual sheep at three specific DNA sites encoding amino acids within the prion protein sequence is a major factor in determining the degree of disease susceptibility and/or resistance. Like all TSEs, scrapie has an extremely long incubation period from infection to the onset of clinical signs, ranging roughly from 24 to 60 months. The progression of clinical signs is directly correlated with the progressive accumulation and spread of PrP^{Sc} throughout the CNS, and is accompanied by a unique pattern of degenerative and vacuolar lesions in the CNS that is shared by all TSEs.

Scrapie is spread by direct contact with infected sheep, probably through oral infection (i.e., ingestion) of PrP^{Sc}. It is also possible that natural infection could occur infrequently by direct inoculation, such as through scarified mucous membranes. Scrapie can be experimentally transmitted by inoculation, including transmission through large volume blood transfusions from infected sheep. This suggests there is a low level of PrP^{Sc} in the blood of scrapie-infected sheep that cannot be detected by other means. Natural contact transmission occurs most frequently when naive sheep or goats are exposed to infected ewes shedding PrP^{Sc} at, or soon after, lambing, and this transmission likely results from the expulsion of PrP^{Sc} infected placenta and/or contaminated fetal/uterine fluids. There is as yet no clear evidence of true vertical transmission (either true genetic transmission or in utero transmission). Lambs appear to be more susceptible to infection than adults. The term "maternal transmission" has been adopted to define transmission from infected ewe to offspring at, or shortly after, lambing and to differentiate it from vertical transmission. Epidemiologic studies suggest that indirect transmission of scrapie also occurs, through exposure to contaminated environments where scrapie-infected sheep have previously been kept. This likely occurs more often where there has been previous high-density confinement of scrapie-infected animals and especially where previous lambing has taken place. One study suggests that scrapie can be transmitted via hay mites in contaminated environments.

The clinical signs of scrapie are progressive and consist of one or more of the following CNS signs: behavioral changes, locomotor problems (incoordination, paresis, proprioceptive limb deficits, hypermetria), mild head or neck tremors, hyperesthesia, and pruritis, often resulting in patchy wool loss from rubbing or biting. Behavioral changes include withdrawal from the flock, nervousness, or aggression. Scrapie-infected sheep also progressively lose body condition. A classic behavior often used to aid in clinical diagnosis of scrapie consists of upward extension of the head and neck with an accompanying licking, nibbling motion, or teeth grinding in response to rubbing the sheep's rump region. However, it should be emphasized that the particular clinical signs seen in any individual infected animal are highly variable.

Etiologic Agent

It is generally accepted that the etiology of scrapie is a prion, an abnormal isoform of a normal host protein of sheep (PrP^{Sc}). PrP^{Sc} is very similar in its size and shares many similarities in its amino acid sequence and biochemical physicochemical properties to abnormal prion proteins responsible for other TSEs. Much of the following expanded discussion of PrP^{Sc} (and scrapie) also holds true for other abnormal prions and the respective disease they cause. In the following discussion the abbreviation *PrP^{Res}* (referring to "resistant" PrP) will be used to reference all abnormal prion proteins as a group, and *PrP^{Sc}* to reference the specific abnormal prions causing scrapie.

Prion Origin, Structure, and Biochemistry

PrP^{Res} is derived from normal cellular proteins ("cellular prion protein" or PrP^{C}) that are found in multiple tissues

of all mammalian species. They are cell membrane-associated proteins found as a constituent part of a larger surface sialoglycoprotein. PrP^{C} is a 35–36 kDa protein that is especially abundant in the CNS (approximately 50 times more than other tissues) within neurons and glial cells. It also occurs in cells of the mononuclear phagocytic system (macrophages, dendritic cells, follicular dendritic cells). The precise function of PrP^{C} is uncertain. Possible functions include aspects of copper metabolism, interactions with the extracellular matrix, and apoptosis and signal transduction. PrP^{C} does not cause disease. PrP^{Res}s are identical in amino acid sequence and length to PrP^{C} of the host species where they have replicated, and differ only in their secondary and tertiary spatial conformation from their originating PrP^{C}. The tertiary conformational change in PrP^{Res} is the putative basis for transformation into an infectious pathogen that propagates and spreads within host tissues to cause disease. PrP^{Res} has a protease-resistant core (27–30 KDa; 142 amino acids) designated PrP27-30, which has been found in brains from humans and animals with prion diseases. This smaller portion of the PrP^{Res} retains infectivity. An even smaller segment of the PrP^{Res}, consisting of only 106 amino acids, is sufficient for replication of PrP^{Res}. These smaller segments of PrP^{Res} are termed miniprions. The PrP27–30 segment of PrP^{C} is derived from a single copy mammalian gene in humans and animals (PRNP and Prnp, respectively). While the precise nature of these structural changes between PrP^{C} and PrP^{Res} is difficult to determine, the central feature thought to be responsible for the physicochemical and infectious transformation of PrP^{Res} is a change in the portion of an alphahelical and coil structure of PrP^{C} to a larger percentage of refolded and rigid beta-pleated sheets in PrP^{Res} (the percentage of beta-pleated sheets increases from 3% to 43% with the transformation to PrP^{Res}). Once in a susceptible host, the propagation of new PrP^{Res} occurs by a post-translational event (not involving DNA or RNA), whereby existent host PrP^{C} is transformed to PrP^{Res}. Experimental evidence suggests that the PrP^{Res} actually serves as a physical template for refolding of PrP^{C} when the latter approximates the PrP^{Res} template. The process also appears to require the presence of a second species-specific host protein ("X") that binds to PrP^{C} and facilitates the transformation to new PrP^{Res}. Once completed, the new PrP^{Res} releases from the template and can then serve as a new template for further propagation of PrP^{Res}. In the case of inherited TSEs of humans, mutations or insertions in the human PRNP gene are postulated to cause the resultant altered PrP^{C} to spontaneously convert to new PrP^{Res}.

Biochemically, PrP^{C} is labile and can be destroyed relatively easily by a variety of insults, such as enzyme destruction and heat. In contrast PrP^{Res} is very resistant to insults like enzyme digestion, heat, ultraviolet light, ionizing radiation, acids, bases, certain autoclaving procedures, formalin fixation, and disinfectants. Because of the resistance of PrP^{Res} to destruction or inactivation, effective procedures to inactivate PrP^{Res}s are extremely limited in number and very severe in nature, including autoclaving at 134–138°C for 18 minutes for porous-load and gravity-displacement autoclaving, autoclaving at 132°C for 1 hour, exposure to 1N NaOH for 1 hour, or both. One authority suggests that the only means to effectively achieve complete decontamination involves either exposure of PrP^{Res} to strong sodium hypochlorite solutions or to hot solutions of NaOH. This resistance to destruction explains the potential longevity of PrP^{Res} in the environment. It also allows for transmission of the TSEs even through contaminated feeds that are cooked or processed, as well as transmission through the use of inadequately autoclaved and contaminated surgical instruments, or via human/veterinary biologicals derived from tissues or fluids harvested from infected animals/humans.

Evidence suggests that not all PrP^{Sc} causing scrapie is the same; rather, there are multiple PrP^{Sc} strains. Initially, PrP^{Sc} strains were discovered through experimental inoculation studies in laboratory animals where differences were noted in the laboratory animal susceptibility profile, disease incubation periods, and the CNS lesion profile within these laboratory animals. Similar differences have also been noted following experimental transmission studies in sheep.

Host-Prion Relationship

The host-prion relationships for scrapie and other TSEs are complex, as expected with diseases caused by infectious agents that actually represent modification of the host proteins.

Host Genetic Polymorphisms

The susceptibility of sheep to contract scrapie following PrP^{Sc} exposure appears to be controlled by a poorly understood complex of factors that include the sheep genotype (referred to as its genetic polymorphism), the strain of the scrapie PrP^{Sc} to which it is exposed, and other poorly understood factors such as sheep breed. One major factor that affects both the incubation period and the susceptibility of sheep to scrapie is the sheep's genetic makeup at codons 136, 154, and 171 of the PrP gene. Each possible genotype at these sites is referred to as a genetic polymorphism. At codon 136, valine (V) is associated with susceptibility and alanine (A) with resistance. At codon 154, histidine (H) is linked to susceptibility and arginine (R) with resistance, and at codon 171, glutamine (Q) and histidine (H) are associated with susceptibility and arginine (R) with resistance. Of the possible polymorphic combinations at these three codons, only five have been found with any frequency in nature, including: $A_{136}R_{154}R_{171}$, $A_{136}R_{154}Q_{171}$, $A_{136}H_{154}Q_{171}$, $A_{136}R_{154}H_{171}$, and $V_{136}R_{154}Q_{171}$. Codon 171 appears to be the most significant in determining sheep susceptibility or resistance, at least within North America, while codon 136 is next in importance and codon 154 seems to be less of a factor. In particular the Q/Q polymorphism at codon 171 is linked with a high degree of susceptibility for scrapie, while Q/R and R/R polymorphisms at codon 171 are associated with resistance to scrapie. In North America, scrapie is diagnosed most commonly in sheep with the Q/Q polymorphism at codon 171. Scrapie has only been very rarely diagnosed in Suffolk sheep with the Q/R polymorphism at codon 171, and only one

scrapie-positive Suffolk sheep has ever been diagnosed with the R/R polymorphism at codon 171. Further data suggests that when scrapie sheep are found with the Q/R polymorphism at codon 171, these sheep also are more likely to have the A/V polymorphism at codon 136. In North America, the "United States Department of Agriculture scrapie flock clean up program" has used these genetic susceptibility patterns to establish criteria for removal or movement-restriction of scrapie-exposed sheep. The criteria are based first on determining the polymorphism of the positively diagnosed scrapie-infected sheep. This helps establish information on the potential strain of scrapie present. Once the scrapie-infected genotype pattern is known, criteria are established for removal or restriction of remaining sheep in the flock with susceptible genetic polymorphisms, as a means for disease eradication. These criteria are lengthy and complex, but salient features include the following: If positive scrapie sheep are Q/Q at codon 171, all remaining Q/Q sheep in the flock are removed or under restricted movement. In rare instances where scrapie is diagnosed in a Q/R sheep, it has been found almost entirely in sheep with A/V_{136} Q/R_{171} polymorphisms. Therefore if scrapie infections are detected in A/V_{136} Q/R_{171} sheep, then all A/V_{136} Q/R_{171} sheep, in addition to the Q/Q_{171} sheep, are targeted for removal or restricted movement.

PrP genetic polymorphisms are also documented in goats, although there is much less data regarding the impact of specific polymorphisms on susceptibility/resistance of goats to scrapie.

Prion Strains

Data from various animal studies indicates that strains of prions can exist within a single prion disease. Only one strain however has been identified for many prion diseases. Different strains of scrapie are reported. The data supporting different PrP^{Res} strains initially came from two observations: experimental inoculation of different PrP^{Sc} isolates into susceptible hosts resulted in variable disease incubation times and the brain lesions induced by these isolates also differed in both distribution and nature. Subsequent studies have shown that these isolates consist of different isoforms of the PrP^{Res}, although the specific factors responsible for "strain" differences are unclear. The strain of prion, which seems to be enciphered in the conformation of PrP^{Sc}, conspires with the PrP sequence, which is specified by the recipient, to determine the tertiary structure of the nascent PrP^{Sc}. This infers that each strain has a unique tertiary structure, but also suggests that the affect each strain has on a host is dependent to some degree on the PrP^{C} amino acid sequence of the host, which is dictated by the host genome, and which takes part in determining the final conformational structure of the PrP^{Res}.

Scrapie Disease Pathogenesis

The putative pathogenesis of scrapie includes the following: PrP^{Sc} is first detected in follicular dendritic cells and macrophages within the tonsils and gut-associated lymphoid tissues (GALT; especially ileal Peyer's Patches) after oral exposure of genetically susceptible sheep. PrP^{Sc} multiplies at these sites and then spreads through the lymph vascular system to peripheral lymph tissues, including the spleen, and numerous lymph nodes where it is next detected. PrP^{Sc} may be detected at this time in the retropharyngeal lymph nodes and in lymph follicles of the third eyelids of sheep. PrP^{Sc} also is found in spinal ganglia of the autonomic nervous system, the adjacent thoracic spinal cord, and in the dorsal vagal nucleus of the vagus nerve within the caudal brain stem. This early CNS invasion likely occurs through invasion of nerve endings within the lymph follicles of the ileum or elsewhere in the gastrointestinal tract and travels through these nerves of the autonomic nervous system and vagus nerve to the thoracic cord and vagal nucleus of the brain stem, respectively. Once within the CNS, the PrP^{Sc} multiplies and spreads. The increased PrP^{Sc} production within the CNS is directly related to the progressive development of CNS degenerative lesions and the onset of clinical signs.

There is no humoral or cellular immune response to the PrP^{Sc} because the protein is identical in its amino acid sequence to the host PrP^C. Thus, there is no serum antibody test to allow for antemortem detection of exposure, and cellular infiltrates are not present within the CNS of affected sheep. Lesions associated with scrapie or any other TSE are found only within the CNS (aside from secondary lesions such as hair loss). These lesions are bilateral in distribution and limited to the gray matter areas. They consist of three basic changes: spongiform change, which refers to vacuolation within the neuropil of gray matter that represents intracytoplasmic vacuolation of nerve processes; neuronal degeneration/loss, which includes intracytoplasmic vacuolation of neurons, shrunken, dark, angular neurons, rare necrotic neurons, and neuronal loss; and astrocytosis or the hypertrophy and hyperplasia of astrocytes within the gray matter (see Fig 71.4). The lesions occur first in the caudal brain stem and progress from there to other regions of the brain stem, cerebellum, and cerebral cortex. PrP^{Sc} can be illustrated even prior to detection of CNS lesions by the use of immunohistochemistry. The PrP^{Sc} deposits around and within neurons and glial cells within the neuropil.

Recent studies in pregnant scrapie-infected sheep indicate that fetal genetic susceptibility plays a major role regarding both maternal transmission of infection to the fetus and the potential spread of scrapie within a flock. The results indicate that in utero fetal infection does not occur in infected ewes. However, the fetal membranes can become infected with PrP^{Sc} during gestation, serving as a source for shedding of PrP^{Sc} into the environment both at and for some time after lambing. Whether the placenta becomes infected is controlled by the fetal genetic polymorphism. As an example, PrP^{Sc} was found in placenta of infected ewes where the fetal genotype was QQ at codon 171 but was not detected in the placenta if the fetus was a resistant QR genotype at codon 171. At lambing, placental PrP^{Sc} is a high risk source for infection, and very young lambs with susceptible genetic polymorphisms are at the highest risk for infection. The reason for this increased susceptibility of young animals is unknown, but it is theo-

rized that the more developed GALT in young animals (which atrophies in older animals) may be responsible.

Cross Species Barriers

For most TSEs, the susceptible host species range is very limited and specific. The barrier limiting cross species transmission is termed the *cross species barrier*. Experimentally, these cross species barriers can often be overcome, albeit with some difficulty. The factors that are used to promote transmission across these barriers are direct intracerebral inoculation of the candidate PrP^{Res} into the resistant host species and multiple serial passages of infected CNS tissue through the resistant species. The exact basis for these species barriers is poorly understood and probably very complex, but contributing factors known to affect the species barrier include:

1. The degree of homology in the amino acid sequence of the donor and recipient of PrP. This genetically determined host PrP^C amino acid sequence is important as it is thought to have a direct affect on the ability of PrP^C to refold in a manner that mimics the PrP^{Res} tertiary conformation.
2. The strain of prion. As mentioned above this is enciphered in the conformation of the PrP^{Res}.
3. The species specificity of the helper "X" protein. This may also be an important determinant in the species barrier.

As a side note, evidence now suggests that the process of experimentally adapting the candidate PrP^{Res} across the previous cross species barrier actually creates resultant modifications of the original PrP^{Res}, and thus essentially creates a new strain of PrP^{Res}. For this reason, PrP^{Res} isolates are now designated not only according to their original natural host, but also by any species through which it has been adapted experimentally.

Subclinical Carriers of Infection

There is some experimental evidence to suggest that, under certain circumstances, and with certain PrP^{Res}s from certain TSEs, PrP^{Res} infections can result in subclinical carriers that do not develop disease. In addition, it may be very difficult to detect the PrP^{Res} in these carriers except by bioassay. As an example, experimental infection across the species barriers in rodents may require multiple serial passages through that rodent species. In such instances following initial inoculation of the resistant host, the PrP^{Res} may not be detected, and the host may live its entire life without contracting a TSE. However, when brain material from such a host is subsequently serially passed through that same species, a TSE disease may eventually result as the cross species barrier adaptation results.

Laboratory Diagnosis

Several diagnostic tests for prion disease have been developed for specific detection of PrP^{Res} in tissues. These tests rely on the use of polyclonal or monoclonal antibodies to the PrP protein. Since these antibodies cannot differentiate between PrP^C and PrP^Res, the test methodologies utilize the biochemical differences between PrP^C and PrP^Res to first destroy the PrP^C epitopes using digestion or denaturing procedures (i.e., proteinase K or formic acid digeston, and/or denaturation by autoclaving), leaving only PrP^Res with its intact antigenic epitopes. This group of tests, which includes immunohistochemistry (IHC) and enzyme-linked immunosorbent assay (ELISA) methodologies, has been utilized successfully for detection of PrP^Res in a variety of TSE diseases.

Scrapie can be diagnosed antemortem by immunohistochemical (IHC) detection of PrP^Sc in third eyelid biopsies. The biopsy consists of a small aggregate of the lymphoid follicles that can be visualized and excised on the inner surface of the third eyelid. A negative test result does not completely ensure the animal is scrapie free for the following reasons: the animal may be in the early incubation stages of infection, or represent one of the small percentage of clinically affected sheep where PrP^Sc is not present/detected in lymph tissue prior to CNS infection; or there may not be sufficient lymphoid tissue present (this seems to occur more in very aged animals and possibly in some sheep breeds more than others).

The postmortem diagnosis in clinically affected animals is often made by histopathologic evaluation of the brain (see Fig 71.4). The extent of the lesions, and therefore the accuracy in diagnosis through routine histology, is directly related to the severity of the clinical disease at death.

Treatment and Control

There is no treatment available for scrapie, so the disease is handled by prevention, control, or eradication. In North America there is a federally regulated program to eradicate the disease, which includes:

1. A "Scrapie Flock Certification Program" that monitors flock disease status over an extended period with the goal of assigning status to flocks with no evidence of scrapie. The program has requirements for individual animal identification, record keeping, reporting, and restrictions on flock additions to ensure scrapie is not introduced into flocks free from detectable scrapie.
2. The eradication of scrapie through disease surveillance, and diagnosis, identification of infected/exposed flocks, elimination of positive or susceptible/exposed animals, and monitoring of sheep movement to control potential spread of scrapie and to allow for successful trace-back from positively diagnosed animals to their flocks of origin.

Within an individual flock, determination of the flock status and strict limitations on the addition of new animals are the best means for prevention and control. Initial determination of the flock status can best be obtained through the Scrapie Flock Certification Program. Maintenance of a disease-free flock is achieved by maintaining a closed flock, particularly a closed ewe flock. If new introductions are to be made, care should be taken to ensure that new additions come from flocks with disease-free status as can best be determined (often difficult). Third eyelid testing of animals over 14 months of age can be considered in making this assessment but is not foolproof. Genotype testing to select for new additions with resistant genotypes is also useful, although research has not eliminated the possibility of a resistant genotype carrier animal. The feeding of ruminant meat and bonemeal to ruminants is prohibited in many countries.

BOVINE SPONGIFORM ENCEPHALOPATHY

Disease

Bovine spongiform encephalopathy (BSE or "mad cow disease") is a chronic, progressive, and uniformly fatal degenerative CNS disease that occurs naturally in cattle, exotic ungulates, and domestic and exotic felids, and is the likely cause of vCJD, a newly recognized TSE in humans. BSE emerged as a newly recognized TSE in England in 1986. The incidence of BSE in cattle rapidly increased, largely in dairy cattle throughout the United Kingdom (U.K.) over the next few years. Shortly thereafter, additional new TSE diseases were then recognized in both captive exotic ungulates and felids from zoos in England, and also in domestic cats in the U.K. Experimental studies and characterization of the PrP^Res from this latter group of prion diseases established that PrP^BSE was the cause, indicating that BSE, unlike other TSEs, had an unusually wide susceptible host range. Significantly, vCJD also emerged in a small number of young human patients in England at the same time. Unlike sporadic CJD, vCJD occurs in humans at a much younger age and has a different time course, EEG pattern, and pattern of clinical CNS signs. Sheep, pigs, primates (macaques), marmosets, lemurs, and mice are experimentally susceptible to BSE infection, although natural occurrence of disease has not been described in these species. Sheep are susceptible experimentally to oral inoculation with BSE, which raises substantial concerns as to how it would be differentiated from scrapie. Because of the association with vCJD, BSE is considered a major threat to public health, which is the basis for national eradication programs in all countries where it exists, and extensive national surveillance and prevention programs in countries where the disease does not.

Following the widespread detection of BSE in the U.K., cases of BSE occurred in other countries through the export of infected meat and bonemeal, infected live animals, and possibly other infected animal products. As of August 2003 a total of 23 countries had reported cases of BSE. These include several countries in Europe, as well as Japan, Israel, and Canada.

Epidemiologic analyses strongly suggest that the primary mode of natural BSE transmission is through the ingestion of contaminated meat and bonemeal containing infected offal. Horizontal transmission from animal to animal does not occur to any significant extent. Young cattle appear more susceptible to infection than adults, and there is an increased risk for BSE among calves born from BSE-affected cows, suggesting a low level of maternally associated transmission. However the mechanism responsible for this increased calf risk is unknown (i.e., what role does direct cow-to-calf maternal infection vs. genetic predisposition vs. feed-borne exposure play?). There is no strong evidence to suggest transmission from a contaminated environment, although the occurrence of a small number of new BSE cases in the U.K. following the enforced animal protein feed ban in animals born after August 1, 1996 is disconcerting.

The initial source of the infected material responsible for the emergence of BSE in the U.K. may never be known. Two theories have been offered to explain the emergence of BSE: 1) BSE arose from the feeding of meat and bonemeal containing sheep offal contaminated with scrapie to cattle or 2) BSE arose from a single spontaneous case of BSE in cattle that was then rendered and fed as contaminated meat and bonemeal to other cattle. A third theory—that BSE arose from the feeding of infected offal from some other mammalian species—has also been proposed. Epidemiologic evidence suggests that a change in the rendering process in England in the late 1970s may have allowed for increased survival of PrP^{Res}s, regardless of the source (offal from infected sheep, bovine, or other species), increasing exposure of cattle to these PrP^{Res}s. Additional epidemiologic data supporting scrapie as the initial source for BSE include the following: the sheep population increased significantly in the 1980s, when BSE likely emerged, possibly increasing the prevalence of endemic scrapie in the U.K.; and meat and bonemeal was a cheap feed source listed for dairy calf starter feeds. However, it is difficult to explain by these point source theories (whether it arose initially from scrapie-infected sheep or a BSE-infected cow) how BSE simultaneously emerged at multiple sites in the U.K., unless this single source was widely distributed. Once BSE infections were established in the cattle population, transmission could be easily amplified by repeated recycling of BSE-infected bovine tissue into meat and bonemeal fed to cattle. BSE soon reached epidemic proportions in the U.K. The epidemic peaked in 1992–93 with 37,280 cases diagnosed in 1992. Disease eradication and prevention programs that were established (see "Treatment and Control," below) have been successful in greatly reducing the numbers of cases. Transmission of BSE to felids and exotic ungulates is thought to have occurred through feeding of infected animal protein, and although the source for vCJD (human) is not proven, ingestion of contaminated animal products is considered the most likely source.

BSE has a long incubation period with a mean incubation period of 4–5 years. Clinical signs include a loss of condition or weight loss, coupled with one more CNS signs that include behavioral changes (apprehension, fear, easily startled, depression), hyperesthesia, hyperreflexia, muscle fasciculations, tremors, myoclonus, ataxia, hypermetria, pruritis, and autonomic dysfunctions (reduced rumination, bradycardia).

Etiologic Agent

BSE is caused by PrP^{BSE} prion with physicochemical properties common to all abnormal prions. Only one strain of BSE (PrP^{BSE}) has been identified. Unlike scrapie, susceptibility to BSE has not yet been associated with any cattle PrP gene polymorphisms. There are no detectable differences in age susceptibility or incubation periods reported for various cattle breeds. PrP^{BSE} has not been found in sheep naturally infected with scrapie, although the potential risk of BSE-infected sheep is recognized. No strains of PrP^{Sc} have been found that are similar to PrP^{BSE}, although the number of strain comparisons has been limited.

Host-Prion Relationship

While polymorphisms in the PrP gene of cattle have been identified, there is no evidence suggesting these polymorphisms have an affect on disease susceptibility. Unlike scrapie, PrP^{BSE} is not readily detected in lymph tissues prior to the onset of CNS infectivity and clinical disease. PrP^{BSE} has been detected only in the CNS (brain and spinal cord) and retina of naturally infected cattle. Experimental studies indicate that it does track through lymph tissues, but it is detected inconsistently and in relatively small amounts as compared to scrapie. The following is a brief summary of experimental studies in cattle.

Following oral inoculation of cattle, PrP^{BSE} is first detected in lymphoid follicles of the distal ileum at 6 months postinoculation (PI). It can be occasionally found in the ileum at later PI dates. It also has been detected in the tonsil between 6–14 months PI in one study. It is first detected in the CNS and dorsal root ganglia at 32 months PI, followed by trigeminal ganglia at 36 months PI. PrP^{BSE} has not been detected in either retropharyngeal, mesenteric, or popliteal lymph nodes of naturally infected cattle. Within the CNS, it progressively accumulates and is associated with degenerative CNS lesions that are generally similar to other TSEs. As with other TSEs, there is no immunologic response to the PrP^{BSE} by the host.

Laboratory Diagnosis

There is no antemortem test currently available for diagnosis of BSE. Postmortem diagnostic tests on the brain are available that are similar to those for scrapie (immunohistochemistry, ELISA, and western blot tests on CNS, not lymph tissue). These tests are utilized in BSE-infected countries as part of their national eradication programs. Routine histopathology of the brain of clinically affected animals will show lesions compatible with BSE, but confirmation of the diagnosis requires confirmatory testing. In the United States, a national surveillance program for BSE is conducted by Animal Plant Health Inspection Service (APHIS) of the United States Department of Agriculture (USDA). The surveillance samples include field cases of cattle exhibiting neurologic disease, cattle condemned at slaughter for neurologic reasons, rabies-negative cattle submitted to public health laboratories, neurologic cases submitted to veterinary diagnostic laboratories and teaching hospitals, cattle that are "nonambulatory" ("downers"), and cattle dying on farms.

Treatment and Control

There is no treatment for BSE. Countries with confirmed BSE cases are attempting to eradicate it, and countries where it is not present institute preventative/surveillance programs to prevent its occurrence. In the U.K., a series of key regulatory measures were taken by the government to stop the food-borne transmission of BSE. These measures, coupled with detection, diagnosis, and eradication programs have proven to be very successful in stemming the epidemic and drastically reducing the number of bovine cases. The first of these measures was a ban on the use of meat and bonemeal in ruminant feed in July of 1988. This was followed in September of 1990 by a further ban on the use of specified bovine offal in feed stuffs of any species; these were bovine tissues thought to harbor the highest concentration of infective material. While these measures resulted in a reduction in new cases, evidence suggested that new feed-borne cases continued in animals, and in March 1996, the feed ban was extended to a total ban on the use of mammalian proteins in feed produced for any farm animals.

CHRONIC WASTING DISEASE

Disease

Chronic Wasting Disease (CWD) is a fatal chronic progressive degenerative CNS disease of mule deer, white tail deer, and elk that is found primarily in North America. There are no reported human TSE cases associated with CWD. CWD was first diagnosed in 1967 in Colorado. The disease was subsequently recognized as an endemic disease in deer and elk in an area that encompassed portions of Colorado, Wyoming, and Nebraska. The range and incidence of the disease began to increase after 1990. The reasons for this sudden spread are not clear, but both unique features of the disease and the husbandry of captive cervids likely contributed. CWD can spread laterally via direct contact transmission, in distinct contrast to BSE where contact transmission does not appear to occur. The lateral transmission of CWD appears to be even more efficient than that of scrapie. The source of the shedding PrP^{CWD} from infected animals and mode of inoculation of uninfected animals are not known, although oral inoculation is considered the most likely route of natural infection. Modeling studies suggest that lateral transmission through shedding of PrP^{CWD} probably begins even before the onset of clinical signs in infected deer and elk. CWD spreads from infected to uninfected deer or elk when comingled in confined surroundings. In addition to direct contact transmission, indirect transmission from contaminated pastures or paddocks occurs, and this indirect transmission also appears to be more efficient than is reported with scrapie. This relative ease of both direct and indirect contact transmission likely explains the very high prevalence of CWD in some infected captive herds (more than 90% of mule deer over a 2-year period in one herd). The prevalence of CWD in free-ranging cervids from endemic areas can also be high (<1–15%).

Aside from the relative ease of transmission, geographical spread of the disease has also been facilitated through transportation of farmed deer and elk between farms. In North America (as of 2002), the disease had been detected in free-ranging deer in Colorado, Wyoming, Nebraska, Wisconsin, South Dakota, New Mexico, Illinois, and Saskatchewan, Canada, and in farmed cervids in South Dakota, Nebraska, Colorado, Oklahoma, Kansas, Minnesota, Montana, Wisconsin, and the Canadian provinces of Alberta and Saskatchewan. It has also been diagnosed in farmed cervids exported to the Republic of Korea. Maternal transmission may occur (there apparently is no direct evidence whether maternal transmission does or does not occur), although modeling studies suggest that CWD epidemics cannot be explained solely by maternal transmission. In the wild, it is possible that transmission might also occur from decay of CWD-infected carcasses, with release of the PrP^{CWD} into the environment through scavenging, and maggots, exposing foraging cervids.

Experimental CWD infections have been documented in cattle, sheep, and goats, but only following intracerebral inoculation. There appears to be a substantial species barrier between these host species and infection with PrP^{CWD}. Natural transmission from deer or elk to these species has not been documented. There is no evidence of experimental transmission to cattle either by direct contact or oral inoculation more than five years following exposure.

Based on examination of natural cases, CWD is thought to have a minimum incubation period of 16–17 months, which is an appreciably shorter incubation period than either scrapie or BSE. The clinical signs in deer or elk with CWD include loss of body condition and one or more of the following CNS abnormalities: behavioral changes (changes in interactions with handlers, walking patterns, depression, lowered head and ears), polydipsia, polyuria, increased salivation or drooling, incoordination, ataxia, head tremors, wide-based stance, and hyperexcitability. However, because clinical signs may not be observed in free-ranging deer, the salient findings at necropsy may include loss of condition and death due to aspiration pneumonia, possibly due to dysphagia or ptyalism.

Etiology

CWD is caused by the PrP^{CWD} prion, which has physicochemical properties similar to other abnormal prions. The origin of PrP^{CWD} will probably never be known, but might include a spontaneous mutation in a cervid or cross species adaptation following initial exposure of deer or elk to scrapie. Strain-typing studies in mice indicate that PrP^{CWD} is unique from several strains of scrapie, BSE, and Transmissible Mink Encephalopathy (TME) agents. There is no current information regarding PrP^{CWD} strains.

Host-Prion Relationship

Multiple deer PrP gene polymorphisms have been described, but the affects of these polymorphisms on disease susceptibility is unknown. The rather uniform CWD susceptibility noted in captive deer would suggest that resistant genotypes, if present, are infrequent.

Like scrapie, PrP^{CWD} is readily detectable in lymphoid tissues throughout the body of infected deer and elk, and the pathogenesis of tissue distribution shares many similarities to scrapie. Following oral exposure, PrP^{CWD} is detected first in lymph tissues prior to detection in the brain. Experimentally it has been found in the Peyer's patches of the ileum, ileocecal lymph node, tonsil, and retropharyngeal lymph node by 42 days after infection. It is first detected in the brain within the dorsal nucleus of the vagus nerve located in the caudal brain stem (obex), similar to scrapie. In one study, PrP^{CWD} was first detected in the obex 3 months following first detection in the GALT. Lesions specific for CWD are confined to the CNS and are similar in overall nature to other TSEs.

Laboratory Diagnosis

There is no antemortem diagnostic test for CWD. Postmortem diagnostic tests available are similar to those used for scrapie, and some of the monoclonal antibodies used for detection of scrapie in the United States also are utilized for detection of PrP^{CWD}. A presumptive diagnosis can also be made based on routine histopathology in clinically affected animals if sufficient CNS lesion development has occurred. Confirmation of the diagnosis through additional tests confirms the diagnosis.

Treatment and Control

There is no treatment for CWD. The long incubation period, resistant etiologic agent, absence of reliable ante-mortem diagnostic tests, and incomplete understanding of the mode of transmission all complicate efforts to control or eradicate CWD. Quarantine and depopulation of affected herds are primary means for control in farmed facilities. Even with depopulation of infected farmed facilities, there is concern of reinfection following placement of new uninfected stock, due to possible environmental contamination. There also are concerns for spread from infected farmed facilities to contiguous free-ranging populations across fence lines or, conversely, from endemic-free populations to farmed facilities. An active, efficient surveillance program is therefore recommended in farmed facilities, not only to identify and remove infected animals, but also to prevent movement of infected animals to other farmed facilities. Management of free-ranging populations is even more problematic. Current management involves active surveillance to determine prevalence, coupled with containment and reduction of prevalence through culling in focused endemic areas. Human-facilitated relocation, or feeding of free-ranging cervids, is banned in endemic areas. Selective culling of clinical animals by itself has not significantly affected prevalence in endemic areas. A program of localized population reduction in Colorado has been instituted, but the effectiveness of this program has yet to be determined. It is thought that an aggressive program of selective culling or general population reduction may be effective in regions where new cases of free-ranging infection are detected early, and prior to establishment of endemic population infections. The potential for transport of hunter-killed infected carcasses to uninfected areas and subsequent contamination of these new environments via discarded infected offal also represents a significant concern for potential spread of CWD to new regions. There is a USDA program currently in place to eradicate CWD from farmed elk operations in the United States.

PART IV

Clinical Applications

67

Circulatory System and Lymphoid Tissues

RICHARD L. WALKER

The circulatory system includes the blood-vascular and lymphatic systems. The blood-vascular system is composed of the heart, arteries, capillaries, veins, and components of blood itself. Infections involving the pericardial sac, which encloses the heart, are also included in this chapter. The lymphatic system includes lymphatic capillaries, afferent lymphatic vessels that drain interstitial fluid and cells from tissues, lymph nodes, and efferent lymphatics that recirculate lymph and cells (primarily lymphocytes) from lymph nodes to the blood-vascular system. Because of the functional association with and cellular trafficking through the circulatory system, infections involving other lymphoid tissues (spleen, bone marrow, and thymus) are included in this chapter. Mucosa-associated lymphoid tissues, although less organized, are included with other lymphoid tissues. The role of mucosa-associated lymphoid tissues in immune surveillance and as potential entry sites for some pathogens into the host are specifically discussed in those chapters on systems where they are found or chapters covering specific agents involved.

While functionally similar, there are anatomic differences in the organization of lymphoid tissues of animals and birds. Birds possess a Bursa of Fabricius, a lymphoepithelial organ, which is dorsal to and communicates with the cloaca. It is a primary lymphoid organ serving as the main site of B lymphocyte differentiation. For the most part, poultry do not have lymph nodes but rather rely on cecal tonsils, Peyer patches, and Meckel's diverticulum in the intestines; lymphoid follicles in various organs; the spleen; and a special paranasal concentration of lymphoid tissue (Harderian gland) for secondary immune functions.

Antimicrobial Properties

Phagocytic cells in the spleen and liver provide the primary defense for the vascular system by removing potential pathogens from circulation. Depending on the location in the vascular system and severity of injury caused directly by an infectious agent or its toxin or as a result of the subsequent inflammatory response, ability to repair damage is variable. Cardiac muscle has little regenerative capability following infectious processes that result in myocardial cell death. Such injury leads to scar formation. Injuries to small vessels that destroy endothelial cells can result in thrombus formation in those vessels. Unaffected vascular endothelial cells at the periphery of the lesion are able to proliferate and reendothelialize those areas that affected vessels supplied.

The lymphoid tissue plays a major role in defense of the body from infection. It is central to the development of the animal's immune system (primary lymphoid tissues) and plays an ongoing role in immune surveillance and defense. Details on mechanisms of immune defense provided by lymphoid tissues are covered in Chapter 2. Because of the surveillance role it plays, lymphoid tissue is exposed to numerous potentially pathogenic microbes, which if not contained may involve the lymphoid tissue in the disease process or cause a systemic infection.

Transient and Persistent Microbes

As a rule, the circulatory system and lymphoid tissues are not recognized to have a normal microbial flora. Transient bacteremias do occur, often as a result of traumatic or invasive events (e.g., dental extractions, endoscopic procedures of the digestive tract, and urethral catheterization) or subsequent to treatments that compromise mucosal barriers (e.g., chemotherapy, radiation therapy). This allows normal mucosal inhabitants to enter the bloodstream. Chronic conditions, such as severe gingival disease, that compromise the normal host barriers may also lead to spontaneous bacteremia. In some instances, no predisposing event or condition is recognized to account for a bacteremic episode. The resulting bacteremia is usually transient, lasting only a short period of time (less than 30 minutes) before removal by phagocytes in the liver and spleen. Not all microorganisms appear to be removed that rapidly and may persist in the vascular system for longer periods. For example, a persistent but subclinical bacteremia with *Bartonella* species occurs in some cats. Bacteremias can serve as a source of microorganisms for serious infections of the circulatory system (e.g., infectious endocarditis, bacterial sepsis).

Microscopic and molecular-based studies suggest that the bloodstream may in fact be colonized with specific microbes rather than just being periodically exposed to organisms through transient bacteremias, and that these "residents" persist in the blood in a benign fashion. However, evidence that a true normal microbial flora of the bloodstream exist remains to be conclusively demonstrated.

Some viruses, particularly retroviruses, persistently infect cells in the lymphoid tissue and blood for the life of the animal.

Infections

Access of microbial pathogens to the circulatory system occurs through a number of mechanisms, including direct inoculation into the blood (e.g., insect bites, contaminated needles, blood transfusions) or by spread from initial site of infection via the vascular system or the lymphatics draining that site.

Microbial agents that enter via the lymphatic system may be eliminated or, at least, arrested at regional lymph nodes, or, if they avoid containment at the lymph nodes, they spread to the bloodstream and can disseminate to other sites in the body. The circulatory system, therefore, provides a means for delivery of many microbial agents from their site of entry to their ultimate target organ(s) in the body. Depending on the agent involved, the circulatory system itself may or may not be affected. For many viral infections a viremia is the primary means of dissemination in the host but is often a clinically inapparent event. Similarly, some bacteria and fungi in animals reach their primary or secondary target organs via the circulatory system without obvious or major clinical signs of circulatory system involvement.

The focus of this chapter is on infections in which the circulatory system and/or lymphoid tissues are one of the primary sites affected in the infectious process. In addition to specific lesions or clinical signs directly related to the circulatory system and/or lymphoid tissues, many of these agents also cause systemic, nonspecific signs that include fever, anorexia, depression, prostration, and weight loss. Some infections of the blood-vascular system present as rapidly fatal infections with few or no premonitory signs (e.g., anthrax, blackleg). Some of the most common and/or important infectious agents affecting the circulatory system and lymphoid tissues of domestic animals and poultry are listed in Tables 67.1–67.7. Specific chapters on each of these pathogens should be referred to for more details on pathogenesis, spectrum of clinical signs, and the pathology they cause.

Bacterial Sepsis

Bacterial sepsis and septic shock are characterized by vascular collapse and multiorgan failure. In addition to the signs specifically related to altered organ perfusion, clinical signs of sepsis include fever, tachypnea, and hypothermia. The most common agents involved in sepsis are gram-negative bacteria belonging to the family *Enterobacteriaceae*, although other gram-negative pathogens (e.g., *Pseudomonas aeruginosa*, members of the Family *Pasteurellaceae*) and gram-positive cocci (e.g., staphylococci, streptococci) also cause sepsis and septic shock. Sepsis frequently occurs in neonates, and is especially important in production animals, horses, and poultry. In veterinary medicine, the increasing level of intensive care afforded animals with debilitating conditions has increased the risk for acquiring nosocomial infections and thus the potential for bacterial sepsis to develop in those patients.

Central to the development of septic shock is lipopolysaccharide in gram-negative organisms or other major cell wall components in gram-positive organisms (e.g., peptidogylcan, lipoteichoic acid). These pathogen-associated molecules bind to receptor signaling complexes on monocytes and macrophages. Toll-like receptors, transmembrane signal transducing coreceptors, play a central role in this process. Exposure of cells to these microbial products results in a dysregulation of the immune response and the produc-

Table 67.1.   Common and/or Important Infectious Agents of Circulatory System and Lymphoid Tissues of Dogs

Agent	Disease	Circulatory/Lymphoid Associated Findings
Viruses		
Canine adenovirus 1	Infectious canine hepatitis	Disseminated intravascular coagulopathy, oral petechial hemorrhages, lymphadenopathy
Canine distemper virus	Canine distemper	Leukopenia, myocarditis in neonates
Canine herpesvirus 1	Canine herpesvirus disease	Generalized ecchymotic hemorrhages in neonatal puppies, lymphoid necrosis
Canine parvovirus	Canine parvovirus disease	Leukopenia, lymphoid necrosis, myocarditis
Bacteria		
Bartonella species[a]	Infectious valvular endocarditis	Heart murmur, valvular endocarditis
Borrelia burgdorferi	Canine Lyme borreliosis	Cardiac arrhythmias, myocarditis
Ehrlichia canis[b]	Canine ehrlichiosis	Anemia, bleeding tendencies, limb edema, lymphadenopathy, splenomegaly
Erysipelothrix spp.	Infectious valvular endocarditis	Heart murmur, emboli formation, valvular endocarditis
Leptospira spp.	Leptospirosis	Generalized hemorrhages, icterus, septicemia
Neorickettsia helminthoeca	Salmon poisoning	Lymphadenopathy, splenomegaly
Rickettsia rickettsii	Rocky Mountain spotted fever	Edema, hemorrhages, lymphadenopathy, myocarditis, vascular obstruction

[a]Includes *B. vinsonii* subsp *berkhoffi* and *B. clarridgeiae*.
[b]Other *Ehrlichia* species cause clinical signs related to anemia, leukopenia, and thrombocytopenia.

Table 67.2. Common and/or Important Infectious Agents of Circulatory System and Lymphoid Tissues of Cats

Agent	Disease	Circulatory/Lymphoid Associated Findings
Viruses		
Feline immunodeficiency virus	Feline immunodeficiency	Anemia, leukopenia, lymphadenopathy, secondary infections
Feline infectious peritonitis virus	Feline infectious peritonitis	Immune complex vasculitis/perivasculitis, lymphadenopathy, pericardial effusion
Feline leukemia virus	Feline leukemia	Anemia, lymphoid depletion, lymphosarcoma, myeloproliferative disease, secondary infections
Feline panleukopenia virus	Feline panleukopenia	Leukopenia, mesenteric lymphadenopathy
Feline sarcoma virus	Feline sarcoma	Fibrosarcomas
Bacteria		
Mycoplasma haemofelis	Feline infectious anemia	Anemia, icterus, splenomegaly
Francisella tularensis	Tularemia	Leukopenia, lymphadenopathy, lymph node abscesses, splenomegaly
Streptococcus canis	Cat strangles	Cervical lymphadenitis, lymph node abscesses
Yersinia pestis	Plague	Cervical/submandibular lymphadenitis, lymph node abscesses, septicemia

Table 67.3. Common and/or Important Infectious Agents of Circulatory System and Lymphoid Tissues of Horses

Agent	Disease(s)	Circulatory/Lymphoid Associated Findings
Viruses		
African Horse Sickness virus[a]	African Horse Sickness	Vasculitis with pulmonary, subcutaneous and eyelid edema
Equine infectious anemia virus	Equine infectious anemia	Anemia, hemorrhages, icterus, splenomegaly
Equine viral arteritis virus	Equine viral arteritis	Edema, hemorrhages, leukopenia, vessel infarction
Venezuelan equine encephalitis virus[a]	Venezuelan equine encephalitis	Cellular depletion of lymph nodes, spleen and bone marrow
Bacteria		
Actinomyces spp.	Actinomycosis	Mandibular lymph node abscesses
Anaplasma phagocytophila	Equine ehrlichiosis	Anemia, edema of the legs, hemorrhages
Agents of neonatal septicemia[b]	Neonatal septicemia	Septicemia, hypotension, organ failure
Burkholderia mallei[a]	Farcy, glanders	Lymphangitis, lymphadenitis, splenic abscesses
Corynebacterium pseudotuberculosis	Ulcerative lymphangitis	Lymphangitis
Neorickettsia risticii	Potomac horse fever	Leukopenia, mesenteric lymphadenopathy
Streptococcus equi subsp. *equi*	Strangles	Pharyngeal/submandibular lymphadenitis/abscesses
	Purpura hemorrhagica	Immune-complex vasculitis, edema
Fungi		
Histoplasma farciminosum[a]	Epizootic lymphangitis	Lymphangitis, regional lymphadenitis
Sporothrix schenckii	Sporotrichosis	Lymphangitis

[a]Classified as a foreign animal disease agent in the United States.
[b]Includes *Actinobacillus equuli, Escherichia coli, Salmonella, Streptococcus equi* subsp. *zooepidemicus.*

tion of excessive levels of proinflammatory cytokines (TNF-alpha, IL-1, IL-6), which are largely responsible for the systemic effects observed in sepsis. Toll-like receptors are also found on endothelial cells lining blood vessels.

Some gram-positive organisms produce superantigens that nonspecifically activate large populations of T lymphocytes to produce excessive amounts of proinflammatory cytokines. Coagulation abnormalities, specifically disseminated intravascular coagulation, can also be a consequence of sepsis.

During a bacterial septicemia, rarely are organisms present in high enough numbers to be detected by direct microscopic examination. Some bacteria are, however, present in large enough numbers in the blood in the terminal stages of disease to be detected in direct smears. *Bacillus anthracis*, the etiologic agent of anthrax, causes an overwhelming septicemia, predominately in ruminants, and results in large numbers of organisms being found in the blood during the time just prior to death (Fig 67.1). *Pasteurella multocida*, the agent of fowl cholera, and *Borrelia anserina*, the agent of avian spirochetosis, can also be found in large numbers in the blood of affected birds.

Table 67.4.   Common and/or Important Infectious Agents of Circulatory System and Lymphoid Tissues of Cattle

Agent	Disease	Circulatory/Lymphoid Associated Findings
Viruses		
Alcelaphine herpesvirus-1[a]	Malignant catarrhal fever	Hemorrhages, leukopenia, lymphoid proliferation, lymphadenopathy
Bovine leukemia virus	Bovine leukemia	Lymphosarcoma
Ovine herpesvirus- 2	Malignant catarrhal fever	Hemorrhages, leukopenia, lymphoid proliferation, lymphadenopathy
Rift Valley fever virus[a]	Rift Valley fever	Splenomegaly, widespread hemorrhages
Rinderpest[a]	Rinderpest	Leukopenia, destruction of lymphoid organs
Bacteria		
Anaplasma marginale	Anaplasmosis	Anemia, icterus, splenomegaly
Arcanobacterium pyogenes	Traumatic reticulopericarditis	Pericarditis (often polymicrobial)
	Infectious valvular endocarditis	Heart murmur, heart failure, valvular endocarditis
Bacillus anthracis	Anthrax	Edema, septicemia, splenomegaly, bleeding from orifices
Clostridium chauvoei	Blackleg	Myocarditis, pericarditis
Clostridium haemolyticum	Bacillary hemoglobinuria	Icterus, intravascular hemolysis, hemorrhages
Ehrlichia ruminantium[a]	African heartwater disease	Edema, hemorrhages, hydropericardium, splenomegaly
Leptospira spp.	Leptospirosis	Anemia, icterus, intravascular hemolysis
Mycobacterium avium subsp. paratuberculosis	Johnes disease	Granulomatous lymphangitis of mesenteric lymph vessels
Mycobacterium bovis	Bovine tuberculosis	Granulomatous tracheobronchial/mediastinal lymphadenitis
Pasteurella multocida serotypes B:2 or E:2[a]	Hemorrhagic septicemia	Edema, hemorrhages, hemorrhagic lymphadenopathy
Salmonella spp.[b]	Salmonellosis	Septicemia, splenomegaly

[a]Classified as a foreign animal disease agent in the United States.
[b]Common serotypes includes Dublin and Typhimurium.

Table 67.5.   Common and/or Important Infectious Agents of Circulatory System and Lymphoid Tissues of Goats and Sheep

Agent	Disease	Circulatory/Lymphoid Associated Findings
Viruses		
Bluetongue virus	Bluetongue	Edema of head and neck, hemorrhages, hyperemia
Peste des petits virus[a]	Peste des petits	Generalized lymphadenopathy, leukopenia, splenomegaly
Rift Valley fever virus[a]	Rift Valley fever	Splenomegaly, widespread hemorrhages
Rinderpest virus[a]	Rinderpest	Leukopenia, destruction of lymphoid organs
Bacteria		
Anaplasma ovis	Anaplasmosis	Anemia
Bacillus anthracis	Anthrax	Edema, septicemia, splenomegaly, bleeding from orifices
Corynebacterium pseudotuberculosis	Caseous lymphadenitis	Lymphadenitis, lymph node abscesses
Mycoplasma haemovis	Eperythrozoonosis	Anemia
Mannheimia haemolytic (S)	Septicemic pasteurellosis	Hemorrhagic septicemia in lambs
Mycoplasma mycoides subsp. mycoides (G) (large colony type)	Septicemic mycoplasmosis	Septicemia, pericarditis
Pasteurella trehalosi (G)	Septicemic pasteurellosis	Hemorrhagic septicemia in lambs
Staphylococcus aureus	Tick pyemia of lambs	Lymphadenopathy, septicemia

(G) = goats, (S) = sheep
[a]Classified as a foreign animal agent disease in the United States.

Infections Involving the Heart and Pericardium

The major infectious processes of the heart are infectious valvular endocarditis (usually bacterial) and myocarditis (bacterial or viral). Infections of the pericardium occur either as a result of a systemic infection, from a focus within the heart (e.g., endocarditis) or by extension of an infec-tious process from adjacent tissues (e.g., pleuropulmonary infections).

Infectious Valvular Endocarditis.   Valvular endocarditis results from bacteria from another site in the body seeding one of the heart valves. Preexisting injury or a functional ab-

Table 67.6. Common and/or Important Infectious Agents of Circulatory System and Lymphoid Tissues of Pigs

Agent	Disease	Circulatory/Lymphoid Associated Findings
Viruses		
African swine fever virus[a]	African swine fever	Generalized edema/hemorrhages/infarctions, hemorrhagic lymph nodes, pericarditis, skin cyanosis, splenomegaly
Encephalomyocarditis virus	Encephalomyocarditis	Hydropericardium, myocarditis, pericarditis
Hog cholera virus[a]	Hog cholera, Classical swine fever	Generalized hemorrhages/infarctions, hemorrhagic lymph nodes, lymphoid depletion, skin cyanosis, splenic infarcts
Lelystad virus	Porcine reproductive and respiratory syndrome	Secondary infections due to macrophage depletion
Porcine circovirus 2	Post-weaning multisystemic wasting syndrome	Lymphadenopathy, myocarditis, poor growth
Bacteria		
Bacillus anthracis	Anthrax	Pharyngeal lymphadenopathy and edema, septicemia
Burkholderia pseudomallei[a]	Melioidosis	Lymph node and splenic abscesses
Erysipelothrix rhusiopathiae	Erysipelas	Hemorrhages, splenomegaly, skin cyanosis, infectious valvular endocarditis
Escherichia coli	Septicemia	Septicemia in unweaned pigs, skin cyanosis, congested organs, lymphadenopathy
Escherichia coli (Shiga-like toxin positive)	Edema disease	Edema in subcutaneous tissues/stomach mucosa due to vasculitis
Haemophilus parasuis	Glasser's disease	Pericarditis, septicemia
Mycobacterium avium[b]	Swine mycobacteriosis	Granulomatous cervical, pharyngeal, and mesenteric lymphadenitis
Mycoplasma spp.[c]	Mycoplasma polyserositis	Pericarditis with other serositides
Mycoplasma haemosuis	Porcine eperythrozoonosis	Anemia, icterus, splenomegaly
Salmonella[d]	Salmonellosis	Lymphadenopathy, skin cyanosis, septicemia, splenomegaly
Streptococcus porcinus	Jowl abscess	Cervical lymphadenitis
Streptococcus suis	Streptococcal septicemia	Pericarditis, septicemia

[a]Classified as a foreign animal disease agent in the United States.
[b]Proposed that swine strains of *Mycobacterium avium* be included in the subspecies *hominissuis*. Other mycobacterial species involved include *M. kansasii, M. xenopi,* and *M. fortuitum. Rhodococcus equi* is also occasionally involved.
[c]Includes *Mycoplasma hyopneumoniae, M. hyorhinis,* and *M. hyosynoviae*.
[d]Most common serotypes are Choleraesuis var Kunzendorf and Typhimurium.

normality of heart valve allows for platelet and fibrin deposition. These deposits provide sites for attachment for bacteria that are present in the circulation, often as a result of one of the mechanisms of transient bacteremia previously described. Attachment to the heart valve is mediated through a number of bacterial surface adhesins that include surface glucans and fibronectin-binding proteins. Exposed extracellular matrix on the valve may also serve as a receptor favoring bacteria expressing fibrinogen- or laminin-binding proteins. A preexisting heart valve lesion is not an absolute requirement for infectious valvular endocarditis to develop. Other cardiac abnormalities (e.g., subaortic stenosis in dogs) or invasive vascular procedures, including catheterization, also predispose to heart valve infections. Sequelae to valvular endocarditis include embolization, multiorgan infarction, and sudden death.

Bacteria involved in infectious endocarditis are predominantly, but not exclusively, gram-positive organisms and include streptococci, enterococci, staphylococci, *Corynebacterium,* and *Arcanobacterium* spp. The genus *Erysipelothrix* is specifically associated with valvular endocarditis in some animals (swine, dogs, poultry). When gramnegative organisms are involved, they are usually members of the families *Enterobacteriaceae* or *Pseudomonaceae*. *Bar-*

tonella, another gram-negative organism, is increasingly being recognized as a cause of infectious valvular endocarditis in dogs.

Myocarditis. Myocarditis, an inflammation of the heart muscle, usually is the result of systemic infection with foci of infection in the heart. Damage occurs directly to myocytes or to vascular endothelial vessels supplying heart muscle. The mechanisms of injury to the heart muscle vary and include 1) direct toxic action of an agent on myocytes, 2) effects of circulating toxic products, or 3) immune-mediated mechanisms. A wide variety of infectious agents have potential to cause myocarditis. Some common microbial agents specifically associated with myocarditis in animals include canine parvovirus, encephalomyocarditis virus in pigs, *Clostridium chauvoei* in cattle, and *Listeria monocytogenes* in ruminants and poultry.

Infections Involving the Pericardium. *Hydropericardium,* a serous fluid accumulation in the pericardial cavity, in conjunction with other systemic signs is a characteristic of certain infectious diseases (e.g., heartwater in cattle, African Horse Sickness, chicken anemia virus infection) and is the result of vascular damage. Fluid accumulations in the

Table 67.7. Common and/or Important Infectious Agents of Circulatory System and Lymphoid Tissues of Poultry

Agent	Disease	Circulatory/Lymphoid Associated Findings
Viruses		
Avian influenza virus-H5 or H7[a] (highly pathogenic)	Avian influenza, fowl plague	Generalized hemorrhages; edema of head, wattles, and comb; lymphoid necrosis; myocarditis
Avian leukosis viruses (C)	Lymphoid leukosis	Anemia, hemangiomas, lymphoid tumors, sarcomas
Chicken anemia virus (C)	Chicken anemia	Anemia, hemorrhages, hydropericardium, hypoplasia of lymphoid and hemopoetic tissues
Exotic Newcastle disease virus[a]	Exotic Newcastle disease	Generalized hemorrhages (especially intestinal), edema
Infectious bursal disease virus (C)	Infectious bursal disease, Gumboro disease	Enlarged/hemorrhagic bursa of Fabricius, lymphoid necrosis, B lymphocyte deficiency, immunosuppression
Marek's disease virus (C)	Marek's disease	Lymphoid tumors of heart, bursa, thymus, spleen
Reticuloendotheliosis virus (T)	Reticuloendotheliosis	Lymphoreticular neoplasia, lymphomas
Turkey adenovirus 2 (T)	Hemorrhagic enteritis of turkeys	Immunosuppression, intestinal hemorrhage, splenomegaly
Bacteria		
Borrelia anserina	Avian spirochetosis	Anemia, hemorrhages, splenomegaly
Chlamydophila psittaci (T)[b]	Ornithosis, chlamydiosis	Pericarditis, splenomegaly, fibrin exudates
Erysipelothrix rhusiopathiae	Erysipelas	Generalized hemorrhages, splenomegaly with infarcts, valvular endocarditis
Escherichia coli	Colisepticemia	Pericarditis, omphalitis, septicemia, splenomegaly
Mycobacterium avium	Avian tuberculosis	Splenic granulomas
Pasteurella multocida	Fowl cholera	Generalized hemorrhages, pericarditis, septicemia
Salmonella[b]	Salmonellosis[c]	Myocarditis, omphalitis, pericarditis, splenitis

(C) = chicken, (T) = turkey
[a]Classified as a foreign animal disease agent in the United States.
[b]Includes serovars Pullorum, Gallinarum, and Typhimurium.
[c]Includes Pullorum disease, Fowl Typhoid, and Paratyphoid.

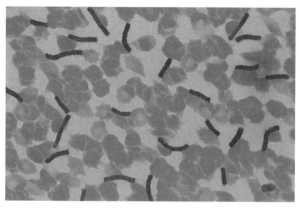

FIGURE 67.1. *Blood smear from a cow with anthrax. Blood was collected 1 hour prior to the cow's death. Numerous, large, squared-end rods typical of* Bacillus anthracis *are present in the smear. Wright's stain.*

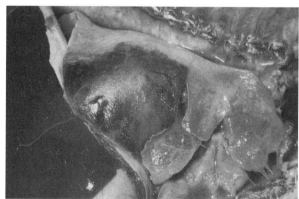

FIGURE 67.2. *Pericarditis and pleuritis in a goat caused by a* Mycoplasma mycoides *subsp.* mycoides *(large colony variant) septicemia.*

pericardial sac also result from damage due to immune-complex deposition in vessels (e.g., feline infectious peritonitis).

Pericarditis denotes an inflammation of the pericardium. Like myocarditis, a number of viral and bacterial agents can be involved. Pericarditis is often part of a systemic infection involving other serosal surfaces and cavities (e.g., Glasser's disease in pigs, mycoplasma septicemia in goats) (Fig 67.2).

The most common traumatic pericardial infection in animals is traumatic reticulopericarditis (hardware disease) in cattle. This is most often associated with the extension of an ingested linear metallic object (e.g., wire, nail) through the reticulum and diaphram into the pericardial sac. It provides bacteria the necessary access to the pericardial space in order for infection to establish. Such infections are usually polymicrobial, with *Arcanobacteium pyogenes* and *Fusobacterium necrophorum* frequently involved.

Infections Affecting Blood Vessels

In general, the endothelium of blood vessels plays an interactive role in most inflammatory reactions through endothelial-leukocyte interaction, pro-coagulation activity, and release of mediators (cytokines, chemokines). Microbes that specifically infect endothelial cells of small vessels and capillaries can cause necrosis with increased vascular permeability resulting from direct vascular endothelial injury by an agent or its toxin (e.g., Shiga-like toxin) or by immune-complex deposition and an ensuing inflammatory response. Disruption of the endothelial barrier leads to edema and/or hemorrhages in affected organs. Clinical signs depend on the agent and vascular site(s) in the body primarily affected (e.g., African Horse Sickness and the pulmonary vasculature with an ensuing pulmonary edema). Central nervous system signs in dogs as a result of bleeding into the brain are attributed to *Rickettsia rickettsii*, the Rocky Mountain spotted fever agent, and the vascular damage it causes. Similarly, damage to the integrity of vessels walls due to immune-complex deposition in feline infectious peritonitis in cats results in the fluid accumulations in serosal cavities, as is found in the "wet form" of the disease. In addition to severe hepatic necrosis, Rift valley fever virus causes massive generalized endothelial damage resulting in widespread hemorrhages. Loss of endothelial anticoagulant activity and platelet activation may cause thrombosis of blood vessels and infarction in some systemic infections ultimately leading to tissue necrosis at the affected site (e.g., skin lesions of erysipelas in swine). Details on the pathogenesis of these and other infectious diseases that affect the blood vasculature and associated pathology are covered in greater detail in chapters on the specific agent or system(s) involved.

Omphalitis, an inflammation of the umbilicus of neonates, deserves special attention. Both the umbilical arteries and veins can be involved. It is especially important in farm animals and horses. The bacteria responsible are either of enteric origin, inhabitants of mucosal surfaces, or environmental contaminants (e.g., *Actinobacillus* sp, *Arcanobacterium pyogenes*, *E. coli*, streptococci). Umbilical infections can lead to local abscess development or, sometimes, serve as a site for establishment of *Clostridium tetani* and the development of tetanus. A septicemia may also develop from umbilical infections (navel ill), which can lead to infections elsewhere in the body, including polyarthritis and meningitis. Failure of passive transfer is a common predisposing factor in these cases. In poultry, yolk sac infection and omphalitis is also a serious problem. A variety of organisms are involved, *E. coli*, *Salmonella*, and *Pseudomonas* being prominent etiologic agents.

Infections Involving Red Blood Cells

Anemia is a common finding in many infectious processes. A number of mechanisms lead to anemia and include suppression of erythropoiesis, sequestration of red blood cells (RBCs), antibody-mediated hemolysis, erythrophagocytosis, direct lysis of RBCs, and alterations in RBC membranes that decrease overall lifespan.

Anaplasma marginale specifically infects RBCs in cattle

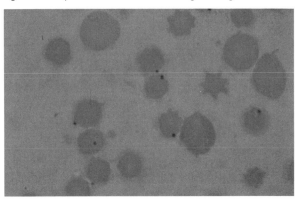

FIGURE 67.3.   *Blood smear from a cow with anaplasmosis. Anisocytosis and polychromasia are evident. A number of* Anaplasma *organisms are present in red blood cell margins. Wright's stain.*

(Fig 67.3). Infections elicit an immune response that results in removal of both infected and uninfected RBCs and may lead to a packed cell volume as low as 6%. The anemia observed with chicken anemia virus disease and FeLV infections in cats are examples of anemia due, at least in part, to decreased erythropoiesis. The bacterial hemoparasite, *Mycoplasma haemofelis*, causes anemia in cats by multiple mechanisms including RBC sequestration and antibody-mediated hemolysis. Immune-mediated hemolytic anemia is also important in FeLV infections and canine ehrlichiosis. Immune-mediated hemolysis can be the result of 1) presence of microbial antigens on the RBCs, 2) cross-reactions between antigens of normal RBC proteins and an infectious agent, or 3) exposure of usually unexposed RBC antigens during the infectious process. Intravascular hemolysis resulting in anemia can be the result of action of certain bacterial toxins (e.g., phospholipase C). *Leptospira* spp. and *Clostridium hemolyticum* are notable agents that destroy RBCs by this mechanism. Anemia in these cases is often accompanied by hemoglobinuria.

Infections Involving White Blood Cells

A number of viruses affect cells of the myeloid and lymphoid series. Venezuelan equine encephalitis virus is a prominent example of a virus that destroys hemopoetic and lymphoreticular cells leading to cellular depletion in bone marrow, lymph nodes, and the spleen. Many viral infections that target cells in these series predispose animals to secondary infections consequent to the immunosuppressive effects that occur. One of the main targets of infectious bursal disease virus in chickens is the cloacal bursa, which initially is enlarged and edematous but eventually becomes atrophied (Fig 67.4). The resulting B lymphocyte deficiency leads to secondary infections. Feline leukemia virus, feline immunodeficiency virus in cats, and porcine circovirus in pigs similarly make animals more susceptible to secondary infections through immunosuppresive effects. These effects can be long-term; however, other viral infections (e.g., distemper virus, hog cholera virus, par-

FIGURE 67.4.   *Enlarged edematous bursa in a chicken with infectious bursal disease. (Courtesy Dr. H. Shivaprasad.)*

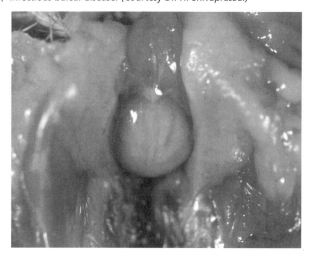

FIGURE 67.5.   *Swollen mandibular lymph node in a cat with Streptococcus canis lymphadenitis. (Courtesy Dr. P. Blanchard.)*

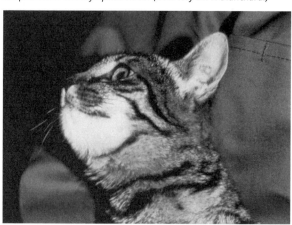

voviruses) cause temporary leukopenias and the immunosuppressive effect is short-term.

Bacterial agents may also infect white blood cells. Certain members of the genera *Anaplasma, Ehrlichia,* and *Neorickettsia* are pathogens of cells belonging to the myeloid or megakaryocyte series. Fungal agents are not commonly associated with infections of the myeloid or lymphoid cell series. However, the systemic fungal agent *Histoplasma capsulatum* specifically infects macrophages and, therefore, histoplasmosis is considered a disease of the monocyte-macrophage system.

Infections of Lymph Nodes, Lymphatics, and Other Lymphoid Tissues

The lymph nodes play a major role in filtering primary sites of infection via the lymphatic vessels and, therefore, act as principle sites for containment of potential pathogens. Many viral infections are dispersed to other parts of the body (target organs) by this route.

Lymphadenitis, an inflammation of the lymph node, can occur in a single lymph node or multiple lymph nodes draining a common region (regional lymphadenitis) or manifest as a generalized lymphadenitis in systemic infections. Depending on the agents involved, the inflammatory response can be non-suppurative, suppurative, necrotizing, or granulomatous. In some cases, depending on the agent and the host response, lymph node abscessation occurs. Microbial agents causing lymph node abscesses are usually but not exclusively bacterial or fungal. Particular organisms consistently associated with lymph node abscesses include *Corynebacterium pseudotuberculosis* in sheep and goats (caseous lymphadenitis) and *Streptococcus equi* subsp. *equi* in horses (strangles). Although less common nowadays, *Streptococcus porcinus* was an important cause of cervical lymph node abscesses in swine (jowl abscess). *Yersinia pestis* should always be considered when mandibular lymph node abscesses (often bilateral) are detected in

cats from geographic regions where plague is endemic. *Francisella tularensis* causes lymphadenopathy with abscessation in cats, along with generalized signs of infection. *Streptococcus canis* also causes purulent inflammation of lymph nodes on the head and neck in cats (Fig 67.5). Outbreaks, presumably via oral transmission, have been described in cats kept in colonies.

Generalized or regional lymphadenitis is encountered with the systemic mycotic infections (blastomycosis, coccidioidomycosis, cryptococcosis, histoplasmosis) and typically results in a caseous-type necrosis in the affected lymph node.

Lymphangitis is an acute or chronic inflammation of the lymphatic channels that results when infections are not contained locally. Infections mostly involve subcutaneous lymphatics. Lymphangitis is not common in animals, but when it occurs the etiologic agents are most often bacterial or fungal. Parasitic agents should also be considered as causes of lymphangitis in animals but are not within the scope of this book. Inflammation of the lymphatic walls can result in lymphatic obstruction and persistent lymphedema in sites drained by the affected lymphatics. Lymphatic vessels may be swollen (corded), with sporadic discharging abscesses occurring along the lymphatic tracts. Lymphangitis is most commonly recognized in horses. *Sporothrix schenckii,* a dimorphic fungus, and *Corynebacterium pseudotuberculosis* are classical causes of equine lymphangitis. Although considered foreign animal disease agents in the United States, *Burkholderia mallei* (agent of glanders) and *Histoplasma farciminosum* (agent of epizootic lymphangitis) should also be considered as potential causes of lymphangitis in horses in countries where these agents are found. *Mycobacterium avium* subsp. *paratuberculosis,* the agent of Johnes disease in ruminants, causes a granulomatous lymphangitis in the mesentery of the intestines in conjunction with granulomatous enteritis.

The spleen plays an active role in antigen trapping as well as removal of defective erythrocytes. Splenitis com-

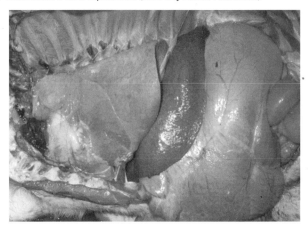

monly occurs as a consequence of generalized infections due to acute congestion and/or reactive hyperplasia. *Salmonella* septicemia is a common cause of splenomegaly in many animals (Fig 67.6). In cattle, anthrax and anaplasmosis also should be considered. In pigs, African swine fever and erysipelas, along with *Salmonella,* are potential agents to consider when splenomegaly is detected.

The thymus is an uncommon site for infections to occur in animals. Viruses that infected T lymphocytes (e.g., feline leukemia virus, feline immunodeficiency virus) cause thymic atrophy. A lymphohistiocytic thymusitis with depletion of cortical thymocytes is a major pathologic feature in epizootic bovine abortion, a disease limited to the western United States. It is caused by an infectious agent of, as yet, unknown etiology.

Neoplasias of the Hemopoetic and Lymphoid Tissues with Infectious Etiologies. Various viral-induced neoplasia involving hemopoetic and lymphatic tissues occur in animals. Marek's disease virus, a herpesvirus, causes a lymphoproliferative disease that affects predominately nervous tissues but also causes lymphoid tumors in a number of other tissues including the heart, bursa, thymus, and spleen. A number of animal retroviruses exist and are able to integrate proviral v-*onc* genes into host cellular DNA. The ability of feline leukemia virus to infect different hemopoetic cells accounts for the variety of disorders of the hemopoetic system seen in infected cats. In addition, solid neoplasias including lymphosarcoma (e.g., thymic lymphosarcoma) can occur. The bovine leukemia virus, also a retrovirus, causes lymphosarcoma that can involve a number of organs including heart, kidney, spleen, lymph nodes, and brain. Avian retroviruses of the leukosis/sarcoma group cause various neoplasias of hemopoetic origin (erythroblastosis, myeloblastosis, myelocytomatosis), as well as lymphoid leukosis and endothelial tumors (hemangiomas). Viruses of reticuloendotheliosis group cause lymphoid leukosis and reticuloendotheliosis in turkeys.

68 Digestive System and Associated Organs

RICHARD L. WALKER

The primary function of the digestive system is to process food in order to provide nutrition for the body. This is performed by a series of complex physical, secretory, and absorptive processes. An in-depth description of all of the varied and interactive functions of the digestive system is well beyond the scope of this chapter. Because the digestive system in its simplest term represents an open tube to the environment, the opportunity for exposure of the digestive system to potential pathogens is great.

The anatomy of the digestive system varies markedly among different animals. In carnivorous animals, it includes the oral cavity, esophagus, stomach, and small and large intestines. The digestive system of herbivores is substantially different from carnivores both anatomically and functionally. Among the herbivorous animals there is also great variation in the digestive system makeup depending on the digestive mechanisms employed (e.g., rumination, cecal digestion). In poultry, further specialization of the digestive system is seen by the presence of a crop (a diverticulum of the esophagus for storage of food) and the division of the stomach into a glandular stomach (proventriculus) and muscular stomach (ventriculus or gizzard). Some of these anatomic differences selectively predispose to specific infectious processes. Infectious diseases of the accessory organs of the digestive system are also covered in this chapter and include common diseases of the liver, gall bladder, and pancreas.

Antimicrobial Properties of the Digestive System

There are a number of anatomic, physiologic, and immunologic mechanisms in place to protect the digestive system from infection by potentially pathogenic microbes. Following are the major protective features of the digestive system.

Gastric Acidity

Acid production in the stomach provides a major protective barrier against pathogens reaching distal sites in the digestive system. The normal acidic environment in the stomach effectively inactivates some viruses and kills most enteric bacteria. Its importance is evident in humans by the increased risk for enteric infections observed in individuals with achlorhydria or in individuals when stomach acid has been neutralized.

Peristalsis

Peristaltic activity in the digestive system is a mechanism whereby nonadhering microorganisms are swept distally. In the small bowel, peristaltic activity plays a major role in host defense. Likelihood of disease is directly related to size of a population of a pathogenic species of bacteria in the small intestine. The most important regulator of the size of this population is peristaltic activity, since there are few other regulators such as those that exist in the large bowel (Eh, fatty acids, and pH). Peristalsis also has an indirect protective role by maintaining distribution and numbers of the normal bacterial flora.

Mucus and Mucosal Integrity

The mucus layer and the integrity of mucosal surface are important factors in providing a barrier to infection in the digestive system, as well as to systemic infections that originate through the digestive system. The mucus barrier, composed of mucin glycoproteins secreted by goblet cells, binds organisms thereby blocking interaction with underlying epithelial cells and, along with peristalsis, promotes their removal. The monolayer of epithelial cells lining the digestive system provides an additional barrier to entry by luminal organisms. Intestinal enterocytes are zippered together by intercellular junctional complexes. Damage to intestinal epithelium allows for intercellular translocation of potentially pathogenic microbes. Some microbes are able to translocate across intestinal mucosa by intracellular means.

Bacterial Interference

Once the normal flora is established, it gives the animal a very potent defense against microorganisms that might cause disease, if they establish. An example of the effectiveness of this "colonization resistance" is the exclusion of *Salmonella* from the intestinal tract of poultry by "cocktails" containing normal flora microorganisms. Disrupting colonization resistance puts the animal at risk by exposing receptors on potential target cells and eliminating a mechanism for regulating the population size of facultative organisms, including species or strains with pathogenic potential. Products of normal bacterial flora, especially the anaerobes that make up the majority of the oral and colonic flora, are important in controlling pathogen establishment (see "Microbial Flora of the Digestive System," below).

The newborn animal is particularly susceptible to enteric disease because, besides being immunologically naive, it is devoid of established flora. The most vulnerable area is the midjejunum and distal ileum.

Immune Defense

Passive protection is afforded the neonate by colostrum. Immunoglobulins in colostrum, specific for antigenic determinants on adhesins used by pathogens for attachment, combine with these structures to block attachment of the pathogen to its target cell. Failure of passive transfer and thus the absence of these protective immunoglobulins is one of the major factors leading to the increased susceptiblity of neonates to enteric infections.

The active immune defense mechanisms in the digestive system rely on patrolling phagocytes and humoral and cell-mediated immunity. There is a normal background of neutrophils, macrophages, plasma cells, and lymphocytes found in the lamina propria indicating a continuous surveillance activity. When stimulated by potential pathogens, inflammatory mediators and chemotactic agents are produced and result in an influx of additional inflammatory cells. As part of the body's mucosal immune system, the gut-associated lymphoid tissue (GALT) is composed of lymphoid tissue in Peyer's patches and lymphocytes in the lamina propria. The microfold (M) cells overlying follicles of Peyer's patch play a role in antigen sampling for the immune system but may also provide a portal of entry for some pathogens. The benefits of GALT and antigen sampling in the digestive system are not just local but rather benefit the entire host through the common mucosal immune system. Secretory IgA and associated secretory piece, which provides resistance to luminal degradation, has a role in osponization and neutralizing. Specific IgM antibodies are also involved.

Commensal bacteria play an important role in the development of the mucosal immune system of the gastrointestinal tract by promoting lymphoid follicle development; however, the immune system responds more vigorously to pathogenic organisms than it does to commensal organisms. This is possibly due to the closer attachment of pathogens to mucosal cells or that commensal organisms, being more permanent residents, temper the immune response directed toward them by blocking proinflammatory responses. Inappropriate inflammatory response to normal commensal bacteria is hypothesized to be an underlying cause for inflammatory bowel disease in humans.

In parts of the digestive tract, the normal flora is integral to maintaining an active innate host surveillance system. In the mouth, for instance, the periodontal microbiota stimulates the formation of an interleukin-8 (IL-8) gradient that promotes migration of neutrophils to bacterial/epithelial interfaces. Thus these commensal microbial communities in the oral cavity provide for an active surveillance in the gingival crevices against potential oral pathogens.

As an associated organ of the digestive system, the liver plays a major role in removal of pathogens from the bloodstream. This innate host defense is accomplished by a complex neutrophil-Kupffer cell (resident liver macrophage) interaction.

Other Antimicrobial Products

Saliva, along with providing an important flushing effect, contains a number of potential antimicrobial agents, including antibodies, complement, lysozyme, lactoferrin, peroxidases, and defensins. In the intestines, bile salts and antimicrobial peptides contribute to limiting and influencing the microbial makeup. Both alpha and beta defensins are produced by cells of the intestinal tract (e.g., Paneth cells). Lactoferrin and peroxidase from the pancreas may also affect bacterial growth in the intestine. In addition to the antibodies in colostrum, the presence of other factors such as lactoferrin and lysozyme provide additional protection for the digestive system in neonates.

Microbial Flora of the Digestive System

A microbial flora that is part of a complex ecosystem inhabits the digestive tract. In addition to its role in protection against the establishment of pathogens, the normal flora plays an important role in physiological health of the host through functions that include promoting functional intestinal villi formation, synthesis of nutrients (e.g., vitamin K), and contributing to the establishment of a functional intestinal mucus consistency by degradation of the secreted glycoproteins.

Establishment

The result of interactions between host and microbe is an ecosystem comprised of many thousands of niches, each inhabited by the species or strains of microbes most aptly suited to that location, to the exclusion of others. The host contributes to the establishment of a normal flora by furnishing receptors for adhesins on the surface of prospective niche dwellers. The niche dweller is the one that has successfully competed for that particular site.

The fetus is microbiologically sterile as it starts down the birth canal. Microorganisms are acquired from the birth canal and, after birth, from the environment. The immediate environment of the newborn is populated with microorganisms excreted by the dam and other animals. These microbes are ingested, compete for niches, and with time become established as part of the normal flora. During the first days to months after birth, the flora is in a state of flux due to the interplay between the various microbes, the niches of the host, and the changing diet. Diet influences the nutritional environment at the level of the niche, which in turn influences the kinds of microbes that will successfully compete for these nutrients. Throughout its life the host's normal flora is influenced by a number of other factors (e.g., aging of the host) and adapts accordingly.

Members of the normal flora establish themselves in a particular niche utilizing various bacterial and host properties in the process. A powerful way for bacteria to secure a particular niche against other species is to secrete antibiotic-like substances such as bacteriocins (cationic membrane-active compounds that form pores in the target cells) and microcins (similar to bacteriocins but smaller than 10 kDa and active against gram-negative microorganisms). Both of these substances are significant, especially in the communities living in the oral cavity. Microcins probably play a significant role in regulating the population composition in the gastrointestinal portion of the digestive system. The role of bacteriocins in this region is less clear.

An important mechanism for regulating population size and ensuring niche security is fatty acid excretion by obligate anaerobes. In the gingival crevice, dental plaque, and the large bowel, the obligate anaerobes in this manner play a central role in regulating the size and composition of the normal facultative flora, the members of which may include potential pathogens. Under the conditions of the bowel (low Eh {<500 mv} and pH of 5 to 6), butyric, acetic, and lactic acids are extremely toxic to facultative anaerobes, especially members of the family *Enterobacteriaceae*. Another way for bacteria to compete successfully is to acquire nutrients more successfully than competitors.

Disruption

Antimicrobial drugs are the single most efficient agents at decreasing colonization resistance. Most antimicrobial agents affect the microbial flora of the oral cavity by depleting the number of streptococci that inhabit the surface of the cheeks and tongue. As a result, these areas are usually repopulated with resistant (to the antimicrobial agent being administered) members of the family *Enterobacteriaceae* within 24 to 48 hours. Resistant members of the environmental flora are also found. Members of the genus *Pseudomonas* are notorious examples of this group.

Antimicrobials also affect the members of the obligate anaerobic communities that inhabit the gingival crevice and dental plaque in the mouth and the large bowel. Overgrowth of various members of the family *Enterobacteriaceae* results because of decreases in levels of fatty acids. Colonization by potential pathogens (e.g., *Salmonella*) is enhanced by antibiotics affecting obligate anaerobes living in the bowel.

Composition

Bacterial species as well as some protozoal and fungal species constitute the bulk of the microflora in the alimentary canal of animals. The overwhelming majority of the normal flora is obligately anaerobic bacteria (up to 99.9%). Viruses are typically only transient residents of the alimentary canal.

The microbial flora of the mouth is roughly uniform among domestic mammals. No information is available

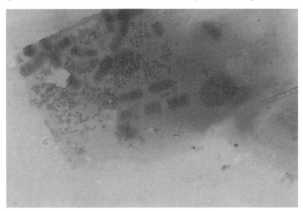

FIGURE 68.1. *Pharyngeal swab from a dog. Simonsiella, showing characteristic monoseriate filaments, are attached to an epithelial cell. Other bacterial rods are also present. Wright's stain.*

for fowl. The description that follows is general and applies to carnivores and herbivores. The buccal surface, tongue, and teeth (plaque) are inhabited by facultative and obligate aerobes. These include streptococci (alpha and nonhemolytic), members of the family *Pasteurellaceae*, *Actinomyces* spp., enterics (*Escherichia coli* being the most common), *Neisseria* spp., CDC group EF-4 ("eugonic fermenter"), and *Simonsiella* (a unique oral commensal that forms characteristic monoseriate filaments) (Fig 68.1). The flora of the gingival crevice is composed almost entirely of obligate anaerobes, the most common genera being *Bacteroides*, *Fusobacterium*, *Peptostreptococcus*, *Porphyromonas*, and *Prevotella*. Saliva contains a mixture of facultative and obligate species of anaerobes and aerobes. The esophagus does not possess a normal flora but is contaminated with organisms found in saliva.

In ruminants, rumen flora is composed of a complex microbial community that includes bacteria (eubacteria and archaea), fungi, and protozoa. The rumen flora is in a delicately balanced symbiotic relationship with the host that is necessary to maintain rumen health for its proper fermentative function. The bulk of the flora are obligate anaerobes, with *Prevotella* spp. and *Butyrivibrio* spp. being among the most common genera found. Also included are bacteria (*Ruminococcus*, *Fibrobacter*) specifically required for digestion of cellulose-rich forage. Disruptions in the normal rumen flora can lead to serious metabolic and physiological problems (see "Infections of the Stomach, Ruminant Forestomach, and Abomasum," below). The flora of the rest of the alimentary canal varies substantially among different animals, as is shown in Tables 68.1–68.5.

Digestive system–associated organs (liver, gall bladder, and pancreas) are not generally considered to have a normal flora but may be transiently seeded as a result of asymptomatic bacteremia. Clostridial spores are readily found in the liver of many animals but remain dormant unless tissue oxygen tension becomes low enough to allow spores to germinate and vegetative cells to proliferate.

Table 68.1. Microbial Flora of the Chicken

	Number of Viable Microorganisms/Gram of Contents[a]					
	Stomach		Small Intestine		Cecum	Feces
	Crop	Gizzard	Upper	Lower		
Total	6	6	8–9	8–9	8–9	8–9
Anaerobes	3	5–6	<2	<2	8–9	7–8
Enterobacteriaceae[b]	6	<2	1–2	1–3	5–6	6–7
Streptococci/Enterococci	2	<2	4	3–5	6–7	6–7
Lactobacillus	5–6	2–3	8–9	8–9	8–9	8–9

[a]Expressed as $\log_{10}$ of the number of organisms cultured.
[b]Mainly *E. coli.*

Table 68.2. Microbial Flora of the Bovine

	Number of Viable Microorganisms/Gram of Contents[a]				
		Small Intestine			
	Abomasum	Upper	Lower	Cecum	Feces
Total	6–8	>7	6–7	8–9	9
Anaerobes	7–8	NA[c]	5–6	8–9	6–9
Enterobacteriaceae[b]	3–4	>7	5–6	4–5	5–6
Streptococci/ Enterococci	6–7	2–3	3–4	4–5	4–5
Yeasts	2–3	—	<3	2	—

[a]Expressed as $\log_{10}$ of the number of organisms cultured.
[b]Mainly *E. coli.*
[c]Not available.

Table 68.3. Microbial Flora of the Horse

	Number of Viable Microorganisms/Gram of Contents[a]				
		Small Intestine			
	Stomach	Upper	Lower	Cecum	Feces
Total	6–8	NA[c]	6–7	8–9	8–9
Anaerobes	3–5	3–4	4–6	3–4	3–5
Enterobacteriaceae[b]	6–7	5–6	5–6	6–7	5–6
Streptococci/ Enterococci	—	—	—	—	<3
Yeasts	6–8	NA[c]	6–7	8–9	8–9

[a]Expressed as $\log_{10}$ of the number of organisms cultured.
[b]Mainly *E. coli.*
[c]Not available.

Table 68.4.   Microbial Flora of the Pig

| | Number of Viable Microorganisms/Gram of Contents[a] | | | | |
| | | Small Intestine | | | |
	Stomach	Upper	Lower	Cecum	Feces
Total	3–8	3–7	4–8	4–11	10–11
Anaerobes	7–8	6–7	7–8	7–11	10–11
Enterobacteriaceae[b]	3–5	3–4	4–5	6–9	6–9
Streptococci/ Enterococci	4–6	4–5	6–7	7–10	7–10
Yeasts	4–5	4	4	4	4
Spiral organisms	NA[c]	NA[c]	NA[c]	NA[c]	8

[a]Expressed as $\log_{10}$ of the number of organisms cultured.
[b]Mainly *E. coli.*
[c]Not available.

Table 68.5.   Microbial Flora of the Dog

| | Number of Viable Microorganisms/Gram of Contents[a] | | | | |
| | | Small Intestine | | | |
	Stomach	Upper	Lower	Cecum	Feces
Total	>6	>6	>7	>8	10–11
Anaerobes	1–2	>5	4–5	>8	10–11
Enterobacteriaceae[b]	1–5	2–4	4–6	7–8	7–8
Streptococci/ Enterococci	1–6	5–6	5–7	8–9	9–10
Spiral organisms (relative amounts)	1+	1+	1+	4+	0

[a]Expressed as $\log_{10}$ of the number of organisms cultured.
[b]Mainly *E. coli.*

Infections of the Digestive System and Associated Organs

Infections of the digestive system and associated organs are important in all domestic animals. Some digestive system pathogens (e.g., enterotoxigenic *E. coli*, rotaviruses) are specific for a particular animal family while others affect a wide variety of animals (e.g., *Salmonella enterica* serovar Typhimurium). In addition to differences in animal susceptibility—age, immune status, and genetic susceptibility—individuals within a species may also predispose to infection by specific pathogens. Some of the most common and/or important pathogens of the digestive system of major domestic animals and poultry are listed in Tables 68.6–68.12.

Infections of the Oral Cavity

The oral cavity of animals is susceptible to infection by a various endogenous (usually bacterial or fungal) and exogenous microbes (usually viral). Viral pathogens are often contagious and may, therefore, affect large populations of animals at a time. Infections from endogenous microbes tend to involve one or a limited number of animals.

A number of viruses cause diseases of the oral cavity. The viruses that cause the vesicular stomatides variously affect ruminants, horses, and swine. Included in this group are foot-and-mouth disease virus (picornavirus), vesicular stomatitis virus (rhabdovirus), swine vesicular disease virus (enterovirus), and vesicular exanthema of swine virus (calicivirus—now believed to be extinct). These are contagious viruses. Lesions initially present as vesicles that eventually rupture and leave painful ulcers in oral mucosa. The coronary band and heel junctions of the digits may also be involved, causing moderate to severe lameness. The exotic nature of some of the vesicular viruses makes them of substantial economic importance in countries free of these diseases. Other viruses are important causes of erosive stomatitis and include bovine viral diarrhea virus in cattle, feline calicivirus, rinderpest virus in sheep and cattle, bluetongue virus in sheep, and the malignant catarrhal fever viruses in cattle. Clinical signs and

Table 68.6. Common and/or Important Infectious Agents of the Digestive System of Dogs

Agent	Major Clinical Manifestations (Common Disease Name)	Age Group(s) Commonly Affected
Viruses		
Canine adenovirus 1	Diarrhea, jaundice, vomiting	Typically less than 6 mos
Canine coronavirus	Diarrhea, vomiting	Any age, typically in puppies
Canine distemper virus	Diarrhea, vomiting, dental enamel hyoplasia (distemper)	Any age, most susceptible at 4–6 mos
Canine oral papillomavirus	Oral cavity warts (oral papillomatosis)	Typically less than 1 yr
Canine parvovirus	Diarrhea, vomiting	Any age, most susceptible at 2–4 mos
Bacteria		
Campylobacter jejuni/coli.	Diarrhea with or without blood	Any age, typically less than 6 mos
Leptospira spp.[a]	Hepatitis, vomiting (leptospirosis)	Any age
Neorickettsia helminthoeca	Diarrhea, vomiting (salmon poisoning)	Any age
Salmonella spp.	Diarrhea, vomiting	Any age, young and old most susceptible
Fungi		
Histoplasma capsulatum	Diarrhea with or without blood, oral ulcers, weight loss (histoplasmosis)	Any age, typically less than 4 yrs
Algae		
Prototheca spp.	Bloody diarrhea (protothecosis)	Any age

[a]Includes *Leptospira* serovars canicola, grippotyphosa, and icterohemorrhagiae.

Table 68.7. Common and/or Important Infectious Agents of the Digestive System of Cats

Agent	Major Clinical Manifestations (Common Disease Name)	Age Group(s) Commonly Affected
Viruses		
Feline calicivirus	Ulcerative stomatitis	Typically less than 1 yr of age
Feline immunodeficiency virus	Secondary gingivitis/stomatitis, diarrhea	Any age
Feline infectious peritonitis virus	Ileal or colonic granulomas with vomiting or constipation	Any age, typically less than 2 yrs of age
Feline leukemia virus	Secondary gingivitis/stomatitis, diarrhea, vomiting/diarrhea due to alimentary lymphoma	Any age
Feline panleukopenia virus	Diarrhea, vomiting	Any age, typically kittens 2–12 mos
Feline rotavirus	Diarrhea	1–8 wks of age
Bacteria		
Campylobacter jejuni/coli	Diarrhea	Any age, typically less than 6 mos
Salmonella	Diarrhea	Any age, young and old most susceptible

Table 68.8. Common and/or Important Infectious Agents of the Digestive System of Horses

Agent	Major Clinical Manifestations (Common Disease Name)	Age Group(s) Commonly Affected
Viruses		
Equine rotavirus	Diarrhea	1–8 wks of age
Vesicular stomatitis virus	Oral ulcers/vesicles	Any age
Bacteria		
Clostridium perfringens (Types A,B,C)	Bloody diarrhea (hemorrhagic enterocolitis)	Less than 1 wk of age
Clostridium difficile	Diarrhea	Adults and foals less than 2 wks
Clostridium piliforme	Diarrhea, hepatitis, sudden death (Tyzzer's disease)	1–8 wks of age
Neorickettsia risticii	Diarrhea (Potomac horse fever)	Typically in adult animals
Rhodococcus equi	Diarrhea, mesenteric lymphadenitis	2–6 mos of age
Salmonella spp.[a]	Diarrhea with or without blood	Any age

[a]Common serotypes include *Salmonella* serotypes Typhimurium, Anatum, and Agona.

Table 68.9.   Common and/or Important Infectious Agents of the Digestive System of Cattle

Agent	Major Clinical Manifestations (Common Disease Name)	Age Group(s) Commonly Affected
Viruses		
Alcelaphine herpesvirus 1[a]	Oral ulcers, diarrhea (malignant catarrhal fever)	Any age
Bovine coronavirus	Diarrhea	1–4 wks of age
Bovine papular stomatitis virus	Oral ulcers	Less than 6 mos of age
Bovine rotavirus	Diarrhea (white scours)	1–3 wks of age
Bovine viral diarrhea virus	Oral/esophageal ulcers, diarrhea	Typically 6 mos–2 yrs of age
Ovine herpesvirus 2	Oral ulcers, diarrhea (malignant catarrhal fever)	Any age
Rinderpest virus[a]	Oral ulcers, diarrhea (rinderpest)	Any age
Vesicular viruses[b]	Vesicles/ulcers on tongue, oral mucosa	Any age
Bacteria		
Actinobacillus ligniersii	Oral pyogranulomas (wooden tongue)	Adult animals
Actinomyces bovis	Granulomas of mandible or maxilla (lumpy jaw)	Adult animals
Arcanobacterium pyogenes	Liver abscesses, weight loss	Adult animals
Clostridium haemolyticum (*C. novyi* Type D)	Hepatic necrosis, sudden death(bacillary hemoglobinuria, red water disease)	Any age
Clostridium perfringens-Types B&C	Bloody diarrhea (hemorrhagic enterocolitis)	Less than 2 wks of age
E. coli-enterotoxigenic[c]	Diarrhea (ETEC diarrhea)	Less than 1 wk of age
E. coli-attaching and effacing	Diarrhea (AEEC diarrhea)	Calves
Fusobacterium necrophorum	Liver abscesses, weight loss	Adult animals
	Necrotic lesions of oral cavity (necrotic stomatitis)	Calves
Mycobacterium avium subsp paratuberculosis	Diarrhea, weight loss (Johnes disease)	Greater than 2 yrs of age
Salmonella spp.[d]	Cholecystitis, diarrhea with or without blood (salmonellosis)	All ages affected, calves 2 wks–2mos most susceptible
Yersinia pseudotuberculosis	Diarrhea, weight loss	Calves, adults
Fungi		
Agents of mycotic rumenitis[e]	Decreased appetite and weight gain (mycotic rumenitis)	Ruminating animals

[a]Considered a foreign animal disease agent in the United States.
[b]Includes foot-and-mouth[a] and vesicular stomatitis viruses.
[c]Includes fimbrial types K99 (also designated F5) and F41.
[d]Common serotypes include *Salmonella* serotypes Dublin, Montevideo, Newport, and Typhimurium.
[e]Includes *Absidia, Aspergillus, Mucor,* and *Rhizopus* species.

pathogenesis of infections are described in detail in specific chapters related to these viruses. Other common viral infections of the oral cavity are bovine papular stomatitis, which causes papules on various structures throughout the oral cavity and canine oral papillomatosis, which in turn presents with cauliflower-like growths (papillomas) that can be widespread throughout the oral cavity.

Bacterial causes of oral infections typically originate endogenously from normal oral flora. Infections such as actinobacillosis (woody tongue) and actinomycosis (lumpy jaw) in cattle are initiated by some preceding trauma that breaches the normal mucosal barrier and allows the introduction of *Actinobacillus lingniersii* and *Actinomyces bovis,* respectively.

Gingival and periodontal diseases are more common problems in dogs and cats than other animals. Multiple bacterial species, predominately gram-negative anaerobes, are involved. Spirochetes also make up a large percent of the bacterial population found in gingivitis and periodontal diseases, but their role in disease pathogenesis is unclear. In cats secondary bacterial gingivitis can be the result of underlying immunosuppressive viral infections (FeLV, FIV).

Mycotic oral infections are uncommon in most animals. Oral candidiasis (thrush) caused by *Candida* species (usually *C. albicans*) is the most common mycotic oral infection encountered. Prior antibiotic treatment, stressful conditions or debilitating diseases that disrupt normal oral flora all predispose to infection. It occurs in all animals but with varying frequency. Candidiasis is especially common in poultry, where it frequently also involves other parts of the digestive system. Lesions in the mouth appear as ulcer-like plaques. In dogs, oral granulomas as a result of disseminated *Histoplasma capsulatum* infections, one of the systemic mycoses, occur with enough frequency to be worth noting. Other fungal infections of the oral cavity are rare.

Infections of the Esophagus

Infections of the esophagus are relatively uncommon, probably due to the rapid passage of material through the

Table 68.10.   Common and/or Important Infectious Agents of the Digestive System of Goats and Sheep

Agent	Major Clinical Manifestations (Common Disease Name)	Age Group(s) Commonly Affected
Viruses		
Bluetongue virus (S)	Cyanosis of mucous membranes, oral ulcers	Any age
Nairobi sheep disease virus[a] (S)	Bloody diarrhea	Any age
Peste des petits virus[a]	Diarrhea, necrotic stomatitis	Any age
Rotavirus	Diarrhea	Typically 1–8 wks of age
Rift Valley Fever Virus[a]	Hepatic necrosis, diarrhea	Any age
Rinderpest virus[a]	Oral ulcers, diarrhea (rinderpest)	Any age
Vesicular viruses[b]	Vesicles/ulcers on tongue, oral mucosa	Any age
Bacteria		
Clostridium haemolyticum (S)	Hepatic necrosis, sudden death (bacillary hemoglobinuria, red water disease)	Any age, usually adults
Clostridium novyi-Type B	Hepatic necrosis, sudden death (infectious necrotic hepatitis, Black disease)	Any age, usually adults
Clostridium perfringens-Type B	Bloody diarrhea (lamb dysentery)	Less than 2 wks of age
Clostridium perfringens-Type C	Bloody diarrhea (necrotic enteritis)	Less than 1 wk of age
Clostridium perfringens-Type D	Diarrhea, sudden death (enterotoxemia)	Rapidly growing animals
Clostridium septicum (S)	Hemorrhagic abomasitis (braxy)	Usually young animals
E. coli-enterotoxigenic[c]	Diarrhea	Less than 1 wk of age
Mycobacterium avium subsp *paratuberculosis*	Hypoproteinemia, weight loss (Johnes disease)	Greater than 2 yrs of age
Salmonella spp.	Diarrhea	All ages affected

G = goats, S = sheep
[a]Considered a foreign animal disease agent in United States.
[b]Includes foot-and-mouth virus[a] and vesicular stomatitis virus.
[c]Includes fimbrial types K99 (also designated F5) and F41.

Table 68.11.   Common and/or Important Infectious Agents of the Digestive System of Pigs

Agent	Major Clinical Manifestations (Common Disease Name)	Age Group(s) Commonly Affected
Viruses		
African swine fever virus[a]	Diarrhea, vomiting (african swine fever)	Any age
Hemagglutinating encephalomyelitis virus	Vomiting (vomiting and wasting disease)	Up to 3 weeks of age
Hog cholera virus[a]	Diarrhea, vomiting (classical swine fever)	Any age
Porcine circovirus type 2	Diarrhea, icterus	Nursery and growing pigs
Porcine epidemic diarrhea virus	Diarrhea, vomiting	Typically piglets postweaning
Swine rotavirus	Diarrhea	1–8 wks of age
Transmissible gastroenteritis virus	Diarrhea and vomiting (transmissible gastroenteritis)	All ages, most severe in piglets
Vesicular viruses[b]	Vesicles/ulcers in oral cavity	Any age
Bacteria		
Brachyspira hyodysenteriae	Bloody diarrhea (swine dysentery)	Growers and finishers
Brachyspira pilosicoli	Diarrhea (colonic spirochetosis)	Weaners, growers, and finishers
Clostridium perfringens (Type A)	Diarrhea	Sucklings, weaners, and growers
Clostridium perfringens (Type C)	Bloody diarrhea (necrotizing enteritis)	Typically less than 1 wk of age
E. coli—attaching and effacing	Diarrhea	1–8 wks of age
E. coli—enterotoxigenic[c]	Diarrhea (colibacillosis)	1 day to 8 wks of age
E. coli—Shiga-like toxin positive	Diarrhea, edema of stomach wall (edema disease)	Typically recent postweaning
Fusobacterium necrophorum	Necrotic ulcers in oral cavity (oral necrobacillosis)	1–3 wks of age
Lawsonii intracellularis	Diarrhea (intestinal adenomatosis)	6–20 wks of age
	Bloody diarrhea (proliferative hemorrhagic enteropathy)	Finishers, breeders
Salmonella species[d]	Diarrhea with or without blood, rectal strictures	Typically postweaning

[a]Considered a foreign animal disease agent in United States.
[b]Includes foot-and-mouth,[a] vesicular stomatitis, swine vesicular disease[a], and vesicular exanthema of swine viruses.
[c]Includes fimbrial types K88, K99, 987P (also designated F4, F5, and F6, respectively), and F41. F18 is associated with postweaning diarrhea and edema disease.
[d]Usual serovars are Typhimurium var Copenhagen or Choleraesuis var kunzendorf.

Table 68.12. Common and/or Important Infectious Agents of the Digestive System of Poultry

Agent	Major Clinical Manifestations (Common Disease Name)	Age Group(s) Commonly Affected
Viruses		
Hemorrhagic enteritis virus (T)	Bloody droppings	4–9 wks of age
Avian rotavirus	Watery droppings	Up to 5 wks of age
Turkey coronavirus (T)	Watery dropping, weight loss (bluecomb disease)	Any age, typically 1–6 wks
Exotic Newcastle disease virus[a]	Stomatitis, esophagitis, necrohemorrhagic enteritis	Any age
Bacteria		
Borrelia anserina	Greenish diarrhea (avian spirochetosis)	Any age
Chlamydophila psittaci (T)	Green gelatinous droppings, hepatitis (ornithosis)	Any age
Clostridium colinum	Watery droppings, liver necrosis (ulcerative enteritis)	3–12 wks of age
Clostridium perfringens Types A&C (C)	Diarrhea, sudden death (necrotic enteritis)	2–16 wks of age
Salmonella serotype Pullorum[b]	Diarrhea, liver necrosis	Typically less than 3 wks
Salmonella serotype Gallinarum[b]	Diarrhea, liver necrosis	More common in adult birds
Fungi		
Candida albicans	Diphtheritic membrane on crop, esophagus, and mouth (thrush, sour crop)	Young birds more susceptible

C = chickens, T = turkeys
[a] Considered a foreign animal disease agent in United States.
[b] Other *Salmonella* serotypes (paratyphoid infections) are usually asymptomatic except in very young birds (<2 wks of age).

esophagus and the tough stratified squamous epithelium that lines it. Some viral infections, typically as part of a systemic infection, cause esophageal erosions or ulcers. Most notable among these are bovine viral diarrhea virus in cattle and exotic Newcastle disease virus in poultry. Mucocutaneous candidiasis in birds most commonly involves the crop (sour crop, crop mycosis) but can also involve the esophagus proper and proventriculus. A pseudomembrane composed of necrotic material overlying mucosal surfaces is the typical presentation (Fig 68.2).

FIGURE 68.2. *Crop mycosis in a turkey caused by* Candida albicans. *Pseudomembranous patches and necrotic material on the mucosal surface are evident. (Courtesy Dr. H. Shivaprasad.)*

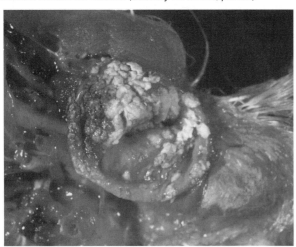

Infections of the Stomach, Ruminant Forestomach, and Abomasum

Because its contractile nature causes relatively rapid transit of ingested material, as well as its mucus coating and acidic environment, the stomach does not provide a very hospitable environment for pathogens. Recently, much attention has been paid to *Helicobacter* species, an organism that has adapted to live in the stomach, as the cause of gastritis and gastric ulcers in humans. Many *Helicobacter* species have been identified in animals; however, their role in disease remains to be clearly established, in part due to their frequent colonization of clinically normal animals. In sheep, a severe hemorrhagic abomasitis (braxy) caused by *Clostridium septicum* occurs and is related to particular feed types. A *Sarcina*-like organism has been associated with abomasal tympany in lambs and goats.

In ruminants, damage to mucosal surface of the forestomach or disruption in the rumen flora can lead to serious and potentially fatal consequences. In dairy cattle, if integrity of the reticulum is penetrated by foreign linear objects such as ingested wire (hardware disease), peritonitis and pericarditis may develop. These infections are polymicrobial with *Arcanobacterium pyogenes* and *Fusobacterium necrophorum* commonly involved.

Sudden dietary changes to carbohydrate rich feeds, which are easily fermentable, leads to a decrease rumen pH. The lower pH kills acid-sensitive rumen flora and damages rumen mucosa. Bacterial rumenitis may develop and can serve as a source of organisms for embolic hepatitis that eventually result in liver abscessation. Common agents recovered from liver abscesses are the familiar abscess producers of ruminants, *A. pyogenes* and *F. necrophorum*. Mycotic rumenitis also develops subsequent to ruminal acidosis or prior antibiotic treatment that has disrupted rumen flora. The fungal agents involved in mycotic rumenitis are often angioinvasive, causing a severe vasculitis, which leads to further tissue necrosis. The zygomycetes (*Mucor, Rhizopus,* and *Absidia*) and *Aspergillus* spp. are the fungi most frequently involved. Mycotic rumenitis may also serve as a source for hematogenous dissemination of fungal elements leading to mycotic abortion.

Infections of the Small and Large Intestines

Microbial infections of the small and large intestines affect all domestic animals. Effective vaccination against many of the major viral enteric pathogens (e.g., parvoviruses, distemper virus) in dogs and cats has substantially decreased the incidence of contagious enteric diseases in companion animals. When dogs and cats are held in close confinement such as kennels, shows, and animal shelters, the risk for contracting contagious enteric diseases increases.

Intestinal infections of both bacterial and viral origin remain of great clinical and economic significance in horses, production animals, and poultry due to intensive rearing conditions, management factors (e.g., failure to insure adequate passive transfer or proper manure management), and the absence of effective vaccines against some of the major pathogens. Host age susceptibility exists for some enteric pathogens (e.g., *Clostridium perfringens* Type C, enterotoxigenic *E. coli*, rotavirus). Neonates, in general, are most susceptible.

The major clinical manifestations of microbial infections of the intestinal tract are diarrhea and vomiting. Vomiting often occurs in enteric infections as part of the enteric defense response and is regulated by the vomition center in the brain. Diarrhea is defined as increase in frequency, fluidity, or volume of feces due to an increase in water content. Insults to the intestines that cause increased secretion or decreased absorption can result in diarrhea. Severity, duration, and characteristics (watery, bloody, etc.) of diarrhea differ depending on the agent involved. Whether diarrhea is actually a benefit to the host, pathogen, or both is unclear. Diarrhea not only serves the host as means to eliminate a buildup of pathogens but also serves the pathogen by providing a means for dissemination and, thereby, maximizes potential for the pathogen to infect other hosts.

Viral infections involving the small and large intestines may be limited to the digestive tract (e.g., rotaviruses, coronaviruses) or be part of a multisystem infectious process (e.g., African swine fever virus, canine distemper virus, and parvoviruses). Intestinal viral infections may be acquired directly via the oral route or as a result of a viremia with localization to intestinal epithelial cells. Some viruses acquired by the oral route are acid resistant, which allows their passage through the stomach, while others are acid-sensitive but can be protected by the buffering action and fats in milk or in feedstuffs with a rapid gastric transit time. Attachment to intestinal epithelial cell receptors (e.g., sialic acid-containing oligosaccharides) via viral attachment proteins is the initial step in establishing infection. This is followed by uptake of the virus into the cell, often through receptor-mediated endocytosis, and replication within the cell. Subsequent destruction of ep-

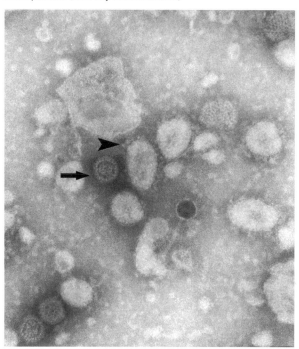

FIGURE 68.3. *Transmission electron micrograph of feces from a 10-day-old Holstein calf with diarrhea. Both rotavirus (arrow) and coronavirus (arrowhead) particles are present. A phage particle is also present. (Courtesy R. Nordhausen.)*

ithelial cells resulting in loss of absorption and resorption capacity and disruption in osmotic equilibrium is manifest by diarrhea. Rotavirus and coronavirus are common causes of viral enteritis in many animals (Fig 68.3) and affect predominantly villus epithelial cells. The time course from exposure to manifestation of clinical signs is usually short. Other viruses affect crypt epithelial cells (e.g, Rinderpest virus in sheep, canine parvovirus) and cause more severe tissue damage. The spectrum of clinical signs and details on pathogenesis associated with specific viral agents that affect the intestines of domestic animals are found in the specific chapters on those agents.

Bacteria are also major pathogens of the small and large intestines. To produce disease in the intestinal tract, potentially pathogenic bacteria must first adhere to *target cells.* If the target cell is part of a niche occupied by normal flora, the microorganisms will encounter "colonization resistance," which they must overcome before adhering. Adherence results from the interaction (*selective adsorption*) of microbial surface structures (*adhesins*) with receptors on target cells. Adhesins are considered virulence factors because most pathogens cannot produce disease without first adhering to a target cell. Fimbrial adhesins are protein in nature and protrude from the surface of the bacterial cell. They are responsible for adherence of some bacteria to carbohydrate moieties that are part of glycoproteins on the surface of host cells. The most commonly found fimbriae (*Type 1 fimbriae*) on the surface of gram-negative bacteria have affinity for mannose-containing glycoproteins on the surface of cells. Bacteria expressing

Type 1 fimbriae, when mixed with red blood cells, agglutinate these cells; this agglutination is inhibited by mannose (mannose-sensitive). Intestinal epithelial cells display structures that serve as receptors for fimbriae expressed by enteropathogenic strains of bacteria.

Other structures on the surface of bacterial cells influence how the bacterium will interact with host cells. These structures are carbohydrates and influence the interaction by rendering the surface of the bacterial cell relatively hydrophilic. This hydrophilic property imparts a repulsive force relative to the host cell surface, since the host cell surface is somewhat hydrophobic. On the other hand, protein receptors on the surface of some host cells have affinity for these surface carbohydrates. The outcome of the latter interaction is adhesion.

After adherence, the pathogen may produce disease by 1) secretion of an exotoxin, resulting, for example, in disruption of fluid and electrolyte regulation of the target cell; 2) invasion of the target cell, causing its death, usually by the action of a toxin (a cytotoxin); or 3) invasion of the target cell and the lymphatics, resulting in a systemic infection. The mechanisms by which the host is affected by different bacterial enteric pathogens are varied and complex. In some cases, as in the enteroxigenic *E. coli*, the diarrhea is solely a result of the production of enterotoxin and little to no pathology is observed (Fig 68.4). Other pathogens (e.g., *Salmonella*) use complex communication systems to translocate effector proteins into host cells (e.g., Type III secretion systems) as well as produce both enterotoxic and cytotoxic effects. Still other pathogens, such as *Mycobacterium avium* subsp. *paratuberculosis*, exert their effect on the intestinal tract by translocating through mucosal epithelial cells and existing in macrophages in the lamina propria and regional lymph nodes. A granulomatous enteritis results, however, the severity of the lesion does not necessarily correlate with the severity of clinical signs. Specific details on the mechanism of pathogenesis and resulting pathology of the important bacterial pathogens of the intestines of domestic animals are covered in the respective chapters on each agent.

FIGURE 68.4. *Enterotoxigenic (K99)* Escherichia coli *infection in a 1-day-old calf. Numerous gram-negative rods are adhered to intestinal villus. Brown & Brenn stain.*

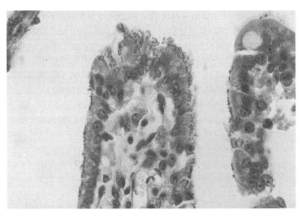

Organisms known to be pathogens of the intestinal tract in certain animals may be found as normal flora in others. Their role in causing disease in some animals, if any, remains to be established. As an example, *Campylobacter jejuni* is the most common cause of diarrhea in humans and is commonly found in the intestinal tract of companion and domestic animals—but its ability to cause disease in some animals is unclear. There is a high carriage rate of *C. jejuni* in chickens with no apparent adverse effects on birds greater than 2 weeks of age.

Various factors predispose or make more likely that an enteric pathogen will establish and cause disease. The importance of antimicrobials on the disruption of normal flora and in allowing pathogens to establish has already been discussed. Other factors that create stress for the host will also result in changes in the intestinal flora, mainly resulting in a drop in the anaerobic component. The level of coliform bacteria will be higher after a decrease in concentration of fatty acids produced by anaerobic flora. The actual reason for the decrease in the number of obligate anaerobes is not known. In addition to these changes, the amount of fibronectin (a glycoprotein) coating epithelial cells in the oral cavity decreases. Since this glycoprotein possesses receptors for gram-positive species in the oral cavity, decrease in this population occurs with a corresponding increase in gram-negative species, especially members of the family *Enterobacteriaceae*.

Fungal infections of the intestines are not common. Of those encountered, granulomatous enteritis in dogs caused by *Histoplasma capsulatum* is among the most common. *Pythium insidiosum*, an oomycete, causes granulomas in the submucosa or muscularis mucosae of the small intestine (and sometimes stomach) in dogs, and it is manifest by vomiting, diarrhea, and weight loss. Rare algal infections caused by *Prototheca* species result in an intractable diarrhea as part of a more generalized process (usually with ocular involvement) in dogs.

Infections of Digestive System–Associated Organs

Infections of the liver occur through a number of routes and include the 1) portal vein, 2) hepatic artery, 3) ascension through the biliary system, and 4) contiguous spread from adjacent infectious processes (e.g., reticulitis).

The liver may be a target for a number of viruses, often as part of a systemic infection. Liver damage can occur by infection of endothelial cells (e.g., canine adenovirus 1) causing vascular stasis and hypoxia as well as through infection of parenchymal cells resulting in hepatocellular necrosis.

A number of bacterial genera and species can affect the liver. Clostridial species are among the most important. Clostridial spores of *C. haemolyticum* (*C. novyi* Type D) and *C. novyi* Type B, the agents of bacillary hemoglobinuria and infectious necrotic hepatitis, respectively, are present in the liver of cattle and sheep. They germinate when local liver necrosis results subsequent to immature fluke migration or when some other event damages the liver (e.g., liver biopsies). Upon germination under this anaerobic environment, a number of cytolytic toxins are produced that further damage the liver. The agent of Tyzzer's disease,

FIGURE 68.5. *Modified Steiner silver stain of a liver lesion from a foal that died of Tyzzer's disease. Silver-stain positive* Clostridium piliforme *organisms are evident in the typical "pick up sticks" arrangement. Modified Steiner silver stain.*

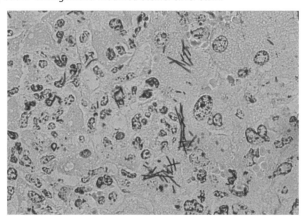

FIGURE 68.6. *Intestinal ulcer in a chicken with ulcerative enteritis caused by* Clostridium colinum. *Liver necrosis was also present.* Clostridium colinum *was isolated from the liver.*

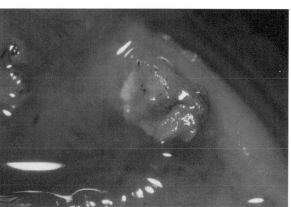

Clostridium piliforme, causes a rare but acute and highly fatal infection in a number of animals. It is most important in laboratory animals. Foals are most commonly affected among domestic animals. Characteristic spindle-shaped bacilli are found in the liver along the edge of areas of hepatic necrosis (Fig 68.5). *Clostridium colinum* causes hepatic necrosis along with ulcerative lesions in the intestines of chickens and turkeys (ulcerative enteritis) (Fig 68.6).

Certain serovars of *Leptospira* will cause a nonspecific reactive hepatitis. Severity of the lesions can vary from severe chronic hepatitis to mild diffuse hepatocellular vacuolation. Often renal involvement also occurs.

As already mentioned, rumenitis provides a source of bacteria through the portal system that can result in liver abscesses. Miliary liver abscesses, most commonly in ruminants, results from hematogenous seeding by a number of different bacteria. Common agents include *Yersinia pseudotuberculosis* and *Rhodococcus equi*. In poultry, liver granulomas are periodically reported to be caused by a gram-positive anaerobic rod, *Eubacterium tortuosum*, and are thought to be of intestinal origin.

The gall bladder infections can be viral (e.g., canine infectious hepatitis virus, Rift Valley fever virus in sheep) and bacterial (e.g., *Salmonella enterica* serotype Dublin in calves) in etiology. Infections of the pancreas are rarely reported in domestic animals.

Diseases of the Digestive System of Unknown but Suspected Infectious Etiology

It is not uncommon for the cause of diarrhea in domestic animals to go undiagnosed. There are a number of important conditions of the digestive tract of domestic animals that are believed to be infectious in origin; however, no specific agent has been conclusively demonstrated to be the cause. In some cases multiple agents are likely involved and/or some interplay between host and environment is necessary for clinical signs to develop. Some major diseases of suspected infectious etiology, but where the specific agent(s) has not been conclusively identified, include poult enteritis mortality syndrome in turkeys, colitis X in horses, hemorrhagic gastroenteritis in dogs, and winter dysentery in cattle (possibly caused by bovine coronavirus).

69

Integumentary System

RICHARD L. WALKER

The integument is the largest organ of the body. It plays a major role in temperature regulation, sensory perception, and protection against fluid loss, and provides a barrier from external insults, including potentially pathogenic microorganisms. It is composed of epidermis, dermis, subcutis, hair follicles, and glandular structures. Glandular structures include sweat and sebaceous glands as well as specialized structures such as anal sacs. Hair type and density vary on the body according to functional need, including sensory, thermoregulatory, and protective functions. Birds have evolved feathers, probably originating from scales, in place of hair. Footpads, horns, hooves, nails, and beaks are all specialized keratinized structures of the integumentary system.

The epidermis is in continual contact with the surrounding environment and provides a home for a resident flora. The outer layer of the epidermis, keratinized stratum corneum, is held together by a lipid cement, and together they form the major physical barrier of the skin. Epidermal thickness varies among animals, among breeds, and at different sites on individual animals. The dermis, through collagen and elastic fibers, provides tensile strength and elasticity to the integumentary system and also varies substantially in thickness throughout the body. The hypodermis provides additional flexibility along with insulation through adipose tissue.

The external ear canal is included in this chapter because the external surface is covered with skin (pinna) or epithelium and glandular structures (external auditory meatus). Overall, the lesions found in otitis externa are similar to those found in skin infections, and some of the important pathogens responsible for otitis externa are the same ones that cause infections elsewhere on the skin.

The mammary gland, although technically not part of the integumentary system, is also included in this chapter because of its direct communication with the skin. Mammary gland pathogens, some of which are resident or transient flora of the skin, primarily enter through the streak canal of the teat. The teat sphincter and a keratin plug produced by epithelial cells lining the teat canal provide the primary physical barrier for the mammary gland.

Antimicrobial Properties of the Skin

The skin provides a less favorable environment for microbial growth than do mucous membranes of the alimentary, respiratory, and urogenital systems owing to properties presented in the following sections.

Dryness

The normal dryness of the skin surface limits the ability of many microbes to survive and establish. Conditions that interfere with the normal evaporative process cause proliferation of resident and transient skin flora through increased moisture retention and changes in temperature, pH, and CO_2 tension. Excessive folding of the skin in certain animal breeds and obese individuals is a prime example of an anatomic condition that increases hydration and temperature of the stratum corneum, providing a more hospitable environment for bacterial proliferation.

Desquamation

Continuous shedding of superficial skin layers eliminates transient organisms. Resident flora numbers are also reduced but are promptly replenished from the residual population.

Secretions and Excretions

Holocrine sebaceous glands secrete lipids, including long-chain fatty acids, many of which inhibit bacteria. They and the apocrine sweat glands contribute to an intercellular seal in superficial epidermal layers, limiting microbial access. Apocrine and eccrine sweat glands excrete lactate, propionate, acetate, caprylate, and high concentrations of sodium chloride. Interferon, lysozyme, transferrin, and all classes of immunoglobulins are also present. Keratinocytes synthesize the antimicrobial peptides—cathelicidins and beta-defensins. All these substances contribute to the self-sterilizing action of the skin—that is, its resistance to colonization by transient microorganisms.

Microbial Interactions

Resident bacteria exclude intruders by excreting inhibitory metabolites (e.g., volatile fatty acids) and bacteriocins, and by occupying available niches.

Immune System

A skin immune system responds to local antigenic stimuli, including microbial ones, and comprises cell types corresponding functionally to those operating on mucosal surfaces. Langerhans cells, an antigen-presenting cell, and intraepithelial T lymphocytes are prominent constituents of the system. Keratinocytes participate in immune defense by producing immune-modulating substances. The interactions between these cells constitutes the skin-associated lymphoid tissue. Complement, cytokines, and immunoglobulins are found in the emulsion layer of the skin and are important to overall integumentary immunocompetence.

Microbial Flora of the Skin

The microbial flora of the skin plays an important role in defense and is probably acquired at birth from the dam. These microorganisms are limited to the superficial epidermal layers, where intercellular cohesion is relaxed prior to desquamation, and to the distal portions of gland ducts and hair follicles. The microbial flora exists predominately in microcolonies, rather than being evenly distributed over the skin. Bacterial adhesion, through lipoteichoic acids in gram-positive cocci, is critical to the establishment and persistence of resident flora. Keratinization defects, as found in seborrhea, provide additional attachment sites and allow for increased numbers of resident flora, as well as changes in overall flora makeup.

Bacteria and yeast variably colonize sites on the skin of animals. The greatest numbers are found in moist, protected areas such as the axilla, inguinal region, interdigital spaces, and ear canals. Their concentration is lower than on colonized mucous membranes, rarely exceeding $10^5/cm^2$ and, in some areas, $10^2/cm^2$.

Gram-positive organisms predominate among resident flora. Among the gram-positives, coagulase-negative staphylococci constitute the majority. Certain strains of coagulase-positive staphylococci are also considered to be resident organisms in some animals. Facultatively anaerobic diphtheroids (*Corynebacterium* and *Propionibacterium* spp.) are consistently present, as are *Micrococcus* spp. and viridans streptococci. Of gram-negatives, only *Acinetobacter* spp. are considered a major part of the resident flora. The main fungal resident is a lipophilic yeast, *Malassezia*, which resides on the skin and in the external ear canal. Viruses are not generally considered part of the normal skin flora. Viral agents that directly infect the skin are maintained in animal populations by persistently infected individuals but are also capable of surviving for extended periods in the environment, which can serve as an alternate source for infecting other animals.

Various transient microbial flora can be encountered. Beta-hemolytic streptococci (generally Lancefield group G) on cat or dog skin are usually associated with abnormal conditions. Members of the family *Enterobacteriaceae*, particularly *Escherichia coli* and *Proteus mirabilis*, and enterococci are common transients. The feet of farm animals carry fecal bacteria, some of which participate in foot infections, most notably *Fusobacterium necrophorum* and *Prevotella melaninogenica*. The agent of ovine footrot, *Dichelobacter nodosus*, although hardly a normal commensal, is limited to epidermal tissues.

Transient fungal flora of the skin represent contaminants of airborne or soil origin. Many genera can be isolated from the skin. Common transient fungal genera found on the skin include *Aspergillus*, *Chrysosporium*, *Cladosporium*, *Penicillium*, and *Scopulariopsis*.

Sterilization of the skin is impossible due to the physical inaccessibility to much of the skin flora. Thorough cleansing of shaved skin with soap and water, followed by soaking with 70% alcohol, will remove 95% of the flora. More than 99% removal of skin flora is claimed for repeated povidone iodine applications and rinses with chlorhexidine (0.5%) in alcohol. Following such treatment there is rapid repopulation, usually by the same organisms.

Infections of the Skin

Susceptibility of skin to infection is inversely related to thickness and compactness of the stratum corneum. Specific animal breeds, because of anatomic conformations, physiologic factors, or genetic factors, are more predisposed to skin infections than others.

Integumentary infections are often secondary, requiring a disruption in the host's innate defense mechanisms. Factors such as trauma, excessive moisture, irritants, insect or animal bites, and burns are all predisposing causes for skin infections to develop. Underlying diseases, including preexisting skin conditions, and immunological disorders also predispose to secondary skin infections. Deep dermal and subcutaneous infections typically require some form of traumatic implantation that allows for the introduction of microbial pathogens that would otherwise not persist on the external epidermal layer.

Systemic infections sometimes involve the integumentary system. Agents with trophism for vascular endothelium or epithelial cells can cause focal or generalized lesions in the skin.

Viral Infections of the Skin

A number of viruses gain entry to the host via the skin, either through abrasions, insect or animal bites or by exposure to contaminated equipment (e.g., needles, harnesses). Some of these viruses simply use the integumentary system as a route for entry into the host and cause either systemic infections or have primary targets that are organs or systems other than the skin (e.g., rabies virus). Details on mechanisms used for entry, replication, and spread via the integumentary system for specific viruses are covered in chapters on those individual viruses.

For some viruses the skin is the primary site of infection or is one of the principal sites where clinical signs manifest. The papillomaviruses and poxviruses are prominent viral pathogens of the integumentary system in animals. The papillomaviruses are introduced through skin abrasions and infect epithelial cells. Infected epithelial cells become hyperplastic. Hyperkeratosis is the result. The lesions (papillomas) are typically raised and filiform, and may be pedunculated. The papillomaviruses are fairly host-specific, although bovine papillomaviruses 1 and 2 are associated with equine sarcoids.

Members of the family *Poxviridae* also affect a number of animals and birds. Many viruses in this family have a limited host range, although some are zoonotic. Transfer occurs through contact with skin lesions, scabs from infected animals, or mechanically by biting insects. The parapox virus that causes sore-mouth in sheep and the fowlpox virus in poultry can be transmitted by respiratory droplets, as well as by direct contact with lesion material or contaminated equipment. Depending on the virus involved, clinical disease can be mild to severe. Generalized signs include fever and anorexia. The skin lesions are typically papulonodular and become pustular or proliferative, eventually resulting in the production of scabs that leave scars.

Cutaneous manifestations are part of the overall clinical presentation of some generalized or multisystem viral infections. Viruses that cause vesicular diseases (foot-and-mouth disease, swine vesicular disease, vesicular exanthema of swine, and vesicular stomatitis viruses) produce vesicles that variably affect the teats, coronary bands, and interdigital areas of the skin. The vesicles readily rupture leaving ulcerative lesions that may become secondarily infected with bacteria. In addition to the lymphoreticular and neurological lesions it produces, the Marek's disease virus of chickens causes nodules to develop in the feather follicles and uses feather follicle dander as a primary means of spreading virus to other birds. Canine distemper virus causes nasal and footpad hyperkeratosis in dogs as a late clinical manifestation.

Bacterial Infections of the Skin

Bacteria associated with skin infections primarily originate from the environment or direct or indirect contact with carrier animals, or are resident flora of the skin, oral cavity, genital tract, or lower digestive tract of the affected animal. Bacterial skin infections are classified as superficial pyodermas (e.g., impetigo, superficial bacterial folliculitis) or deep pyodermas (e.g., folliculitis, furunculosis, cellulitis, and subcutaneous abscesses). Coagulase-positive staphylococci (e.g., *S. aureus*, *S. intermedius*, *S. hyicus*) are the primary agents of superficial pyodermas. They produce a myriad of enzymes and toxins that contribute to the disease process. Along with cell wall components, some of these microbial products have potent chemotactic effects that account for the pyogenic inflammatory response observed in staphylococcal infections. *Staphylococcus hyicus*, the cause of greasy pig disease, produces an exfoliative toxin that specifically causes separation of intraepidermal layers resulting in focal erosions in the epidermis. In neonatal pigs, this generalized epidermitis is associated with substantial mortality.

Dermatophilus congolensis, an actinomycete, also causes a superficial dermatitis, most often in horses and ruminants. Infection stimulates an intense inflammatory response that is characterized by alternating waves of inflammatory cells followed by newly generated epidermis (Fig 69.1). In contrast to the abundance of products produced by coagulase-positive staphylococci, few virulence factors are recognized in *Dermatophilus*. It produces an extracellular serine protease that may contribute to the overall disease process; however, environmental factors are key to the development of disease. Persistent wetting of the skin or insect bites are needed for *Dermatophilus* to initially invade the epidermis. Once invasion occurs, an inflamma-

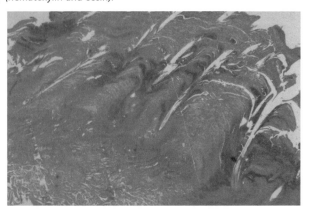

FIGURE 69.1. *Waves of inflammatory exudate and regenerated epidermis from a cow with dermatophilosis (hematoxylin and eosin).*

tory reaction is induced, which results in profuse cellular exudation. If predisposing conditions remain to promote invasion of newly generated epidermis, the infection/inflammatory cycle repeats, giving rise to the characteristic histopathology; otherwise, the infection resolves.

Deep bacterial pyodermas involve the dermis and sometimes the subcutaneous tissue. Injury or trauma almost always precede the development of deep pyodermas. In some cases, deep skin infections occur as a result of the extension of a superficial pyoderma. Again, coagulase-positive staphylococci are frequently involved, although other bacteria may be secondarily involved. Furunculosis (inflammation of the dermis and subcutis) and folliculitis (inflammation of the hair follicle) are most commonly recognized in dogs but also occur with some frequency in horses, goats and sheep.

Subcutaneous abscesses are typically the result of a bite wound or penetrating foreign body. The bacteria introduced usually represent members of the oral flora and cause an accumulation of purulent exudate in the dermis and subcutaneous tissue. Subcutaneous abscesses most commonly occur in cats and most frequently involve *Pasteurella multocida* and obligate anaerobic bacteria. Subcutaneous abscesses are also common in ruminants, with *Arcanobacterium pyogenes* frequently being recovered. *Corynebacterium pseudotuberculosis* causes subcutaneous abscesses in sheep and horses. In cattle it manifests as an ulcerative dermatitis rather than forming abscesses.

Cellulitis is a loose purulent inflammation of the subcutaneous tissue. It is generally poorly contained and extends rapidly along tissue planes from the site of initiation. A variety of bacterial agents cause cellulitis. Among the most serious forms of cellulitis is the anaerobic cellulitis caused by one of a number of histotoxic clostridial species. Under anaerobic environments these species produce potent and highly destructive toxins. Horses, ruminants, swine, and poultry are most commonly affected by clostridial cellulitis. Infections have a high fatality rate, even in the face of aggressive treatment. An *E. coli*–associated cellulitis in broiler chickens is an especially economically important disease for the poultry industry, accounting for a substantial percentage of condemnations at slaughter plants. *Staphylococcus aureus* causes an acute cellulitis in horses that spreads rapidly and causes necrosis of the overlying skin. Thoroughbred racehorses are most commonly affected.

Other bacterial infections of the skin include mycobacterial granulomas. Cats are most commonly affected by these organisms, although infections also occur in swine, cattle, and dogs. The saprophytic mycobacteria responsible are introduced by some trauma. If they establish, infections are characterized by chronic, nonhealing wounds with draining fistulas. A specific entity in young cats referred to as *feline leprosy* is caused by *Mycobacterium lepraemurium* and presents as cutaneous nodules of the head and extremities that sometimes ulcerate. A regional lymphadenopathy is often present. A second, more generalized form of the disease caused by an unidentified mycobacterium has been described in older cats. Pyogranulomatous dermatitis caused by *Actinomyces* spp. occurs in dogs (*A. viscosus* or *A. hordeovulneris* associated with plant awns) and cattle (*A. bovis*). Draining tracts and the presence of yellow granules composed of bacterial colonies, sometimes surrounded by a homogenous eosinophilic material, are found in the draining material (Fig 69.2).

Some bacterial skin infections involve two or more bacteria working in concert. In contagious ovine footrot, *Fusobacterium necrophorum* causes an interdigital dermatitis in macerated skin, which allows *Dichelobacter nodosus* to establish by fimbrial attachment and proliferate. Production of a number of serine and basic proteases by *D. nodosus* results in an underrunning of the sole and, thereby, allows for additional opportunistic bacteria to invade, further aggravating the condition.

A substantial integumentary component is part of certain systemic bacterial infections. The urticarial plaques and diffuse erythematous lesions in the skin of swine, resulting from cutaneous infarctions, are characteristic of erysipelas. The effects on vascular endothelium of bacterial toxins or hypersensitivity reactions to bacterial antigens may also manifest in the skin. Subcutaneous swelling of the eyelids, lips, and forehead occur in edema disease in pigs, caused by Shiga-like toxin producing strains of *E. coli*.

The dependent edema resulting from the vasculitis that occurs in purpura hemorrhagica in horses is a sequelae to infection with *Streptococcus equi* subsp. *equi*.

Fungal Infections of the Skin

Fungal infections of the skin are classified as superifical cutaneous mycoses or subcutaneous mycoses. In addition, fungal agents that cause systemic mycoses (*Blastomyces dermatitidis*, *Coccidioides immitis*, *Cryptococcus neoformans*, *Histoplasma capsulatum*) cause pyogranulomatous lesions in the integumentary system subsequent to disseminated infection.

The most important of the superficial mycotic infections is dermatophytosis or ringworm. It denotes a specialized dermatomycosis caused by fungi that specifically attack keratinized structures. These fungi (*Microsporum* spp, *Trichophyton* spp.) produce enzymes (keratinases) that digest keratin and infect growing hair and stratum corneum (Fig 69.3). Lesions are inflamed, crusty, or scaly and often circular to oval in shape due to the centripetal progression of the lesion. Affected hair is brittle, leaving areas of alopecia. Dermatophytes are not always pathogens and can represent transient flora of the skin (usually geophilic dermatophytes) or be carried inapparently (zoophilic dermatophytes).

Malassezia, a lipohilic yeast, is the other main fungal agent involved in superficial mycotic infections of the skin (Fig 69.4). It causes an erythematous, scaly lesion. Since it can be found in low numbers on normal skin, clinical relevance of its isolation must be decided based on clinical signs.

The subcutaneous mycoses involve the dermis and subcutaneous tissues and may be localized lesions or spread via the lymphatics. Most of the fungal agents involved are from an environmental source (e.g., soil, plant material) and gain entry by traumatic introduction. A number of different subcutaneous mycotic infections are recognized and classified by their gross and histopathologic characteristics. These different conditions include chromoblastomycosis, phaehyophomycosis, and eumycotic mycetoma. They are described in more detail in the chapter on agents of subcu-

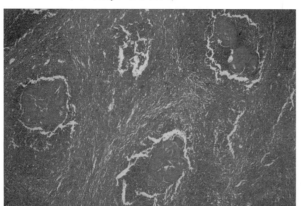

FIGURE 69.2.   *Numerous granules from* Actinomyces bovis *lesion in a cow (hematoxylin and eosin).*

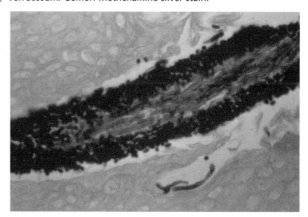

FIGURE 69.3.   *Fungal hyphae and arthroconidia on the hair shaft from a goat with dermatophytosis caused by* Trichophyton verrucosum. *Gomori methenamine silver stain.*

FIGURE 69.4.   *(A) Skin of pig with* Malassezia *dermatitis (hematoxylin and eosin). (B) Numerous broad-based budding yeast, characteristic of Malassezia are found in stratum corneum. Periodic acid-Schiff reaction.*

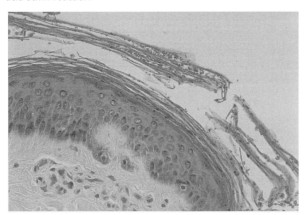

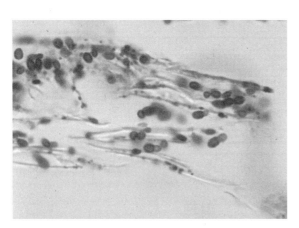

FIGURE 69.5.   *Grain from a eumycotic mycetoma in the skin of a horse. The grain, composed of aberrantly shaped fungal hyphae, is surrounded by a mixture of neutrophils, macrophages, plasma cells, and giant cells. Gomori methenamine silver stain with hematoxylin counterstain.*

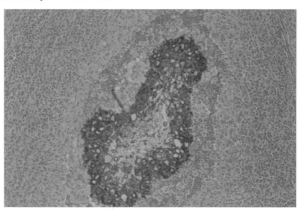

FIGURE 69.6.   *Numerous yeast forms of* Histoplasma capsulatum *are present in skin from a dog with disseminated histoplasmosis. Gomori methenamine silver stain with hematoxylin counterstain.*

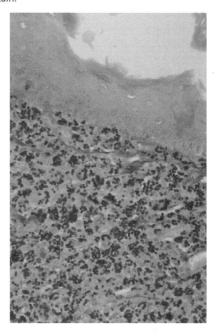

taneous mycoses. More than one fungal agent may be responsible for each of these conditions. For example, eumycotic mycetomas—which are characterized by 1) localized swelling at the infection site (tumefaction), 2) draining sinus tracts, and 3) the presence of granules or grains composed of colonies of the causative agent (Fig 69.5)—are caused by over 14 species of dematiaceous (pigmented) fungi and over 9 species of hyaline (colorless) fungi. They produce dark- and white-grained mycetomas, respectively.

Sporotrichosis is a subcutaneous mycosis caused by the dimorphic fungus, *Sporothrix schenckii*. Lesions of sporotrichosis are ulcerative nodules or recurrent draining tracts in the skin. Infections may also involve the lymphatics causing a lymphangitis, in addition to the skin lesions. Cats, horses, and dogs are most commonly affected.

Cutaneous pythiosis is caused by an oomycete, *Pythium insidiosum*, and therefore is not a true fungal infection. It is found in swamps and ponds, and the disease is associated with exposure to those environments. Skin infections are characterized by firm or spongy, ulcerated lesions that often have draining fistulous tracts. Necrotic masses of tissue (kunkers) may be found in the lesion. Although uncommon, horses and dogs are most frequently affected. An additional genus, *Lagenidium*, has also been reported to be involved in such lesions.

When one of the systemic mycotic agents involves the integumentary system, the lesions are typically ulcerative nodules that may develop draining tracts. These pyogranulomatous skin lesions (Fig 69.6) may be the initial clinical manifestation of an infection even though organisms responsible for the skin lesions almost always originate from disseminated respiratory tract infections.

Common and/or important agents of the integumentary system of domestic animals and poultry are listed in Tables 69.1–69.7.

Table 69.1. Common and/or Important Infectious Agents of the Integumentary System of Dogs

Agent	Major Clinical Manifestations (Common Disease Name)
Viruses	
Canine distemper virus	Nasal and footpad hyperkeratosis (distemper)
Canine papillomavirus	Cutaneous papillomas (canine papillomatosis)
Bacteria	
Actinomyces viscosus, A. hordeovulneris	Draining tracts, subcutaneous abscesses
Brucella canis	Scrotal dermatitis
Staphylococcus intermedius[a]	Cellulitis, folliculitis, furunculosis, impetigo
Fungi	
Malassezia pachydermatis	Exfoliative dermatitis
Microsporum canis, M. gypseum Trichophyton mentagrophytes	Circular, scaly, crusty, alopectic skin lesions (dermatophytosis, ringworm)
Pythium insidiosum	Ulcerative and pyogranulomatous skin lesions (cutaneous pythiosis)
Systemic mycotic agents[b]	Papules, nodules, abscesses, draining tracts

[a]Other coagulase-positive *Staphylococcus* sp. involved in pyoderma include *S. aureus* and *S. schleiferi* subsp *coagulans.*
[b]Includes *Blastomyces dermatitidis, Coccidioides immitis, Cryptococcus neoformans,* and *Histoplasma capsulatum.*

Table 69.2. Common and/or Important Infectious Agents of the Integumentary System of Cats

Agent	Major Clinical Manifestations (Common Disease Name)
Viruses	
Cowpox virus[a]	Macules, papules, nodules (cowpox virus infection)
Feline sarcoma virus	Cutaneous and subcutaneous nodules
Bacteria	
Mycobacterium spp[b]	Chronic nodular dermatitis, draining tracts, panniculitis (atypical mycobacteriosis)
Mycobacterium lepraemurium	Noduloulcerative skin lesions with lymphadenopathy (feline leprosy)
Obligate anaerobic bacteria[c]	Subcutaneous abscesses
Pasteurella multocida	Subcutaneous abscesses
Fungi	
Cryptococcus neoformans	Draining tracts, nodules, ulcers (cryptococcosis)
Microsporum canis	Alopectic annular skin lesions (dermatophytosis, ringworm), pseudomycetoma
Sporothrix schenckii	Draining tracts, ulcerative nodules (sporotrichosis)

[a]Not seen in the United States.
[b]Includes *M. fortuitum, M. chelonei, M. xenopi, M. smegmatis,* and *M. phlei.*
[c]Includes *Peptostreptococcus* spp., *Fusobacterium* spp., *Porphyromonas* spp., and *Clostridium* spp.

Table 69.3.   Common and/or Important Infectious Agents of the Integumentary System of Horses

Agent	Major Clinical Manifestations (Common Disease Name)
Viruses	
Bovine papillomaviruses 1&2	Verrucous, fibroblastic or flat and thickened skin lesions (equine sarcoid)
Equine papillomavirus	Cutaneous papillomas of lips and nose (equine papillomatosis)
Equine viral arteritis virus	Edema of distal limbs, scrotum, and ventrum
Vesicular stomatitis virus	Vesicles/ulcers on coronary band
Bacteria	
Bacillus anthracis	Diffuse subcutaneous and dermal edema (anthrax)
Burkholderia mallei[a]	Subcutaneous nodules that ulcerate, lymphangitis (farcy)
Clostridium perfringens[b]	Cellulitis
Corynebacterium pseudotuberculosis	Pectoral (pigeon breast) or inguinal abscesses, lymphangitis (ulcerative lymphangitis)
Dermatophilus congolensis	Exudative dermatitis (dermatophilosis, rain rot)
Rhodococcus equi	Cutaneous abscesses, cellulitis
Staphylococcus aureus[c]	Cellulitis, folliculitis, furunculosis
Fungi	
Histoplasma farciminosum[a]	Nodules of head, neck, and leg; lymphangitis (histoplasmosis farciminosi)
Pythium insidiosum	Ulcerative pyogranulomatous lesions (cutaneous pythiosis, swamp cancer)
Sporothrix schenckii	Ulcerative nodules on legs, lymphangitis (sporotrichosis)
Trichophyton equinum, T. mentagrophytes, M. equinum	Crusty skin lesions; hair loss often involving head, shoulders, and back (dermatophytosis, ringworm)

[a]Considered a foreign animal disease agent in the United States.
[b]Other clostridial species include *C. septicum, C. sordellii,* and *C. sporogenes.*
[c]Other coagulase-positive species affecting horses include *S. intermedius* and *S. hyicus* subsp. *hyicus.*

Table 69.4.   Common and/or Important Infectious Agents of the Integumentary System of Cattle

Agent	Major Clinical Manifestations (Common Disease Name)
Viruses	
Bovine herpesvirus 2	Mammary vesicles and ulcers (bovine mammilitis)
Bovine papillomavirus	Cutaneous papillomas (bovine papillomatosis, warts)
Lumpy skin disease virus[a]	Generalized or local papules and nodules that ulcerate (lumpy skin disease)
Pseudocowpox virus	Mammary vesicles, papules, and scabs (pseudocowpox)
Pseudorabies virus	Uncontrolled pruritis (pseudorabies)
Vesicular viruses[b]	Vesicles and ulcers on coronary band and interdigital areas
Bacteria	
Actinobacillus ligniersii	Head and neck abscess, draining fistulas
Actinomyces bovis	Draining tracts, subcutaneous abscesses (actinomycosis, lumpy jaw)
Arcanobacterium pyogenes	Subcutaneous abscesses
Clostridium septicum	Cellulitis (malignant edema)
Corynebacterium pseudotuberculosis	Ulcerative dermatitis
Dermatophilus congolensis	Exudative epidermitis (dermatophilosis)
Fusobacterium necrophorum/ Prevotella melaninogenicus[c]	Interdigital dermatitis, cellulitis (interdigital necrobacillosis, footrot)
Salmonella Dublin	Gangrene of distal extremities, ears, and tail due to terminal endarteritis
Fungi	
Trichophyton verrucosum	Round to oval, crusty skin lesions with alopecia (dermatophytosis, ringworm)

[a]Considered a foreign animal disease agent in the United States.
[b]Includes foot-and-mouth disease virus[a] and vesicular stomatitis virus.
[c]Agents act synergistically.

Table 69.5.   Common and/or Important Infectious Agents of the Integumentary System of Sheep/Goats

Agent	Major Clinical Manifestations (Common Disease Name)
Prions	
Scrapie prion	Pruritus, excoriations, self-mutilation (scrapie)
Viruses	
Bluetongue virus	Erythema, edema of ears and muzzle, coronitis (bluetongue)
Goat pox, sheep pox viruses[a]	Papules, vesicles, pustules (goat pox, sheep pox)
Parapoxvirus	Crusting proliferative mucocutaneous lesions, teat lesions (contagious ecthyma, soremouth)
Vesicular viruses[b]	Vesicles and ulcers on teats, coronary bands, and interdigital areas
Bacteria	
Clostridium novyi	Edema of the head, neck, and thorax (big head in rams)
Corynebacterium pseudotuberculosis	Skin abscesses (caseous lymphadenitis)
Dermatophilus congolensis	Exudative dermatitis (dermatophilosis, lumpy wool disease, strawberry footrot)
Dichelobacter nodosus/Fusobacterium necrophorum[c]	Interdigital dermatitis, underrunning of the sole (contagious footrot)
Staphylococcus aureus[d]	Pustular dermatitis of face, udder, teats, and ventral abdomen (staphylococcal dermatitis)
Fungi	
Trichophyton verrucosum, T. mentagrophytes	Crusting, circular skin lesions with alopecia (dermatophytosis, ringworm, club lamb fungus)

[a]Considered a foreign animal disease agent in the United States.
[b]Includes foot-and-mouth disease virus[a] and vesicular stomatitis virus.
[c]Agents act synergistically.
[d]*Staphylococcus aureus* subsp. *anaerobius* is associated with subcutaneous abscesses in sheep.

Table 69.6.   Common and/or Important Infectious Agents of the Integumentary System of Pigs

Agent	Major Clinical Manifestations (Common Disease Name)
Viruses	
African swine fever virus[a]	Reddish-purple discoloration of skin (African swine fever)
Hog Cholera virus[a]	Erythema, purple discoloration of skin, necrosis of ears and tail (hog cholera)
Swinepox virus	Macules, papules, pustules (swinepox)
Vesicular viruses[b]	Vesicles and ulcers on coronary band and interdigital areas
Bacteria	
Bacillus anthracis	Diffuse subcutaneous and dermal edema of neck and thorax (anthrax)
Erysipelothrix rhusiopathiae	Congested raised skin lesions, rhomboidal-shaped necrotic skin lesions (erysipelas)
Escherichia coli (Shiga-like toxin positive)	Subcutaneous edema of lips and eyelids (edema disease)
Salmonella Choleraesuis	Reddish-purple discoloration of the skin
Streptococcus equi subsp. *zooepidemicus,* *S. dysgalactiae* subsp. *equisimilus*	Pustular dermatitis, subcutaneous abscesses
Staphylococcus hyicus	Generalized exudative dermatitis (exudative epidermitis, greasy pig disease)
Fungi	
Microsporum nanum, Trichophyton spp.	Reddish circular skin lesions with crusting at periphery (dermatophytosis, ringworm)

[a]Considered a foreign animal disease agent in the United States.
[b]Includes foot-and-mouth,[a] vesicular stomatitis virus, swine vesicular disease, and vesicular exanthema of swine viruses.

Table 69.7.   Common and/or Important Infectious Agents of the Integumentary System of Poultry

Agent	Major Clinical Manifestations (Common Disease Name)
Viruses	
Fowlpox virus	Papules and nodules of beak, comb, and wattles (avian pox)
Marek's disease virus (C)	Nodular lesions of feather follicles (Marek's disease)
Bacteria	
Staphylococcus aureus	Plantar abscesses (bumblefoot), gangrenous dermatitis
Clostridium septicum, C. perfringens	Gangrenous dermatitis
Erysipelothrix rhusiopathiae	Turgid/red-purple snood, erythema (erysipelas)
Escherichia coli (C)	Cellulitis
Fungi	
Microsporum gallinae	White, powdery lesions of comb, wattles, and legs (dermatophytosis, favus)

(C) = chickens predominantly

Table 69.8.   Common Agents of Canine Otitis Externa and Key Organism Characteristics

Agent	Typical Colonies On: Blood Agar (24-48 hrs)	MacConkey Agar	Ancillary Tests Gram stain	Oxidase	Catalase
Staphylococcus intermedius	White or off-white, often with double-zone hemolysis	No growth	Positive cocci	NA	Positive
Staphylococcus schleiferi subsp. coagulans	White, hemolytic	No growth	Positive cocci	NA	Positive
Proteus mirabilis	Swarms, no discrete colonies	Colorless	Negative rods	Negative	NA
Pseudomonas aeruginosa	Gray to greenish, fruity odor, hemolytic	Colorless, sometimes pigment detected	Negative rods	Positive	NA
Streptococcus canis	Small, white, ß hemolytic	No growth	Positive cocci	NA	Negative
Escherichia coli	Smooth, grey, some strains are hemolytic	Pink to red with red haze	Negative rods	Negative	NA
Klebsiella pneumoniae	Mucoid, whitish-grey	Mucoid, pink without red haze	Negative rods	Negative	NA
Malassezia pachydermatis	No growth or tiny colonies[a]	No growth	Variable staining, budding yeast	NA	NA

NA = not applicable
[a]May require prolonged incubation. Best recovery on Sabouraud's dextrose agar at 37°C under microaerophilic conditions.

Otitis Externa

Otitis externa in dogs is one of the most common dermatological problems encountered. There is a direct relation between ear conformation and otitis externa, with pendulous-eared dogs being predisposed to infection. The L-shaped configuration of the external meatus is a further complicating factor because it limits aeration and drainage. An abundance of lipid-rich earwax and heavy ear canal hair additionally contribute to development of otitis externa. A breed predilection (e.g., cocker spaniels) for development of otitis externa is also evident.

The agents of canine otitis externa are endogenous in origin and are not thought to play the initiating role in the disease process, but rather act as opportunists once other factors are in place. Infections are frequently polymicrobial. Commonly recovered agents from canine otitis externa are listed in Table 69.8.

Mastitis

Mastitis, an inflammation of the mammary gland, occurs in all animal species. It is most common in dairy cattle and is of greatest economic significance to the dairy industry. For mastitis to develop, the innate physical barriers must be breached. Once that occurs, both innate immunity (lactoferrin, complement, resident immune cells) and specific immunity play a role in preventing microbial pathogens from establishing. If a pathogen does establish in the mammary gland, chemotactic gradients formed by inflammatory cytokines and chemokines result in rapid re-

FIGURE 69.7. *Lactophenol aniline blue wet mount preparation of a* Prototheca *isolate from a cow with mastitis. Sac-like structures (thecae) containing variable numbers of daughter cells (autospores) are seen.*

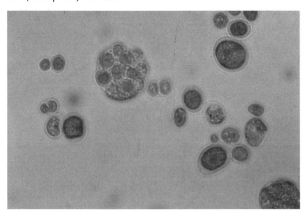

cruitment on inflammatory cells in an effort to control the infection. Most of the clinical signs associated with mastitis are a consequence of the inflammatory response.

Bacteria are the main infectious agents of mastitis, although viruses are important mammary pathogens in some animals (Maedi-visna, sheep; CAE, goats). Fungi (e.g., *Candida, Aspergillus, Pseudallescheria*) and an achloric algae, *Prototheca* (Fig 69.7), are rare causes of mastitis in cattle but can occasionally cause herd outbreaks.

Different organisms predominate as mastitis pathogens depending on the animal involved. Coliforms (dogs, swine), *Staphylococcus aureus* (sheep, goats), beta-hemolytic streptococci (horses), *Mannheimia haemolytica* (sheep), and *Mycoplasma* species (sheep, goats) are the most commonly encountered bacteria.

The agents associated with mastitis in cattle are extensive and are classified as either "contagious" pathogens where the mammary gland is the source or as "environmental" pathogens when they originate from transient skin flora or environmental reservoirs. Cow age, parity, stage of lactation, milking operation management methods, and environmental sanitation control (housing and bedding) are underlying factors in most cases of mastitis. Common agents of bovine mastitis are listed in Table 69.9.

Table 69.9. Agents of Bovine Mastitis

Agent[a]	Frequency	Specific Features
Arcanobacterium pyogenes	Occasional	Associated with teat injury or cannula/dilator use, poor treatment response
Clostridium perfringens	Rare	Causes gangrenous mastitis
Coagulase-negative *Staphylococcus* spp.	Frequent	Source is skin, many infections transient
Escherichia coli	Frequent	Environmental source, acute infections, may cause systemic illness
Klebsiella pneumoniae	Occasional	Severe mastitis, associated with sawdust/wood shaving bedding
Mycoplasma spp.[b,c]	Frequent	Cow is source, spread by milking, destructive mastitis, cow not usually systemically ill, can be eradicated
Mycobacterium spp	Rare	Spread by contaminated treatment equipment or materials
Nocardia spp.	Rare	Spread by contaminated treatment equipment or materials
Pasteurella multocida	Rare	Sporadic infections, suggests cross-contamination during treatment
Prototheca spp.	Rare	Achloric algae, associated with poor environmental hygiene, not treatable
Staphylococcus aureus[b]	Frequent	Source is infected udder, spread by milking, rare cause of gangrenous mastitis, can be eradicated
Streptococcus agalactiae[b]	Occasional	Causes high bulk tank somatic cell count, can be eradicated
S. dysgalactiae subsp. *dysgalactiae*	Frequent	Bovine origin, survives in environment
Streptococcus uberis	Frequent	Found on bovine skin and environment

[a]Also consider *Corynebacterium bovis, Serratia, Bacillus, Pseudomonas,* and various other *Enterobacteriaceae.*
[b]Contagious pathogens.
[c]Most common species recovered are *M. bovis, M. californicum,* and *M. canadense.*

70 Musculoskeletal System

RICHARD L. WALKER

The musculoskeletal system provides a structural framework for the body, protects vital organs, and provides the capacity for locomotion. It is composed of the axial and appendicular skeleton and associated ligaments, muscles, and tendons. Joint spaces and bursas and their synovial membranes are included in this system.

The musculoskeletal system does not have a normal flora per se, although seeding from transient bacteremias or "trafficking" through supposed sterile sites may occur. Bacterial spores (*Clostridium* sp.) may be found dormant in muscle, particularly in ruminants, subsequent to entry through the digestive tract and hematogenous distribution.

Antimicrobial Defenses of the Musculoskeletal System

The antimicrobial defenses of the musculoskeletal system predominately rely on the circulating immune defenses.

Normal healthy bone is considered fairly resistant to infection. Even direct inoculation of bone with pathogenic bacteria does not usually lead to infection unless predisposing factors are present. Bone undergoes constant remodeling, and injured/infected bone can be resorbed and replaced with new bone.

Muscle has a rich blood supply and, therefore, benefits from its intimate association with circulating innate immune defenses. Skeletal muscle also has great ability to regenerate necrotic muscle segments resulting from inflammatory/infectious processes.

In synovial membrane-lined sites (synovial joints, bursas, and tendon sheaths), the synovium lining is composed of a thin cellular surface layer of predominately macrophages and fibroblast-like synoviocytes and an underlying rich vascular layer. Production of proinflammatory cytokines by cells at these sites (chondrocytes, synoviocytes, synovial macrophages) promotes a strong inflammatory response in the face of infection. The rich blood supply to synovial membranes predisposes to localization of microbial agents but also allows for rapid recruitment of vascular immune defenses. While the inflammatory response is important for controlling infection, it can also lead to degradative changes to articular cartilage in synovial joints by stimulating production of catabolic metalloproteinases and inhibiting synthesis of collagen and proteoglycans. As inflammation resolves, fibrosis may lead to decreased functionality.

Infections of the Musculoskeletal System

Infections of the musculoskeletal system are initiated by introduction of microbial agents through 1) direct inoculation from traumatic or iatrogenic events, 2) extension of infectious processes from contiguous focuses, or 3) hematogenous seeding from distantly infected sites or during septicemia. Within the musculoskeletal system sites of traumatic injury, areas of active growth with increased vascularity or sites with specific vascular features (e.g., discontinuous epithelium in capillaries in vertebral end plates and metaphyses) are predisposed to infection. Viral, bacterial, and fungal agents can be involved. Parasite infections of muscle are also important but are not within the context of this book. As a rule, bacteria are the most common microbial agents involved among the three groups of agents discussed here. Specific bacterial factors are important for infection to develop. Adherence factors (e.g., fibrinogen or fibronectin-binding proteins), toxins that promote inflammatory response and tissue damage (e.g., superantigens, cytotoxins), and factors that aid in evasion of the immune system (e.g., capsules, protein A) all provide an advantage to establishment and persistence.

The major infectious processes in the musculoskeletal system are 1) infections of bone including vertebral body and associated intervertebral disk infections; 2) infections involving articular surfaces or bursas including their synovial membranes; and 3) infections of skeletal muscle, tendons, and surrounding fascia. These infectious processes do not necessarily occur as distinct entities (e.g., infection of metaphyseal bone and associated joint infections in neonatal septicemia in some animals). Diseases of neurologic origin that affect muscle activity as a result of inhibition of neurotransmitter release (tetanus and botulism) are covered in chapter 71. Microbial agents causing cellulitis may overlap with musculoskeletal infections and are also covered in chapter 69. Common and/or important agents associated with musculoskeletal infections of domestic animals and poultry are listed in Tables 70.1–70.6.

Infections of Bone (Including Vertebral Body and Intervertebral Disk Infections)

Osteitis is an inflammation of the bone. Osteomyelitis and periostitis denote involvement of the medullary cavity and periosteum, respectively. Osteomyelitis can be further divided into hematogenous or post-traumatic osteomyelitis.

Table 70.1. Common and/or Important Infectious Agents of Musculoskeletal System of Dogs and Cats

Agent	Major Clinical Manifestations (Common Disease Name)
Viruses	
Feline syncytium-forming virus (C)	Arthritis
Bacteria	
Actinomyces spp.[a]	Diskospondylitis, osteomyelitis
Beta-hemolytic Streptococcus spp. (D)	Arthritis, diskospondylitis, myositis, necrotizing fasciitis
Borrelia burgdorferi (D)	Arthritis (Lyme disease)
Brucella canis (D)	Diskospondylitis, osteomyelitis
Leptospira spp	Polymyositis
Obligate anaerobes[b]	Myositis
Pasteurella multocida (C)	Myositis
Staphylococcus intermedius	Arthritis, diskospondylitis, myositis, osteomyelitis
Fungi	
Aspergillus spp. (D)	Diskospondylitis, osteomyelitis
Blastomyces dermatitidis (D)	Osteomyelitis
Coccidioides immitis (D)	Osteomyelitis

(C) = cats, (D) = dogs
[a]Includes *A. viscosus* and *A. hordeovulneris.*
[b]Includes *Fusobacterium, Bacteroides, Porphyromonas,* and *Peptostreptococcus.*

Table 70.2. Common and/or Important Infectious Agents of Musculoskeletal System of Horses

Agent	Major Clinical Manifestations (Common Disease Name)
Bacteria	
Actinobacillus equuli ssp. equuli	Arthritis, osteomyelitis (joint ill)
Brucella abortus	Atlantal or supraspinous bursitis (poll evil/fistulous withers), osteomyelitis
Escherichia coli	Arthritis, osteomyelitis (joint ill)
Histotoxic Clostridium spp.[a]	Myositis (clostridial myositis)
Salmonella spp.	Arthritis, osteomyelitis (joint ill)
Staphylococcus aureus	Arthritis, atlantal or supraspinous bursitis (poll evil/fistulous withers), myositis, osteomyelitis, tenosynovitis
Streptococcus equi subsp. equi	Muscle infarction—immune complex–mediated
Streptococcus equi subsp. zooepidemicus	Arthritis, osteomyelitis (joint ill)

[a]Includes *C. perfringens, C. sordellii,* and *C. septicum.*

Table 70.3. Common and/or Important Infectious Agents of the Musculoskeletal System of Cattle

Agent	Major Clinical Manifestations (Common Disease Name)
Bacteria	
Actinobacillus lignieresii	Myositis (actinobacillosis)
Actinomyces bovis	Osteomyelitis (lumpy jaw), myositis
Arcanobacterium pyogenes	Arthritis, diskospondylitis, fasciitis, myositis, osteomyelitis
Clostridium chauvoei	Myositis (blackleg)
Escherichia coli	Arthritis, osteomyelitis
Fusobacterium necrophorum	Arthritis, diskospondylitis, osteomyelitis
Histotoxic Clostridium spp[a]	Myositis (malignant edema)
Mycoplasma spp.[b]	Arthritis, bursitis, tenosynovitis
Salmonella spp.	Arthritis, osteomyelitis

[a]Includes *C. perfringens, C. novyi, C. septicum,* and *C. sordellii.*
[b]Includes *M. bovis, M. californicum, M. alkalescens,* and *M. arginini.*

Table 70.4. Common and/or Important Infectious Agents of the Musculoskeletal System of Sheep and Goats

Agent	Major Clinical Manifestations (Common Disease Name)
Viruses	
Bluetongue virus (S)	Muscle infarction
Caprine arthritis-encephalitis virus (G)	Arthritis
Bacteria	
Arcanobacterium pyogenes (S)	Diskospondylitis, myositis
Chlamydophila percorum	Arthritis
Corynebacterium pseudotuberculosis	Myositis
Erysipelothrix rhusiopathiae (S)	Arthritis (erysipelas)
Histotoxic Clostridium spp[a]	Myositis
Mycoplasma spp. (G)[b]	Arthritis, tenosynovitis

(G) = goats, (S) = sheep
[a]Includes *C. perfringens, C. novyi, C. septicum,* and *C. sordellii.*
[b]Includes *M. mycoides* subsp. *mycoides* (large colony type), *M. capricolum* subsp. *capricolum,* and *M. putrefaciens.*

Most bone infections are bacterial in nature. While a variety of bacteria can cause bone infections, a select number predominate within animal groups. In companion animals and poultry, coagulase-positive *Staphylococcus* species (*S. intermedius, S. aureus, S. hyicus*) are frequently involved. Other organisms encountered include enterics (*E. coli, Proteus* spp.) and obligate anaerobes. In horses, the agents most commonly isolated from osteomyelitis in neonates are *Actinobacillus equuli* subsp. *equuli, E. coli, Streptococcus equi* subsp *zooepidemicus,* and *Salmonella,* while coagulase-positive staphylococci predominate in adults. In ruminants and pigs, *Arcanobacterium pyogenes* and *Salmonella* are major causes of osteomyelitis. Others of note in production animals are *E. coli* and *Fusobacterium necrophorum.*

The microvasculature (discontinuous epithelium and lack of basement membrane) and possibly the slow blood flow through capillaries in areas of active growth favor the establishment of infections (hematogenous osteomyelitis). Macrophages associated with vascular endothelium

Table 70.5. Common and/or Important Infectious Agents of Musculoskeletal System of Pigs

Agent	Major Clinical Manifestations (Common Disease Name)
Bacteria	
Arcanobacterium pyogenes	Arthritis, osteomyelitis
Beta-hemolytic *Streptococcus* spp.	Arthritis
Brucella suis	Arthritis, diskospondylitis (brucellosis)
Clostridium septicum	Myositis (malignant edema)
Erysipelothrix rhusiopathiae	Arthritis, diskospondylitis (erysipelas)
Haemophilus parasuis	Arthritis (Glasser's disease)
Mycoplasma hyorhinis	Arthritis
Mycoplasma hyosynoviae	Arthritis
Pasteurella multocida	Atrophy of nasal turbinate bones (atrophic rhinitis)
Streptococcus suis (Type 2)	Arthritis

Table 70.6. Common and/or Important Infectious Agents of Musculoskeletal System of Poultry

Agent	Major Clinical Manifestations (Common Disease Name)
Viruses	
Reovirus	Arthritis, bursitis, tenosynovitis
Bacteria	
Arcanobacterium pyogenes (T)	Osteomyelitis
Erysipelothrix rhusiopathiae (T)	Arthritis (erysipelas)
Escherichia coli	Arthritis, bursitis, osteomyelitis, tenosynovitis
Mycoplasma meleagridis (T)	Bowing of tibiotarsal bone, cervical vertebrae deformation
Mycoplasma synoviae	Arthritis, bursitis, tenosynovitis (infectious synovitis)
Staphylococcus aureus, S. hyicus	Arthritis, bursitis, osteomyelitis, tenosynovitis

(T) = turkeys

Use of synthetic material in reconstructive or replacement surgeries (e.g., hip replacements) may also disrupt the innate resistance of bone to infection by providing an avascular surface and protection from immune defenses. Bone cement used in some replacement surgeries may itself inhibit phagocytosis and complement activity. Host fibronectin deposited on implant material allows for bacterial attachment, which is followed by production of exopolysaccharides (glycocalyx) by bacteria. Along with host products, the glycocalyx forms biofilms that provide bacteria protection from host defenses and killing by antibiotics.

Bite wounds, penetrating foreign bodies, orthopedic surgical procedures, and traumatic injuries are possible initiating events for development of osteomyelitis in companion animals. The long bones are most commonly affected.

In production animals, hematogenous osteomyelitis is a frequent event. Hematogenous osteomyelitis in neonatal ruminants is associated with failure of passive transfer. Infections begin at the metaphysis or the epiphysis beneath articular cartilage and often occur in conjunction with or subsequent to infectious synovitis. In neonatal infections, vessels that cross the growth plates are important for spreading infection to the metaphysis from joints. Epiphyseal osteomyelitis in conjunction with arthritis in calves is commonly caused by *Salmonella* serovar Dublin. *Arcanobacterium pyogenes* osteomyelitis in older calves and adults more commonly begins on the metaphyseal side of the growth plate. *Arcanobacterium pyogenes* also causes a hematogenous vertebral osteomyelitis in pigs associated with tail biting or foot lesions. Commercial turkeys develop focal areas of osteomyelitis caused by *S. aureus* or *E. coli*. The proximal tibiotarsus and proximal femur are most often affected and infections are associated with a green discoloration of the liver in adolescent male turkeys (turkey green-liver osteomyelitis complex) (Fig 70.1). Hematogenous osteomyelitis is uncommon in dogs and cats.

Post-traumatic osteomyelitis is also common in production animals, usually in adults. In cattle a chronic pyo-

are the main defense in these areas. Infections also occur in areas of bone with poor or interrupted vascular supply from trauma (post-traumatic osteomyelitis) or when adjacent tissue infections result in ischemic injury. If both the medullary and periosteal vascular supply to bone becomes compromised during an infectious process, a sequestration of necrotic bone may result. In some cases, persistent drainage from sinus tracts develops. Under these conditions, bacteria are better able to establish and more difficult to eliminate because they become inaccessible to immune defenses and refractory to antibiotic treatment. Host cellular products, and perhaps some bacterial products, stimulate monocytes and fibroblast to produce osteolytic cytokines and stimulate osteoclastic activity, causing greater separation of living from dead bone.

FIGURE 70.1. *Osteomyelitis in the femur of a 17-week-old turkey with green-liver osteomyelitis complex. Staphylococcus hyicus was isolated from the bone lesion. (Courtesy Dr. H. Shivaprasad.)*

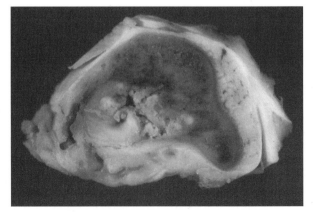

granulomatous inflammation involving the mandible ("lumpy jaw") or maxilla is caused by *Actinomyces bovis*.

Viral agents rarely cause inflammatory bone disease. Distemper virus in dogs may damage osteoblasts and cause growth retardation. Canine hepatitis virus can cause metaphyseal hemorrhage and necrosis.

Fungal bone infections occur but at a low frequency. Fungal osteomyelitis is usually the result of dissemination from another site, most often the lung. Many of the systemic mycotic agents are capable of causing fungal osteomyelitis. *Coccidioides immitis* is notable for disseminating to the appendicular skeleton in dogs. Disseminated *Blastomyces dermatitidis* infections in dogs can involve the bones in up to 30% of the cases with vertebrae, and long bones are most commonly affected.

Diskospondylitis, an inflammatory process of the intervertebral disk and adjacent vertebrae, is a particularly common site for bone infections to occur. It usually begins at the vertebral end plates. The discontinuous capillary epithelium and slow-flowing venous channels predispose this area to bacterial seeding. Diskospondylitis is most common in dogs and ruminants and often results via hematogenous dissemination. The L7–S1 region is a commonly affected site in the dog but any vertebral body can be affected. *Staphylococcus intermedius* is the most common agent identified.

Vertebral infections of T13–L3 in the dog are associated with migration of foreign bodies (e.g., plant awns). *Actinomyces* spp. are the usual agents involved. Diskospondylitis associated with *Brucella* species deserves particular attention. The persistent bacteremia that occurs with some *Brucella* species predisposes to infection at extragenital sites and *Brucella* should always be considered as a potential agent in diskospondylitis in dogs (*B. canis*) and pigs (*B. suis*). Calves with diskospondylitis caused by hematogenous dissemination of either *A. pyogenes* or *Fusobacterium necrophorum* present with paresis or paralysis.

German shepherd dogs are particularly prone to developing diskospondylitis and osteomyelitis of fungal origin caused by *Aspergillus* spp. *Aspergillus terreus* and *A. deflectus* are the most common species recovered.

Infections Involving Articular Surfaces, Bursas, and Synovial Membranes

Arthritis denotes an inflammatory process of a joint space. Most joint infections are bacterial, but viral and fungal infections do occur. Monoarticular infections typically arise from direct inoculation or spread from a contiguous site (e.g., distal interphalangeal joint infection in cattle following sole abscessation). Hematogenous infections frequently result in polyarthropathies. In neonates, the umbilicus or gastrointestinal tract are common entry points. Arthritis is a common sequelae to septicemia, especially in young animals and especially where there is failure of passive transfer. In adult animals, joint abnormalities, immunosuppressive diseases, infections at other sites in the body, intra-articular injections, surgery, and joint prostheses all predispose to joint infections.

Infection of the joint usually begins in synovial tissue—in part, because of the rich vascular supply and lack of basement membrane. Infection results in expression of a cascade of inflammatory mediators (TNF, IL-1, IL-6, and NO) that result in increased blood flow to the area, increased capillary permeability, and an influx of inflammatory cells. The agent involved dictates the type and intensity of inflammatory response. Synovitis in unchecked infections results in increased synovial fluid containing cellular exudates that subsequently progresses to involve the articular surfaces. Alone or in combination, bacterial products, products resulting from the inflammatory response, and proteases already present or produced by cells in the joint damage articular cartilage. Once damaged, articular cartilage has limited capacity for repair.

Current evidence suggests that when viable bacteria are no longer detectable in cases of septic arthritis, the inflammatory response continues and further destruction to articular cartilage ensues. This is likely due to residual bacterial products such as peptidoglycan-polysaccharide complexes that continue to promote an inflammatory response. Even bacterial DNA, specifically unmethylated CpG motifs, appears to stimulate a variety of cell types to produce pro-inflammatory cytokines leading to further tissue destruction. Joint functionality may be further affected by fibrosis that results during resolution of the inflammatory process. In some cases ankylosis of the joint occurs.

Post-infective arthritis, which is associated with microbial fragments localizing in the joint during a septicemia but without microbial replication in the joint itself, is less well recognized in veterinary medicine than it is in human medicine. When it occurs, joint damage results solely from immune mechanisms.

Morphologic variants of bacteria have also been associated with joint infections. Bacterial L- forms, which are wall-less bacteria, which have "turned off" the genes responsible for cell wall synthesis, and small colony variants of bacteria, which have decreased growth rates presumably due to defective respiratory metabolism, have been associated with persistent joint infections.

In species where transphyseal vessels provide a direct connection between the metaphyses and the epiphyseal cartilage (e.g., ruminants, horses), both acute osteomyelitis and joint infections are common. This is also true when metaphyseal bone is included within the joint capsule. Sometimes synovitis represents only one of a number of clinical manifestations of systemic infectious processes (e.g., polyserositis in pigs caused by *Mycoplasma hyorhinis* or *Haemophilus parasuis*).

Bacterial arthritis is uncommon in companion animals. When it occurs, coagulase-positive *Staphylococcus* species and *Streptococcus* species are the most common agents involved. Infections result from direct inoculation from trauma or surgery. The canine stifle joint appears particularly predisposed to post-surgical infections. Recurrent lameness, sometimes involving multiple joints, is associated with a chronic and progressive arthritis due to *Borrelia burgdorferi*, the Lyme disease agent.

Arthritis is common in production animals and horses, and a variety of organisms can be involved. In neonates, *Salmonella* and *E. coli* are the main agents. *Mycoplasma* arthritis in ruminants is also an important entity in feed-

FIGURE 70.2.   *Polyarthritis involving the carpal joints of a Holstein dairy calf.* Mycoplasma bovis *was isolated from the joint fluid. (Courtesy Dr. P. Blanchard.)*

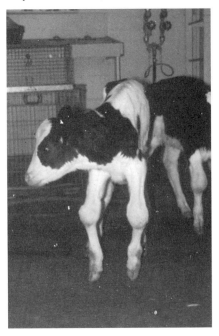

FIGURE 70.3.   *Gram stain of exudate from a fistulous withers lesion in a horse. Clusters of gram-positive cocci are present.* Staphylococcus aureus *was isolated.*

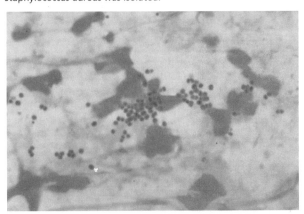

The digital flexor and metatarsal extensor tendons and hock joints are most commonly affected. The stability of the virus, potential for horizontal and vertical transmission and high-density rearing practices used today make it a potentially serious flock problem.

Infections of Skeletal Muscle, Tendons, and Fascia

Infections of skeletal muscles are uncommon. While viral and fungal agents occasionally cause muscle infections, bacteria again are the most frequent of the three groups involved. Myositis can be in the form of a localized abscess, granuloma or diffuse inflammatory process that spreads along fascial planes. Preceding events include trauma, injections, bite wounds, or a contiguous infectious process (e.g., cellulitis, subcutaneous abscess, osteomyelitis). Pyogenic bacteria cause localized abscesses (e.g., *Pasteurella multocida* in cats). Granulomatous and pyogranulomatis myositis are associated with bacterial species known to evoke granulomatous pyogranulomatis inflammatory responses (e.g., *Mycobacterium bovis, Actinomyces* spp., *Actinobacillus lignieresii*). Clostridial myositis is typically a more diffuse infectious process and spreads rapidly along fascial planes. It is the most severe and aggressive form of the infectious myositides due to the production of potent histotoxins. Myositis may occur subsequent to or in conjunction with clostridial cellulitis. Most animal species are affected; however, clostridial myositis is most common in ruminants and horses. Clostridial agents usually reach affected sites by direct penetration (e.g., penetrating wound, injections) or, in the case of *Clostridium chauvoei*, the agent of blackleg, are already present in muscle as dormant spores. When tissue becomes devitalized, producing an anaerobic environment, the spores germinate and vegetative cells proliferate (Fig 70.4). Numerous cytotoxic exotoxins produced by these clostridial species contribute coagulative muscle necrosis.

Hemolytic *Streptococcus* spp. have been associated with severe necrotizing fasciitis in dogs. In horses, immune complex vasculitis is the supposed mechanism by which

lot cattle and dairy calves. In addition to arthritis, which usually involves carpal and hock joints (Fig 70.2), tenosynovitis and bursitis occur. *Mycoplasma bovis* is the usual species recovered. In goats, mycoplasma arthritis affects both kids and adults. *Mycoplasma mycoides* subspecies *mycoides* (large colony type) and *M. capricolum* subsp. *capricolum* are principal species isolated. *Mycoplasma* arthritis is also important in pigs. Chlamydial joint infections (*Chlamydophila percorum*) are commonly recognized in goats and sheep ("stiff lamb disease"). Infections can present in conjunction with conjunctivitis. The chlamydial species involved is different from the species associated with goat and sheep abortions. In horses, joint infections in neonates are caused by organisms also associated with neonatal osteomyelitis and include *E. coli, Salmonella, Actinobacillus,* and *Streptococcus* spp. In adult horses, *Staphylococcus* or *Streptococcus* spp. are usually involved.

Bursitis refers to an inflammation of the synovial lined bursas and can be affected in a manner similar to synovial membranes in joints. Of specific importance are *Brucella abortus* and *S. aureus* infections of the atlantal and supraspinous bursas in horses (Fig 70.3). These infections may spread to involved spinous processes of adjacent vertebrae.

Although bacteria are responsible for most cases of infectious arthritis, viral agents are sometimes involved. Feline syncytium-forming virus infections cause both proliferative and erosive forms of joint involvement in cats. Caprine arthritis-encephalomyelitis virus is of substantial importance in goats causing a hyperplastic polysynovitis, usually in goats older than 12 months. Avian reovirus causes arthritis and tenosynovitis in turkeys and chickens.

FIGURE 70.4. *Direct fluorescent antibody test using fluorescein-labeled, anti-*Clostridium chauvoei *antisera on an impression smear from muscle of a cow with a fibrinohemmorhagic, necrotizing myositis. Fluorescent* C. chauvoei *organisms are apparent.*

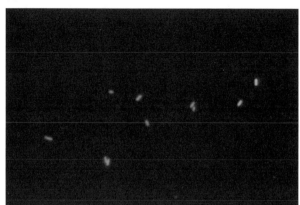

muscle damage due to vessel infarction and hemorrhage results post-*Streptococcus equi* subsp. *equi* infections.

Tendon sheaths have an inner synovial membrane and may become infected as a result of hematogenous dissemination, trauma (e.g., bite wounds), treatments (e.g., sheath injections in horses) or spread from a contiguous focus. Tenosynovitis is especially important in horses, most commonly involving digital tendons. Infections typically result from a wound with a variety of bacteria being involved or subsequent to sheath injection, where *S. aureus* is usually the cause.

71

Nervous System

RICHARD L. WALKER

The nervous system is divided into the central and peripheral nervous systems. The central nervous system includes the brain and spinal cord, the cerebrospinal fluid that bathes it, and the meningeal layers that cover it. The peripheral nervous system is comprised of nerves that arise from the central nervous system (cranial or spinal nerves) and innervate muscles or effector organs. The peripheral nervous system is further divided into somatic-sensory and autonomic divisions.

Nervous system infections most commonly involve the central nervous system. In some cases, peripheral nerves are the targeted site for infectious or immunological processes or microbial toxin action, or serve as the site for entry of infectious agents or toxic products that act on the central nervous system. The nervous system does not have a normal microbial flora. Some viruses (e.g., herpesviruses, distemper virus) can cause latent infections, and in some cases viruses integrate into the host genome as proviruses (e.g., visna virus).

Antimicrobial Defenses

Sensitivity of the nervous system to injury makes exclusion of microbial pathogens or their toxins of paramount importance. Anatomic and immunological defenses are the primary defense mechanisms available; the following sections present these defenses.

Anatomic Defenses

The skull and vertebrae provide rigid coverings that protect the brain and spinal cord from traumatic or penetrating injuries that might lead to introduction of microbial pathogens. The meningeal layers (pia, arachnoid, and dura) provide further anatomic barriers that act to contain or prevent infectious processes from progressing into the nervous system parenchyma.

The blood brain barrier provides the major anatomical separation between the nervous system parenchyma and components of the vascular system. It protects the central nervous system from agents disseminated via the blood stream from other sites in the body. Central to the blood brain barrier are the capillary endothelial cells, which form tight intercellular junctions that prevent movement of blood constituents into the central nervous system. Movement of substances across the endothelial cells is further controlled by specialized carrier transport systems.

Astrocyte processes and pericytes, a subclass of microglial cells, that surround capillaries and an extracellular matrix contribute to the overall makeup of the blood brain barrier. Not all areas are protected by the blood brain barrier (e.g., pituitary, choroid plexus). The secretory selectivity of choroid plexus epithelial cells and ependymal cells contribute to a barrier between the blood and cerebrospinal fluid. Nerves of the peripheral nervous system are protected from inflammatory reactions and immune responses by a blood nerve barrier, although it is not as restrictive as the blood brain barrier.

Immunological Defenses

Much of our knowledge of immune defense of the nervous system is based on studies in rodents and humans. The central nervous system has long been considered an immunologically privileged site because it lacks an organized lymphatic system for antigen delivery to lymph nodes and normally has greatly reduced expression of major histocompatibility complex determinants. Current evidence indicates that the nervous system has a much more advanced immunological defense system than was previously thought. Antigens from the cerebrospinal fluid are able to access lymph nodes (cervical) by lymphatic drainage along cranial nerves. Major histocompatibility antigens are expressed by cells in the central nervous system parenchyma (e.g., astrocytes and microglial cells) under proper conditions. The blood brain barrier contributes to the relative immune privilege of the healthy central nervous system by excluding entry of large molecules from the blood and by restricting immune cell entry. This restriction is not absolute and, although few immune cells are normally found, both activated and naive T lymphocytes can penetrate the blood brain barrier and are present in the absence of inflammation, suggesting a "patrolling" function. While an active immune system is in place, it is geared to provide a degree of protection and yet minimize innocent bystander damage. This is meant to avoid inflammatory responses that lead to profound or irreversible disturbances in neuronal function. Local inflammatory responses are regulated by immunosuppressive mechanisms. Subclasses of glial cells express cytokines (e.g., IL-6, TGFß2) that help restrict the inflammatory response. An ability to induce T lymphocyte apoptosis is also present.

The central nervous system possesses certain innate immune capabilities. Complement plays an essential role in innate immune defense. Both neuronal cells and astrocytes have ability to produce complement components. A number of nervous system pathogens will induce complement component synthesis (e.g., exotic Newcastle disease virus, *Listeria monocytogenes*), which plays both a direct role in pathogen killing by membrane attack complex formation, as well as in recruitment of leukocytes. Uncontrolled complement activation, resulting from progressing infectious processes, contributes to pathology when host cell membrane complement inhibitors are overwhelmed.

Various cell types are also critical to central nervous system defense. Microglia cells are myeloid bone marrow–derived cells. When activated, they produce various chemokines and cytokines, act as macrophages, and potentially have a role in antigen presentation. Dendritic cells, which are potent antigen-presenting cells, have also been demonstrated in the brain. Astrocytes have been shown to be involved in antigen presentation and chemokine/cytokine production. In the face of an inflammatory response, astrocytes become activated and can form glial scars to insulate damaged areas of the brain parenchyma. Nerve cells, themselves, are capable of producing certain cytokines (interferon γ).

During infectious processes, migration of inflammatory cells from the vascular system to affected sites is important for controlling progressing infectious processes. Inflammatory cell migration is mediated, as elsewhere in the body, through production of chemokines and expression of adhesion ligands (selectin and integrins).

Infections of the Nervous System

For microbial pathogens to affect the nervous system, they or their products must reach the nervous system (route of infection), be able to penetrate or interrupt anatomic barriers, and establish and persist by evading or subverting immune defenses. Clinical signs resulting from infection depend on whether and where the infection is localized, what agent is involved and the type and degree of inflammatory response induced. Most nervous system infectious processes have a rapid progression, requiring timely intervention. Most infections involve the brain or meninges; however, other areas can be involved concomitantly or serve as the principal targeted site. The decreased frequency of spinal cord involvement is most likely due to reduced blood flow to the spinal cord rather than some greater inherent resistance to infection than the brain. In some cases, the major or sole clinical manifestation is related to spinal cord lesions. For example, equine herpesvirus 1 infections may result in immune complex–related vasculitis causing necrosis that affects both the brain and spinal cord. Lesions in the spinal cord are sometimes the source for the predominant clinical signs. Peripheral nerve involvement is less frequent but is the site for important neurological diseases (e.g., Marek's disease in chickens).

The presence or growth of a microbial agent in the nervous system is not necessary for signs to develop. Microbial toxins ingested or produced at another site in the host (e.g., *C. perfringens* epsilon toxin, botulinum toxin, and tetanus toxin) and immune-mediated events af-

fecting vessels supplying the central nervous system (e.g., feline infectious peritonitis virus, equine herpesvirus 1) are responsible for important nervous system diseases.

The role of infectious agents in autoimmune diseases is still poorly understood. In humans, cross-reacting pathogen and host antigens results in molecular mimicry and has been associated with certain nervous system diseases. Notable is the mimicry between lipopolysaccharide structures of selected serotypes of *Campylobacter jejuni* and gangliosides (e.g., GM1, GD1a) of motor neurons. This is thought to account for the association between antecedent *Campylobacter* infections and some cases of Guillain-Barré syndrome, an acute demyelinating polyneuropathy, in humans. Some cases of acute canine polyradiculoneuritis (coonhound paralysis) may similarly be associated with immune reactions to viral or bacterial infections.

Some of the most common and/or important microbial agents associated with nervous system infections in domestic animals and poultry are listed in Tables 71.1–71.7.

Routes of Infection

The hematogenous route is the most common route of entry for microbial pathogens. Other important routes include retrograde movement within neurons or extension of the infectious processes from contiguous sites. Some pathogens appear capable of using more than one of these routes (e.g., *Listeria*).

Hematogenous Route. Systemic infections or infectious processes that involve multiple organ systems typically reach the nervous system by this route. Infection occurs when pathogens enter through vessels of the choroid plexus, meninges, or parenchyma, or from septic emboli that lodge in vessels and result in direct damage to vascular endothelial cells. Some viruses are able to cross the blood brain barrier themselves or are carried across in infected immune cells, while others directly infect the endothelium of capillaries or cells of the choroid plexus or ependyma.

Studies with *E. coli* show that 1) a high degree of bacteremia, 2) invasion of brain microvascular endothelial cells, 3) host cell actin cytoskeletal rearrangement, and 4) specific signaling mechanisms promote translocation of *E. coli* across the blood brain barrier. Different bacteria use different signaling mechanisms. Cytokines produced by astrocytes and microglial cells and nitric oxide from inflammatory cells in response to insults contribute to disruption of vascular barrier and further loss of ability to exclude entry of pathogens.

Retrograde Movement Within Neurons. Some infections result when an agent infects peripheral nerves and moves in a retrograde fashion to reach the central nervous system (e.g., rabies virus, pseudorabies virus). Binding to specific cell receptors is necessary for entry. For example, rabies viruses use nicotinic acetylcholine and low-affinity nerve–growth-factor receptors to attach and penetrate cells. In some cases cell-to-cell junctions, including synaptic junctions, are crossed. Some herpesviruses latently infect sensory ganglia and are later activated and may extend

Table 71.1. Common and/or Important Infectious Agents of the Nervous System of Dogs

Agent	Disease(s)	Neurological Signs
Viruses		
Canine adenovirus 1	Infectious canine hepatitis	Seizures
Canine distemper virus	Canine distemper	Ataxia, seizures
Canine herpesvirus	Canine herpes virus disease	Depression, opisthotonus, seizures
Pseudorabies virus	Pseudorabies	Intense pruritus, seizures
Rabies virus	Rabies	Temperament change, aggressive behavior, paralysis
Bacteria		
Agents of otitis externa[a]	Otitis media-interna	Vestibular dysfunction
Ehrlichia canis	Ehrlichiosis	Ataxia, cerebellar and vestibular dysfunctions, seizures
Clostridium botulinum	Botulism	Flaccid paralysis, paresis
Clostridium tetani	Tetanus	Opisthotonus, seizures, tremors
Rickettsia rickettsii	Rocky Mountain spotted fever	Ataxia, depression, seizures, vestibular dysfunctions
Fungi		
Cryptococcus neoformans	Cryptococcosis	Ataxia, head tilt, paresis, seizures

[a]Includes *E. coli*, *Proteus* spp., *Pseudomonas* spp., *Staphylococcus* spp., and *Streptococcus* spp.

Table 71.2. Common and/or Important Infectious Agents of the Nervous System of Cats

Agent	Disease	Neurological Signs
Prions		
BSE prion[a]	Feline spongiform encephalopathy	Ataxia, behavioral changes, muscular tremors
Viruses		
Feline panleukopenia virus[b]	Cerebellar hypoplasia	Ataxia
Feline immunodeficiency virus	Feline acquired immunodeficiency syndrome	Aggressive or psychotic behavior, seizures
Feline infectious peritonitis virus	Feline infectious peritonitis	Ataxia, paresis, seizures
Feline leukemia virus	Epidural lymphoma	Posterior paresis
	Feline leukemia	Abnormal vocalization, hyperesthesia, paresis
Pseudorabies virus	Pseudorabies	Hyperexcitability, paralysis, paresis
Rabies virus	Rabies	Aggressive behavior, paralysis
Fungi		
Cryptococcus neoformans	Cryptococcosis	Ataxia, paresis, cranial nerve deficits, seizures

[a]Classified as a foreign animal disease agent in the United States.
[b]Congenital infection.

into the central nervous system. Tetanus toxin moves in a retrograde fashion in the peripheral nerves to reach the central nervous system.

Extension of Infectious Process from Contiguous Sites. Parenchymal or meningeal infections may result from extension of infectious processes involving paranasal sinuses, tooth roots, or the middle ear (e.g., otitis media-interna in calves). Infections of the epidural and subdural spaces usually result by direct invasion of pathogens subsequent to trauma or surgery (e.g., tail-docking in sheep). Bacterial infections of vertebrae or intervertebral disks can involve the spinal cord by direct extension or as a result of pressure from epidural abscessation.

Infections of the Central Nervous System

Once a pathogen establishes, injury results from either direct cytotoxic effects by the pathogen or as a result of injury due to the inflammatory response directed at the pathogen, or a combination of both. Clinical signs associated with infections are varied and typically progressive. Specific clinical signs may aid in localizing the infections

Table 71.3.   Common and/or Important Infectious Agents of the Nervous System of Horses

Agent	Disease	Neurological Signs
Viruses		
Equine encephalomyelitis viruses (WEE, EEE, VEE[a])	Equine encephalomyelitides	Ataxia, drowsiness, head-pressing, paralysis
Equine herpesvirus 1	Myeloencephalitis	Ataxia, tetra or paraplegia
Rabies virus	Rabies	Ascending paralysis, ataxia, depression, vocalization
West Nile virus	West Nile encephalitis	Ataxia, muscle tremor, paresis, seizures, somnolence
Bacteria		
Clostridium botulinum[b]	Botulism (shaker foal disease, forage disease)	Flaccid paralysis, muscle fasciculations, paresis
Clostridium tetani	Tetanus	Muscle spasms, prolapsed third eyelid, rigid "sawhorse" stance, seizures
Streptococcus equi subsp. *equi*	Brain abscess, meningitis	Blindness, circling, coma, head-pressing, seizures
	Guttural pouch infection	Dysphagia, head-shaking
Fungi		
Aspergillus fumigatus	Guttural pouch mycosis	Dysphagia, head-shaking

[a]Classified as a foreign animal disease agent in the United States.
[b]Most commonly Types B and C.

Table 71.4.   Common and/or Important Infectious Agents of the Nervous System of Cattle

Agent	Disease	Neurological Signs
Prions		
BSE prion[a]	Bovine spongiform encephalopathy	Aggressive or apprehensive behavior, ataxia, ear twitching
Viruses		
Akabane virus[a,b]	Hydranencephaly, neurogenic arthrogryposis (Akabane disease)	Sensory and motor deficits at birth
Alcephaline herpesvirus 1[a]	Malignant catarrhal fever (wildebeest)	Ataxia, head-pressing, paralysis, tremors, seizures
Bovine viral diarrhea virus[b]	Cerebellar hypoplasia	Head tremors, incoordination
Infectious bovine rhinotracheitis	IBR encephalitis	Ataxia, hyperexcitability, tremors
Ovine herpesvirus 2	Malignant catarrhal fever (sheep)	Ataxia, head-pressing, paralysis, tremors, seizures
Pseudorabies virus	Pseudorabies	Intense pruritus, salivation, seizures, vocalization
Rabies virus	Rabies	Ataxia, paralysis
Bacteria		
Arcanobacterium pyogenes	Brain/pituitary abscess	Ataxia, blindness, depression, fascial paralysis
Histophilus somni[c]	Thromboembolic meningoencephalitis, otitis media-interna	Ataxia, blindness, opisthotonus, stupor
Clostridium botulinum[d]	Botulism	Flaccid paralysis, loss of tongue withdrawal and blink responses, muscle fasciculations, paresis
Clostridium tetani	Tetanus	Opisthotonus, seizures, tremors
Escherichia coli	Meningitis	Blindness, head-pressing, seizures, somnolence
Fusobacterium necrophorum	Brain/pituitary abscess	Ataxia, blindness, depression, facial paralysis
Listeria monocytogenes	Listeriosis	Ataxia, circling, facial palsy, head tilt
Mycoplasma bovis	Otitis media-interna	Ataxia, droopy ear, head tilt
Pasteurella multocida	Otitis media-interna	Ataxia, droopy ear, head tilt

[a]Classified as a foreign animal disease agent in the United States.
[b]Congenital infection.
[c]"*Haemophilus somnus*" is the obsolete name for this organism.
[d]Most commonly Types B, C, and D.

Table 71.5. Common and/or Important Infectious Agents of the Nervous System of Sheep and Goats

Agent	Disease	Neurological Signs
Prions		
Scrapie prion	Scrapie	Ataxia, exaggerated nibbling reflex, intense pruritus, muscle tremors
Viruses		
Akabane virus[a,b]	Hydranencephaly, neurogenic arthrogryposis (Akabane disease)	Sensory and motor deficits at birth
Bluetongue virus[a]	Cerebellar hypoplasia, hydranencephaly	Blindness at birth, inability to walk
Border disease virus[a]	Hypomyelinogenesis	Ataxia, tremors
Caprine arthritis-encephalitis virus (G)	Caprine arthritis-encephalitis	Paralysis, paresis, tremors
Louping ill virus[b]	Louping ill	Ataxia, muscle tremors
Rabies virus	Rabies	Ataxia, constipation, paralysis
Visna virus (S)	Visna	Abnormal gait, ataxia, paralysis, paresis
Bacteria		
Arcanobacterium pyogenes	Cerebral abscess, pituitary abscess	Ataxia, head pressing, head tilt, blindness
Clostridium botulinum	Botulism	Ataxia, flaccid paralysis
Clostridium perfringens Type D	Focal symmetrical encephalomalacia	Coma, depression, head-pressing, opisthotonus
Clostridium tetani	Tetanus	Opisthotonus, seizures, tremors
Escherichia coli	Meningitis	Blindness, head-pressing, seizures, somnolence
Listeria monocytogenes	Listeriosis	Ataxia, circling, facial palsy, head tilt

(G) = goats, (S) = sheep.
[a]Congenital disease.
[b]Classified as a foreign animal disease agent in the United States.

Table 71.6. Common and/or Important Infectious Agents of the Nervous System of Pigs

Agent	Disease	Neurological Signs
Viruses		
Hemagglutinating encephalomyelitis virus	Vomiting and wasting disease	Depression, jerking movements, paralysis, seizures
Encephalomyocarditis virus	Encephalomyocarditis	Ataxia, depression, tremors
Porcine enterovirus 1	Porcine polioencephalomyelitis (Talfan/Teschen)	Ataxia, paresis, coma, paralysis, seizures
Hog cholera virus[a,b]	Cerebellar hypoplasia	Ataxia, seizures
Nipah virus[a]	Nonsuppurative meningitis	Paresis, tetanic spasms, seizures
Pseudorabies virus	Pseudorabies	Ataxia, tremors, seizures
Rabies virus	Rabies	Aggressive behavior, ataxia, paralysis, seizures
Bacteria		
Clostridium tetani	Tetanus	Opisthotonus, muscle rigidity, seizures, stiff gait, tremors
Escherichia coli (Shiga toxin positive)	Edema disease	Ataxia, edema of face, paralysis, stiffness
Haemophilus parasuis	Meningitis (Glasser's disease)	Ataxia, paddling, tremors
Listeria monocytogenes	Listeriosis	Ataxia, hyperexcitability, trembling
Streptococcus suis (Type 2)	Meningitis	Ataxia, depression, paralysis, seizures, tremors

[a]Classified as a foreign animal disease agent in the United States.
[b]Congenital infections cause congenital tremors in piglets.

to the meninges (nuchal rigidity, depressed mental status), cerebrum (circling, behavioral changes, seizures), brainstem (cranial nerve deficits, head tilt), cerebellum (ataxia, tremors), or spinal cord (tetra or paraplegia).

Mechanism of Central Nervous System Injury

Vascular Damage. Damage to blood vessels may be the initiating factor in disease. Microbial toxins can cause vaso-genic cerebral edema through effects on the blood brain barrier and resultant leakage of proteins into extracellular spaces. This is the proposed mechanism of action of *C. perfringens* Type D epsilon toxin, which produces a focal symmetrical encephalomalacia, especially involving the thalamus, hippocampus, and midbrain in sheep (Fig 71.1) and the Shiga-like toxin of toxigenic *Escherichia coli* strains associated with edema disease in swine. Viral effects on the vascular system include immune-mediated vasculitis and

Table 71.7.   Common and/or Important Infectious Agents of the Nervous System of Poultry

Agent	Disease	Neurological Signs
Viruses		
Avian encephalomyelitis virus	Avian encephalomyelitis	Ataxia, paralysis, tremors
Avian influenza virus[a]	Avian influenza	Ataxia, depression
Eastern equine encephalitis virus (T)	Eastern equine encephalitis	Ataxia, depression, paralysis
Exotic Newcastle disease virus[a]	Exotic Newcastle disease	Depression, paresis, torticollis, tremors
Marek's disease virus (C)	Marek's disease	Ataxia, leg or wing paresis/paralysis
Bacteria		
Clostridium botulinum[b]	Botulism (Limberneck)	Flaccid paralysis, inability to support head
Listeria monocytogenes	Listeriosis	Ataxia, opisthotonus, torticollis
Salmonella enterica subsp. *arizonae* (T)	Meningitis/encephalitis (Arizonosis)	Ataxia, paralysis, seizures
Fungi		
Aspergillus fumigatus	Mycotic encephalitis	Loss of equilibrium, torticollis
Ochroconis gallopavum[c]	Mycotic encephalitis	Loss of equilibrium, torticollis

(C) = chickens, (T) = turkeys.
[a]Classified as a foreign animal disease agent in the United States.
[b]Most commonly Type C.
[c]*Dactylaria gallopava* is the obsolete name for this organism.

FIGURE 71.1.   *Focal symmetrical encephalomalacia in a sheep brain. Lesions are associated with enterotoxemia due to* Clostridium perfringens *Type D. (Courtesy of Dr. F. Uzal.)*

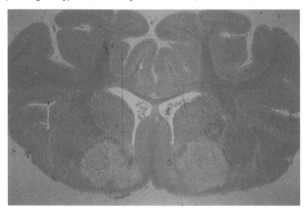

perivascular inflammation (e.g., feline infectious peritonitis, equine herpesvirus 1). Rickettsial agents (*Ehrlichia* and *Rickettsia)* induce endothelial damage and vasculitis that lead to bleeding in the brain. Thrombosis of vessels may cause malacia of brain parenchyma (e.g., *Histophilus somni* in calves, *Salmonella enterica* subsp. *arizonae* in turkeys). Septic emboli may result in brain abscesses.

Injury to Brain Parenchyma or Meninges.   Injury to cells in the central nervous system is by direct action of the pathogen or from the resulting inflammatory response. The inflammatory response can be suppurative, nonsuppurative, granulomatous, or some combination of these and is predominately influenced by the agent involved. Inflammatory processes of the brain parenchyma (encephalitis), meninges (meningitis), or spinal cord (myelitis) occur independently or in combination. Disorder in myelin for-

mation results in some cases (e.g., distemper, visna). Movement of infectious agents may occur within the cerebrospinal fluid or interstitium, or within different cell types.

Viral Infections.   Viruses with neurotrophic properties affect all animal species (see Tables 71.1–71.7). Some viruses specifically affect the nervous system (e.g., rabies virus in all species, pseudorabies in most species), and other viruses involve the nervous system as part of a multisystem disease process (e.g., malignant catarrhal fever virus in cattle, exotic Newcastle disease virus in poultry, distemper virus in dogs). Viruses usually reach the central nervous system via the blood stream, often as the result of a secondary viremia. Entry is via one of the methods described previously (see the section "Routes of Infection," above). Effects on specific cell types in the nervous system are either due to direct viral cytocidal effects or damage resulting for the ensuing inflammatory response. Gliosis, perivascular cuffing, and neuronal degeneration typically characterize viral encephalitis. Viral infections in the central nervous system only rarely serve as the primary mechanism for transmission between hosts. Typically transmission relies on infection at other sites in the body.

Some viral infections in the dam affect the fetal nervous system and lead to developmental problems, including cerebellar hypoplasia (bovine viral diarrhea virus, panleukopenia virus), hydranencephaly (bluetongue virus), and hypomyelinogenesis (Border disease virus).

Bacterial Infections.   Bacterial meningitis in dogs and cats is relatively uncommon and often associated with primary infections at other sites (e.g., urinary tract infection, endocarditis). Involvement of the nervous system may also arise from local extension of infectious processes (e.g., ear infections, tooth root abscesses, sinus infections). Organisms involved are usually endogenous and include aerobes (*Staphylococcus, Streptococcus, Pasteurella, Actinomyces*) and anaerobes (*Bacteroides, Porphyromonas, Fusobacterium, Peptostreptococcus*).

Bacterial meningitis is more common in neonates, with horses and production animals most commonly affected. In these animals, the etiology agent is often an enteric organism (e.g., *E. coli*) and is associated with failure of passive transfer of maternal immunoglobulins. *Haemophilus, Pasteurella, Salmonella,* and *Streptococcus* are other genera encountered with some frequency in bacterial meningitis. Prolonged bacteremia and the total bacterial numbers appear directly related to the likelihood that the blood brain barrier will be crossed. In bacterial meningitis, a fibrinopurulent response typically results.

Brain abscesses are also more common in horses and ruminants than in companion animals and develop as a result of bacteremia, trauma (direct implantation), or spread from a contiguous site. *Streptococcus equi* subsp. *equi* is the most common cause of brain abscesses in horses, a form of so-called "bastard strangles," and is related to a bacteremic event subsequent to rhinopharyngitis and lymph node abscessation (strangles). Brain abscesses in cattle are also associated with primary extraneural infections (e.g., hardware disease). The pituitary gland is an especially common site in ruminants, possibly due to the anatomy and close association of the rete mirabilis with the pituitary gland. Common ruminant pyogenic agents (*Arcanobacterium pyogenes, Fusobacterium necrophorum)* are the usual suspects in these cases. Infections involving vertebrae and intervertebral disks, especially in dogs, ruminants, and swine, may involve the spinal cord and manifest as posterior paralysis/paresis. Some bacterial species exhibit a greater degree of neurotropism than others (e.g., *Listeria* in ruminants, *Histophilus somni* ["*Haemophilus somnus*" is the obsolete name] in beef cattle). Lesions associated with *Listeria* encephalitis typically are in the form of microabscesses in the brainstem (pons, medulla oblongata) and are almost pathognomonic for *Listeria* encephalitis (Fig 71.2).

As already mentioned, bacterial toxins rather than the agent itself may be responsible for clinical signs and pathology. Some bacterial toxins directly affect the vasculature of the central nervous system (e.g., epsilon toxin of *C. perfringens* in enterotoxemia and Shiga-like toxin of *E. coli* in edema disease). On the other hand, tetanospasmin (tetanus toxin), the toxin produced by *Clostridium tetani,* binds to peripheral nerves and travels to the central nervous system where it blocks release of inhibitory neurotransmitters from presynaptic inhibitory motor nerve endings.

Fungal Infections. As a general rule, fungal infections of the central nervous system are infrequent. When they occur, the inflammatory response is typically granulomatous. Most of the systemic mycotic agents (*Blastomyces, Coccidioides, Cryptococcus, Histoplasma*) have the potential to be involved in nervous system disease, but this usually occurs secondarily and late in the course of the infection. Most fungal infections result from hematogenous dissemination. *Cryptococcus neoformans* is the most common fungus encountered in nervous system disease and most commonly affects dogs and cats (Fig 71.3). It produces a number of virulence factors, including a large polysaccharide capsule, which allows it to persist (see Fig 45.1). Evidence suggests it uses monocytes and endothelial cells to cross the blood brain barrier. Granulomatous encephalitis with focal caseonecrotic lesions caused by *Aspergillus* sp. has been described in poultry. Outbreaks of mycotic encephalitis in poultry flocks caused by a thermophilic fungus, *Ochroconis gallopavum* (*Dactylaria gallopava*—obsolete name), have also been reported.

Prion Diseases

Transmissible spongiform encephalopathies or prion diseases (bovine spongiform encephalopathy [BSE], scrapie, feline spongiform encephalopathy) are rare but important nervous system diseases because they are largely untreatable, may cross species barriers, and can have substantial economic impact because of public health concerns. An abnormal conformer of normally present prion protein (PrP^c) designated PrP^{Res} (for "resistant" PrP) is believed to cause conversion of normal PrP^c into the pathological iso-

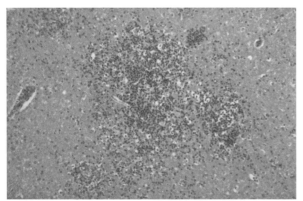

FIGURE 71.2. *Microabscess in the brainstem of a cow that died from* Listeria *encephalitis.* Listeria monocytogenes *was isolated. Hematoxylin eosin stain.*

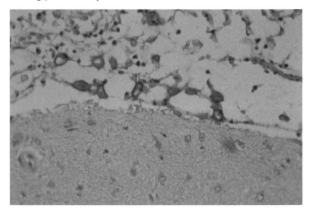

FIGURE 71.3. Cryptococcus neoformans *meningitis in a cat. Numerous yeast cells are present. Spaces around stained yeast bodies are the result of shrinkage of the polysaccharide capsule during the staining process. Mayer's mucicarmine stain.*

FIGURE 71.4. *Spongiform encephalopathy characterized by vacuolation of neurons and neuropil in the brain of a sheep with scrapie (H&E). (Courtesy Dr. B. Barr.)*

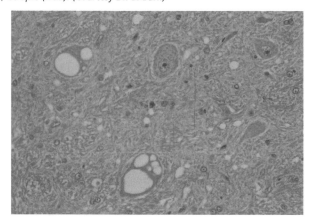

FIGURE 71.5. *Botulism in a cow. Flaccid paralysis of the tongue has resulted in an inability of the cow to retract its tongue. Clostridium botulinum type C was the cause of botulism in this case. (Courtesy Dr. R. Moeller.)*

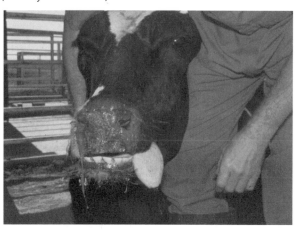

form. Acquired principally through ingestion of PrP^Res-contaminated material (e.g., meat and bone meal in BSE and possibly infected placenta or feces in scrapie) prions are able to pass from the digestive tract and are potentially amplified in the lymphoreticular system before moving up the peripheral nervous system to the brain. The accumulation of PrP^Res is responsible for the pathology (neuronal intracellular spongiosis) associated with transmissible spongiform encephalopathies (Fig 71.4).

Infections of the Peripheral Nervous System

As noted previously, the peripheral nervous system is less frequently involved in infectious processes than the central nervous system, however some important diseases specifically or predominantly involve the peripheral nervous system. The toxin of *Clostridium botulinum* affects peripheral nerves, specifically components of the synaptic vesicle docking and fusion complex at peripheral motor nerve terminals. This blocks the release of acetylcholine resulting in the flaccid paralysis characteristic of the disease (Fig. 71.5). Involvement of peripheral nerves, usually sciatic and brachial nerve plexuses, is a characteristic feature of Marek's disease virus. Grossly enlarged nerves with both inflammatory and neoplastic histologic characteristics, as well as myelin degeneration, are found. Mycotic and bacterial infections of the guttural pouch of horses may involve the glossopharyngeal and vagus nerves, resulting in swallowing difficulties or laryngeal hemiplegia.

72 Ocular Infections

Richard L. Walker

The primary function of the eye is vision. Factors that affect vision impact overall animal well-being. In this chapter, the ocular system includes the eyelids, lacrimal apparatus, conjunctiva, the eye itself, and the surrounding fascia. The eye includes the cornea, sclera, lens, uveal tract, retina, optic nerve, and aqueous and vitreous chambers. The major sites for infectious ocular disease to develop are the conjunctiva, cornea, and uveal tract.

Antimicrobial Properties of the Eye

Considering the frequent exposure to environmental elements, the eye is remarkably resistant to infection. Mechanical, anatomical, antimicrobial, and immunological factors all play roles in protecting the eye from infection. The following sections detail these specific factors.

Mechanical and Anatomic Factors

The eyelids, including the cilia, and blink (menace) and corneal reflexes provide a barrier to external insults that may traumatize the eye and predispose to infection by endogenous or exogenous microbes. Intact conjunctiva and cornea epithelium provide additional barriers to infection. Precorneal tear film, a complex multilayered fluid, continuously coats exposed surfaces of the eye without impairing vision. The tear film has a number of functions including lubrication, retarding evaporation, and nutrient transport. Meibomian and lacrimal glands, the conjunctiva, and cornea all contribute to the composition of the tear film. Tears provide overall protection for the eye surface through the uniform coating effect and by mechanically rinsing the eye of noxious materials and microbes.

Protection for internal structures of the eye comes from tight junctions of endothelial and epithelial cells that form the blood-aqueous and blood-retinal barriers. The blood aqueous barrier is formed by ciliary epithelial cells between capillaries in the ciliary stroma and aqueous fluid in the posterior chamber of the eye. The blood-retinal barrier is composed of tight junctions of endothelial cells of retinal capillaries and cells of the pigmented retinal epithelium. These barriers afford protection to intraocular structures of the eye from microbes of hematogenous origin. When microbes from systemic infections do involve intraocular sites, it is these areas where infection typically initiates. Breakdown of blood-ocular barriers is largely the result of inflammatory processes that disrupt tight junctions.

Antimicrobial Factors

In addition to serving as an interface to ameliorate the effects of external stimuli; tears contain nonspecific antimicrobial substances that include:

1. *Lactoferrin.* Lactoferrin is a substantial protein component of tears (up to 25%). By binding free iron, lactoferrin makes this essential enzyme component unavailable to bacteria, thereby limiting bacterial growth. In addition, lactoferrin may have a role in enhancing natural killer cell function and inhibiting formation of C3 convertase.
2. *Lysozyme.* Tears are rich in lysozyme (up to 40% of tear protein). The enzymatic action of lysozyme on the glycan chain of the peptidoglycan of bacterial cell walls provides nonspecific protection from exogenous and resident bacteria. Variation in lysozyme concentration occurs among different animals and may, in part, account for variation in susceptibility of different animals to external ocular infections. Decrease in the lysozyme concentration in tears correlates with increased ocular infections.
3. *Antimicrobial Peptides.* Broad-spectrum cationic antimicrobial peptides are innately produced by ocular surface tissues. These peptides act as natural antibiotics through interactions with bacterial cell surfaces. They may also play a role in signaling that activates host cell processes involved in immune defense. Antimicrobial peptides can be detected in the conjunctiva, cornea and tears.

Immunological Factors

The conjunctiva is part of the common mucosal immune system, which includes gastrointestinal, respiratory, urogenital, and mammary mucosa. It is unclear if antigen-presenting capabilities exist in the conjunctiva or lacrimal gland lymphoid tissue. It is plausible that ocular immunization occurs by passage of antigen through the nasal lacrimal duct to GALT or BALT sites. Plasma cells in the lacrimal glands are derived by clonal expansion and differentiation of IgA committed B lymphocytes that localize in the lacrimal gland. IgA is produced, which in turn combines with secretory pieces. Secretory IgA is resistant to proteolytic enzymes in tears and constitutes the major immunoglobulin in tears. Its role in microbial defense includes preventing bacterial attachment and neutralization of viruses. A functional complement system is also present in tears.

Because of its rich vascular supply, an aggressive inflammatory response, predominately composed of neutrophils, occurs in the conjunctiva. The cornea, due to its avascular nature, is suppressed or delayed in its inflammatory response.

The intraocular immune response is programmed to prevent an overexuberant response that may irreparably damage intraocular structures and ultimately vision. Subsets of T lymphocytes that cause substantial bystander injury are suppressed, and the immune response is more localized.

Competitive Inhibition Effect of Microbial Flora

It is possible that the normal flora, as elsewhere in the body, plays a protective role in the ocular system by inhibiting establishment of more pathogenic species.

Microbial Flora of the Eye

A normal conjunctival flora is present but varies by animal, breed, geography, housing conditions, and time of year. The most commonly recovered flora are gram-positive organisms and include staphylococci, micrococci, streptococci, diphtheroids, and *Bacillus* spp. Less frequently nonenteric, gram-negative bacteria are isolated and include predominately *Moraxella*, *Neisseria*, and *Pseudomonas* species. In ruminants, *Moraxella* species may be the predominant bacterial type in normal eyes. *Mycoplasma* species are also found as conjunctival flora in some animals. Few studies have been done to actually quantitate the relative numbers of each of the different species that constitute normal flora. Not all conjunctival specimens from normal animals yield microbial growth, indicating that the conjunctiva is not heavily populated by normal flora. Internal structures of the eye are normally sterile.

Ocular Infections

Ocular infections can be primary infections or part of multisystem infectious processes (e.g., upper respiratory tract infections). The organisms involved are often contagious and may affect populations of animals rather than individuals. In other cases, ocular infections are secondary to insults that comprise the integrity and innate defenses of the eye. Compromising factors in these cases include decreased tear production, excess ultraviolet radiation, immunosuppressing diseases, trauma or penetrating injuries, anatomic defects (e.g., entropions), or surgical interventions. In such situations, normally benign ocular or other endogenous flora can cause serious infections once they gain entry to unprotected sites. A number of systemic infectious diseases also include ocular manifestations as a consequence of dissemination from the initial focus of infection.

Depending on the microbial agent involved, the agent's tissue trophism, route of exposure, and the host's ability to contain infection, ocular infections may or may not be limited to specific parts of the eye. The inflammatory

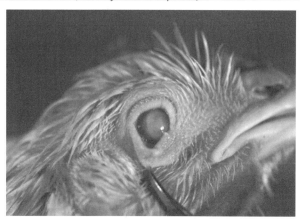

FIGURE 72.1. *Endophthalmitis in a chicken caused by Escherichia coli. (Courtesy Dr. H. Shivaprasad)*

process can and frequently does involve structures in the eye adjacent to the site of initial infection or, especially in uncontrolled infections, becomes widespread to involve intraocular cavities and surrounding structures (endophthalmitis, panophthalmitis) (Fig 72.1). Route of exposure of the eye to infectious agents is through surface contact with endogenous or exogenous microbes or via the blood stream or lymphatic system and, perhaps, by extension from nervous tissues.

Common and/or important infectious agents of the ocular system in domestic mammals and poultry are listed in Tables 72.1–72.7.

Infectious processes of the eye frequently include those presented in the following sections.

Eyelid and Lacrimal Apparatus Infections

Bacteria are the most common cause of infections of eyelid margins (blepharitis) and lacrimal glands. The source for bacteria is endogenous, with staphylococci and streptococci being the most common agents. In dogs, a purulent blepharitis occurs in conjunction with juvenile pyoderma. Dermatophyte infections may extend to involve eyelids.

Conjunctival Infections

Infections of the conjunctiva induce an inflammatory response characterized by hyperemia, chemosis, and cellular exudate. Conjunctivitis occurs both as a local infection (e.g., *Chlamydophila* infections in cats) or as part of a systemic disease (e.g., distemper in dogs).

Viral-induced conjunctivitis (e.g., alphaherpesviruses conjunctivitis) often occurs in conjunction with upper respiratory or digestive tract infections when virus specifically attaches to and replicates in surface epithelial cells. Cytopathic effects caused by viruses and induction of an inflammatory response account for clinical signs observed. Conjunctival infections may spread to or concurrently involve the cornea (keratoconjunctivitis).

Bacterial infections of the conjunctiva may begin in the

Table 72.1. Common and/or Important Infectious Agents of the Ocular System of Dogs

Agent	Major Clinical Manifestations (Common Disease Name)
Viruses	
Canine adenovirus 1	Corneal edema, immune-complex uveitis, keratitis (blue eye)
Canine distemper virus	Chorioretinitis, conjunctivitis, optic neuritis (distemper)
Canine papillomavirus	Papillomas of eyelids and conjunctiva
Bacteria	
Beta-hemolytic streptococci	Conjunctivitis, dacryocystitis
Brucella canis	Anterior uveitis, endophthalmitis
Coagulase-positive staphylococci	Blepharitis, conjunctivitis, dacryocystitis
Ehrlichia spp.	Anterior uveitis, conjunctival hyperemia, chorioretinitis
Leptospira spp.	Anterior uveitis
Rickettsia rickettsii	Anterior uveitis, chorioretinitis, conjunctival hyperemia, retinal hemorrhage
Fungi	
Blastomyces dermatitidis	Anterior uveitis, chorioretinitis, endophthalmitis
Cryptococcus neoformans	Chorioretinitis, optic neuritis
Algae	
Prototheca spp.	Anterior uveitis, chorioretinitis

Table 72.2. Common and/or Important Infectious Agents of the Ocular System of Cats

Agent	Major Clinical Manifestations (Common Disease Name)
Viruses	
Feline herpesvirus 1	Conjunctivitis, corneal ulcer, stromal keratitis (feline viral rhinotracheitis)
Feline immunodeficiency virus	Anterior uveitis, chorioretinitis
Feline infectious peritonitis virus	Anterior uveitis, chorioretinitis, keratic precipitates, keratitis (feline infectious peritonitis)
Feline leukemia virus	Anterior uveitis, uveal lymphosarcoma, retinal hemorrhage
Feline panleukopenia virus	Retinal degeneration, retinal dysplasia (feline panleukopenia–in utero infection)
Bacteria	
Chlamydophila felis	Conjunctivitis (feline pneumonitis)
Mycoplasma felis[a]	Conjunctivitis
Fungi	
Cryptococcus neoformans	Chorioretinitis, optic neuritis (cryptococcosis)

[a]Role as an ocular pathogen is uncertain.

Table 72.3. Common and/or Important Infectious Agents of the Ocular System of Horses

Agent	Major Clinical Manifestations (Common Disease Name)
Viruses	
African Horse Sickness virus[a]	Conjunctivitis, eyelid and periorbital edema
Equine arteritis virus	Conjunctivitis, periorbital edema
Equine herpesvirus 2	Conjunctivitis, keratitis
Equine influenza virus	Conjunctivitis
Bacteria	
Leptospira spp.	Panuveitis (equine recurrent uveitis)
Pseudomonas aeruginosa	Keratitis, corneal ulcer
Fungi	
Aspergilllus spp.	Keratitis, corneal ulcer
Fusarium spp.	Keratitis, corneal ulcer

[a]Classified as a foreign animal disease agent in the United States.

Table 72.4. Common and/or Important Infectious Agents of the Ocular System of Cattle

Agent	Major Clinical Manifestations (Common Disease Name)
Viruses	
Alcelaphine herpesvirus 1[a]	Anterior uveitis, conjunctivitis, corneal edema, eyelid edema, keratitis (malignant catarrhal fever)
Bovine herpesvirus 1	Conjunctivitis, corneal edema/opacity (infectious bovine rhinotracheitis)
Bovine papillomavirus	Papillomas of eyelid and conjunctiva
Bovine viral diarrhea virus	Cataracts, retinal atrophy, optic neuritis (bovine virus diarrhea–in utero infection)
Ovine herpesvirus 2	Anterior uveitis, conjunctivitis, corneal edema, eyelid edema, keratitis (malignant catarrhal fever)
Bacteria	
Arcanobacterium pyogenes	Orbital cellulitis
Histophilus somni[b]	Retinal hemorrhages, retinitis (thromboembolic meningoencephalitis)
Listeria monocytogenes	Conjunctivitis, keratitis, uveitis
Moraxella bovis	Conjunctivitis, keratitis, corneal ulcer, panophthalmitis (infectious bovine keratoconjunctivitis or pinkeye)
Mycoplasma bovoculi	Conjunctivitis

[a]Classified as a foreign animal disease agent in the United States.
[b]"Haemophilus somnus" is the obsolete name for this organism.

Table 72.5. Common and/or Important Infectious Agents of the Ocular System of Sheep and Goats

Agent	Major Clinical Manifestations (Common Disease Name)
Prions	
Scrapie prion	Retinal detachment
Bacteria	
Chlamydophila pecorum[a]	Conjunctivitis, keratitis
Listeria monocytogenes	Conjunctivitis, keratitis, uveitis
Moraxella spp. *Branhamella ovis*[a]	Conjunctivitis, keratitis
Mycoplasma conjunctivae	Conjunctivitis, keratitis (infectious keratoconjunctivitis)

[a]Role as an ocular pathogen is uncertain.

Table 72.6. Common and/or Important Infectious Agents of the Ocular System of Pigs

Agent	Major Clinical Manifestations (Common Disease Name)
Viruses	
African swine fever virus[a]	Conjunctivitis (African swine fever)
Classical swine fever virus[a]	Conjunctivitis (Classical swine fever, hog cholera)
Porcine rubulavirus	Corneal opacity/edema, keratitis (blue eye disease)
Pseudorabies virus	Conjunctivitis, keratitis
Swine influenza virus	Conjunctivitis
Bacteria	
Chlamydia suis	Conjunctivitis
Escherichia coli (Shiga toxin positive)	Palpebral edema (edema disease)
Pasteurella multocida	Conjunctivitis, nasolacrimal duct occlusion (atrophic rhinitis)

[a]Classified as a foreign animal disease agent in the United States.

Table 72.7. Common and/or Important Infectious Agents of the Ocular System of Poultry

Agent	Major Clinical Manifestations (Common Disease Name)
Viruses	
Avian encephalomyelitis virus (C)	Cataracts, uveitis
Infectious laryngotracheitis virus	Conjunctivitis, keratitis
Marek's disease virus (C)	Loss of iris pigmentation, panuveitis
Newcastle disease virus[a]	Conjunctival edema, hemorrhage
Bacteria	
Bordetella avium (T)	Conjunctivitis
Chlamydophila psittaci	Conjunctivitis
Escherichia coli	Conjunctivitis, endophthalmitis
Haemophilus paragallinarum	Conjunctivitis, periorbital edema
Mycoplasma gallisepticum	Conjunctivitis,
Pasteurella multocida	Conjunctivitis, eyelid edema, orbital cellulitis
Salmonella spp.[b]	Endophthalmitis
Fungi	
Aspergillus spp.	Endophthalmitis, keratitis

(C) = Chicken, (T) = Turkey
[a]Classified as a foreign animal disease agent in the United States.
[b]Includes *Salmonella arizonae*.

conjunctiva or may result from extension of eyelid or lacrimal gland infections. *Chlamydia/Chlamydophila* conjunctivitis occurs in a number of animal species and can be a primary conjunctivitis or, in addition, involve other sites. Bacterial conjunctivitis may develop secondary to primary viral conjunctival infections. As with viral conjunctivitis, concurrent corneal involvement may occur. Fungal infections of the conjunctiva are rare.

Corneal Infections

Corneal inflammation (keratitis) with or without loss of the epithelium and part of the stroma (corneal ulcer) is a common condition in most animals. Keratitis can begin externally on the epithelial surface or internally at the level of the endothelium. Because it is avascular, the initial inflammatory response in the cornea results from migration of neutrophils from the conjunctiva or limbic sclera. In chronic disease the cornea becomes vascularized and directly participates in the inflammatory response.

Among the most common causes of viral keratitis are members of the herpesviruses. Cats and cattle are most frequently affected. In some herpesvirus infections, recurrence sometimes results from reactivation of latent infections in sensory ganglia (e.g., trigeminal ganglia) following stress.

Primary bacterial keratitis is rare. However, once the cornea is breached a number of bacterial species will readily establish and spread to involve the corneal stroma. These opportunistic bacteria include staphylococci, streptococci, and *Pseudomonas* species. Damage to the cornea due to bacterial toxins and enzymes (e.g., proteolytic enzymes of *Pseudomonas*) is further exacerbated by enzymes from recruited neutrophils (e.g., collagenases, elastases). *Pseudomonas aeruginosa* can be an especially virulent corneal pathogen once it is established and is associated with so-called "melting ulcers" but still requires a break in the corneal epithelial barrier in order to establish. *Moraxella bovis* is one of the few bacteria in veterinary medicine that cause a primary bacterial keratitis. It produces specific virulence factors including adhesins (fimbria) for adherence to epithelial cells and toxins that cause necrosis of epithelial cells (Fig 72.2).

Mycotic keratitis (keratomycosis) is of greatest significance in horses. Exposure of the eye to plant material often introduces the fungus, although some studies have found various fungi on the conjunctiva from normal

FIGURE 72.2.   *Corneal ulcer in a cow with "pinkeye" caused by* Moraxella bovis. *(Courtesy Dr. J. Angelos.)*

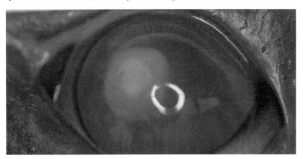

equine eyes. These most likely represent transient flora as a result of random environmental exposure. The intact corneal epithelium provides an excellent barrier to fungal infections, thus requiring trauma to the corneal epithelial as a preceding event to the development of keratomycosis. Corticosteroid use enhances the likelihood of fungal infections of the equine cornea and exacerbates the condition once present. Typically, mycotic infections of the cornea do not have a concurrent conjunctivitis.

Intraocular Infections

Intraocular infections are frequently the consequence of a systemic infection with exogenous organisms that localize in the uveal tract (iris, ciliary body, choroid). The infection may initiate and/or predominate at a particular site in the uveal tract; however, involvement of other sites in the tract is common. At some level, at least histologically, widespread involvement of the uveal tract occurs in most infections. Uveitis can be divided on the basis of the anatomic site most prominently involved in the inflammatory process (e.g., anterior uveitis) and whether adjacent sites are also involved (e.g., chorioretinitis). In intraocular infections, extension to other parts of the eye occurs due to proximity of other structures (e.g., retinal involvement), the fluid nature inside the eye, and the open communication between intraocular chambers. Depending on the agent, stage of the inflammatory response and even the animal involved, the inflammatory response in the uveal tract can be suppurative, lymphoplasmacytic, granulomatous, or some combination of these responses.

The pathogenesis of viral-induced uveitis is either by direct infection of the uveal tract and subsequent inflammatory response or through deposition of immune complexes resulting in immune-mediated Type III hypersensitivity reactions. Likewise, bacterial uveitis occurs subsequent to bacterial (e.g., *Brucella*) localization to the uveal tract or in some cases from immune complex deposition (e.g., *Leptospira*). Nonspecific bacterial uveitis can result subsequent to other preexisting bacterial conditions (e.g., gingivitis, prostatitis). All of the systemic mycoses agents (*Blastomyces, Histoplasma, Coccidioides, Cryptococcus*) have the capability of causing a panuveitis. Most present clinically as a chorioretinitis, with dogs and cats predominately affected. In dogs, *Prototheca*, an achlorophyllous alga, causes a granulomatous chorioretinitis in conjunction with other systemic manifestations (e.g., bloody diarrhea, paresis).

Congenital defects of ocular structures in utero infections, usually viral in origin, occur in some animal species. Bovine viral diarrhea virus infections in pregnant cows have been linked to retinal atrophy and cataracts in calves. Panleukopenia in cats is associated with dysplastic ocular development in kittens.

Infections of the Orbit

Infections in the orbit can be the result of a foreign body, penetrating wound from the oral cavity or hematogenous dissemination. Purulent infections in the form of orbital cellulitis and retrobulbar abscesses most often result. All animal species can develop orbital infections, although most occur in dogs and cats. The etiology is usually a mixture of bacterial agents, often including *Pasteurella* species.

73 | Respiratory System

RICHARD L. WALKER

The primary function of the respiratory system is gaseous exchange. The structure of the respiratory tract is such that noxious substances, particulate material, and microbial pathogens are prevented from entering and compromising the distal portions of respiratory tract where gaseous exchange occurs. Innate protective properties are present at all levels of the respiratory tract.

In most vertebrates the respiratory system is composed of the nasal cavity, sinuses, larynx, pharynx, trachea, bronchi and bronchioles, and lungs. In birds, the respiratory system is more complex and markedly different from other vertebrates. Most notably, birds possess large, subcutaneous, infraorbital sinuses that communicate with the nasal cavity and are especially predisposed to infection—in part, because of poor drainage. The lungs of birds are fairly rigid compared to other vertebrates. Air sacs are present that communicate with the lungs and are located in the coelom and medullary cavity of some bones.

Antimicrobial Properties of the Respiratory System

The act of breathing involves exposure of the respiratory tract to airborne microorganisms, including potentially pathogenic ones. Resident microorganisms are present in most upper parts of the tract, while various defense mechanisms operate to exclude or eliminate them from other sites.

Different protective mechanisms operate in the nasopharyngeal, tracheobronchial, and pulmonary portions of the respiratory tract. Aerodynamic filtration operates through different forces at these levels in depositing variously sized airborne particles. Inertial forces deposit larger particles (>5 μm in diameter) in the nasopharyngeal and upper tracheobronchial sections through impaction. In small bronchi and beyond, where air velocity is reduced, gravity acts to sediment particles 5 to 1 μm in size. In the smallest bronchioles and alveoli, particles measuring less than 1 μm gain contact with membranes through Brownian movement.

The mucus lining covering airway epithelium contains numerous substances with antimicrobial properties or that provide protective effects. Lysozyme, which is selectively bactericidal by its action on peptidoglycan, is present in varying quantities throughout the respiratory tract. Broad spectrum antimicrobial peptides, beta-defensins, produced by ciliated epithelial cells are active against viruses, bacteria, and fungi. Their expression is increased upon exposure to microbial components (e.g., lipopolysaccharide). The antimicrobial reactive nitrogen species, nitric oxide, is also produced by ciliated epithelial cells, primarily by inducible nitric oxide synthetase (iNOS). Bacterial products modulate the expression of iNOS. Nitric oxide plays an important role as a biological mediator in the regulation of host defense and inflammation, producing both pro- and anti-inflammatory effects. Also present in the mucus are immunoglobulins and interferon and lactoferrin, which by binding iron, makes it unavailable to most bacteria. Alpha-1 antitrypsin, an enzyme inhibitor that reduces the destructive effect of inflammatory reactions, plays a protective role.

Nasopharyngeal Compartment

Protective mechanisms in the nasopharyngeal compartment include vibrissae (guard hairs) around the nostrils of some animals that arrest the largest inhaled particles (15 μm in diameter) and the nasal conchae. The nasal conchal arrangement creates a turbulent airflow that increases the chances that particles will impact mucosal surfaces. Once impinged on the mucus-lined nasal turbinates or the nasopharyngeal wall, they encounter mucociliary action (see "Mucociliary Apparatus," below) and are transported to the caudal pharynx to be swallowed and eliminated via the digestive tract.

In the humid, warm nasal passages, particles swell through hydration, becoming more likely to impinge on a mucous membrane. Warming of air in the nasal passages also benefits cold-sensitive clearance mechanisms in the lower tract. Pharyngeal lymphoid tissues act in the filtration of microorganisms and initiation of the immune responses as a constituent of the mucosa-associated lymphoid tissue.

The resident flora provides colonization resistance as well as production of antibacterial substances. The sneeze reflex aids in clearing infectious particles from this area.

Tracheobronchial Compartment

The tracheobronchial compartment includes the larynx, trachea, bronchi, and bronchioles. Closure of the glottis during swallowing protects this area from contamination. Coughing removes gross accumulations of fluid. The tracheobronchial compartment is lined by mucociliary epithelium, which traps particles and transports them cranially to the pharynx (see "Mucociliary Apparatus," below). Deposition of particles on airway membranes is favored by bronchial branching due to directional airflow changes.

Bronchiolar-associated lymphoid tissue (BALT) is distributed along the airways and is concentrated at bronchial bifurcations, which corresponds to sites where the greatest trapping of inhaled particles occurs. BALT includes both cellular and humoral immune responses. Epithelial cells mediate the active transport of IgA from the lamina propria to the airway lumen.

Pulmonary Compartment

Clearance mechanisms of the pulmonary compartment (alveoli) consist of pulmonary alveolar macrophages (PAMs), neutrophils, and monocytes recruited from the blood. Particles are disposed of by phagocytosis. Susceptible microorganisms are killed and digested. Phagocytes migrate to sites where mucociliary transport occurs or via the lymphatics to remove other engulfed particles. The same protective substances as in tracheobronchial secretions operate at the pulmonary level, supplemented by those derived from alveolar macrophages.

Mechanisms

Overall, the mucociliary apparatus and PAMs constitute the main clearance mechanisms of the respiratory tract and are described in greater detail below.

Mucociliary Apparatus

The mucociliary apparatus is composed of ciliated and secretory cells. Ciliated cells are pseudostratified in the nasal and cranial tracheobronchial portions of the tract, simple columnar in the smaller bronchi, and simple cuboidal in the smallest bronchioles. The cilia, some 250 per cell, measuring 5.0 x 0.3 μm, resemble eukaryotic flagella and beat up to 1000 times a minute. The density of ciliated cells decreases gradually from the proximal to distal bronchioles. Alterations in cilia activity or deciliation of the epithelial cells hinder clearance activity and promote invasion by opportunistic pathogens. In addition, loss of ciliated epithelial cell function results in decreased production of antimicrobial substances and cytokines that mediate the inflammatory response.

The secretory components of the mucociliary apparatus are goblet cells, interspersed with ciliated cells, and, in the nose, trachea, and larger bronchi, submucosal serous and mucous glands. Serous fluid bathes the cilia, while a viscid mucus layer engages their tips. Mucus is propelled, along with particles trapped in it, caudally in the nasopharynx and cranially in the tracheobronchial compartment toward the pharynx by cilia beating at a rate of up to 20 mm/min. The particle clearance rate is fastest in the trachea and slowest in the smallest airways, where goblet cells are absent, mucus is sparse, and cilia beat more slowly—an arrangement that prevents logjams in the large airways. The trachea (e.g., cat) can be cleared within an hour, and all airways within a day.

Mucociliary clearance is inhibited by temperature extremes, respiratory viruses, some bacteria (e.g., *Bordetella*), dryness, general anesthetics, dust, noxious gases (sulfur dioxide, carbon dioxide, ammonia, tobacco smoke), and hypoxia. Mucus production through disruption of goblet cell integrity increases in response to irritant exposure.

Pulmonary Alveolar Macrophage

The pulmonary alveolar macrophage (PAM) is a monocyte adapted to the lung environment and located in the alveolar space. It is recruited from the blood when needed. The pulmonary alveolar macrophage is a pleomorphic cell, 20 to 40 μm in diameter, with many lysosomal granules containing numerous bioactive substances. Also produced by PAMs are mediator substances—complement components, interleukin 1, and tumor necrosis factor—which enable additional cellular and humoral defenses to be mobilized. Complement and IgG receptors on PAMs enhance its phagocytic capability. PAMs are motile and usually exist in the alveolus less than a week. Energy is obtained mainly by oxidative phosphorylation. The absence of ciliated epithelial cells and mucus-producing cells in the alveolus requires that PAMs remove particles that reach the alveoli.

Particles ingested by PAMs—other than susceptible bacteria killed upon ingestion—are removed via the mucociliary escalator or via interstitial centripetal or centrifugal lymphatics. The centripetal route leads directly to the hilar lymph nodes and may require two weeks. The centrifugal route goes via the pleura and may take months. Agents that cannot be removed are sequestered by inflammatory processes (abscesses, granulomas).

PAM activities are inhibited by sulfur dioxide, ozone, nitrogen oxides, and respiratory viruses. Bacterial leukotoxins and hemolysins destroy PAMs and are major virulence factors produced by some important bacterial respiratory pathogens (e.g., *Mannheimia haemolytica* in cattle, *Actinobacillus pleuropneumoniae* in swine).

Microbial Flora

The density and constituency of the microbial flora of the respiratory tract varies among animals and within the respiratory tract itself. Resident flora are limited to the nasal cavity and pharynx where a highly diverse flora can be found. For example, over 30 different gram-positive bacterial species alone can be recovered from the nasal conchae and tonsils of unweaned and weaned piglets. Overall, the nasal flora consistently includes viridans streptococci and coagulase-negative staphylococci along with potential pathogens that vary with the animal host. Although not usually considered a respiratory tract pathogen, coagulase-positive staphylococci can colonize the nose and be carried at a high rate in some populations. There they serve as a source for infections elsewhere in the body (e.g., integumentary infections). Some of the resident flora of the upper respiratory tract and oropharynx represent major respiratory bacterial pathogens (e.g., members of the *Pasteurellaceae* and *Streptococcus* and *Mycoplasma* species) if they are able to establish in lower parts of the tract. Many potentially pathogenic mycoplasmas are normal residents of the upper respiratory tract of the host they affect or are carried there by persistently infected individuals. They play a prominent role as pathogens at most levels in the respiratory tract, contributing to "respiratory disease complexes," or under the proper circumstances are by themselves significant pathogens.

As with the digestive tract, the resident flora of the respiratory system confer colonization resistance that is reduced by antibiotic treatment and environmental changes that alter its composition.

Nonresident organisms include both potential pathogens and harmless transients. Transient flora are comprised of microbes that enter during the breathing process and, therefore, reflect the environment in which the animal is maintained. Environmental factors, such as dry, dusty environments or confined environments where ventilation is poor, increase the microbial load and types of transient flora an animal is exposed to. It is not uncommon to isolate *E. coli* and other enteric bacteria from the upper respiratory tract as transient flora. The significance of their presence in the nasopharynx is difficult to assess without corresponding clinical and pathologic information.

The larynx, trachea, bronchi, and lungs lack a resident flora. However, the lower portion of the respiratory tract is continually being exposed to microbes that are present in the upper portion. In the uncompromised respiratory tract, these organisms are quickly removed by the natural host defense mechanisms. Fluid from the distal tract may contain up to 10^3 bacteria/ml in normal animals (e.g., cats).

Infections of the Respiratory System

Respiratory tract infections are of substantial importance in all animals. Some of the most common and/or important agents responsible for respiratory tract diseases in major domestic animals and poultry are listed in Tables 73.1–73.7. Agent characteristics, route of infection, host susceptiblity, and host immune response determine the location(s) in the respiratory tract affected, severity of the infection, and associated pathology. Pathogens of the respiratory tract covered in this chapter include viral, bacterial, and fungal agents, as well as one aquatic protistan parasite, *Rhinosporidium*.

Potential respiratory viral pathogens belong to a range of families (e.g., *Adenoviridae, Caliciviridae, Coronaviridae, Herpesviridae, Paramyxoviridae, Orthomyxoviridae*). The majority of the bacterial respiratory tract pathogens belong to the family *Pasteurellaceae* or to the genera *Bordetella, Mycoplasma,* and *Streptococcus*. Some important respiratory tract pathogens are associated with specific, well-defined clinical entities (e.g., *Rhodococcus equi* and pyogranulomatous pneumonia in foals). Under the proper conditions, a number of opportunistic bacteria (e.g., *Actinomyces* spp., members of the family *Enterobacteriaceae*, obligate anaerobes) from the oral cavity and lower digestive tract can cause or contribute to respiratory disease (e.g., aspiration pneumonia). Fungal agents of the respiratory tract are pre-

Table 73.1. Common and/or Important Infectious Agents of the Respiratory System of Dogs

Agent	Major Clinical Manifestations (Common Disease Name)
Viruses	
Canine adenovirus 2	Nasal discharge, tracheobronchitis (kennel cough syndrome), bronchointerstitial pneumonia
Canine distemper virus	Nasopharyngitis, laryngitis, bronchitis, bronchointerstitial pneumonia (distemper)
Canine parainfluenza virus 2	Nasal discharge, tracheobronchitis (canine kennel cough syndrome)
Bacteria	
Actinomyces spp.	Pyogranulomatous pneumonia, pleuritis
Bordetella bronchiseptica	Tracheobronchitis (infectious tracheobronchitis, kennel cough), bronchopneumonia
Escherichia coli	Bronchopneumonia
Nocardia spp.	Pyogranulomatis pleuritis
Obligate anaerobes[a]	Bronchopneumonia
Pasteurella multocida	Bronchopneumonia
Fungi	
Agents of systemic mycoses[b]	Granulomatous pneumonia
Aspergillus fumigatus	Rhinitis, sinusitis (nasal aspergillosis)
Cryptococcus neoformans	Granulomatous nasal masses (cryptococcosis)
Protist	
Rhinosporidium seeberi	Nasal granulomas (rare)

[a]Includes *Bacteroides, Peptostreptococcus, Fusobacterium,* and *Porphyromonas* species.
[b]Includes *Blastomyces dermatitidis, Coccidioides immitis, Cryptococcus neoformans,* and *Histoplasma capsulatum.*

Table 73.2. Common and/or Important Infectious Agents of the Respiratory System of Cats

Agent	Major Clinical Manifestations (Common Disease Name)
Viruses	
Feline calicivirus	Rhinitis, interstitial pneumonia, tracheitis (feline calicivirus disease)
Feline herpesvirus 1	Rhinotracheitis (feline viral rhinotracheitis)
Feline infectious peritonitis virus	Pleural effusion, pyogranulomatous pleuritis
Bacteria	
Bordetella bronchiseptica	Tracheobronchitis, bronchopneumonia (feline bordetellosis)
Chlamydophila felis	Pneumonia (feline pneumonitis), rhinitis
Obligate anaerobic bacteria	Pleural empyema (pyothorax)
Pasteurella multocida	Pleural empyema (pyothorax)
Fungi	
Cryptococcus neoformans	Rhinitis, granulomatous nasal masses, sinusitis, pneumonia

Table 73.3.   Common and/or Important Infectious Agents of the Respiratory System of Horses

Agent	Major Clinical Manifestations (Common Disease Name)
Viruses	
African Horse Sickness virus[a]	Pulmonary edema (African horse sickness)
Equine adenovirus 1	Bronchiolitis, interstitial pneumonia (equine adenovirus disease)
Equine herpesvirus 1	Rhinitis, pneumonitis (equine rhinopneumonitis)
Equine herpesvirus 4	Rhinitis, pneumonitis
Equine influenza virus	Rhinitis, tracheobronchitis, interstitial pneumonia (equine influenza)
Equine viral arteritis virus	Rhinitis, interstitial pneumonia
Hendra virus[a]	Pulmonary edema with respiratory distress
Bacteria	
Actinobacillus equuli ssp. *haemolytica*	Bronchopneumonia, pleuritis
Burkholderia mallei[a]	Rhinitis, pyogranulomatous nasal nodules (glanders)
Burkholderia pseudomallei[a]	Abcesses in nasal mucosa, embolic pneumonia, pulmonary abscesses
Escherichia coli	Bronchopneumonia, pleuritis
Mycoplasma felis	Pleuritis
Obligate anaerobes[b]	Bronchopneumonia, pleuritis
Rhodococcus equi	Pyogranulomatous pneumonia
Streptococcus equi subsp. *equi*	Guttural pouch empyema, rhinopharyngitis, retropharyngeal lymph nodes abscesses (strangles), sinusitis
Streptococcus equi subsp. *zooepidemicus*	Bronchopneumonia, pleuritis, sinusitis
Fungi	
Aspergillus species	Guttural pouch mycosis
Protist	
Rhinosporidium seeberi	Nasal granulomas (rare)

[a]Considered a foreign animal disease agent in the United States.
[b]Includes *Fusobacterium*, *Peptostreptococcus*, and *Prevotella*.

Table 73.4.   Common and/or Important Infectious Agents of the Respiratory System of Cattle

Agent	Major Clinical Manifestations (Common Disease Name)
Viruses	
Bovine herpesvirus 1	Rhinotracheitis (infectious bovine rhinotracheitis)
Bovine respiratory coronavirus	Interstitial pneumonia
Bovine respiratory syncytial virus	Interstitial pneumonia (bovine respiratory syncytial virus disease)
Parainfluenza virus 3	Rhinitis, interstitial pneumonia (parainfluenza virus 3 infection)
Bacteria	
Arcanobacterium pyogenes	Embolic pneumonia, lung abscesses
Fusobacterium necrophorum	Necrotic laryngitis (calf diphtheria)
Histophilus somni[a]	Bronchopneumonia, otitis media
Mannheimia haemolytica	Bronchopneumonia (enzootic pneumonia, shipping fever)
Mycobacterium bovis	Granulomatis pneumonia, pleuritis (bovine tuberculosis)
Mycoplasma bovis	Bronchopneumonia, otitis media
Mycoplasma dispar	Pneumonia—alveolitis
Mycoplasma mycoides subsp *mycoides*—small colony type[b]	Bronchopneumonia, pleuritis (contagious bovine pleuropneumonia)
Pasteurella multocida	Bronchopneumonia (enzootic pneumonia, shipping fever), otitis media
Salmonella Dublin	Interstitial pneumonia
Fungi	
Mortierella wolfii	Embolic pneumonia

[a]"*Haemophilus somnus*" is the obsolete name of this organism.
[b]Considered a foreign animal disease agent in the United States.

dominately the agents of systemic mycoses (*Blastomyces dermatitidis, Coccidioides immitis, Cryptococcus neoformans, Histoplasma capsulatum*) and *Aspergillus* spp. Individual chapters on particular respiratory tract pathogens should be consulted for details on pathogenesis and pathology specific to a particular agent.

Many infectious respiratory diseases are multifactorial, requiring environmental, host, and agent factors to be in play. Respiratory infections commonly involve sequential infection with different pathogens (e.g., viral pneumonia leading to secondary bacterial pneumonia). Respiratory tract infections can initiate either by the aerogenous or hematogenous route. A factor predisposing to infection of hematogenous origin, especially in cats, pigs, and rumi-

nants, is the role played by pulmonary intravascular macrophages in removing bloodborne pathogens.

Infections of the Nasopharyngeal Compartment

The major infectious diseases of the nasopharyngeal compartment are rhinitis and sinusitis, which can occur independently or concomitantly. Rhinitis is an inflammation of the nasal mucosa. Common signs of rhinitis are sneezing and nasal discharges of varying composition. The characteristic of the exudate in rhinitis is the result of serous or mucus secretions, alterations in vascular permeability (fibrinogen deposition), and influx and type of inflammatory cells.

Viral rhinitis can be caused by a number of viruses (e.g., herpesviruses, adenoviruses, influenza viruses) and occurs, to some degree, in most animals. In general, ciliated epithelial cells are infected, sloughed, and subsequently replaced. Clinical signs reflect the associated inflammatory response. Secondary bacterial infections can be a complication of a primary viral rhinitis (e.g., rhinotracheitis virus and calicivirus infections in cats predispose

Table 73.5.   Common and/or Important Infectious Agents of the Respiratory System of Sheep and Goats

Agent	Major Clinical Manifestations (Common Disease Name)
Viruses	
Caprine arthritis/encephalitis virus (G)	Interstitial pneumonia
Jaagsiekte sheep retrovirus (S)	Interstitial pneumonia, pulmonary carcinoma (ovine pulmonary adenocarcinoma)
Maedi/visna virus (S)	Interstitial pneumonia (ovine progressive pneumonia, maedi)
Parainfluenza virus 3	Interstitial pneumonia
Bacteria	
Arcanobacterium pyogenes	Pulmonary abscesses, traumatic pharyngitis
Fusobacterium necrophorum	Necrotic laryngitis, traumatic pharyngitis
Mannheimia haemolytica	Bronchopneumonia, pleuritis (pneumonic pasteurellosis)
Mycoplasma capricolum subsp *capripneumoniae* (G)[a]	Bronchopneumonia, pleuritis (contagious caprine pleuropneumonia)
Mycoplasma mycoides subsp *mycoides*—large colony type (G)	Pneumonia, pleuritis
Mycoplasma ovipneumoniae (S)	Interstitial pneumonia (ovine nonprogressive pneumonia)
Pasteurella trehalosi	Bronchopneumonia

(S) = sheep, (G) = goats.
[a]Considered a foreign animal disease agent in the United States.

Table 73.6.   Common and/or Important Infectious Agents of the Respiratory System of Pigs

Agent	Major Clinical Manifestations (Common Disease Name)
Viruses	
Lelystad virus	Interstitial pneumonia (porcine reproductive and respiratory syndrome)
Nipah virus[a]	Alveolitis, bronchointerstitial pneumonia
Porcine herpesvirus 1	Rhinopharyngitis, tracheitis (pseudorabies, Aujeszky's disease)
Porcine herpesvirus 2	Rhinitis (inclusion body rhinitis)
Swine influenza virus	Rhinitis, tracheobronchitis, bronchointerstitial pneumonia (swine influenza)
Bacteria	
Actinobacillus pleuropneumoniae	Bronchopneumonia, pleuritis (porcine pleuropneumonia)
Bordetella bronchiseptica[b]	Rhinitis (atrophic rhinitis), bronchopneumonia
Fusobacterium necrophorum	Necrotic nasal cellulitis (necrotic rhinitis, bull nose)
Haemophilus parasuis	Bronchopneumonia, polyserositis (Glasser's disease)
Mycoplasma hyopneumoniae	Bronchopneumonia (enzootic pneumonia)
Mycoplasma hyorhinis	Polyserositis
Pasteurella multocida[b]	Rhinitis (atrophic rhinitis), bronchopneumonia
Salmonella species	Bronchointerstitial pneumonia
Streptococcus suis	Bronchopneumonia, pleuritis, embolic pneumonia

[a]Considered a foreign animal disease agent in the United States.
[b]*B.bronchiseptica* and *P. multocida* sometimes act synergistically.

to bacterial rhinitis and sinusitis). Latently infected animals that periodically shed virus (e.g., infectious bovine rhinotracheitis virus) are a common source for infections in naive animals.

Bacterial infections of the nasopharyngeal compartment, while not as frequent as viral infections, are still significant. Notable among these are atrophic rhinitis in pigs, contagious rhinopharyngitis (strangles) in horses, and sinus infections in poultry (see below). In atrophic rhinitis in pigs, the dermonecrotic toxin of *Pasteurella multocida* (Type D) induces osteolysis of nasal turbinates and distortion of the nasal cavity (Fig 73.1). To a lesser extent, the dermonecrotic toxin of *Bordetella bronchiseptica* is also involved. Pigs present with sneezing and a clear to cloudy nasal discharge. The disease can be a mild, nonprogressive, or more active, progressive form. Reduced weight gain, poor feed conversion, and increased susceptibility to other respiratory infections are the main consequences of atrophic rhinitis.

Streptococcus equi subspecies *equi,* the cause of contagious rhinopharyngitis (strangles) in horses, typically also involves submandibular and/or retropharyngeal lymph nodes. The resulting intense inflammatory response produces a thick, bilateral, purulent nasal discharge. Strangles is considered highly contagious. Serious consequences can

result from strangles infections including guttural pouch empyema (see below), "bastard strangles," and purpura hemorrhagica.

Sinusitis is an inflammation of one of the nasal sinuses. It can result from extension of a nasal cavity infection into sinuses or be related to other problems of the oral-nasal cavities (e.g., extension of infection from an infected tooth). It is an occasional occurrence in most animals. Agents involved are typically resident flora of the nasal cavity or those involved in rhinitis.

In poultry, sinusitis is an especially common problem that has major economic consequences due to the contagious nature of some of the agents involved and potential for large numbers of birds to be affected (Fig 73.2). A number of microbial agents can infect the sinuses of birds, and typically sinusitis is found in conjunction with clinical signs in other areas of the respiratory system (e.g., Gallid herpesvirus 1 in chickens, avian influenza viruses). *Mycoplasma gallisepticum* in turkeys (infectious sinusitis) and *Haemophilus paragallinarum* in chickens (fowl coryza) are among the most economically important causes of sinusitis in poultry. Poor growth performance and decreased egg

Table 73.7.   Common and/or Important Infectious Agents of the Respiratory System of Poultry

Agent	Major Clinical Manifestations (Common Disease Name)
Viruses	
Avian infectious bronchitis virus (C)	Air sacculitis, tracheobronchitis (avian infectious bronchitis)
Avian influenza virus	Air sacculitis, sinusitis, tracheitis (avian influenza)
Avian paramyxovirus 1[a]	Hemorrhagic tracheitis (exotic Newcastle disease)
Avian pneumovirus	Rhinotracheitis, sinusitis (turkey rhinotracheitis), periorbital and infraorbital sinus swelling in chickens (swollen head syndrome)
Avian poxvirus	Diphtheritic lesions of nares, pharynx, larynx and trachea (pox-diphtheritic form)
Gallid herpesvirus 1 (C)	Laryngotracheitis (infectious laryngotracheitis)
Bacteria	
Bordetella avium	Rhinotracheitis, sinusitis (bordetellosis, turkey coryza)
Escherichia coli	Colisepticemia, secondary pneumonia
Haemophilus paragallinarum (C)	Rhinitis, sinusitis (fowl coryza)
Mycoplasma gallisepticum	Air sacculitis (chronic respiratory disease), rhinitis, sinusitis (infectious sinusitis) (T)
Mycoplasma synoviae	Air sacculitis, sinusitis
Ornithobacterium rhinotracheale	Air sacculitis, bronchopneumonia, sinusitis
Pasteurella multocida	Air sacculitis, pneumonia
Fungi	
Aspergillus fumigatus	Tracheitis, air sacculitis, pneumonia (brooder pneumonia)

(C) = chickens only.
[a]Considered a foreign animal disease agent in the United States.

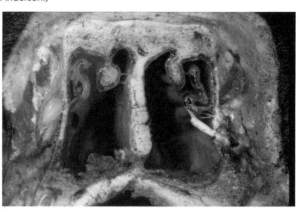

FIGURE 73.1.   *Atrophic rhinitis in a pig. Cross section of snout showing severe atrophy of nasal turbinates. (Courtesy Dr. M. Anderson.)*

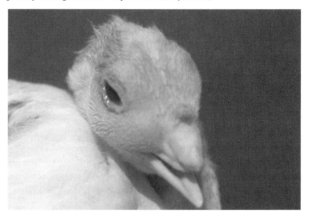

FIGURE 73.2.   *Sinusitis in a 5-week-old turkey. Sinus cavity is greatly enlarged. (Courtesy Dr. H. Shivaprasad.)*

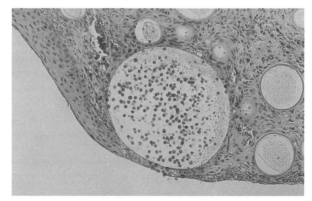

FIGURE 73.3.   *Rhinosporidiosis in a dog. Section of a nasal polyp showing the variable-sized spherules. Mature spherules (up to 300 μm in diameter) contain numerous endospores. One large spherule is present near the surface of the lesion (H&E).*

production are among the main reasons for economic losses.

Fungal infections of the nasopharyngeal compartment are infrequent and when they occur they evoke a granulomatous inflammatory response. *Aspergillus* rhinitis and sinusitis in dogs and nasal cryptococcosis in cats are among the most important fungal infections of the nasal cavity.

Rhinosporidium seeberi, a protist in the class Mesomycetozoea, is a rare cause of granulomatous nasal masses containing large spherules and endospores of *Rhinosporidium* (Fig 73.3). Grossly the nasal lesions resemble multilobed granular polyps. Although any animal including poultry can be infected, most cases are reported in dogs and horses. Infections are associated with exposure to freshwater ponds, lakes, or rivers.

Sites that communicate with the upper respiratory tract may be affected by the direct extension of an infectious process in the nasopharyngeal compartment or become infected independent of other nasopharyngeal disease by residents of the nasopharyngeal compartment. Guttural pouch empyema in horses, caused by *S. equi* subsp. *equi*, develops as a sequel to primary rhinopharyngitis or rupture of an abscessed retropharyngeal lymph node (strangles). Unilateral nasal discharge, especially when the head is down, is a common way for guttural pouch infections to present. Incomplete drainage from the guttural pouch, scarring of the pharyngeal opening, and development of concretions (chondroids) on the floor of the guttural pouch interfere with resolution of the infection. Fungal infections also occur in the guttural pouch of horses (guttural pouch mycosis), typically involving the dorsal wall of the medial compartment. *Aspergillus* species (especially *A. nidulans*) are the most common etiologic agents. The initiating factor(s) for guttural pouch mycosis has not been clearly elucidated. When guttural pouch infections involve neural or vascular structures, serious (dysphagia, laryngeal hemiplegia and Horner's syndrome due to nerve injury) or even fatal (rupture of the internal carotid artery) consequences may result.

Otitis media in calves is commonly caused by respiratory pathogens (e.g., *Mycoplasma bovis, Pasteurella multocida, Histophilus somni*) harbored as residents of the upper respiratory tract. The likely route of infection is via the auditory tube into the middle ear. Calves present with a head tilt, nystagmus, and droopy ear(s). The tympanic bullae are typically partially or completely filled with caseous debris and serosanguineous fluid. In some cases the disease progresses and results in otitis interna and meningitis, where calves may exhibit severe neurologic signs. Other species of animals are similarly but less commonly affected.

Infections of the Tracheobronchial Compartment

The major diseases of the tracheobronchial compartment are laryngitis, tracheitis, and bronchitis. Viral and bacterial agents are the primary causes of infectious diseases of the tracheobronchial compartment. *Aspergillus* infections in poultry can, however, involve the trachea and bronchi.

Viral infections of the trachea and bronchi (e.g., equine influenza, infectious bovine rhinotracheitis, infectious laryngotracheitis in chickens) damage respiratory epithelial cells and interrupt the mucociliary apparatus. Tracheal lesions caused by many different viruses may not have particularly distinguishing features; however, inclusions in some infections assist in identifying the particular virus involved (e.g., infectious laryngotracheitis in chickens, avian pox viruses). Viral tracheitis is often sufficiently destructive to predispose to secondary bacterial infections.

Necrotic laryngitis in young feedlot cattle is one of the most common bacterial laryngeal diseases (Fig 73.4). *Fusobacterium necrophorum*, the etiologic agent, establishes in preexisting contact ulcers found on the laryngeal mucosa, which are suspected to originate from some preceding trauma (e.g., reflex coughing). Once established, *F. necrophorum* causes a severe necrotic laryngitis that can be fatal if untreated. Other ruminants are affected but less frequently.

In dogs, the kennel cough syndrome, an infectious tracheobronchitis, involves multiple potential etiologic agents, sometimes working in concert. Kennel cough in

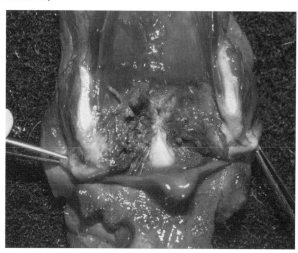

FIGURE 73.4. *Necrotic laryngitis in a calf. Fibrinonecrotic material is covering the arytenoid cartilages. (Courtesy of Dr. M. Anderson.)*

dogs is considered contagious and is associated with dogs maintained in confined, close-contact environments (e.g., kennels, animal shelters). Viral agents include canine adenovirus 2 and parainfluenza virus 2. *Mycoplasma* species have been implicated, but their involvement is unproven. The bacterium, *Bordetella bronchiseptica,* is also associated with the kennel cough syndrome. It is considered a primary pathogen of the respiratory tract because of its ability to adhere to ciliated epithelial cells and affect epithelial cell functions. Infections involving *B. bronchiseptica* tend to be more productive than those caused by viral agents. Evidence is growing that *B. bronchiseptica* is also a significant respiratory pathogen in cats.

In poultry, *Bordetella avium* is a common cause of upper respiratory infections (rhinitis, sinusitis, tracheitis) in turkeys and to a lesser extent in chickens. Sneezing is the most common sign, along with an oculonasal discharge. After colonization, damage to ciliated respiratory epithelial cells and ciliostatic effects occur. Collapse of the trachea due to softening of tracheal rings may also result. Infections with *B. avium* predispose birds to other infections, such as colibacillosis.

Some microorganisms that affect the tracheobronchial compartment concurrently involve other parts of the respiratory system (e.g., feline viral rhinotracheitis, infectious bovine rhinotracheitis, *Bordetella avium* in turkeys). Additionally, systemic infections may involve epithelial cells in the tracheobronchial compartment (e.g., fibrinohemorrhagic tracheitis in exotic Newcastle disease in poultry) (Fig 73.5), along with sites in the host outside the respiratory system.

Infections of the Pulmonary Compartment

The major infectious disease of the pulmonary compartment is pneumonia. Pneumonia can be classified morphologically as a(n) bronchopneumonia, interstitial pneumonia, granulomatous pneumonia, embolic pneumonia, or a

FIGURE 73.5.   *Exotic Newcastle disease in a chicken. Exposed larynx and tracheal lumen are covered with a fibrinohemorrhagic exudate. (Courtesy Dr. H. Kinde.)*

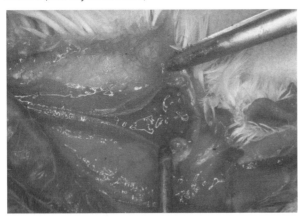

mixture of these types. The agent, route of infection, and immune response determine the type of pneumonia that develops. Viruses, bacteria, and fungi are all potentially important pathogens of the pulmonary compartment. Chapters on specific pathogens should be consulted for details on pathogenesis and pathology associated with that particular agent.

Infections of the pulmonary compartment often require a preceding event(s) that impairs the innate antimicrobial factors. Confined housing environment, ammonia build-up (noxious gas), and transportation stress would typify the type of factors that sufficiently impair defenses and allow pathogens that would otherwise be rapidly cleared by innate host defense mechanisms to establish in the lower respiratory tract.

Some of the same viruses found in the upper respiratory tract cause mild lower respiratory tract disease (e.g., parainfluenza virus, adenoviruses). Serologic evidence indicates that a large percent of populations are inapparently or subclinically infected by these organisms. Other viruses are substantial pathogens of the pulmonary compartment in their own right, sometimes causing fatal infections (e.g., African Horse Sickness virus, Hendra virus). Viral respiratory pathogens in animals with the potential to be transmitted from animal to humans (e.g., influenza viruses, Hendra virus, Nipah virus) are of substantial public health concern.

While some bacterial pathogens are considered primary pathogens of the pulmonary compartment (e.g., *Rhodococcus equi* in horses, *Actinobacillus pleuropneumoniae* in pigs), viral infections often precede bacterial infections and create an environment that allows bacteria to establish by damaging the mucociliary escalator system or altering the immune response by impairing phagocytic function. Once predisposing factors are in play, it is not uncommon to find multiple bacterial pathogens involved in lower respiratory tract infections.

The bovine respiratory disease complex is an example of the complex and, as yet, incompletely understood interactions of environmental factors along with specific infec-

tious agents and host response. It constitutes one of the most economically significant disease complexes of cattle. Environmental or management-related stresses (weather, transportation) and/or viral infections (e.g., adenovirus, bovine respiratory syncytial virus, infectious bovine rhinotracheitis virus, parainfluenza virus 3) are believed to alter respiratory tract epithelium and innate defenses. Possible immunosuppressive effects related to bovine viral diarrhea virus may also contribute to increasing susceptibility to bacterial infections. These factors allow one of the primary bacterial agents in bovine respiratory disease complex, *Mannheimia haemolytica,* to establish in the pulmonary compartment. Armed with a number of virulence factors, *M. haemolytica* is able to engage the host defenses. Endotoxin activates pulmonary intravascular macrophages, neutrophils, and lymphocytes, and precipitates an inflammatory response that ultimately determines the degree of pulmonary injury and whether the pathogen is contained. In addition, leukotoxin from *M. haemolytica* destroys phagocytic cells and, at lower concentrations, further enhances the inflammatory response (Fig 73.6). If pulmonary defenses are compromised sufficiently, more opportunistic bacterial pathogens are established and further aggravate the condition. It is common to recover *Arcanobacterium pyogenes*, a major abscess-former of ruminants, from more chronic bovine respiratory disease complex lesions (Fig 73.7).

The systemic mycoses (coccidioidomycosis, cryptococcosis, blastomycosis, and histoplasmosis), for the most part, begin in the lower respiratory tract causing a granulomatous pneumonia and an associated lymphadenopathy. Severity of respiratory infection varies based on individual animal immune status, breed, and animal species. Dogs, horses, and cats most commonly develop clinical disease. Inability of the animal to contain these infections to the respiratory tract leads to disseminated infections involving other systems in the body. Other than the systemic mycoses, fungal pneumonias are not common in animals. The exception is aspergillosis in poultry where pneumonia, often with concurrent tracheitis and air sacculitis, is a major respiratory tract disease. This is a disease of substan-

FIGURE 73.6.   *Bronchopneumonia in a calf caused by* Mannheimia haemolytica. *Cranioventral lung lobes are predominantly involved. (Courtesy Dr. M. Anderson.)*

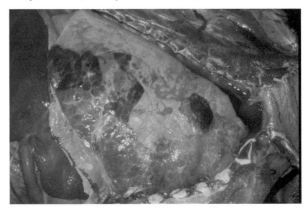

FIGURE 73.7. *Chronic bronchopneumonia in a calf. Multiple areas of abscessation are apparent. (Courtesy Dr. M. Anderson.)*

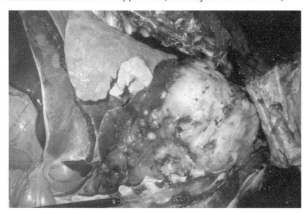

FIGURE 73.8. *Aspergillosis in a turkey. Conidiophores, vesicles, and phialides are evident in material from lumen of the trachea. Numerous conidia are dispersed throughout the field. Hematoxylin-eosin stain.*

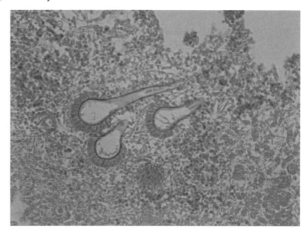

tial economic significance to the poultry industry, especially the turkey industry. Closed environments that allow for increased concentration of aerosolized asexual reproductive structures (conidia) and/or moldy feeds are common predisposing factors. Growth in aerated air sacs, bronchi, and trachea permit the production of large numbers of conidia that are not typically produced in solid tissues (Fig 73.8).

Aspiration pneumonias in most cases are polymicrobial in nature, and bacteria are usually the microbial agents involved. Aspiration pneumonia in animals results when impaired airway protection allows fluids or material to enter the lower respiratory tract, initially causing a chemical pneumonia. Common events leading to aspiration pneumonia are improper treatment procedures (e.g., drench-

ing, improper stomach tubing), bottle or bucket feeding of young animals, poor sucking reflexes, nasopharyngeal tube feeding, choke, or aspiration of gastric or rumen fluids that might occur during the anesthesia recovery period. In newborns, aspiration of meconium may also lead to aspiration pneumonia. The bacteria most frequently involved in aspiration pneumonia typically reflect organisms found in the upper respiratory or digestive tracts and include *E. coli, Bordetella, Klebsiella, Pasteurella, Pseudomonas, Streptococcus,* and obligate anaerobes (*Fusobacterium, Peptostreptococcus, Prevotella, Porphyromonas*).

74 Urogenital System

RICHARD L. WALKER

The urinary and genital tracts are included together in this chapter because of their anatomical proximity, shared structures (urethra in males), and some overlapping disease processes. Common and/or important urogenital tract agents of domestic animals and poultry are listed in Tables 74.1–74.7.

The Urinary Tract

The urinary tract has a number of important functions, including elimination of metabolic wastes, acid-base regulation, maintenance of the extracellular potassium ion concentration, and endocrine functions (vitamin D conversion and production of erythropoietin and renin). The mammalian urinary system includes the kidneys, ureters, bladder and urethra. The functional filtration unit of the kidney is the nephron, which includes the glomerulus, proximal and distal tubules, loop of Henle, and collecting duct. In birds, the urinary tract differs from mammals. The kidneys are divided into lobes. A bladder is absent and ureters enter the cloaca, medial to the deferent duct in the male and dorsal to the oviduct in the female. Urine, concentrated as a slurry, is voided with feces.

Antimicrobial Defenses

Because it is primarily an excretory system, the urinary tract is not subject to massive microbial exposure but has developed specific antimicrobial defenses to counter occasional exposure to potential pathogens. Protective features include:

1. *Washout by Urine.* The flow of urine—its direction, diluting effect, and frequent periodic removal—discourages the establishment of microorganisms in the normally sterile portions of the tract—that is, the kidneys, ureters, bladder, and proximal male urethra. Urine retention is correlated with increased urinary tract infections.
2. *Bacterial Interference.* Colonization of the distal urethra by normal flora may block attachment sites for colonization of the lower urinary tract by potentially pathogenic organisms.
3. *Glycoprotein Slime Layer.* Mucin covering the epithelium may inhibit bacterial adhesion.
4. *Epithelial Desquamation.* Exfoliating epithelial cells promote shedding of uropathogens.

5. *Local and Systemic Immune Defenses.* Cysteine-rich antimicrobial peptides play a role in inhibiting bacteria from establishing. Immune response to urinary tract infections has been studied mostly in humans and laboratory animals. Studies indicate that serum and urinary antibody titers tend to be low in cystitis and asymptomatic infections and high in pyelonephritis. Secretory IgA (sIgA) tends to be most prominent in urine, but IgG and IgM antibodies also occur regularly. Serum IgA, IgG, IgM, and sIgA antibodies are produced in renal infections. The protective function of these antibodies is unclear. The ability to readily mobilize leukocytes promotes rapid clearance of uropathogens from the urinary system.
6. *Antimicrobial Properties of Urine.* Urine itself has properties that may play a role in limiting bacterial growth and include:
   a. *High osmolality:* Urine osmolality (1000 mOsm/kg) reduces growth, particularly of rod-shaped bacteria. It may, however, depress leukocyte activity and preserve bacteria with cell walls damaged by immune reactions or antibiotic therapy. Combined with high concentrations of ammonia, which is anticomplementary, urine osmolality may contribute to the susceptibility of the renal medulla to infection.
   b. *Urine pH:* While extremes in pH discourage multiplication of some bacteria, ranges bactericidal to common urinary tract pathogens are unlikely to be reached.
   c. *Urine constituents:* Urea imparts to urine an unexplained bacteriostatic effect, which is diminished by removal of urea from urine and enhanced by dietary supplementation. Methionine and hippuric and ascorbic acids produce an antibacterial effect largely by acidifying the urine. Urinary ammonium nitrogen also has antibacterial properties.

Normal Flora

For most of the urinary tract there is no resident flora. The distal urethra does have a resident flora and is colonized by bacteria that generally are not associated with urinary tract infection. The flora is predominantly gram-positive and includes coagulase-negative *Staphylococcus* spp., *Streptococcus* spp., *Corynebacterium* spp., and *Enterococcus* spp. but varies

Table 74.1.   Common and/or Important Infectious Agents of the Urogenital System of Dogs

Agent	Major Clinical Manifestations (Common Disease Name)
Viruses	
Canine adenovirus 1	Immune-complex glomerulonephritis (infectious canine hepatitis)
Canine herpesvirus	Abortion, balanoposthitis, infertility in females
Bacteria	
Brucella canis	Abortion, epididymitis (canine brucellosis)
Escherichia coli	Cystitis, epididymitis, orchitis, prostatitis, pyometra, vaginitis
Leptospira spp.	Interstitial nephritis, renal failure (leptospirosis)
Other agents of UTI (see Table 74.8.)	Cystitis

Table 74.2.   Common and/or Important Infectious Agents of the Urogenital System of Cats

Agent	Major Clinical Manifestations (Common Disease Name)
Viruses	
Feline infectious peritonitis virus	Immune-mediated pyogranulomas of kidney
Feline leukemia virus	Immune-complex glomerulonephritis, fetal absorption, abortion, renal lymphoma
Feline panleukopenia virus	Abortion, congenital abnormalities (panleukopenia)
Feline rhinotracheitis virus	Abortion

Table 74.3.   Common and/or Important Iinfectious Agents of the Urogenital System of Horses

Agent	Major Clinical Manifestations (Common Disease Name)
Viruses	
Equine herpesvirus 1	Abortion (equine viral rhinopneumonitis)
Equine herpesvirus 3	Vesicles/erosions on external genitalia (coital exanthema), balanoposthitis
Equine infectious anemia	Immune-complex glomerulonephritis
Equine viral arteritis virus	Abortion (equine viral arteritis)
Bacteria	
Actinobacillus equuli subsp. *equuli*	Glomerulonephritis (sleepy foal disease)
Escherichia coli	Abortion
Leptospira spp.	Abortion
Pseudomonas aeruginosa	Pyometra
Staphylococcus aureus	Post-castration spermatic cord infection (scirrhous cord)
Streptococcus equi subsp. *zooepidemicus*	Abortion, endometritis
Taylorella equigenitalis[a]	Cervicitis, endometritis (contagious equine metritis)
Fungi	
Aspergillus spp.	Abortion
Candida spp.	Endometritis

[a]Considered a foreign animal disease agent in the United States.

according to animal, housing, and hygiene. Small numbers of bacteria may enter the bladder via the urethra, especially in the female, but are normally removed during urination. The significance of asymptomatic bacteriuria is unclear, however, when detected investigation into potential underlying diseases is warranted.

Certain viruses that persistently infect tubular epithelial cells, although not normal flora, may cause a prolonged viruria (e.g., equine rhinitis A virus and arenaviruses).

Diseases

Host Factors.   A number of host factors can predispose an animal to urinary tract infections (UTI):

1. *Animal Susceptibility.* Urinary tract infections are most common and of greatest significance in dogs. In cats, idiopathic lower urinary tract disorders are frequently encountered. Viral, nutritional, and metabolic factors have been implicated in the etiology, particularly of obstructive forms. However, bac-

terial involvement in feline urinary tract disease is uncommon. Infections, particularly cystitis and pyelonephritis, are important in cattle and swine. Urinary tract infections are less common in goats, sheep, poultry, and horses.

2. *Anatomic and Physiologic Factors.* Interference with the free flow of urine and with complete emptying of the bladder predisposes to UTI. This can be due to tumors, polyps, calculi, anatomic anomalies (e.g., ectopic ureters, patent urachus), and neural defects. Vesico-ureteral reflux, the reentry of urine into the ureters during urination, causes bladder urine to reach the renal pelvis, possibly carrying bacteria into a susceptible area. Reflux is aggravated (perhaps initiated) by infection and complicates existing infections by increasing the likelihood of renal involvement.

3. *Other Host Factors.* Other host factors include endocrine disturbances such as diabetes mellitus and hyperadrenocorticism (Cushing's disease). Long-term use of corticosteroids appears to predispose dogs to UTI.

Routes of Infection.   The primary means by which uropathogens reach the urinary tract are the ascending and hematogenous routes. The ascending route via the urethra is most common. The presence of potential pathogens near the urethral orifice and the usual localization of infection

Table 74.4.   Common and/or Important Infectious Agents of the Urogenital System of Cattle

Agent	Major Clinical Manifestations (Common Disease Name)
Viruses	
Bovine papillomavirus	Penile and vaginal fibropapillomas
Bovine viral diarrhea virus	Abortion, congenital abnormalities
Infectious bovine rhinotracheitis virus	Abortion, infectious pustular vulvovaginitis, balanoposthitis
Rift Valley fever virus[a]	Abortion (Rift Valley fever)
Bacteria	
Arcanobacterium pyogenes	Abortion, metritis, pyometra, seminal vesiculitis
Brucella abortus	Abortion, epididymitis, orchitis, seminal vesiculitis
Campylobacter fetus subsp. venerealis	Early embryonic death (bovine venereal campylobacteriosis, vibriosis)
Corynebacterium renale group	Pyelonephritis
Epizootic bovine abortion agent (unidentified)	Abortion (foothill abortion)
Escherichia coli	Interstitial nephritis (white-spotted kidney disease), pyelonephritis, pyometra
Fusobacterium necrophorum, other anaerobes	Post-parturient metritis
Leptospira spp.	Abortion
Listeria monocytogenes, L. ivanovii	Abortion
Mycoplasma spp., Ureaplasma spp.	Granular vulvitis
Fungi	
Aspergillus sp.	Abortion
Mortierella wolfii	Abortion

[a]Considered a foreign animal disease agent in the United States.

Table 74.5.   Common and/or Important Infectious Agents of the Urogenital System of Sheep and Goats

Agent	Major Clinical Manifestations (Common Disease Name)
Viruses	
Akabane virus[a]	Abortion, dystocia due to arthrogryposis of fetus
Bluetongue virus (S)	Abortion, congenital abnormalities (bluetongue)
Border disease and BVD viruses	Congenital abnormalities, stillbirths (Border disease, hairy shaker disease)
Cache Valley virus	Abortion, congenital abnormalities
Rift Valley fever virus[a]	Abortion
Bacteria	
"Actinobacillus seminis"(S)	Epididymitis
Brucella abortus, B. melitensis[a]	Abortion, orchitis
Brucella ovis(S)	Epididymitis, rare abortions
Campylobacter fetus subsp. fetus	Abortion
Campylobacter jejuni	Abortion
Chlamydophila abortus	Abortion (enzootic abortion of ewes)
Corynebacterium renale group	Balanoposthitis (ulcerative posthitis, pizzle rot), pyelonephritis
Coxiella burnetti	Abortion (Q-fever)
Histophilus somni[b] (S)	Epididymitis
Leptospira sp.	Abortion
Listeria monocytogenes, L. ivanovii	Abortion
Salmonella sp.	Abortion, metritis

(G) = goats predominately, (S) = sheep predominately.
[a]Considered a foreign animal disease agent in the United States.
[b]"Histophilus ovis" is the obsolete name.

Table 74.6.   Common and/or Important Infectious Agents of the Urogenital System of Pigs

Agent	Major Clinical Manifestations (Common Disease Name)
Viruses	
African swine fever virus[a]	Abortion, immune-complex glomerulonephritis (African swine fever)
Classical swine fever virus[a]	Abortion, embryonic death, immune-complex glomerulonephritis (classical swine fever, hog cholera)
Lelystad virus	Abortion (porcine reproductive and respiratory syndrome)
Pseudorabies virus	Abortion (pseudorabies)
Swine parvovirus	Embryonic death, mummification
Bacteria	
Actinobaculum suis	Cystitis, pyelonephritis, ureteritis
Brucella suis	Abortion, orchitis
Escherichia coli	Vaginitis (discharging sows)
Leptospira spp.	Abortion (leptospirosis)

[a]Considered a foreign anmial disease agent in the United States.

in the bladder point to it as the portal of entrance. Pyelonephritis is a consequence of retrograde extension of infection from the bladder.

Infection of the urinary tract via the hematogenous route occurs secondary to bacteremia/viremia and primarily affects the kidney, causing glomerulonephritis or interstitial nephritis. It occurs less commonly than lower urinary tract infectious, due probably to the high resistance of the renal cortex, where infection begins. Young animals are especially at risk because of the greater likelihood for septicemia to occur in that age group.

Glomerulonephritis and Interstitial Nephritis. Glomerulonephritis is an inflammation of the glomerulus due to localization of an infectious agent in the glomerulus and ensuing inflammatory response or from deposition of immune complexes. Viral glomerulonephritis is the result of selected viruses (e.g., infectious canine hepatitis virus, equine arteritis virus, nephrotoxic infectious bronchitis virus in chickens) replicating in glomerular capillary endothelial cells, usually as a consequence of a systemic viral

Table 74.7.   Common and/or Important Infectious Agents of the Urogenital System of Poultry

Agent	Major Clinical Manifestations (Common Disease Name)
Viruses	
Avian adenovirus (C)	Soft-shelled or shell-less eggs (egg drop syndrome)
Avian encephalomyelitis virus	Decreased egg production
Avian influenza virus	Decreased egg production, oophoritis
Avian leukosis virus (C)	Nephroblastoma, renal carcinoma
Avian pneumovirus	Decreased egg production
Infectious bronchitis virus (C)	Decreased egg production, decreased hatchability, nephritis (infectious bronchitis-nephrotoxic strains)
Newcastle disease virus[a]	Decreased egg production
Bacteria	
Escherichia coli (C)	Salpingitis
Gallibacterium anatis (C)[b]	Oophoritis, salpingitis
Haemophilus paragallinarum (C)	Decreased egg production (infectious coryza)
Mycoplasma gallisepticum	Decreased egg production, salpingitis
Mycoplasma iowae (T)	Reduced hatchability, increased embryo mortality
Salmonella Pullorum	Oophoritis, salpingitis (pullorum disease)
Salmonella Gallinarum	Oophoritis, salpingitis (fowl typhoid)
Salmonella Enteritidis (phage Type 4)	Oophoritis, salpingitis

(C)= chickens predominately, (T) = turkeys predominately.
[a]Considered a foreign animal disease agent in the United States.
[b]Includes organisms previously identified as *"Actinobacillus salpingitidis,"* *"Pasteurella-haemolytica-like,"* or *"Pasteurella haemolytica-Actinobacillus salpingitidis-complex."*

FIGURE 74.1.   *Embolic nephritis in a foal caused by* Actinobacillus equuli *subsp* equuli. *Microabscesses are scattered throughout the renal cortex (A). Bacterial microcolonies and a suppurative inflammatory response are present (B).*

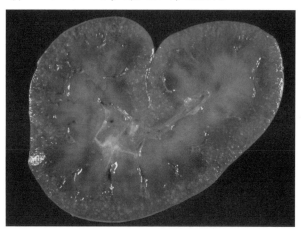

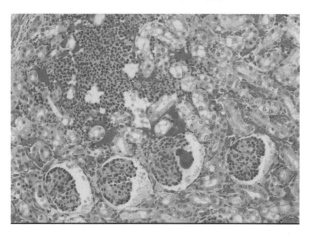

infection. In bacterial glomerulonephritis, bacteria from a septicemia/bacteremia settle in the glomerulus (e.g., *Actinobacillus equuli* subsp. *equuli* in foals). The ensuing inflammatory response is typically suppurative. The result is an embolic nephritis (Fig 74.1).

In some hematogenous infections, the renal tubules rather than the glomeruli are the primary target. Interstitial nephritis is commonly seen with *E. coli* septicemia in neonatal ruminants (white-spotted kidney) and leptospirosis in a number of different animals.

Deposition of immune complexes in the glomeruli in the case of persistent viral infections (e.g., infectious canine hepatitis, equine infectious anemia, feline infectious peritonitis), specific bacterial infections (e.g., *Borrelia* spp.), or chronic bacterial infections at other sites in the body may result in immune-complex glomerulonephritis.

Cystitis. Bacterial cystitis (inflammation of the urinary bladder), especially in dogs, is the most common urinary tract infection encountered by veterinarians. The ability of bacteria to adhere to epithelium is considered a prerequisite to establishment of cystitis. The infection may begin with colonization of the urethral orifice by a potential pathogen that subsequently reaches the bladder through multiplication, extension along the epithelial surface, or migration through active motility or random movement. The resulting infection, after further multiplication, is marked by bacteriuria (Fig 74.2). Pyuria and low-grade proteinuria may be present. Inflammation is triggered by the interaction of lipopolysaccharide (gram-negatives) or muramyl dipeptides (gram-positives) with transitional cells of the bladder that secrete proinflammatory mediators, which attract polymorphonuclear neutrophil leukocytes. Signs, when present, include dysuria or urinary frequency or urgency. There may be hematuria and incontinence. The prevalence of the common agents implicated in canine urinary tract infections and characteristic features are summarized in Table 74.8.

Pyelonephritis. The most serious complication of lower urinary tract infection is pyelonephritis, which is caused by an ascending infection via the ureters. Pyelonephritis is essentially an inflammation of the renal pelvis and renal parenchyma. Once bacteria reach the renal pelvis they are hard to eliminate due to the poor vascular supply and in-

FIGURE 74.2.   *Gram stains of urine sediment from a dog with cystitis. Stain in A is from a dog with* Escherichia coli *cystitis, and the stain in B is from a dog with* Enterococcus *sp. cystitis.*

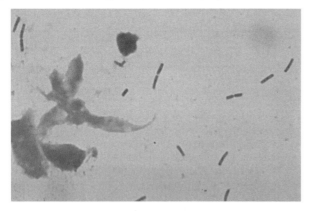

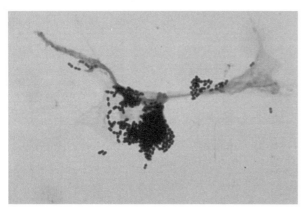

most common cause of pyelonephritis in animals. Other bacterial agents that cause cystitis have the potential to cause pyelonephritis, if they reach the renal pelvis.

Diphtheroid bacteria, belonging to the *Corynebacterium renale* group are specifically associated with pyelonephritis in cattle. They colonize the lower genital tract and pass between animals by direct and indirect contact. Many clinical cases are probably endogenous. The process is an ascending urinary tract infection, beginning with cystitis, which proceeds to ureteritis and pyelonephritis. An anaerobic diphtheroid, *Actinobaculum suis,* causes urinary tract infection of sows (Fig 74.3). Like bovine pyelonephritis, the disease is an apparently ascending infection caused by an urealytic diphtheroid agent, limited to females and often related to breeding operations, pregnancy, and parturition.

Uroliths and Urinary Tract Infections.   Uroliths of dogs are predominantly (70%) the result of infection and consist of struvite or apatite, or various combinations, and are often referred to as *triple phosphate stones*. Urease-producing bacteria are implicated—in dogs, chiefly coagulase-positive staphylococci, and to a lesser extent *Proteus mirabilis*. Inhibition of urease activity by urea analogues (e.g., acetohydroxamic acid) can suppress infectious stone formation. Uroliths in ruminants are related to nutritional factors rather that infectious ones.

Virulence Factors of Bacterial Uropathogens

Bacteria capable of initiating UTI require virulence determinants, the most firmly established of which are adhesins (e.g., the pyelonephritis-associated pilus, Pap). Fimbrial attachment of *E. coli* to surface slime glycoproteins by Type 1 (mannose-sensitive) pili is probably of less significance than that mediated by several mannose-resistant adhesins, one of which is Pap, that attach to cell membrane glycolipids. *Escherichia coli* isolates from different animals appear to maintain the same Pap alleles. Mannose-resistant adhesins occur commonly in uropathogenic *E. coli*, but irregularly in other strains. Other properties associated with uropathogenic *E. coli* include resistance to serum bacterici-

hibitory effects of urine osmolarity and ammonia on immune defenses, as mentioned previously. Signs of pyelonephritis are vague. Fever is transient even during the acute phase. Pain in the thoracolumbar area is not specific unless directly associated with kidney palpation. Urinalysis may reveal lowered specific gravity and casts. In advanced cases, blood urea nitrogen is elevated. *Escherichia coli* is the

Table 74.8.   Leading Bacterial Causes of Urinary Tract Infections in Dogs

Species	Prevalence (%)	Typical Colonies On: Blood Agar	MacConkey Agar	Confirmatory Tests Gram Stain	Oxidase	Catalase
Escherichia coli	42–46	Smooth grey; often hemolytic	Red discrete, surrounded by red haze	Negative rods	Negative	NA
Enterococcus	11–14	Very small (<1 mm)	No growth	Positive cocci	NA	Negative
Coagulase-positive *Staphylococcus*	12	White or off-white (often hemolytic)	No growth	Positive cocci	NA	Positive
Proteus mirabilis	6–12	Swarms; no discrete colonies	Colorless	Negative rods	Negative	NA
Klebsiella	8–12	Large, wet mucoid, whitish-grey	Pink, slimy coalescing; not surrounded by red haze	Negative rods	Negative	NA
Pseudomonas	<5	Gray to greenish-gray; fruity or ammonia odor; often hemolytic	Colorless, surrounded by blue-green pigment	Negative rods	Positive	NA

NA = not applicable.

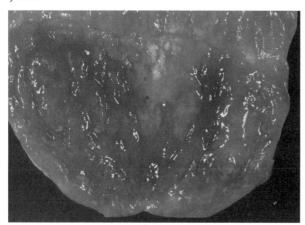

FIGURE 74.3. *Hyperemic mucosal surface of the bladder with white mucinous material from a sow with* Actinobaculum suis *cystitis.*

dal action; hemolytic activity; and possession of certain O-antigens, iron-scavenging proteins, and bacteriocins. These properties are rare in random *E. coli* strains, suggesting that agents of urinary tract infections represent a select subpopulation within their species.

Pili-mediated attachment to urothelium and urea hydrolysis are considered critical virulence factors in pathogenesis of the *Corynebacterium renale* group infections. Urea breakdown with production of ammonia initiates an inflammatory process, high alkalinity in urine (pH 9.0), and suppression of antibacterial defenses, possibly through complement inactivation by ammonia.

Miscellaneous Urinary Tract-Associated Infectious Processes

Fungi are rarely involved in urinary tract infections. Fungal hyphae can be detected in the urine of dogs with disseminated *Aspergillus* infections. Rarely, mycotic cystitis is identified. The yeast *Candida albicans* is sometimes isolated from the urine of dogs with diabetes mellitus.

Kidney tumors are associated with infections with the avian leukosis/sarcoma complex of viruses. Renal lymphoma is associated with feline leukemia virus infections in cats.

The Genital Tract

The primary function of the genital tract is reproduction. The genital tract in mammals includes the ovaries, oviducts, uterus, cervix, vagina, and externa genitalia in females and the testes, ductus deferens, accessory sex organs, penis, and prepuce in males. In poultry, the genital tract differs substantially from mammals. In males the testes are internal and, lacking accessory sex glands and a distinct copulatory organ, the ductus deferens parallels the ureter into the cloaca. Females typically have only a single functional ovary (left) and oviduct with the shell gland (uterus), which empties into the cloaca.

Antimicrobial Defenses

Antimicrobial defenses are in place at all levels of the genital tract and include:

1. *Anatomic Defenses.* Stratified squamous epithelium in the vagina and vulva provide for resistance to infection. The cervix provides a physical barrier to infections of the upper genital tract, especially during pregnancy. The long urethra in males provides a barrier to retrograde infections.
2. *Hormonal Defenses.* Hormones play a part in protecting the genital tract from disease. Estrogens increase the blood supply to the vagina and uterus, the number of polymorphonuclear neutrophil leukocytes in the cervix and uterus, and the myeloperoxidase activity of phagocytic cells in the tract. These activities are important because the vagina and perhaps the uterus may become contaminated with potentially harmful agents during coitus.
3. *Immune Defenses.* The immune system of the genital tract appears to be similar in structure and function to other mucosal surfaces. There are lymphoid follicles in the submucosa from the cervix caudally. These follicles supply cells that will ultimately secrete IgA. IgG and IgM will be found in this area as well, but these isotypes probably arrive through transudation. In the uterus, IgG and IgM, and some sIgA are found. In the prepuce, mainly sIgA is found; it is probably secreted by the accessory glands or locally from cells arising from the lymphoid follicles in this area. The defensive potential of these antibodies depends upon the isotype. Antibodies of the IgA isotype make particles more hydrophilic, thereby negating any surface attraction an organism might have for usually hydrophobic host cell surfaces as well as sterically hindering attachment. IgG and IgM, on the other hand, will opsonize, trigger the complement cascade, and sterically hinder attachment. All immunoglobulins, if specific for epitopes comprising flagella, immobilize bacteria that use motility as a way to ascend the tract from the more caudal regions.

Normal Flora

Lower portions of the genital tract in all animals possess a normal flora. The flora varies by animal and within an individual is dynamic over time. Factors including age, parity, and hormones affect flora makeup. The actual microbial flora of the genital tract is likely to be more complex than presently recognized because optimal culture methods for highly fastidious organisms have not always been employed in past studies on normal flora prevalence. Population density of individual flora members is less well understood, yet it is probably equally or more important than the particular flora makeup in the overall ecology and stability of the microbial population of the genital tract.

In general, the female genital tract possesses a resident microbial flora caudal to the external cervical os. The uterus is normally sterile or transiently contaminated with small numbers of microorganisms. The vagina contains a flora that is mainly composed of species of obligate anaerobic bacteria, including both gram-negative and gram-positive species. The aerobic and facultative anaerobic organisms, about one-tenth the number of obligate anaerobes, include gram-positive and gram-negative species, as well as *Mycoplasma* and *Ureaplasma*.

As is the case with other mucosal surfaces, the flora should be thought of as protective insofar as other, perhaps more pathogenic, strains are excluded through colonization resistance. Mechanisms for exclusion include blocking attachment, efficient use of available substrates, and production of antimicrobial substances. In a more practical sense, the normal or transient flora does include some species that will contaminate the uterus should it become compromised. Some examples include *Streptococcus equi* subsp. *zooepidemicus* in mares with endometritis, *Arcanobacterium pyogenes* along with *Fusobacterium necrophorum* in cows with pyometra, and *Escherichia coli* in bitches with pyometra. All of the organisms mentioned above are part of the normal or transient vaginal flora of the affected animals. The potential for these organisms to cause disease does not simply result from their presence but requires a critical level of replicative dominance over other flora before disease can occur. If the normal flora is disturbed, as during antibiotic treatment of bacterial endometritis in the mare, the vagina will be repopulated with other, more resistant strains, which may ultimately infect the uterus if the underlying compromising condition goes uncorrected.

The resident flora of the external genitalia includes commensal anaerobes, which are largely gram-negative, non–spore-formers; *Mycoplasma* spp.; alpha-hemolytic and beta-hemolytic streptococci; lactobacilli; *Haemophilus* spp. (particularly *H. haemoglobinophilus* in dogs); corynebacteria; propionibacteria; and coagulase-negative staphylococci. *Taylorella equigenitalis,* a venereally transmitted pathogen of mares, may be carried inapparently in the clitoral fossa.

The prepuce and the distal urethra of the male genital tract possess a resident flora that plays a role similar to that played by the flora in the vagina. The origin of organisms responsible for bacterial disease in these areas is almost always endogenous. Some venereally transmitted organisms reside in the prepuce (e.g., *Campylobacter fetus* subsp. *venerealis* in cattle, *Taylorella equigenitalis* in stallions) causing no adverse effects at these sites. The preputial cavity, including the preputial diverticulum of swine, is home for agents of pyelonephritis in cattle (*C. renale* group) and swine (*Actinobaculum suis*).

Diseases

Host and Environmental Factors. For disease to occur in the genital tract frequently some predisposing host and environmental factor(s) must be in place and include:

1. *Anatomic Factors.* Vulvar conformation of mares is a well-known predisposing factor to infection of the vagina and uterus. The more horizontally positioned the vulva, the greater the tendency for fecal contamination of the vagina to occur. Urine pooling in the vagina predisposes to cervicitis and endometritis. Phimosis in males can lead to nonspecific inflammation and infection of the prepuce and penis.
2. *Hormonal Factors.* Hormones play a role in making the genital tract more susceptible to disease. In general, under the influence of progesterone, the uterus is more prone to infection. Neutrophil activity in the genital tract is suppressed under the influence of progesterone, including decreased migration and phagocytic ability. At least in bitches, during the luteal phase, receptors for *E. coli* are expressed. Colonization by *E. coli* expressing appropriate adhesins allows for establishment and can ultimately lead to development of pyometra. Whether the same occurs in other species is unknown.
3. *Other Factors.* Trauma that may occur during parturition can compromise integrity of the epithelial barrier leading to infection. Dystocias and retained fetal membranes increase chances for post-parturient infections. Nutritional factors sometimes influence genital tract disease development. For example, posthitis in sheep occurs typically in animals on rich legume pastures that are high in proteins, which increase urea excretion, and estrogens. This leads to preputial swelling and urine retention in the sheath.

Infectious Processes. For most genital tract pathogens, the routes of exposure are venereal or by ingestion. Localization to the genital tract occurs by ascending or hematogenous routes. In some diseases, although venereally transmitted, pathogens localize to areas in the genital tract by a hematogenous means. Some genital tract pathogens reside in the digestive tract and become blood-borne to cause disease in the genital tract (e.g., *Campylobacter fetus* subsp. *fetus* in sheep).

Female Reproductive Tract. The most common infections of the female reproductive tract involve the vulva, vagina, cervix, and uterus. Vulvitis in cattle is associated with *Ureaplasma* and *Mycoplasma* spp., but a solid etiological link remains to be shown. Infectious bovine rhinotracheitis virus causes vulvovaginitis in cattle. Various coliforms, especially *E. coli*, cause vaginal-vulvar discharge in sows. Such infections are often related to hygiene and management practices. Vaginitis in dogs is most commonly associated with *Staphylococcus* spp, *Streptococcus* spp., or *E. coli*. In prepubertal females, vaginitis tends to resolve on its own as the dog matures. In older bitches, there is usually an underlying factor involved.

Uterine infections are typically related to breeding, pregnancy, or parturition, the nonpregnant uterus being fairly resistant to infection. During breeding or parturition when the cervix is open, infections of the uterus are most often ascending. Infections of the uterus can involve the endometrium (endometritis) or the entire wall of the uterus (metritis). Endometritis occurs in all animals but is most common and of greatest consequence in the horse. Inability of some horses with endometritis to resolve infections is in part due to defects in migration of neutrophils to the site of infection as well as decreased phagocytic ability of the neutrophils. *Streptococcus equi* subsp. *zooepidemicus* is the pathogen most commonly associated with endometritis in mares, although other organisms (enterics, other streptococci, *Pseudomonas*) can be involved.

If prior to resolution of a uterine infection the cervix closes and pus accumulates, a pyometra develops. Pyometras occur in all animals but are most frequent in dogs, cats, and cattle. Overall, *E. coli* is the organism most often associated with pyometra. A number of other organisms, including *Streptococcus* sp. and *Pseudomonas,* can also be involved. In cattle, *Arcanobacterium pyogenes* and obligately anaerobic bacteria are frequently found.

Fetus. Abortion, especially in farm animals and horses, is one of the most common and economically significant genital tract diseases. Abortion is essentially expulsion of the fetus before full development. A number of viral, bacterial, and fungal agents can trigger this process (see Tables 74.1–74.7). During pregnancy, the placenta and/or fetus are infected predominately by the hematogenous route. Mares are an exception; bacterial and fungal placental infections most often originate through the cervical os.

A number of viruses can cause abortion in animals. The herpesviruses are prominent among the viruses involved and affect a number of different animals, most notably horses (equine herpesvirus 1). Viral-induced abortions result subsequent to fetal inflammatory lesions with necrosis, fetal anoxia, or endometrial lesions.

Bacteria responsible for abortion often cause a placentitis or placental edema. If the fetus becomes infected, typically large numbers of organisms are found in the fetal stomach fluid (Fig 74.4). In some bacterial abortions, lesions in the fetus may suggest the likely agent. As an example, the focal areas of hepatic necrosis in the fetus are suggestive of—however, not exclusive to—abortions in sheep caused by *Campylobacter fetus* subsp. *fetus* (Fig 74.5). While most bacterial abortions occur in the last trimester, early fetal death and resorption occurs with some agents. In

FIGURE 74.4. *Gram stain with carbolfuchsin counterstain of abomasal fluid from an aborted bovine fetus due to* Brucella abortus. *Multiple gram-negative rods to coccobacilli are present.*

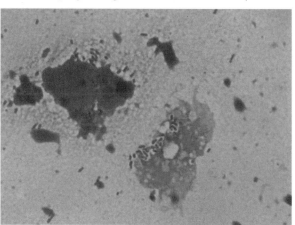

FIGURE 74.5. *Areas of hepatic necrosis in the liver of aborted ovine fetus.* Campylobacter fetus *subsp.* fetus *was isolated.*

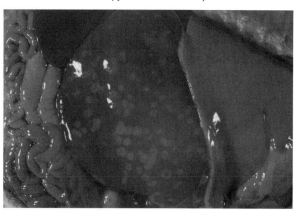

those cases, the infection presents clinically as an infertility problem (e.g., *Campylobacter fetus* subsp. *venerealis* in cattle).

Fungal abortions are most common in horses and cattle and typically are the result of a placentitis. The portal of entry in cattle is either the respiratory or gastrointestinal tract with subsequent hematogenous spread to the placenta. In horses, an ascending infection through the cervix is the most common route. Fetal lesions in cattle, if present, are for the most part limited to focal, hyperkeratotic lesions on the skin; in horses fetal lesions are uncommon. *Mortierella wolffi,* a zygomycete, causes a fulminating pneumonia with a high mortality rate in about 25% of affected cows as a result of a lung-uterus-lung infection cycle. Fungal elements absorbed from the uterus cause a fulminating embolic pneumonia in the cow that typically follows the abortion.

Some viral infections of the fetus result in congenital abnormalities. Factors influencing whether abnormalities develop are dependent on the stage of fetal development, immune competence of the fetus, and the particular viral strains responsible (e.g., feline panleukopenia virus; bovine viral diarrhea virus; and Akabane, Cache Valley, Border disease, and bluetongue viruses in sheep).

Details on the pathogenesis and pathology as it relates to individual abortifacient agents are found in specific chapters on those agents.

Male Reproductive Tract. In males, the predominant genital tract infections are orchitis, epididymitis, and infections of the accessory sex glands (prostatitis, seminal vesiculitis). Orchitis can develop by an ascending or hematogenous route. Occasionally periorchitis develops from descending peritonitis, which subsequently involves the testes. Epididymitis affects all animal species but is most common in rams (Fig 74.6). In younger rams, an ascending infection by age-dependent preputial residents ("*Actinobacillus seminis*", *Histophilus somni* ["*Histophilus ovis*" is the obsolete name]) is the rule. In adult rams, *Brucella ovis* is the main agent involved. It localizes to the epididymal ductules via the hematogenous route. Inflammation and

FIGURE 74.6.   *Epididymitis in yearling ram (ram-lamb epididymitis) caused by* Histophilus somni *("Histophilus ovis" is the obsolete name). Tail of the epididymis is greatly enlarged (A) and contains a greenish purulent material (B).*

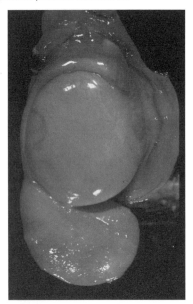

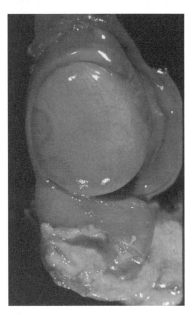

FIGURE 74.7.   *Oophoritis in a chicken with pullorum disease (Salmonella* Pullorum*). (Courtesy Dr. H. Shivaprasad.)*

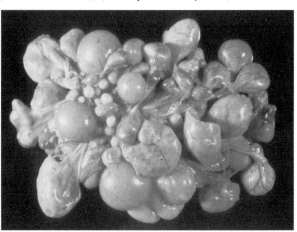

scesses, which can rupture and cause peritonitis. Seminal vesiculitis occurs most commonly in bulls and is the most common cause for inflammatory cells detected during semen examination. Many potential agents have been implicated, with *Arcanobacterium pyogenes* the most frequently recovered.

Infections of the penis or prepuce can be from endogenous or exogenous sources. Various herpes viruses cause balanoposthitis in animals. Members of the *Corynebacterium renale* group cause a necrotizing inflammation of the prepuce and adjacent tissues in wethers or rams. The disease develops in the presence of these urealytic agents in an area constantly irrigated with urine. Ammonia is thought to initiate the inflammatory process. A similar condition occurs occasionally in goats and bulls.

Genital Tract of Poultry.   Infections of the oviduct (salpingitis) in poultry can be the result of an ascending infection from the cloaca or occur in conjunction with colibacillosis when the left abdominal air sac is involved. *Escherichia coli* is the most common pathogen recovered. Although pullorum disease and fowl typhoid have become uncommon diseases in developed countries, oophoritis, salpingitis, and orchitis are all possible consequences of the septicemia associated with infections by *Salmonella* serovars Pullorum and Gallinarum, respectively (Fig. 74.7).

Decreased egg production and/or hatchability can result from a number of systemic infections in poultry. A number of viruses (e.g., avian adenovirus, infectious bronchitis virus, avian influenza virus) and bacteria (e.g., *Mycoplasma, Haemophilus paragallinarum, Salmonella*) can affect overall egg production and hatchability. Some poultry pathogens (e.g., *Mycoplasma, Salmonella*) are transmitted vertically in eggs.

extravasation of sperm lead to development of a spermatic granuloma.

Bacterial prostatitis most commonly occurs in dogs and is, in fact, the most common cause of prostatic disease in dogs. Infections are mostly ascending in origin and can be acute or chronic. Consequences include prostatic ab-

Index